Metastasis of Colorectal Cancer

Cancer Metastasis – Biology and Treatment

VOLUME 14

Series Editors

Richard J. Ablin, *Ph.D., University of Arizona, College of Medicine and The Arizona Cancer Center, AZ, U.S.A.*
Wen G. Jiang, *M.D., Wales College of Medicine, Cardiff University, Cardiff, U.K.*

Advisory Editorial Board

Harold F. Dvorak, *M.D.*
Phil Gold, *M.D., Ph.D.*
Danny Welch, *Ph.D.*
Hiroshi Kobayashi, *M.D., Ph.D.*
Robert E. Mansel, *M.S., FRCS.*
Klaus Pantel, *Ph.D.*

Recent Volumes in this Series

Volume 7: DNA Methylation, Epigenetics and Metastasis
Editor: Manel Esteller
ISBN 978-1-4020-3641-8

Volume 8: Cell Motility in Cancer Invasion and Metastasis
Editor: Alan Wells
ISBN 978-1-4020-4008-3

Volume 9: Cell Adhesion and Cytoskeletal Molecules in Metastasis
Editors: Anne E. Cress and Raymond B. Nagle
ISBN 978-1-4020-5128-X

Volume 10: Metastasis of Prostate Cancer
Editors: Richard J. Ablin and Malcolm D. Mason
ISBN 978-1-4020-5846-2

Volume 11: Metastasis of Breast Cancer
Editors: Robert E. Mansel, Oystein Fodstad and Wen G. Jiang
ISBN 978-1-4020-5866-7

Volume 12: Bone Metastases: A Translational and Clinical Approach
Editors: Dimitrios Kardamakis, Vassilios Vassiliou and Edward Chow
ISBN 978-1-4020-9818-5

Volume 13: Lymphangiogenesis in Cancer Metastasis
Editors: Steven A. Stacker and Marc G. Achen
ISBN 978-90-481-2246-2

Volume 14: Metastasis of Colorectal Cancer
Editors: Nicole Beauchemin and Jacques Huot
ISBN 978-90-481-8832-1

Metastasis of Colorectal Cancer

Edited by

Nicole Beauchemin
Rosalind and Morris Goodman Cancer Research Centre, McGill University, Montreal, QC, Canada

and

Jacques Huot
Le Centre de recherche en cancérologie de l'Université Laval et Centre de recherche du CHUQ, l'Hôtel-Dieu de Québec, Québec, QC, Canada

🄯 Springer

Editors
Dr. Nicole Beauchemin
Rosalind and Morris Goodman
Cancer Research Centre
McGill University
3655 Promenade Sir-William-Osler
Lab 708, Montreal
QC, Canada, H3G 1Y6
nicole.beauchemin@mcgill.ca

Dr. Jacques Huot
Le Centre de recherche en cancérologie de
l'Université Laval et
Centre de recherche du CHUQ, l'Hôtel-Dieu
de Québec, Québec, QC, Canada
G1R 2J6
Jacques.Huot@fmed.ulaval.ca

ISSN 1568-2102
ISBN 978-90-481-8832-1   e-ISBN 978-90-481-8833-8
DOI 10.1007/978-90-481-8833-8
Springer Dordrecht Heidelberg London New York

Library of Congress Control Number: 2010930563

© Springer Science+Business Media B.V. 2010
No part of this work may be reproduced, stored in a retrieval system, or transmitted in any form or by any means, electronic, mechanical, photocopying, microfilming, recording or otherwise, without written permission from the Publisher, with the exception of any material supplied specifically for the purpose of being entered and executed on a computer system, for exclusive use by the purchaser of the work.

Printed on acid-free paper

Springer is part of Springer Science+Business Media (www.springer.com)

This book is dedicated to all colorectal cancer patients. Thanks to our families, friends and colleagues.

Contents

1. **THE METASTATIC PROCESS: AN OVERVIEW** 1
   Nicolas Porquet, Stéphanie Gout and Jacques Huot

2. **PHYSIOPATHOLOGY OF COLORECTAL METASTASIS** 33
   Cristiano Ferrario and Mark Basik

3. **THE GENETICS OF COLORECTAL CANCER** 65
   Andrew M. Kaz and William M. Grady

4. **EPIGENETICS OF COLORECTAL CANCER** 101
   F. Javier Carmona and Manel Esteller

5. **CANCER-INITIATING CELLS IN COLORECTAL CANCER** 127
   Antonija Kreso, Liane Gibson and Catherine Adell O'Brien

6. **EPITHELIAL-MESENCHYMAL TRANSITION IN COLORECTAL CANCER** 147
   Otto Schmalhofer, Simone Brabletz and Thomas Brabletz

7. **CELL ADHESION MOLECULES IN COLON CANCER METASTASIS** 173
   Azadeh Arabzadeh and Nicole Beauchemin

8. **EPITHELIAL CELL SIGNALLING IN COLORECTAL CANCER METASTASIS** 205
   Caroline Saucier and Nathalie Rivard

9. **ANGIOGENESIS AND LYMPHANGIOGENESIS IN COLON CANCER METASTASIS** 243
   Delphine Garnier and Janusz Rak

10 **ROLE OF THE HOST INFLAMMATORY RESPONSE IN COLON CARCINOMA INITIATION, PROGRESSION AND LIVER METASTASIS** 289
Pnina Brodt

11 **MOLECULAR PROGNOSTIC MARKERS IN COLON CANCER** .. 321
Thomas Winder and Heinz-Josef Lenz

12 **THE SENTINEL LYMPH NODE AND STAGING OF COLORECTAL CANCER** 343
Gaetan des Guetz and Bernard Uzzan

13 **TREATMENT OF COLORECTAL CANCER** 359
Eisar Al-Sukhni and Steven Gallinger

14 **DIAGNOSIS AND TREATMENT OF RECTAL CANCER** 389
Té Vuong, Tamim Niazi, Sender Liberman, Polymnia Galiatsatos and Slobodan Devic

15 **FUTURE DIRECTIONS** 409
Jacques Huot and Nicole Beauchemin

Index 413

Contributors

Eisar Al-Sukhni Ontario Cancer Institute, Toronto General Hospital, University Health Network, Toronto, ON, Canada

Azadeh Arabzadeh Rosalind and Morris Goodman Cancer Research Centre, McGill University, Montreal, QC, Canada, H3G 1Y6

Mark Basik Department of Oncology, McGill University, Montreal, QC, Canada; Segal Cancer Center, Jewish General Hospital, Montreal, QC, Canada, mark.basik@mcgill.ca

Nicole Beauchemin Rosalind and Morris Goodman Cancer Research Centre, McGill University, 3655 Promenade Sir-William-Osler, Lab 708, Montreal, QC, Canada, H3G 1Y6, nicole.beauchemin@mcgill.ca

Simone Brabletz Department of Visceral Surgery, University of Freiburg, Freiburg 79106, Germany, simone.spaderna@uniklinik-freiburg.de

Thomas Brabletz Department of Visceral Surgery, University of Freiburg, Freiburg 79106, Germany, thomas.brabletz@uniklinik-freiburg.de

Pnina Brodt Department of Surgery, Medicine and Oncology, McGill University and the McGill University Health Center, Royal Victoria Hospital, Montreal, QC, Canada, pnina.brodt@mcgill.ca

F. Javier Carmona Cancer Epigenetics and Biology Program (PEBC), Bellvitge Institute for Biomedical Research (IDIBELL), 08907 L'Hospitalet, Barcelona, Catalonia, Spain

G. des Guetz Departments of Oncology, APHP, hôpital Avicenne, Bobigny 93009, France, gaetan.des-guetz@avc.aphp.fr

Slobodan Devic Department of Medical Physics, Jewish General Hospital, McGill University, Montréal, QC, Canada

Manel Esteller Cancer Epigenetics and Biology Program (PEBC), Bellvitge Institute for Biomedical Research (IDIBELL), 08907 L'Hospitalet, Barcelona, Catalonia, Spain, mesteller@iconcologia.net

Cristiano Ferrario Department of Oncology, McGill University, Montreal, QC, Canada, cristianoferrario@gmail.com

Polymnia Galiatsatos Department of Gastroenterology, Jewish General Hospital, McGill University, Montréal, QC, Canada

Steven Gallinger Ontario Cancer Institute, Toronto General Hospital, University Health Network, Toronto, ON, Canada, steven.gallinger@uhn.on.ca

Delphine Garnier Montreal Children's Hospital Research Institute, McGill University, Montreal, QC, Canada

Liane Gibson Division of Cell and Molecular Biology, University Health Network, Toronto, ON, Canada

Stéphanie Gout Institut Albert Bonniot Grenoble, Centre de recherche Inserm/UJF U823 Equipe 2, Grenoble, France, stefigout@gmail.com

William M. Grady Fred Hutchinson Cancer Research Center, Seattle, WA, USA, wgrady@fhcrc.org

Jacques Huot Le Centre de recherche en cancérologie de l'Université Laval et Centre de recherche du CHUQ, l'Hôtel-Dieu de Québec, Québec, QC, Canada, G1R 2J6, Jacques.Huot@fmed.ulaval.ca

Andrew M. Kaz Fred Hutchinson Cancer Research Center, Seattle, WA, USA

Antonija Kreso Department of Molecular and Medical Genetics, University of Toronto, Toronto, ON, Canada

Heinz-Josef Lenz Division of Medical Oncology, Los Angeles, CA, USA; Department of Preventive Medicine, Keck School of Medicine, University of Southern California/Norris Comprehensive Cancer Center, Los Angeles, CA 90033, USA, lenz_h@ccnt.usc.edu

Sender Liberman Department of Surgery, McGill University Health Centre, McGill University, Montréal, QC, Canada

Tamim Niazi Department of Radiation Oncology, Jewish General Hospital, McGill University, Montréal, QC, Canada, H3T 1E2

Catherine Adell O'Brien Division of Cell and Molecular Biology, University Health Network, Toronto, ON, Canada; Division of General Surgery, University Health Network, Toronto, ON, Canada; Toronto General Hospital, Toronto, ON, Canada, cobrien@uhnresearch.ca

Nicolas Porquet Le Centre de recherche en cancérologie de l'Université Laval et Centre de recherche du CHUQ, l'Hôtel-Dieu de Québec, Québec, QC, Canada, G1R 2J6, Nicolas.Porquet@unice.fr

Janusz Rak Montreal Children's Hospital Research Institute, McGill University, Montreal, QC, Canada, janusz.rak@mcgill.ca

Nathalie Rivard Département d'Anatomie et de Biologie Cellulaire, Faculté de Médecine et des Sciences de la Santé, Université de Sherbrooke, Sherbrooke, QC, Canada, Nathalie.Rivard@USherbrooke.ca

Caroline Saucier Département d'Anatomie et de Biologie Cellulaire, Faculté de Médecine et des Sciences de la Santé, Université de Sherbrooke, Sherbrooke, QC, Canada, Caroline.Saucier@USherbrooke.ca

Otto Schmalhofer Department of Visceral Surgery, University of Freiburg, Freiburg 79106, Germany, otto.schmalhofer@uniklinik-freiburg.de

B. Uzzan Departments of Pharmacology, APHP, hôpital Avicenne, Bobigny 93009, France

Té Vuong Department of Radiation Oncology, Jewish General Hospital, McGill University, Montréal, QC, Canada, H3T 1E2, tvuong@jgh.mcgill.ca

Thomas Winder Division of Medical Oncology, Los Angeles, CA, USA; Department for Internal Medicine, Academic Teaching Hospital Feldkirch, Feldkirch 6800, Austria

Introduction

Nicole Beauchemin[1] and Jacques Huot[2]
[1] Rosalind and Morris Goodman Cancer Research Centre, McGill University, 3655 Promenade Sir-William-Osler, Lab 708, Montreal, QC, Canada, H3G 1Y6, e-mail: nicole.beauchemin@mcgill.ca
[2] Le Centre de recherche en cancérologie de l'Université Laval et Centre de recherche du CHUQ, l'Hôtel-Dieu de Québec, Québec, QC, Canada, GIR 2J6, e-mail: Jacques.Huot@fmed.ulaval.ca

Over the last decades, considerable efforts have been devoted to understanding the genetic and physiopathological basis of colorectal cancer that remains a very traumatic and deadly disease with 50% of patients eventually succumbing to metastatic spread mainly to the liver but also to the lung, peritoneal cavity and bones. Colorectal cancer (CRC) is now ranked third in the world with respect to the number of patients affected by cancer in their lifetime. An explosion of data has revolutionized how basic and clinical researchers deal with advanced CRC disease with novel treatments and options. We have accepted the challenge of summarizing the knowledge currently available on 'Metastases of Colorectal Cancer' in this book, in the hopes that this knowledge would encourage scientists and clinicians to tackle new challenges in this field and entertain discussions leading to novel therapies. We have convened an impressive cohort of authors, well renowned for their contributions to the field of colorectal cancer. They have devoted time and energy in providing our readers with the most up-to-date information in the field. We sincerely thank them for having accepted our invitation and providing the readers with excellent chapters on 'Metastases of Colorectal Cancer'.

To begin with, Dr. Jacques Huot and his colleagues (Université Laval, Quebec, Canada) introduce us in Chapter 1 to the cancer cell's journey from its original site of cancer development in the colon to its final metastatic niche, generally the liver. A fraction of the initial cancer cells succeed in squeezing through muscle layers, flowing through lengthy blood vessels and entering into liver sinusoids, constantly making contact with the respective microenvironments and adapting to an ever-changing protein array defining these cells. Most tumour cells die in the process, but the few that survive create the metastatic time bomb. The physiopathology of colorectal metastasis being a complex process, how a cancer cell travels through the circulation or moves locally has been discussed in Chapter 2 by Dr. Mark Basik (Jewish General Hospital, McGill University, Montreal, Canada). Many different factors will either facilitate or hinder the CRC cell's migration and adhesion to metastatic sites. Dr. Basik has emphasized the role of tumour factors such as Tissue Factor and Epidermal Growth Factor Receptor (EGFR) status, host immunity and the role of diet, exercise and liver disease as well as iatrogenic factors such as inflammatory state after a surgical trauma or biopsies and liver resection. In Chapter 3,

Drs. Andrew Katz and William Grady (Fred Hutchinson Cancer Research Center, Seattle, WA) have focused on pathological insights into the molecular genetics and epigenetics of colorectal cancer including the multistep nature of carcinogenesis, the central role of tumour suppressor pathways, the role of DNA repair genes and genomic stability in cancer formation, and the role of the Wingless/Wnt, RAS-RAF-MAPK, phosphatidyl inositol 3 kinase (PI3K), p53 and transforming growth factor β (TGF-β) signalling pathways in tumour development. Genome-wide association studies and metastatic genes are also discussed. How these genetic pathways intersect in the metastatic phenotype and how they can be modulated to decrease or completely hinder metastasis remains one of the major challenges in the future. In Chapter 4, Drs. Carmona and Esteller (Bellvitge Institute for Biomedical Research, Barcelona, Spain) summarize novel findings in epigenetic regulation of CRC-associated genes particularly those associated with differential methylation of CpG islands and histone modifications in the promoter of colon cancer progression genes, particularly tumour suppressor genes. The authors also synthesize an ever-expanding sum of data on colon cancer-specific microRNAs as well as metastasis-associated microRNAs. This comprehensive information is now tested clinically; a panel of epigenetic biomarkers, and combinations of the 5-azacytidine drug and histone deacetylase inhibitors are currently being tested in CRC clinical trials. One of the hopes for future treatments of CRC patients lies in the characterization of colon-cancer-initiating cells (CC-ICs). Dr. Catherine O'Brien (University Health Network, Toronto, Canada) has made significant headway in this field and reports in Chapter 5 on preliminary evidence suggesting that CC-ICs are capable of surviving conventional chemotherapy and successfully metastasizing. Current research is focused on understanding the biology of these cells so as to devise novel therapeutics targeting the aberrant biology that underlies their contribution to CRC. In Chapter 6, Dr. Thomas Brabletz (University of Freiburg, Freiburg, Germany) and his colleagues expand on the intricacies of the Wnt signalling pathway and in particular on the E-cadherin, and β-catenin and its target genes in mediating proliferation, stemness, invasion and neo-angiogenesis, all necessary in the metastasic process. In addition, the authors explain how β-catenin-mediated transcription favours induction of epithelial-mesenchymal transition within the tumor cells, thereby activating tumour progression. Some of the latest results are presented regarding the activity of a class of transcriptional repressors that cooperate with β-catenin to induce *E-cadherin* gene repression. In addition to the classical E-cadherin cell adhesion molecule (CAM), Drs. Arabzadeh and Beauchemin (Goodman Cancer Research Centre, McGill University, Montreal, Canada) have examined in Chapter 7 how a number of other cell adhesion molecules are altered in expression at the primary colon tumour site or in the metastatic colonization site. Modulation of these CAMs through specific pharmacological inhibitors or specific antibodies is currently being assessed for its clinical value.

In Chapter 8, Drs. Saucier and Rivard (Université de Sherbrooke, Sherbrooke, Canada) discuss the importance of the crucial EGFR tyrosine kinase signalling pathways in devising novel therapeutic possibilities. The status of PI3K/PTEN, K-RAS and B-RAF mutations are now considered clinically relevant to define those classes of patients that will benefit from anti-EGFR interventions. These studies have become the paradigm to understand how receptor tyrosine kinase (RTK) regulatory signalling may contribute to adaptation of the tumour microenvironment as well as its subversion rendering it permissive for dissemination of tumour cells. This will also help identify promising molecule targets for antimetastatic CRC therapy. A major component of metastasis is the development of new blood and lymphatic vessels through angiogenesis and lymphangiogenesis processes, as described in Chapter 9 by Drs. Garnier and Rak (Montreal Children's Hospital Research Institute, McGill University, Montreal, Canada). Intervention of these processes has met with reasonable success in the last few years. However, it has also become clear that interfering with the central vascular endothelial growth factor (VEGF) that drives most of this signalling does not always produce the desired inhibitory result, with sometimes non-productive and tumour type-, site- and stage-specific effects. Although presumed originally to be local in nature, recent data now point to systemic regulatory network signalling via soluble mediators, circulating bone marrow-derived cells, platelets and microvesicles. This holds promise of offering more effective overall therapy to patients with metastatic CRC. Dr. Pnina Brodt (McGill University and the McGill University Health Center, Montreal, Canada) brings us up-to-date in Chapter 10 on the role of E-selectin and inflammatory cytokine-driven signalling in CRC progression and metastasis. She focuses on a number of inhibitory compounds that have met with success in pre-clinical and sometimes clinical settings. Drs. Winder and Lenz (University of Southern California/Norris Comprehensive Cancer Center, Los Angeles, CA) report on molecular prognostic and predictive markers of CRC in Chapter 11. Currently, the only two established molecular markers in CRC are microsatellite instability (MSI) for prognosis and K-Ras for prediction. With the new technologies of DNA microarrays and proteomics, novel markers will undoubtedly be identified and validated, therefore giving clinical oncologists a better handle in individualized therapies. Similarly, Dr. Des Guetz (Hôpital Avicenne, Bobigny, France) has highlighted in Chapter 12 that sentinel lymph node (SLN) biopsies can serve as a novel tool for better CRC staging as well as defining lymph node involvement in metastasis, although technical difficulties will need to be overcome. In Chapter 13, Drs. Al-Sukhni and Gallinger (University Health Network, Toronto, Canada) describe the most recent surgical, medical and radiation oncology advances in treating CRC patients. In spite of these new developments, patients diagnosed with advanced disease are unlikely to sustain a complete cure of the disease as tumours have invaded the local environment and have spread systemically. Novel considerations in colon cancer stem cells and CRC molecular profiling of individual patients will likely become part of the treatment modalities offered to patients in the future. And finally, in Chapter 14, Dr. Té Vuong and her colleagues (Jewish General Hospital, McGill University, Montreal, Canada) summarize the management of rectal cancer. For patients with locally advanced rectal cancer, neo-adjuvant radiation therapy with or without chemotherapy followed by tumour excision has proven to be fairly successful. But recently, delivery of local radiation with high dose brachytherapy also appears very promising.

Our most sincere wish is that this up-to date information will help both the research and clinical community in pushing forward with new challenges for the benefit of the CRC patients.

The editors would sincerely like to acknowledge the help of Ms. Samantha Benlolo and Mr. François Houle who respectively contributed to the language and figure editing of the chapters in this book.

Abbreviations and Acronyms

CAM	Cell adhesion molecule
CC-IC	Colon-cancer-initiating cells
CRC	Colorectal cancer
EGFR	Epidermal growth factor receptor
MSI	Microsatellite instability
PI3K	Phosphatidyl inositol 3 kinase
RTK	Receptor tyrosine kinase
TGF-β	Transforming growth factor β
VEGF	Vascular endothelial growth factor

Chapter 1

THE METASTATIC PROCESS: AN OVERVIEW

Nicolas Porquet[1], Stéphanie Gout[2] and Jacques Huot[3]

[1] *Le Centre de recherche en cancérologie de l'Université Laval et Centre de recherche du CHUQ, l'Hôtel-Dieu de Québec, Québec, QC, Canada, G1R 2J6, e-mail: Nicolas.Porquet@unice.fr*
[2] *Institut Albert Bonniot Grenoble, Centre de recherche Inserm/UJF U823 Equipe 2, Grenoble, France, e-mail: stefigout@gmail.com*
[3] *Le Centre de recherche en cancérologie de l'Université Laval et Centre de recherche du CHUQ, l'Hôtel-Dieu de Québec, Québec, QC, Canada, G1R 2J6, e-mail: Jacques.Huot@fmed.ulaval.ca*

Abstract: About one third of patients who will receive a cancer diagnostic will die of this disease. In most cases, death results from the formation of secondary neoplasms called metastases. The metastatic process is characterized by the detachment of cancer cells from the primary sites followed by their dissemination throughout the bloodstream and/or lymph stream to distal sites where they proliferate to give rise to secondary tumours. Intriguingly, the metastatic process is rather inefficient and in spite of its clinical significance, it remains poorly understood. Nevertheless, significant progress has been achieved during the past years and the increasing knowledge of the metastatic process is encouraging and raises high therapeutic expectations. Several events that lead to cancer and metastasis are under genetic and epigenetic controls. In particular, cancer initiation is tightly associated with specific mutations that affect proto-oncogenes and tumour suppressor genes. These mutations lead to unrestrained growth of the primary neoplasm and to a propensity to detach and progress through the subsequent steps of metastatic dissemination. Epigenetic alterations are mainly characterized by deregulation of DNA methylation and microRNA (miRNA)-dependent functions, as well as disruption of histone modifiers and chromatin-remodelling factors. In addition to these molecular alterations, several studies highlight that tumour development and

Nicolas Porquet and Stéphanie Gout contributed equally to this review dissemination rely on a continuous crosstalk between cancer cells and their microenvironments. This chapter will provide an overview of the metastatic process as it applies to colorectal cancer.

Key words: Metastasis · Adhesion · Homing · Stroma · Microenvironment

1.1 Introduction

The genome of tumour cells is altered at several sites as a result of point mutations or changes in chromosome integrity (Hanahan and Weinberg, 2000). These changes affect oncogenes, tumour suppressor genes and several metastasis-related genes such as cadherins, laminins, protease inhibitors and hypoxia-inducible factor-1 (Lujambio and Esteller, 2009). However, the dysregulation of these genes is not always a result of mutations. Other factors including epigenetic alterations such as CpG island hypermethylation-associated silencing, disruptions of histone modifiers and chromatin remodelling factors and deregulation of miRNA-mediated control of mRNA functions contribute to the incidence of metastasis (Esteller, 2008). The genetic and epigenetic modifications that affect cancer cells interact to confer six phenotypic traits that constitute the essential hallmarks of cancer (Hanahan and Weinberg, 2000): (1) cancer cells have acquired growth self-sufficiency through mutations or epigenetic alterations that activate proto-oncogenes, which enable cancer cells to generate their own growth signals such as secretion of transforming growth factor-α (TGFα); (2) cancer cells are characterized by their insensitivity to anti-growth signals; (3) cancer cells have gained the capability to escape apoptosis as a result of mutations or epigenetic modifications that inactivate tumour suppressor genes such as p53 or phosphatase and tensin homolog deleted on chromosome 10 (PTEN), or through activation of survival pathways involving insulin-like growth factor-1/2 (IGF1/2) or interleukin-3 (IL-3); (4) cancer cells have lost the cell-autonomous program that limits their multiplication. This loss results mainly from turning on telomerase, thereby impairing senescence and death; (5) the growing neoplasm promotes angiogenesis and becomes capable of sustaining its oxygen and nutritive supplies; (6) cells from the primary neoplasm detach from this site and travel to distant sites that they will colonize to form metastases. More recently, inflammation has been suggested to represent a seventh hallmark of cancer (Solinas et al., 2010).

Recent studies have indicated that during the acquisition of genetic and epigenetic alterations that underlie the inherent hallmarks of cancer, cancer cells need to interact synergistically with their surrounding microenvironment in order to form a neoplasm and progress further to colonize distant organs (Gout and Huot, 2008). Incidentally, several studies support the view that the formation of metastases is not random and is tightly associated with the microenvironment of invaded organs. This gave rise to the homing or 'seed and soil' theory of metastasis. This chapter is a brief overview of the metastatic process as it applies to colorectal cancer. It introduces notions that will be discussed in detail in the other chapters of this book.

1.2 Models of Metastasis

Many hypotheses as well as six models have been proposed to explain the metastatic process and its inefficiency (Hunter et al., 2008). They are outlined in Fig. 1.1 and are briefly discussed below.

1.2.1 The Progression Models

The linear progression model, also known as the clonal evolution model, was initially proposed for colorectal cancer. According to this model, tumours develop by a process of linear clonal evolution that results from the accumulation of somatic genetic alterations leading to a small fraction of cells that acquire a full metastatic potential (Hunter et al., 2008; Khalique et al., 2009; Klein, 2009). Many experimental and clinical observations support this model. Notably, clonal derivatives of cultured cell lines have different metastatic potentials, which is consistent with the existence of metastatic subpopulations (Fidler and Kripke, 1977). On the other hand, most, if not all ovarian cancer metastases are clonally related to the primary tumours (Khalique et al., 2009). However, in that specific case, metastatic progression does not follow a linear-clonal evolution process. Instead, the data support a model in which primary ovarian cancers have a common clonal origin, but become polyclonal, with different clones at both early and late stages of genetic divergence that acquire the ability to progress to metastasis. This gave rise to the parallel progression model (Klein, 2009).

Despite the number of studies that support the progression models, these cannot be applied to all cases of metastasis. Notably, although variant clones with high metastatic potential are identified in populations of metastatic cells, these variants revert to low metastatic capacity after several generations (Harris et al., 1982). The clonal progression model would predict that the metastatic events that confer metastatic potential would be stably inherited, rather than rapidly lost. Hence, even if the progression models may account for most cases of metastasis, they cannot be viewed as universal models. Note that in the linear progression model, the inefficiency of the metastatic potential is explained by the low probability that any given cell within the primary tumours will acquire all the multiple alterations required to traverse the different steps of the metastatic cascade.

Fig. 1.1 Models of metastasis. Several models are proposed to explain the metastatic process (**a**) *Progression model*. The linear progression model proposes that a primary neoplasm gains metastatic features as a result of the accumulation of somatic mutations in a small number of cells that acquire a full metastatic potential (**b**) *Transient compartment model*. In this model, all the viable cells within a tumour may acquire metastatic potential. However, only a small number of them will form metastases due to positional restrictions or epigenetic events (**c**) *Fusion model*. A metastatic cell would result from the formation of a cellular hybrid between a circulating cancer cell and a lymphoid cell. Alternatively, oncosomes containing 'oncogenic material' released from metastatic cells will fuse with non-metastatic cells conferring a metastatic phenotype (not shown)

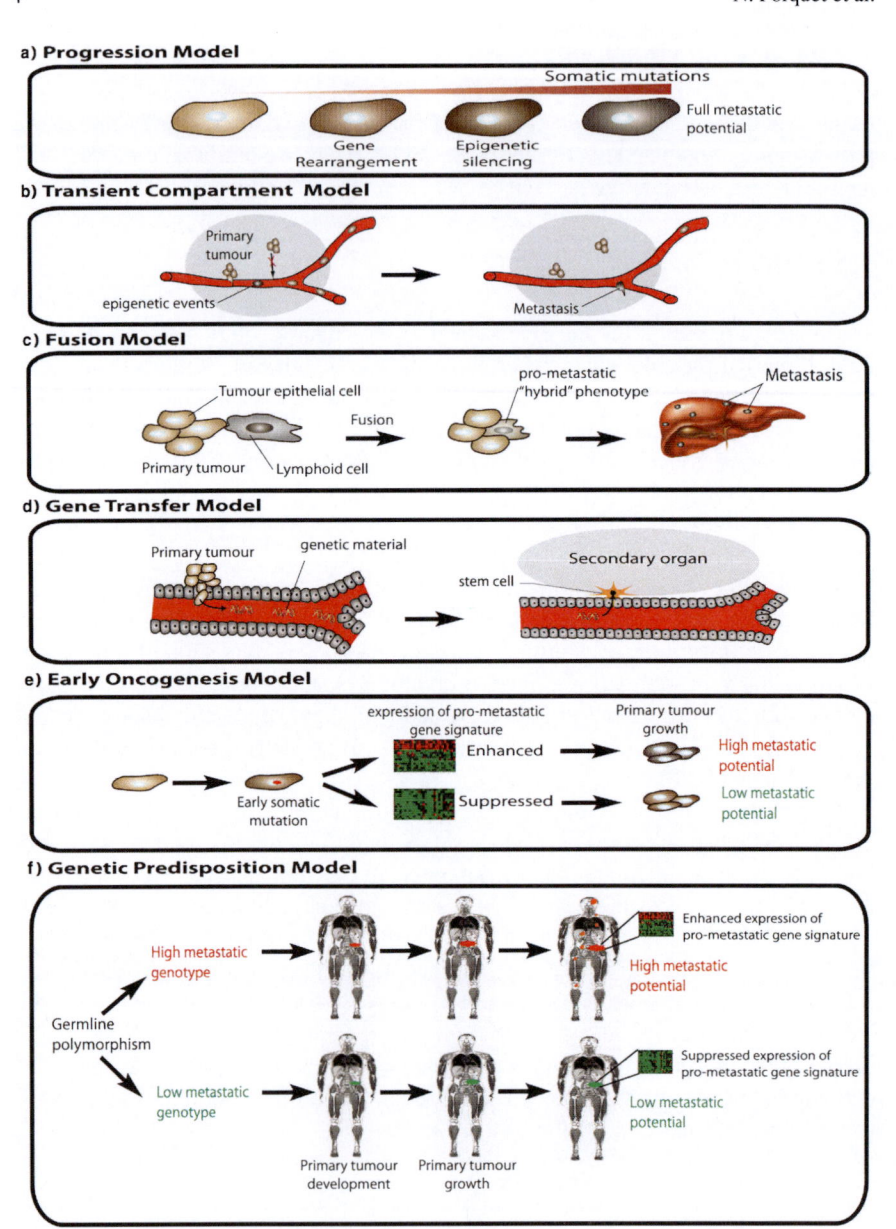

Fig. 1.1 (continued) (**d**) *Gene transfer model*. According to this model, circulating DNA harbouring mutations that confer metastatic potential to parental cancer cells will be taken up by stem cells at the secondary site initiating the formation of metastases (**e**) *Early oncogenesis model*. The metastatic potential of any primary neoplasm is present early in its evolution presumably as a consequence of somatic mutation. This confers a metastatic signature to the tumour and raises the possibility to predict metastasis and even the sites of metastasis (**f**) *Genetic predisposition model*. The metastatic potential of any tumour is influenced by its genetic background. This means that a given individual will be more or less prone to tumour dissemination depending on constitutional polymorphism (Hunter et al., 2008)

1.2.2 The Transient Compartment Model

The transient compartment model of metastasis attempts to explain why the metastatic capacity of secondary tumours is not increased in comparison to that of the primary tumours (Weiss, 1990). In this model, although many cells in a neoplasm possess full metastatic potential, only a few of them will colonize secondary sites. This is due to microenvironmentally-induced random epigenetic events or inadequate access to the vasculature. This model is supported by the findings showing that inhibition of methylation modulates the metastatic capacity of cell lines and also by those showing that angiogenesis is often a prerequisite to metastasis (Hunter et al., 2008; Lunt et al., 2009; Trainer et al., 1988). A major limitation of the model is that global demethylation by inhibitors of methylation cause chromosomal aberrations. This raises the possibility that the modulation of metastatic capacity induced by these inhibitors is due to mutational rather than epigenetic events (Frost et al., 1987). More importantly, the transient compartment model does not explain the clonal nature of metastases.

1.2.3 The Early Oncogenesis Model

Recent findings obtained by microarray technology identified metastatic gene signatures in primary solid tumours. This suggests that metastasis propensity is established early in oncogenesis, even at the time of diagnosis (Ramaswamy et al., 2003). These observations raise the possibility of predicting which tumours may form metastasis at diagnosis (Ellsworth et al., 2009; Wang et al., 2005). Furthermore, they challenge the concept behind the progression models by stating that metastatic capacity is acquired by very few cells harbouring somatic mutations that will later develop as malignant clones with metastatic properties. One of the advantages of the early oncogenic model, in addition to having a predictive potential, is that it may explain metastases of unknown primary origin. Along the same lines, this model can explain how small primary tumours might quickly start to disseminate at secondary sites. However, the model does not easily explain why certain carcinomas of the same origin and size do not necessarily have the same metastatic potential. In that regard, it presupposes that metastatic gene profiles are induced by somatic oncogenic events, but does not account for genomic heterogeneity that results from inherited polymorphism (Hunter et al., 2008).

1.2.4 The Fusion Model

Metastatic cells distinguish themselves from parental cells by gaining several phenotypic features, some of which are lymphoid in nature. This observation is at the origin of the fusion theory. According to this theory, the acquisition of a metastatic phenotype occurs when a healthy migratory leukocyte fuses with a primary tumour cell. A metastatic cell will emerge from the resultant hybrid that keeps both the white blood cell's natural potential to disseminate around the body, and the uncontrolled cell division that characterizes the original cancer cell (Pawelek and Chakraborty, 2008). It is difficult to assess the importance of this model in clinical metastasis. Nevertheless, there is circumstantial evidence that hybrid formation occurs within human tumours. For example, premature chromosome condensation (PCC) occurs in about 6% of 284 human bladders examined. Given that PCC is a property of multinucleated cells, and that increased ploidy is seen in these cells, these observations suggest that fusion occurs between normal plasma and malignant cells of the bladder (Atkin, 1979). Hence, it remains possible that fusion may be responsible for some aspects of metastasis. Intriguingly, a recent study has brought new grounds that expand the concept of the fusion model. Gliomas often express EGFRvIII, a truncated and oncogenic form of the epidermal growth factor receptor. Within each tumour, only a small percentage of glioma cells may actually express EGFRvIII (Biernat et al., 2004). Nevertheless, most cells exhibit a transformed phenotype. Janusz Rak's group showed that glioma cells can share EGFRvIII by intercellular transfer of membrane-derived microvesicles called oncosomes (Al-Nedawi et al., 2008). This leads to the transfer of oncogenic activity, including activation of MAPK and v-akt murine thymoma viral oncogene homologue (Akt), morphological transformations and an increase in anchorage-independent growth capacity. The authors conclude that membrane microvesicles of cancer cells can contribute to a horizontal propagation of oncogenes and their associated transforming phenotype among subsets of cancer cells. This important study re-actualizes the fusion model.

1.2.5 The Gene Transfer Models

Tumour DNA is present in the blood of both animal models and cancer patients (Leon et al., 1977; Bendich et al., 1965). These findings lead to the geno-metastasis hypothesis of metastasis formation (Garcia-Olmo and Garcia-Olmo, 2001). This theory proposes that metastases arise from the horizontal transfer in stem cells of circulating DNA bearing somatic mutations. This would confer metastatic features to recipient cells at secondary sites. In this model, metastasis would not be the progeny of primary tumours, but rather de novo tumours that arise in cancer patients. This model may possibly explain some cases of metastatic dissemination, but it cannot be viewed as a universal or frequent mechanism of metastasis. For example, the model is not compatible with the seed and soil theory discussed below unless it is associated with the improbable uptake of tissue specific genes by the recipient stem cells. In addition, the quantity of circulating 'malignant' DNA uptake should be sufficiently important to reprogram the stem cells to adopt the morphology and the biochemical markers of the cells from the primary tumours (Guy et al., 1992; Kramer et al., 1981).

1.2.6 The Genetic Predisposition Model

Using a highly malignant mammary tumour transgenic mouse strain that they bred to 27 different inbred strains, Hunter et al. (Lifsted et al., 1998) showed that the resulting strains differ in their ability to form lung metastasis and in the kinetics of induction of the primary mammary tumours. These findings demonstrate that the inherited polymorphism is a significant factor of metastatic dissemination, irrespective of the metastatic promoting somatic events present in the tumours. The findings also support the concept that the genetic background of the patients in which a tumour develops is a key determinant of the tumour's ability to form metastases. Later on, the same group identified *Sipa1* as the first polymorphic metastasis efficiency gene in mice (Park et al., 2005). This polymorphism that confers metastatic efficiency is associated with an amino acid polymorphism that results in decreased Sipa1's Rap1GAP activity and ability to bind Aqp2, its cognate partner (Park et al., 2005). Interestingly, polymorphism in the human *SIPA1* gene is associated with markers of poor outcome in a cohort of Caucasian breast cancer patients (Park et al., 2005). Moreover, several recent studies are consistent with this genetic polymorphism predisposition model of metastasis. Notably, the p53 codon 72 polymorphism is associated with susceptibility for colorectal cancer in the Korean population (Cao et al., 2009). Furthermore, there is evidence indicating that the MMP1-1602 2G allele is also associated with increased susceptibility to metastasis in colorectal cancer (Decock et al., 2008; Elander et al., 2006).

Given that cancer and metastasis develop in individuals with different genetic backgrounds, it is obvious that this model may explain certain paradoxes of other models and may even serve as an integrator of those models. In particular, the early oncogenesis model presupposes that the metastatic gene expression profiles are associated with somatic mutations. However, it does not take into account that the basal gene transcription rate is different in individuals of different genetic backgrounds. Reciprocally, it does not take into account that the prognostic profile of some genes may vary from individual to individual. In this context, it is possible that the metastasis predictive gene expression signatures that form the basis of the early oncogenic model may be a measure of inherited metastasis susceptibility segregating throughout the human population in addition to being an indication of somatic mutations driving progression (Hunter et al., 2008). Similarly, it is also clear that the inherited genetic background of an individual may affect (or may be affected by) the clonal expansion of metastatic cells as proposed by the progression model. On the other hand, if a sufficient fraction of metastatic risk is encoded by germline polymorphisms, then any tissue in the body should reflect that risk. In agreement, the genetic predisposition model further raises the possibility of using non-tumour tissues as a possible predictive source of cancer and metastasis. Incidentally, positive results have already been observed in that direction since risk groups of mice have been defined by assessing salivary gland protein profiles (Yang et al., 2005).

1.3 Metastatic Steps

The metastatic process consists of a number of sequential steps, all of which must be successfully completed to give rise to a secondary tumour (Gout and Huot, 2008; Gout et al., 2008; Joyce and Pollard, 2009). These steps include the detachment of cancer cells from the primary tumour followed by their intravasation into the pre-existing or newly formed angiogenic blood or lymphatic vessels. Cancer cells will then aggregate or not with leukocytes or platelets, survive or not in the circulation and arrest in the capillary bed of the new organ. Cancer cells will then

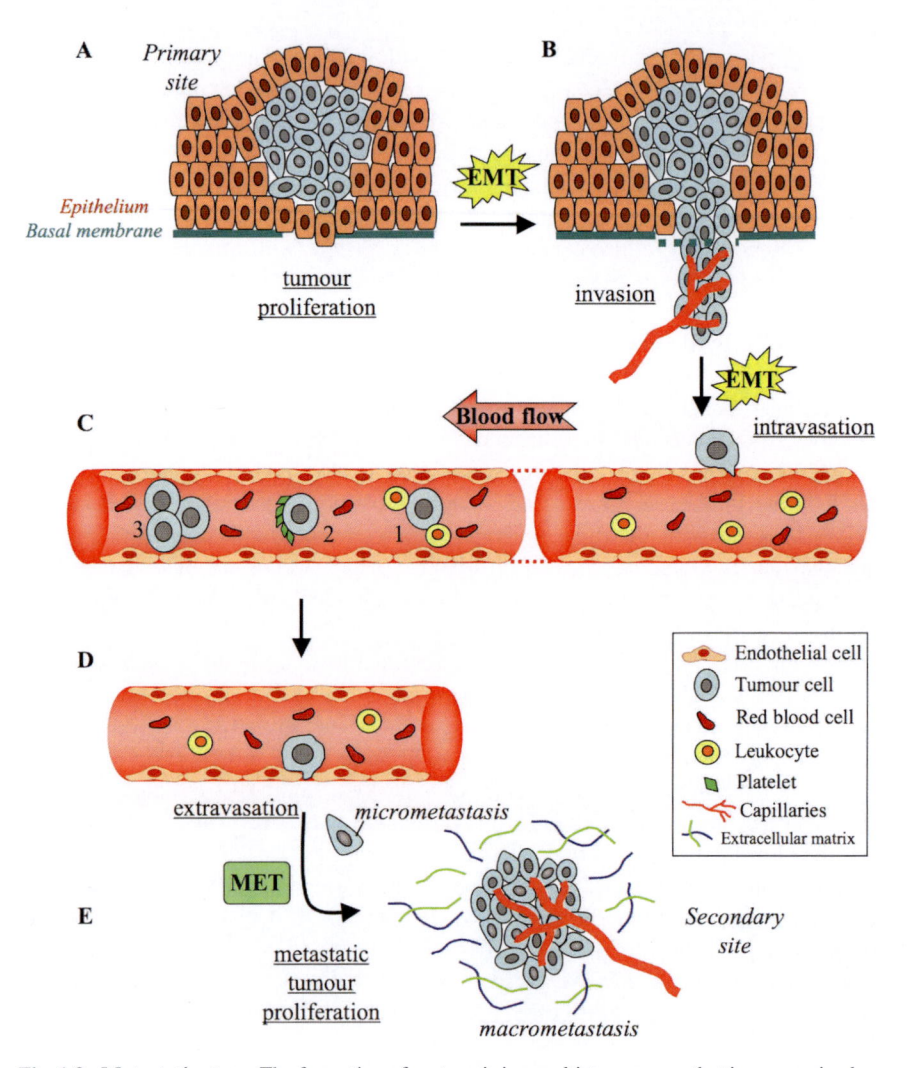

Fig. 1.2 Metastatic steps. The formation of metasasis is a multistep process that is summarized as follows: (**a**) Formation of the primary neoplasm (**b**) Detachment of cancer cells from the primary neoplasm (**c**) Intravasation in a pre-existing or newly formed capillary and tumour cell survival in blood circulation: 1, interaction with leukocytes that may be destructive or not; 2, aggregation with platelets, which protects cancer cells against mechanical stress and lytic leukocytes; 3, tumour cell-cell aggregation, which protects against stress and formation of intra-capillary thrombosis (**d**) Extravasation out of a vessel of the target organ (**e**) Metastatic growth in the new appropriate environment and formation of a secondary neoplasm (Gout and Huot, 2008)

grow locally within vessels, but most of the time they will extravasate into the surrounding tissue where they will proliferate and initiate colonization of the secondary neoplasm (Fig. 1.2). The completion of this series of events is destructive to most cancer cells and the formation of metastases is an intrinsically inefficient process (Bockhorn et al., 2007; Mehlen and Puisieux, 2006). Nevertheless, high resolution in vivo video-microscopy and cell-fate analysis suggest that intravasation into the bloodstream, arrest in the secondary organ and extravasation are completed very efficiently. In contrast, later steps (growth of micrometastases into the secondary organ, vascularization and formation of macrometastases) are inefficient (Cameron et al., 2000; Naumov et al., 2002). This metastatic inefficiency is principally determined by failure of solitary cells to initiate growth, failure of early micrometastases to continue growth into macroscopic tumours and apoptotic regression of micrometastases (Cameron et al., 2000; Luzzi et al., 1998; Wong et al., 2001). Each step of the metastatic process is characterized by intense interactions and crosstalk between cancer cells and their microenvironment; successful metatastic outgrowth depends on the ability of cancer cells to adapt to distinct microenvironments. In some cases, cancer cells lie dormant for many years because the microenvironment suppresses their malignancy. Their re-activation to form a clinically relevant metastasis probably occurs through perturbations in the microenvironment (Joyce and Pollard, 2009; Suzuki et al., 2006). We briefly review here the steps of colon cancer metastasis that we have already described in detail in recent reviews (Gout and Huot, 2008; Gout et al., 2008).

1.3.1 Development of the Primary Colorectal Neoplasm

1.3.1.1 Initiation of the Primary Colorectal Neoplasm

Most colorectal cancers arise from dysplastic adenomatous polyps. The transformation process involves a series of events characterized by the activation of proto-oncogenes (e.g.: *K-ras, N-Ras and c-Myc*) and by the inactivation of tumour suppressor genes (e.g. *APC, DCC, p53*) or DNA repair genes (e.g. *hMSH2, hMSLH1*). These events result from the accumulation of genetic (gene mutations, gene amplification, etc) and epigenetic alterations (aberrant DNA methylation, chromatin modifications, etc) that confer a selective growth advantage to colonic epithelial cells and trigger the transformation of the normal epithelium into pre-cancerous adenomatous polyps. Thereafter, the latter will undergo malignant transformation and subsequently metastasize (Gout and Huot, 2008; Grady and Carethers, 2008; Tischoff and Tannapfel, 2008). Beyond the genetic and epigenetic alterations at the origin of the primary neoplasm, the synergistic crosstalk that occurs between cancer cells and the host cellular and non-cellular microenvironment is required to support cancerous growth and dissemination (Li et al., 2007). We briefly review the influence of the stroma on the development of the primary neoplasm and thereafter, on the formation of colorectal metastases.

1.3.1.2 Influence of Stromal Cells

The primary neoplasm is embedded within a stromal reactive microenvironment that markedly influences its development and progression (Kalluri and Zeisberg, 2006). This reactive stroma is characterized by an increased number of fibroblasts, enhanced capillary density and deposition of a new ECM rich in type-1 collagen and fibrin. Macrophages and other bone marrow-derived cells (BMDC) are also recruited to the reactive stroma in response to the healing process generated by the tumour. Moreover, the tumour microenvironment is rich in blood vessels and lymphatic endothelial cells (Kalluri and Zeisberg, 2006). The reactive stroma influences the initiation and promotion of cancer by secreting cytokines and growth factors or by expressing their receptors (Fig. 1.3). For example, stromal cells within colon carcinoma express high levels of the PDGF receptor (PDGFR). In turn, this has a marked impact in colon cancer progression since pharmacological inhibition of PDGFR signalling in stromal cells inhibits cancer progression (Kitadai et al., 2006). On the other hand, a subset of tumour stromal fibroblasts commonly referred to as cancer-associated fibroblasts (CAFs), acquire several mutations and distinct phenotypic characteristics. These cells share many properties of normal myo-fibroblasts such as expression of α-smooth muscle actin, increased production of growth factors and matrix remodelling proteases which facilitate migration and invasion of tumour cells (Le et al., 2008). These genetically altered fibroblasts may directly be involved in cancer initiation. Notably, when immortalized prostate epithelial cells are grafted in mice together with normal fibroblasts or CAFs taken from the primary site, intraepithelial neoplasia of the prostate emerges only in the presence of CAFs (Olumi et al., 1999). The tumour-induced ability of CAFs relies mainly

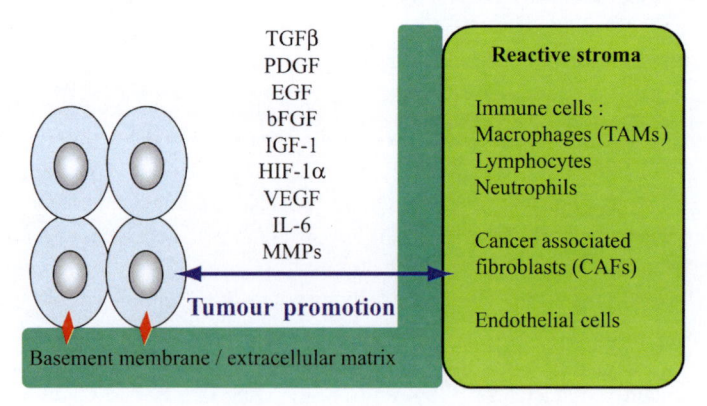

Fig. 1.3 Interaction of cancer cells with their microenvironment. Beyond genetic and epigenetic alterations that affect cancer cells, a dynamic interaction occurs between the cancer cells and the host stromal microenvironment to support cancerous growth and dissemination. The stroma is constituted mainly of cellular elements such as fibroblasts and immune cells and non-cellular elements such as the extracellular matrix (ECM). These stromal elements act in synergy with the cancer cells from the primary sites to sustain cancer growth and metastasis. For example, cancer-associated macrophages and fibroblasts influence cancer initiation/promotion by secreting cytokines, growth factors and chemokines (Gout and Huot, 2008)

on the production of cytokines such as TGFβ that activates cancer cells and triggers their detachment from the primary neoplasm. Interestingly, TGFβ triggers the transformation of lung endothelial cells into CAFs, which favours lung cancer progression in mice. This finding indicates that endothelial cells contribute to the expansion of the pool of CAFs that synergize with cancer cells favouring their progression (Zeisberg et al., 2007). It further highlights the intricate signalling network that exists between a tumour and its microenvironment. As discussed in depth in Chapter 6 by Brabletz et al., in this book, dysregulation of the Wnt/β catenin signalling pathway plays a major role in the development and progression of colon cancer (Le et al., 2008). Along these lines, CAFs are primary candidates for local modulation of the Wnt/β-catenin signalling, resulting in dysregulated patterns of β-catenin intracellular localization within colorectal tumours (Brabletz et al., 2001; Le et al., 2008).

A large proportion of the primary tumour mass is constituted of bone marrow-derived cells (BMDC) including tumour-associated macrophages (TAMs) (Pollard, 2004). The recruitment of BMDC and TAMs to tumours is a response to cancer-associated inflammation and may explain why some cancers respond to anti-inflammatory agents (Balkwill et al., 2005; Mantovani et al., 2008). The importance of TAMs in cancer is supported by the fact that their presence within a tumour correlates with a poor prognosis given that they contribute to stimulate cell migration, invasion and intravasation (Joyce and Pollard, 2009). In the case of colon cancer, it seems that TAMs favour metastasis by secreting vascular endothelial growth factor (VEGF), thereby promoting angiogenesis at the primary site (Barbera-Guillem et al., 2002). Moreover, TAMs promote removal of apoptotic colon cancer cells that express the sulfoglycolipids SM4s. During the process, the phenotype of TAMs is modified, as it is associated with an increased expression of TGFβ1 and secretion of IL-6. This phenotypic modification may putatively contribute to further activate the angiogenic process (Popovic et al., 2007). Neutrophils are also recruited to colorectal cancer and, as is the case with macrophages, this recruitment is associated with poor prognosis, possibly by enhancing angiogenesis and metastasis (Murdoch et al., 2008). On the other hand, infiltration of CD8+ T cells and dendritic cells is associated with a favourable prognosis in colorectal cancer as they destroy cancer cells via perforin- and granzyme-mediated apoptosis (de Visser et al., 2006; Talmadge et al., 2007). Thus, it seems that BDMC have either tumour-suppressive or tumour-promoting properties depending on the nature of BDMC and on the tissue context (Joyce and Pollard, 2009; Ostrand-Rosenberg, 2008).

1.3.1.3 Influence of the Extracellular Matrix

Cells are in contact with an extracellular matrix (ECM) that is constituted by five classes of macromolecules: collagens, laminins, fibronectins, proteoglycans and hyaluronans. There is a continuous exchange between cells and the ECM. These interactions involve cell adhesion receptors such as integrins and cadherins which modulate important cellular functions such as proliferation, migration, gene expression and apoptosis/anoikis (Juliano, 2002). This is discussed in detail in Chapter 7 by Arabzadeh and Beauchemin in this book. The composition and functions of

ECM vary with developmental stage, biological location and diseases. Notably, cancer cells highjack the normal cell/ECM interactions to ensure their survival. Along these lines, de novo synthesis and/or deposition of components of basement membrane (BM), a specialized type of ECM, are associated with different types of tumours, which suggests an active role for BM/ECM molecules in tumour invasion. For example, the expression of laminin-1 in gastric carcinoma is a risk factor for liver metastasis. Moreover, in human gastric and pancreatic carcinomas, laminin-5 is expressed by metastatic malignant cells, and is considered a marker of invasiveness (Pyke et al., 1995). ECM modifications are accompanied by changes in transmembrane adhesive receptors expressed by tumour cells. The best-characterized example of these changes is the 'switch' of function of the α6β4 integrin. This integrin is usually associated with hemi-desmosomes and its usual role is to provide stable adhesion of epithelial cells to BM. However, in colon carcinoma, the α6β4 integrin instead promotes cell migration on laminin-1 by inducing and stabilizing actin-containing motility structures (Rabinovitz and Mercurio, 1997).

Cancer cells of the primary neoplasm secrete a variety of proteins that include growth factors and ECM-degrading proteases. They may also stimulate the host to secrete biomolecules that favour detachment and degradation of the matrix enabling further steps of cancer progression (Fig. 1.3). Matrix degradation takes place in a region close to the tumour cell surface, where the amount of the active enzymes outbalances the natural protease inhibitors present in the matrix or secreted by normal cells (Handsley and Edwards, 2005). Matrix metalloproteinases (MMPs), metalloproteinases (ADAMs) and tissue inhibitors of metalloproteinases (TIMPs) constitute the major ECM proteolytic axis whose dysregulation is associated with cancer. In particular, metastatic colon cancer cells are able to induce the expression and/or secretion of MMP-2 and MMP-9 in stromal cells, either via direct contact or via paracrine regulation (Mook et al., 2004). Moreover, elevated levels of TIMP-4 are associated with colon cancer progression as well as that of breast, ovary, endometrium and papillary renal tumours. In contrast, the expression of TIMP-4 is down-regulated in pancreatic and clear cell renal tumours (Melendez-Zajgla et al., 2008).

In summary, there is increasing evidence indicating that an intense crosstalk occurs between stromal cells, ECM and cancer cells and that this crosstalk plays a major role in influencing tumour cell detachment at the primary site and in initiating the metastatic cascade. Moreover, there is also evidence showing that ECM components secreted at the primary sites may favour establishment of metastases at the secondary site. For example, lysyl oxidase induced by hypoxia in breast cancer cells at the primary site is responsible for their invasive properties by increasing FAK activity (Erler et al., 2006).

1.3.1.4 Epithelial-Mesenchymal Transition

In addition to the role of MMPs in loss of cell-cell adhesion at the primary site, the cellular de-adhesion process is tightly associated with epithelial-mesenchymal transition (EMT). During embryogenesis, EMT is a morphogenetic process where epithelial cells lose their characteristics and gain mesenchymal properties. The earliest EMT event in embryonic development is the formation of the mesoderm from the ectoderm during gastrulation (Yang and Weinberg, 2008). Currently, an increasing amount of evidence indicates that carcinoma cells usurp the mechanism of embryonic EMT to detach from primary neoplasms and migrate to distal sites to form metastases. In particular, the progression of colon cancer is closely connected with EMT (Bates and Mercurio, 2005; Bates et al., 2007) as discussed in detail in Chapter 6.

The hypoxic environment that surrounds the primary tumour is a major condition inducing EMT. Hypoxia-induced EMT results mainly from up-regulation of hypoxia-inducible factor-1α (HIF1α), hepatocyte growth factor (HGF), Snail1, Twist1 as well as from the activation of the Notch or NF-κB pathways, and the induction of DNA hypomethylation (Gort et al., 2008). Hypoxia may also activate self-reinforcing positive-feedback loops that help stabilize the mesenchymal state. As discussed below, hypoxia-induced activation of Snail1 causes repression of E-cadherin transcription. This leads to the release of cytoplasmic β-catenin and activation and stabilization of EMT-inducing transcription factor expression in the nucleus (Polyak and Weinberg, 2009).

TGFβ is a major effector of EMT. Typically, the binding of TGFβ to TGFβR1/TGFβR2 triggers the serine/threonine phosphorylation of the Smad2/Smad3 dimers that dissociate from the receptors to interact with Smad4. They then enter the nucleus to regulate transcriptional modulation (Massague, 2008). Several genes regulated downstream of the TGFβ/SMAD2/SMAD3/SMAD4 axis, including E-cadherin and Slug, are part of the EMT signature in colon cancer (Joyce et al., 2009). In addition to transcriptional regulation, the TGF-β-activated pathways are associated with cytoskeletal remodelling and increased cell motility. In this context, the expression of integrin α6β4, as a consequence of the EMT, enables motile and invasive colorectal cancer cells to interact with interstitial matrices and sustain the activation of TGF-β (Bates et al., 2005). Interestingly, TNFα produced by infiltrating macrophages increases TGFβ-induced EMT of colon cancer cells via paracrine signalling (Bates et al., 2004; Bates and Mercurio, 2003; Massague, 2008).

One of the major characteristics of the EMT of carcinoma cells is the loss of E-cadherin-mediated cell-cell adhesion (Cavallaro and Christofori, 2004; Polyak and Weinberg, 2009). This loss results from mutations in the E-cadherin gene, proteolytic degradation of E-cadherin, and IGF1-mediated internalization of E-cadherin (Cavallaro and Christofori, 2004). In colon cancer, epithelial cell adhesion molecule (EpCAM) functions as a homophilic cell adhesion molecule that also interferes with E-cadherin-mediated cell–cell contact (Litvinov et al., 1997; Maetzel et al., 2009). Loss of E-cadherin further results in a decrease in its expression subsequent to promoter hypermethylation and activation of transcriptional repressors such as Snail and FOXC2 (Dumont et al., 2008; Thiery and Sleeman, 2006). As mentioned above, the loss of E-cadherin expression is concomitantly associated with the release of β-catenin, normally tethered to the E-cadherin cytoplasmic tail. In turn, the freed β-catenin molecules migrate to the nucleus and induce the expression of EMT-inducing transcription factor (Polyak and Weinberg, 2009). In colon cancer cells, deregulation of E-cadherin and induction of EMT are associated with increased cell migration as a consequence of a peripheral accumulation of Src and phospho-myosin and an increased expression of the guanine nucleotide exchange factor TIAM1 (Avizienyte et al., 2004; Minard et al., 2006). Elevated RhoC expression is also associated with an aberrant expression and localization of E-cadherin in colon cancer cells correlating with a poor prognostic (Bellovin et al., 2006). Interestingly, in melanoma, breast and prostate cancers, the disruption of E-cadherin-mediated cancer cell adhesion is associated with the so-called cadherin-switch in which the E-cadherin loss is accompanied by de novo expression of mesenchymal cadherin, such as N-cadherin. Furthermore, by up-regulating N-cadherin expression, cancer cells interact with stromal cells, thereby changing their location and favouring the invasion of the surrounding stroma. N-cadherin confers motility and migration to cancer cells (Hazan et al., 2000). Hence, the cadherin switch is an important component of the EMT that characterizes the early step of cancer progression toward an invasive and metastatic phenotype.

1.3.1.5 Angiogenesis and Lymphangiogenesis

Cancer cells cannot grow when they are located at a distance greater than 110 μm from a blood vessel (Kerbel and Folkman, 2002).In fact, tumour growth and progression are both dependent on angiogenic neo-vascularization to provide cancer cells with oxygen and nutrients. Accordingly, cancer cells begin to promote angiogenesis early in tumourigenesis in order to sustain their growth. At a later stage, angiogenesis is further involved as an important step of metastasis; the cancer cells that detach from the primary site use the new vessels as a path to reach and colonize new sites. A tight balance between pro- and anti-angiogenic agents regulates the angiogenic process. Typically, the 'angiogenic switch' is initiated by tumour-associated hypoxic conditions, which contribute to activate the transcription of HIF-1. In turn, HIF-1 promotes the expression of several angiogenic factors by the cancer cells including VEGF, basic fibroblast growth factor (bFGF) and placental growth factor (PLGF) (Liao and Johnson, 2007). On the other hand, tumour angiogenesis is preserved in HIF-1-deficient colon cancer cells indicating that the expression of these angiogenic agents by cancer cells is also increased through a HIF-1-independent pathway (Mizukami et al., 2005, 2007). Once they are expressed, angiogenic growth factors interact with their respective receptors at the surface of endothelial cells initiating the angiogenic program activation. In particular, VEGF binds to VEGFR2, which triggers signalling cascades involving endothelial nitric oxide synthase (eNOS), phosphatidyl inositol 3 kinase (PI3K), p38 and extracellular signal-regulated kinase (ERK) mitogen-activated protein (MAP) kinases leading to the induction of vasodilation, endothelial cell migration/proliferation and vessel assembly (Lamalice et al., 2007). The angiogenic switch also involves down-regulation of angiogenesis suppressor proteins, such as thrombospondin, and recruitment of progenitor endothelial cells to the tumour (Kerbel and Folkman, 2002). Importantly, angiogenesis is involved in colorectal cancer growth and dissemination. The level of angiogenesis is a survival predictor for diseased patients (Goh et al., 2007). Along these lines, patients who demonstrate a Doppler vascularity index greater than 15% at the primary site have a poorer overall survival than the patients with an index <15% (Chen et al., 2000). The importance of angiogenesis in colon cancer metastasis to the liver is further highlighted by the finding that anti-angiogenic agents such as the anti-VEGF-directed antibody bevacizumab in combination with standard chemotherapy offers stimulating promises in blocking the metastatic process of colon cancer (Ellis and Haller, 2008; Ellis and Hicklin, 2008).

In solid cancers including colorectal cancer, the lymph node status is the most important prognostic indicator for patient clinical outcome (Sundar and Ganesan, 2007; Sundlisaeter et al., 2007). Interesting findings indicate that lymphangiogenesis is present in colorectal cancer and that the lymphatic vessel density of the tumour correlates with depth of invasion and metastasis, not only to regional lymph nodes but also to the liver (Gout and Huot, 2008). It is thought that colon cancer is closely related to lymphangiogenesis because colorectal cancer cells express the CXCR5 chemokine receptor and both lymphatic endothelial cells and the liver express its ligand BCA-1/CXCL13 (Meijer et al., 2006). Hence, it is possible that cancer cells may be directed via lymphangiogenesis to both lymph nodes and liver, which would explain the correlation between lymph node and liver metastasis of colon. As for angiogenesis, the importance of lymphangiogenesis in colorectal cancer will be discussed in detail in Chapter 9.

1.3.2 Intravasation

The detachment of cancer cells from the primary neoplasm is followed by their entry or intravasation into the surrounding blood or lymphatic vessels. Unfortunately, the intravasation process has not been investigated as intensively as other stages of metastasis and is not understood very well in colon cancer. This information deficit is mostly due to the lack of reliable animal models (Vernon et al., 2007). There is a current controversy as to whether distal hematogenous metastases develop as a result of direct blood vessel intravasation at the primary tumour site or whether they are derived from cells that have previously colonized local lymph nodes (Bacac and Stamenkovic, 2008). In the first hypothesis, tumour cells need to degrade vascular BM in order to enter into the blood circulation. Several arguments favour this possibility, as discussed previously. Notably, vascular invasion and penetration by tumour cells is observed by microscopic examination of tissue sections. Moreover, many experimental approaches illustrate that intravasation is associated with ECM degradation by metalloproteinases. In particular, the urokinase-type plasminogen activator (u-PA) system plays a determinant role in the intravasation of colorectal cancers (Leupold et al., 2007). Following its binding to receptor (u-PAR), u-PA activates plasminogen and other proteases such as matrix metalloproteinases-2 (MMP-2) and MMP-9, which contributes to ECM breakdown and favours intravasation. A recent study has shown that u-PAR gene expression is induced downstream of AP-1 promoter Src-mediated activation and Ser73 and Ser63 c-Jun phosphorylation. Src activity continually increases during the transition from benign colonic polyps to primary colon cancers and then to colon cancer metastases, and is associated with an increased in vitro invasion of cultured colon cancer cells (Iravani et al., 1998). Moreover, elevated Src activity is a poor prognostic factor in colorectal cancer patients (Allgayer et al., 1999). Hence, it is possible that Src contributes to ECM breakdown thereby promoting intravasation by regulating the u-PA/u-PAR system activity. Intriguingly, a large number of cancer cells undergo fragmentation when they interact with blood vessels indicating that they must acquire additional capability in order to survive the intravasation process (Wyckoff et al., 2000). In this regard, colon cancer cells overexpress FAK, suggesting that the detached cancer cells can by-pass integrin signalling thereby resisting anoikis and aquiring the potential to survive in the absence of ECM contact (Owens et al., 1995). FAK may contribute to enhanced survival by activating survival-signal pathways, such as ERK or AKT pathways (Mehlen and Puisieux, 2006; Zeng et al., 2002).

In the second case, detached tumour cells first invade lymph nodes and then disseminate from lymph nodes to blood vessels. This could occur via migration of the cells to efferent lymphatic vessels, followed by transport to the *vena cava* from where haematogenous spread would be possible. The cancer cell entry into lymphatic circulation is tightly associated with lymphangiogenesis. The mechanisms by which lymphangiogenesis contributes to colon cancer and cancer metastasis are still unclear. It is possible that VEGF-C-stimulated lymphatic endothelial cells secrete chemotactic or mitogenic factors that attract cancer cells to the newly growing lymphatic vessels enabling their adhesion and intravasation on and through the lymphatic endothelium (Karkkainen et al., 2002). In this context, chemokine C-X-C motif receptor (CXCR4) and chemokine receptor type 7 (CCR7) expression by human breast cancer cells facilitates their migration to the lymph nodes (Muller et al., 2001). Once they have interacted with the endothelium of lymphangiogenic vessels, the entry of cancer cells into these vessels is greatly facilitated by the fact that they are leaky and tortuous (Fig. 1.4). As mentioned earlier, colorectal cancer cells express the CXCR5 chemokine receptor and both lymphatic endothelial cells and liver express its ligand BCA-1/chemokine ligand 13 (CXCL13) (Meijer et al., 2006). It is then possible that cancer cells may be directed to both lymph nodes and liver, via lymphangiogenesis.

Overall, intravasation into the blood stream might occur via direct entry of the cancer cells into the blood vessels or secondarily via lymphatic vessel invasion. In the latter case, haematogenous metastasis may be secondary to cancer cells that have first invaded lymphoid tissue and then gained access to the blood circulation via the thoracic duct and subsequently the *vena cava*. Both mechanisms might be operational and the relative ease of lymphatic vessel invasion and penetration might explain why lymph nodes are usually the first metastatic site in carcinomas.

1.3.3 Circulation of Cancer Cells

A large number of cancer cells can be detected in the blood of cancer patients. However, only 0.01% of metastatic clonal cancer cells injected into the circulation of animal models generate metastases. This suggests that circulation is deleterious

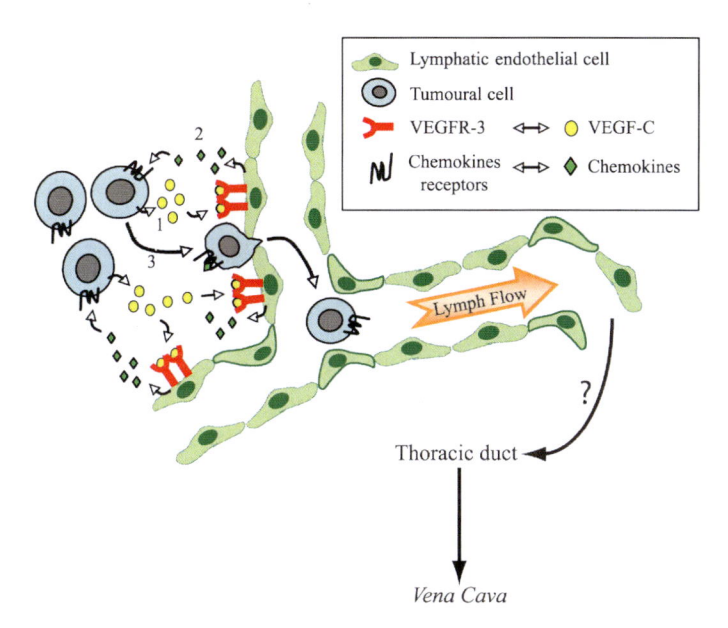

Fig. 1.4 Mechanisms of intravasation of cancer cells across lymphatic vessels. In several human cancers, increased expression of VEGF-C in primary tumours correlates with regional lymph node metastases. A reciprocal cross-talk exists between tumour cells and lymphatic endothelial cells to induce tumour lymphangiogenesis and formation of lymph node metastases. Notably, VEGF-C activates lymphatic endothelial cells (*1*) that may secrete chemotactic factors (*2*). This contributes to attract cancer cells bearing appropriate chemokine receptors to the growing lymph vessels (*3*), and to enable their adhesion and their intra-lymphatic intravasation. Eventually some cancer cells will leave the lymphatic vessel and gain access to the blood stream via the thoracic duct and the *vena cava* (Gout and Huot, 2008)

for most cancer cells. In fact, intravital videomicroscopy studies using radiolabelled or fluorescently-labelled cancer cell lines injected into the circulation support the hypothesis that solitary cancer cells in the circulation are highly sensitive to apoptosis (Chambers et al., 2001; Luzzi et al., 1998; Mehlen and Puisieux, 2006; Wong et al., 2001). Death of solitary cells in the circulation occurs mostly through tumour immune surveillance or destruction by mechanical stresses.

The mechanical stress imposed by the circulation is a major strain that cancer cells must survive to form metastases. It represents the first line of defence of the host against the circulating cancer cells (Gassmann and Haier, 2008). Its influence is especially important in narrow capillaries and within the microvasculature of contracting skeletal and heart muscle, in which sphere-to-cylinder shape transformation is lethal to most cancer cells (Weiss et al., 1992). The deleterious effect of shear stress may also be mediated via NO and reactive oxygen species (ROS) production following endothelial contraction (Mehlen and Puisieux, 2006). Oxyradical production is required for apoptosis of intravenously injected colorectal cancer cells in hepatic sinusoids (Edmiston et al., 1998). Cancer cells have developed several ways to survive the mechanical stresses associated with circulation. Notably, they express high levels of stress proteins such as HSP70, which increases their resistance to shear stress as well as to any other type of stress (Mehlen and Puisieux, 2006). Moreover, tumour cells resist shear stress following their association with platelets and leukocytes. As discussed in detail in Chapter 7, cancer cells often express an altered glycosyltranferase repertoire associated with increased expression of glycosylated proteins, which enables their binding to selectins present on platelets and leukocytes (Kim et al., 1999). This contributes to protect cancer cells by shielding them against external aggression, thereby favouring tumour metastasis (Bacac and Stamenkovic, 2008). Incidentally, platelets may further facilitate metastasis by protecting the vasculature via secretion of their granule contents (Ho-Tin-Noe et al., 2009). Experimental evidence suggests that integrins and adhesion molecules of the immunoglobulin superfamily are also implicated in protecting cancer cells against mechanical stress by enabling their adhesion to the endothelium and allowing them to escape anoikis (Gout and Huot, 2008; Joyce and Pollard, 2009). These survival processes are only effective for a small percentage of circulatory cancer cells, since only 0.01% of them form metastases.

Interleukin-2 (IL-2) is effective in treating patients with metastatic melanoma and kidney cancers, and its anti-tumoural activity is closely related to its ability to expand and activate specific subsets of immune cells, such as T cells and natural killer (NK) cells (Rosenberg, 2001). Stimulation of NK cells by Il-8 and Il-12 is also associated with suppression of metastasis (Kim et al., 2000). Mechanisms of tumour-cell killing by NK cells is mediated either by the NKG2/perforin or Trail pathways (Smyth et al., 2004; Takeda et al., 2001). These findings highlight the fact that immuno-destruction is another process that cancer cells must overcome in order to survive in the circulation (Malmberg and Ljunggren, 2006). In this context, the cancer cell/platelet aggregates protect cancer cells not only against shear stress but also against NK cell-mediated lysis (Nieswandt et al., 1999; Palumbo et al., 2007; Rosenberg, 2001). Furthermore, cancer cells may use inflammation-associated mechanisms to further protect themselves against apoptosis. For example, the level of acute-phase glycoproteins is abnormally high in patients with cancer, which correlates with the extent of the disease. These glycoproteins, synthesized by the liver in response to an inflammatory stimulus, may protect tumours including colorectal cancer from the host's immunological attack (Allin et al., 2009; Samak and Israel, 1982). Intriguingly, there is no direct evidence indicating that human immuno-deficiencies are associated with increased development of metastasis from solid tumours. Hence, it is still difficult to fully understand the specific contribution of tumour cell death induced by the immune system in limiting metastasis. Nevertheless, manipulating the immune system to induce colon cancer or other types of tumour regression presents a great therapeutic interest (Morse et al., 2007).

1.3.4 Extravasation

The tumour microenvironment needs to be permissive for the incoming tumour cells to grow and form metastases (Kaplan et al., 2006). Notably, the adhesive interactions between the cancer cells and target organ endothelial cells are crucial components of metastasis. These interactions determine the arrest of the circulatory cells in the capillaries and initiate the cascade of events that culminate in diapedesis of the cancer cells across the endothelium.

1.3.4.1 The Adhesion to Endothelial Cells and the Homing Concept of Metastasis

Extravasation of circulating tumour cells in the host organ first requires successive adhesive interactions between endothelial cell receptors and their ligands or counter-receptors present on the cancer cells, and second, their passage across the endothelium (Gout et al., 2008; Nicolson, 1988). Several types of cancers have an organ preference to form metastasis. For example, colorectal cancer metastasizes to liver and lungs, and intraocular cancer like uveal melanoma preferentially metastasizes to liver, but rarely to other organs. Additionally, breast cancer preferentially spread to bones, liver, brain and lungs while patients with prostate cancer develop bone metastases (Table 1.1). This organ selectivity leads to the 'seed and soil' hypothesis that was proposed by Stephen Paget (Paget, 1889). According to this theory, the successful adhesive interactions of tumour cells (seed) with the microenvironment of a particular organ (soil) are necessary for the formation of metastases in specific organs. This 'homing concept of metastasis' was challenged by James Ewing who suggested that organ-selectivity of metastasis merely results from mechanical factors involving the first circulatory bed encountered by the circulating cancer cells (Ewing, 1928). However, several clinical observations do not support this view. Notably, metastases often form in low-irrigated organs such as the brain, bone and adrenals whereas cancer cells rarely colonize highly vascularized organs such as heart, muscles and spleen. In fact, Ewing's theory may possibly explain only certain particular types of loco-regional metastasis

Table 1.1 Examples of primary tumors that selectively form metastasis in preferential target organs

Homing of cancer metastasis	
Primary tumors	Metastatic sites
Colon, rectum, stomach	Liver, lung
Breast	Bone, liver, lung, brain, adrenal gland
Lung (small cells)	Brain, liver, bone marrow
Lung (non-small cells)	Liver, bone, brain
Prostate	Bone
Kidney	Lung, bone, adrenal gland
Melanoma (skin)	Liver, brain, colon
Melanoma (uveal)	Liver
Neuroblastoma	Liver, adrenal gland
Thyroid	Bone, lung

(Ribatti et al., 2006). In contrast, Paget's seed and soil theory is supported by several clinical observations and experimental approaches. In particular, the organ selectivity of B16 clonal melanoma cells to form metastasis in the organ from which the parental cells have been isolated is a major support to the seed and soil theory (Fidler, 1996).

Adhesive interactions between the cancer cells and target organ endothelial cells constitute a major mechanism to explain the seed and soil hypothesis. These interactions determine the arrest of the circulatory cells in the capillaries and initiate the cascade of events that culminate in extravasation of the cancer cells in the colonized organs in which they will proliferate to give rise to secondary neoplasms. Circulating tumour cell extravasation in the host organ requires successive adhesive interactions between endothelial cells and their glycosylated ligands or counter-receptors present on cancer cells (Nicolson, 1988). These interactions stimulate selectin-mediated initial attachment and rolling of the circulating cancer cells on the endothelium. Rolling cancer cells then become activated by locally released chemokines present at the endothelial cell surface. This triggers integrin activation on cancer cells allowing their firmer adhesion via members of the Ig-CAM family such as intercellular adhesion molecule (ICAM), initiating the transendothelial migration and extravasation processes (Walzog and Gaehtgens, 2000) (see Chapter 7). Several studies show that cancer cells may initiate endothelial adhesion molecule expression. This is supported, among others, by studies showing that cancer cell culture medium may contain cytokines such as TNFα, IL1-β or IFNγ that will directly activate endothelial cells to express E-selectin, P-selectin, ICAM-2 or vascular endothelial cell adhesion koelcule (VCAM) (Kannagi et al., 2004; Narita et al., 1996). Moreover, highly metastatic human colorectal and mouse lung carcinoma cells trigger a rapid host inflammatory response upon entry into the hepatic micro-circulation by inducing TNFα production in resident Kupffer cells. In turn, this triggers E-selectin expression by endothelial cells enhancing the binding and extravasation of the cancer cells (Khatib et al., 2005).

Since the adhesion of cancer cells to the endothelium requires the presence of endothelial selectins as well as sialyl-Lewis carbohydrates on cancer cells, the level of selectin expression on the vascular wall and the presence of the appropriate ligand on cancer cells are determinant for their adhesion and extravasation into a specific organ. Along these lines, the homing of B16F10 melanoma cells to the liver requires the expression of the E-selectin ligand by melanoma cells and the expression of soluble E-selectin in the liver in mice. This concept is further supported by the fact that endothelial selectins may be expressed differentially in blood vessels from different tissues. For example, LPS and TNFα strongly induce expression of P-selectin on endothelial cells of the leptomeninges, but to a weaker level on blood vessels of the brain parenchyma (Araki et al., 1997). Furthermore, we found that sialylated death-receptor-3 (DR3)-mediated invasive properties of colon cancer cells are activated following their binding to the E-selectin expressed by activated endothelial cells (Gout et al., 2006, 2008). The partners DR3/E-selectin may be important players in the colon cancer metastasis homing to the liver since E-selectin expression in liver sinusoidal endothelial cells is increased by the cancer cell-mediated activation of Kupffer cells and its corresponding inflammatory response (Gout et al., 2008; Khatib et al., 2005). Based on these findings, it can be proposed that the specific interactions that take place between selectins differentially expressed by endothelial cells of potential target organs and their ligands displayed on cancer cells are major determinants underlying the organ-specific metastases distribution. In this context, cancer cells that express DR3 such as uveal melanoma cells and colon cancer cells bind E-selectin and disseminate preferentially to the liver.

Importantly, homing of cancer cells is further determined by the expression of specific metastatic genes. Notably, three groups of genes determine homing: metastasis initiation genes, metastasis progression genes and metastasis virulence genes (Nguyen et al., 2009). Initiation genes group genes that are altered in the primary tumour and that confer features such as cell motility, EMT, ECM degradation, bone marrow progenitor mobilization, angiogenesis or evasion of the immune system. It is assumed that these genes probably continue to express these properties after cancer cells infiltrate distant tissues. In particular, the metastasis-associated colon cancer 1 (*MACC1*) gene is crucial in colorectal carcinoma development (Stein et al., 2009). Metastatic growth of colorectal carcinomas is also initiated by the suppression of *miR-126* (Guo et al., 2008). Initiation metastasis gene expression is associated with poor prognosis and might provide markers that predict organ-specific colonization (Nguyen et al., 2009).

In contrast to the initiation genes, the deregulated expression of the progression metastasis genes generally occurs when the cells have left the primary tumours. In certain circumstances, these genes could already be prominently expressed in a primary tumour, although they might have a unique role at a distant site. Notably, we recently reported that DR3, a member of the TNF family of receptors present in primary colon cancer, may confer metastatic properties to colon cancer cells by increasing their invasive and survival properties (Gout et al., 2006). The expression of the progression genes such as CCL5 and presumably DR3 is associated with processes regulating the infiltration of distant organs by circulating cancer cells. Given that the structure and composition of capillary walls and surrounding parenchyma vary in different organs, the functions required for metastatic infiltration, survival and colonization might also differ depending on the target organ.

On the other hand, the metastasis virulence genes accentuate the metastatic propensity of disseminated cancer cells that have successfully completed the previous steps of metastasis initiation and progression. These genes confer activities that are essential for metastatic colonization of a certain organ. Their expression becomes detectable only in cancer cells that metastasize to those tissues. For example, osteoclast mobilizing factors, such as parathyroid hormone-related protein and interleukin 11 enable breast cancer cells to establish osteolytic metastases in bone. However, they do not provide an advantage to breast cancer cells in primary tumours (Kang et al., 2003). The expression of the virulence genes could become stabilized as it provides a selective advantage to malignant cells in a particular microenvironment. However, their expression would not contribute to the expression signatures that are predictive of metastasis in primary tumours (Nguyen et al., 2009).

1.3.4.2 The Passage Across the Endothelium

Following their adhesion to endothelial cells, cancer cells extend invadipodia into the endothelial cell junctions initiating their retraction and enabling their trans-endothelial migration. The mechanisms by which cancer cells regulate retraction of endothelial cells are not well defined. In the case of Lewis lung carcinoma cells, it may rely on the release of 12(S)-hydroxyeicosatetraenoic acid (Honn et al., 1994) by the cells themselves. On the other hand, we reported that retraction of endothelial cells following E-selectin-mediated adhesion of colon cancer cells results from an ERK-dependent dissociation of the VE-cadherin/β-catenin complex associated with a p38-dependent actin filament retraction (Tremblay et al., 2006, 2008). In some cases, an irreversible retraction of the endothelial layer may be caused by cancer cell-induced apoptosis of endothelial cells, for instance following the transcellular diapedesis of colon cancer cells across individual endothelial cells (Tremblay et al., 2008). The extravasation process also involves the contribution of proteases (collagenases type I and IV) that are located at the invasive front of the cancer cells. These proteases degrade ECM components and also trigger the release of growth factors, stored in the BM, that will induce retraction (Miles et al., 2008). In both cases, extravasation is favoured. Following extravasation, cancer cells adhere to the sub-endothelial BM/ECM via an interaction between BM proteins (laminin, collagen IV and VIII, fibronectin and heparan sulfate) and cancer cell adhesion receptors such as integrins and CD44 (Banerji et al., 2007; Miles et al., 2008). Cancer cells will then grow and initiate the development of a secondary neoplasm. Alternatively, they will move across the ECM and grow at a further distance.

1.3.5 Colonization of the Secondary Sites

Colonization of secondary sites is the final step of the metastatic process and is defined as the lodging and subsequent growth of disseminated cancer cells into detectable metastases (Taylor et al., 2008). Cancer cell metastatic growth at secondary sites is tightly regulated by their interactions with their new environment. In fact, most cancer cells that reach secondary sites die by apoptosis. Moreover, only a small subset of them initiate cell division to form micrometastases and only some of them become vascularized and grow to form macroscopic metastases. In other words, cancer cells successfully colonizing secondary sites are those that will develop mechanisms to escape apoptosis and initiate neo-vascularization. In the case of colon cancer cells, it has been proposed that they release soluble CD44 which acts as a decoy receptor impairing interaction of cancer cells with their hyaluronate ligand within the ECM, thereby conferring resistance to apoptosis (Subramaniam et al., 2007). Several lines of evidence further indicate that ECM, by altering the expression of growth factors and growth factor receptors in colon cancer cells, modulates the liver proliferation of these cancer cells. For example, heparin proteoglycan stimulates colon cancer cell hepatic proliferation via induction of autocrine growth factors and their receptors (Zvibel et al., 1998). Another factor that may limit the proliferation of all the incoming cancer cells at the secondary site is the fact that the latter is poorly vascularized at the onset. This will yield dormant micrometastases that may eventually develop into macrometastases following appropriate remodelling of the microenvironment. Notably, EGF receptor expression coupled to growth factor expression such as TGFα are among the well-known molecular factors that influence the ability of colon cancer cells to grow in the liver (Radinsky, 1995; Radinsky and Ellis, 1996). Moreover, the chemokine receptor CXCR4 is required for outgrowth of colon carcinoma micrometastases in the liver (Zeelenberg et al., 2003).

As described in Section 1.3.1.4, progression of solid tumours involves transition of epithelial transformed cells into mesenchymal cells (EMT), a process by which cancer cells acquire a more invasive and metastatic phenotype. Subsequently, the disseminated mesenchymal cancer cells must undergo the reverse transition, mesenchymal-epithelial transition (MET), at the metastatic site to allow micrometastases to give rise to a secondary neoplasm that has the characteristics of the primary one. In this regard, cancer cells from the secondary site re-express markers of epithelial cells such as E-cadherin (Yang et al., 2009; Yates et al., 2007). Since initiation of tumour growth at the secondary site is the rate-limiting step in metastasis, this suggests that the ability of mesenchymal cells to undergo MET in the appropriate microenvironments, is a key feature of metastasis (Hugo et al., 2007). In the case of colon cancer metastasis, it seems that the liver microenvironment, especially a subpopulation of CAFs, contributes to activate the MET process. This is achieved by promoting the crosstalk between autocrine/paracrine growth factors and cell adhesion molecules expressed by cancer and stromal cells. For instance, CAFs taken from the liver of patients having developed colon metastases overexpress cyclooxygenase-2 (COX2) and TGF-β2 and enhance the proliferation of colon cancer cells in in vitro co-culture systems (Nakagawa et al., 2004). It is possible that the role of CAFs in colorectal metastasis is modulated through the production of IL-8, a chemokine related to invasion and angiogenesis (Mueller et al., 2007a; 2007b).

In summary, the ability of cancer cells to grow at a specific site depends on features inherent to the cancer cell and to the microenvironment of the invaded organ, as well as on the active interplay between these factors. Much remains to be learned about the detailed molecular interactions between cancer cells and the microenvironment of specific secondary sites. However, there is strong evidence indicating that these interactions are important in determining the survival and proliferation potential of a cancer cell in a specific organ.

1.4 Concluding Remarks

The journey of colon cancer cells from the primary to the secondary site is hindered by a destructive and inefficient process. Yet, some cells succeed and traverse all these impediments to generate metastases that will become fatal. In each case, the molecular events that lead to the massive destruction of the cancer cells or that allow their survival during their journey is governed by an intricate interactive crosstalk between the cancer cells and their microenvironment. We have briefly reviewed some of the molecular interactions that characterize colon cancer cell dissemination to the liver. The different topics summarized in this chapter will be reviewed in detail by the contributors to this book.

Acknowledgements The work described in this chapter was supported by the Canadian Cancer Society Research Institute.

Abbreviations and Acronyms

ADAM	A disintegrin and metalloproteinase
Akt	v-akt murine thymoma viral oncogene homologue 1
BDMC	Bone marrow-derived cells
bFGF	Basic fibroblast growth factor
BM	Basement membrane
CAFs	Cancer-associated fibroblasts
COX2	Cyclooxygenase 2
CpG	Cytosine-phosphate-guanine
CXC	Chemokine C-X-C motif
CXCL	Chemokine ligand
CXCR	Chemokine C-X-C motif receptor
DR3	Death receptor-3
ECM	Extracellular matrix
EGFR	Epidermal growth factor receptor
EMT	Epithelial mesenchymal transition
EpCAM	Epithelial cell adhesion molecule
ERK	Extracellular-signal regulated kinase
eNOS	Endothelial nitric oxide synthase
FAK	Focal adhesion kinase
HGF	Hepatocyte growth factor
HIF1α	Hypoxia-inducible factor-1α
ICAM-1	Intercellular adhesion molecule-1
IGF1/2	Insulin-like growth factor-1/2
IL-3	Interleukin-3
MAPK	Mitogen-activated protein kinase
MACC1	Metastasis-associated colon cancer 1
MET	Mesenchymal-epithelial transition
miRNA	microRNA
MMP	Matrix metalloprotease
NK cells	Natural killer cells
PCC	Premature chromosome condensation
PDGFR	Platelet-derived growth factor receptor
PI3K	Phosphatidyl inositol 3 kinase

PLGF	Placental growth factor
PTEN	Phosphatase and tensin homolog deleted on chromosome 10
p38 MAPK	p38 mitogen-activated protein kinase
ROS	Reactive oxygen species
TAMs	Tumour-associated macrophages
TIMP	Tissue inhibitors of metalloprotease
TGFα	Transforming growth factor-α
uPA	Urokinase plasminogen activator
uPAR	uPA receptor
VCAM	Vascular cell adhesion molecule
VEGF	Vascular endothelial cell growth factor
VEGFR	Vascular endothelial cell growth factor receptor

References

Al-Nedawi K, Meehan B, Micallef J, Lhotak V, May L, Guha A et al. (2008). Intercellular transfer of the oncogenic receptor EGFRvIII by microvesicles derived from tumour cells. *Nat Cell Biol* **10**: 619–24.

Allgayer H, Wang H, Gallick GE, Crabtree A, Mazar A, Jones T et al. (1999). Transcriptional induction of the urokinase receptor gene by a constitutively active Src. Requirement of an upstream motif (-152/-135) bound with Sp1. *J Biol Chem* **274**: 18428–37.

Allin KH, Bojesen SE, Nordestgaard BG (2009). Baseline C-reactive protein is associated with incident cancer and survival in patients with cancer. *J Clin Oncol* **27**: 2217–24.

Araki M, Araki K, Biancone L, Stamenkovic I, Izui S, Yamamura K et al. (1997). The role of E-selectin for neutrophil activation and tumor metastasis in vivo. *Leukemia* **11**(**Suppl 3**): 209–12.

Atkin NB (1979). Premature chromosome condensation in carcinoma of the bladder: presumptive evidence for fusion of normal and malignant cells. *Cytogenet Cell Genet* **23**: 217–19.

Avizienyte E, Fincham VJ, Brunton VG, Frame MC (2004). Src SH3/2 domain-mediated peripheral accumulation of Src and phospho-myosin is linked to deregulation of E-cadherin and the epithelial-mesenchymal transition. *Mol Biol Cell* **15**: 2794–803.

Bacac M, Stamenkovic I (2008). Metastatic cancer cell. *Annu Rev Pathol* **3**: 221–47.

Balkwill F, Charles KA, Mantovani A (2005). Smoldering and polarized inflammation in the initiation and promotion of malignant disease. *Cancer Cell* **7**: 211–17.

Banerji S, Wright AJ, Noble M, Mahoney DJ, Campbell ID, Day AJ et al. (2007). Structures of the Cd44-hyaluronan complex provide insight into a fundamental carbohydrate-protein interaction. *Nat Struct Mol Biol* **14**: 234–39.

Barbera-Guillem E, Nyhus JK, Wolford CC, Friece CR, Sampsel JW (2002). Vascular endothelial growth factor secretion by tumor-infiltrating macrophages essentially supports tumor angiogenesis, and IgG immune complexes potentiate the process. *Cancer Res* **62**: 7042–49.

Bates RC, Bellovin DI, Brown C, Maynard E, Wu B, Kawakatsu H et al. (2005). Transcriptional activation of integrin beta6 during the epithelial-mesenchymal transition defines a novel prognostic indicator of aggressive colon carcinoma. *J Clin Invest* **115**: 339–47.

Bates RC, DeLeo MJ 3rd, Mercurio AM (2004). The epithelial-mesenchymal transition of colon carcinoma involves expression of IL-8 and CXCR-1-mediated chemotaxis. *Exp Cell Res* **299**: 315–24.

Bates RC, Mercurio AM (2003). Tumor necrosis factor-alpha stimulates the epithelial-to-mesenchymal transition of human colonic organoids. *Mol Biol Cell* **14**: 1790–800.

Bates RC, Mercurio AM (2005). The epithelial-mesenchymal transition (EMT) and colorectal cancer progression. *Cancer Biol Ther* **4**: 365–70.

Bates RC, Pursell BM, Mercurio AM (2007). Epithelial-mesenchymal transition and colorectal cancer: gaining insights into tumor progression using LIM 1863 cells. *Cells Tissues Organs* **185**: 29–39.

Bellovin DI, Simpson KJ, Danilov T, Maynard E, Rimm DL, Oettgen P et al. (2006). Reciprocal regulation of RhoA and RhoC characterizes the EMT and identifies RhoC as a prognostic marker of colon carcinoma. *Oncogene* **25**: 6959–67.

Bendich A, Wilczok T, Borenfreund E (1965). Circulating DNA as a possible factor in oncogenesis. *Science* **148**: 374–76.

Biernat W, Huang H, Yokoo H, Kleihues P, Ohgaki H (2004). Predominant expression of mutant EGFR (EGFRvIII) is rare in primary glioblastomas. *Brain Pathol* **14**: 131–36.

Bockhorn M, Jain RK, Munn LL (2007). Active versus passive mechanisms in metastasis: do cancer cells crawl into vessels, or are they pushed? *Lancet Oncol* **8**: 444–48.

Brabletz T, Jung A, Reu S, Porzner M, Hlubek F, Kunz-Schughart LA et al. (2001). Variable beta-catenin expression in colorectal cancers indicates tumor progression driven by the tumor environment. *Proc Natl Acad Sci U S A* **98**: 10356–61.

Cameron MD, Schmidt EE, Kerkvliet N, Nadkarni KV, Morris VL, Groom AC et al. (2000). Temporal progression of metastasis in lung: cell survival, dormancy, and location dependence of metastatic inefficiency. *Cancer Res* **60**: 2541–46.

Cao Z, Song JH, Park YK, Maeng EJ, Nam SW, Lee JY et al. (2009). The p53 codon 72 polymorphism and susceptibility to colorectal cancer in Korean patients. *Neoplasma* **56**: 114–18.

Cavallaro U, Christofori G (2004). Cell adhesion and signalling by cadherins and Ig-CAMs in cancer. *Nat Rev Cancer* **4**: 118–32.

Chambers AF, Naumov GN, Varghese HJ, Nadkarni KV, MacDonald IC, Groom AC (2001). Critical steps in hematogenous metastasis: an overview. *Surg Oncol Clin N Am* **10**: 243–55, vii.

Chen CN, Cheng YM, Liang JT, Lee PH, Hsieh FJ, Yuan RH et al. (2000). Color Doppler vascularity index can predict distant metastasis and survival in colon cancer patients. *Cancer Res* **60**: 2892–97.

Decock J, Paridaens R, Ye S (2008). Genetic polymorphisms of matrix metalloproteinases in lung, breast and colorectal cancer. *Clin Genet* **73**: 197–211.

de Visser KE, Eichten A, Coussens LM (2006). Paradoxical roles of the immune system during cancer development. *Nat Rev Cancer* **6**: 24–37.

Dumont N, Wilson MB, Crawford YG, Reynolds PA, Sigaroudinia M, Tlsty TD (2008). Sustained induction of epithelial to mesenchymal transition activates DNA methylation of genes silenced in basal-like breast cancers. *Proc Natl Acad Sci U S A* **105**: 14867–72.

Edmiston KH, Shoji Y, Mizoi T, Ford R, Nachman A, Jessup JM (1998). Role of nitric oxide and superoxide anion in elimination of low metastatic human colorectal carcinomas by unstimulated hepatic sinusoidal endothelial cells. *Cancer Res* **58**: 1524–31.

Elander N, Soderkvist P, Fransen K (2006). Matrix metalloproteinase (MMP) -1, -2, -3 and -9 promoter polymorphisms in colorectal cancer. *Anticancer Res* **26**: 791–95.

Ellis LM, Haller DG (2008). Bevacizumab beyond progression: does this make sense? *J Clin Oncol* **26**: 5313–15.

Ellis LM, Hicklin DJ (2008). Pathways mediating resistance to vascular endothelial growth factor-targeted therapy. *Clin Cancer Res* **14**: 6371–75.

Ellsworth RE, Seebach J, Field LA, Heckman C, Kane J, Hooke JA et al. (2009). A gene expression signature that defines breast cancer metastases. *Clin Exp Metastasis* **26**: 205–13.

Erler JT, Bennewith KL, Nicolau M, Dornhofer N, Kong C, Le QT et al. (2006). Lysyl oxidase is essential for hypoxia-induced metastasis. *Nature* **440**: 1222–26.

Esteller M (2008). Epigenetics in cancer. *N Engl J Med* **358**: 1148–59.

Ewing J (1928). *Neoplastic Diseases. A Treatise on Tumors,* 3rd edn. WB Saunders Company: Philadelphia, p. 1127.

Fidler IJ (1996). Critical determinants of melanoma metastasis. *J Investig Dermatol Symp Proc* **1**: 203–8.

Fidler IJ, Kripke ML (1977). Metastasis results from preexisting variant cells within a malignant tumor. *Science* **197**: 893–95.

Frost P, Kerbel RS, Hunt B, Man S, Pathak S (1987). Selection of metastatic variants with identifiable karyotypic changes from a nonmetastatic murine tumor after treatment with 2'-deoxy-5-azacytidine or hydroxyurea: implications for the mechanisms of tumor progression. *Cancer Res* **47**: 2690–95.

Garcia-Olmo D, Garcia-Olmo DC (2001). Functionality of circulating DNA: the hypothesis of genometastasis. *Ann N Y Acad Sci* **945**: 265–75.

Gassmann P, Haier J (2008). The tumor cell-host organ interface in the early onset of metastatic organ colonisation. *Clin Exp Metastasis* **25**: 171–81.

Goh V, Padhani AR, Rasheed S (2007). Functional imaging of colorectal cancer angiogenesis. *Lancet Oncol* **8**: 245–55.

Gort EH, Groot AJ, van der Wall E, van Diest PJ, Vooijs MA (2008). Hypoxic regulation of metastasis via hypoxia-inducible factors. *Curr Mol Med* **8**: 60–67.

Gout S, Huot J (2008). Role of cancer microenvironmentin metastasis: focus on colon cancer. *Cancer Microenviron* **1**: 69–83.

Gout S, Morin C, Houle F, Huot J (2006). Death receptor-3, a new E-Selectin counter-receptor that confers migration and survival advantages to colon carcinoma cells by triggering p38 and ERK MAPK activation. *Cancer Res* **66**: 9117–24.

Gout S, Tremblay PL, Huot J (2008). Selectins and selectin ligands in extravasation of cancer cells and organ selectivity of metastasis. *Clin Exp Metastasis* **25**: 335–44.

Grady WM, Carethers JM (2008). Genomic and epigenetic instability in colorectal cancer pathogenesis. *Gastroenterology* **135**: 1079–99.

Guo C, Sah JF, Beard L, Willson JK, Markowitz SD, Guda K (2008). The noncoding RNA, miR-126, suppresses the growth of neoplastic cells by targeting phosphatidylinositol 3-kinase signaling and is frequently lost in colon cancers. *Genes Chromosomes Cancer* **47**: 939–46.

Guy CT, Cardiff RD, Muller WJ (1992). Induction of mammary tumors by expression of polyomavirus middle T oncogene: a transgenic mouse model for metastatic disease. *Mol Cell Biol* **12**: 954–61.

Hanahan D, Weinberg RA (2000). The hallmarks of cancer. *Cell* **100**: 57–70.

Handsley MM, Edwards DR (2005). Metalloproteinases and their inhibitors in tumor angiogenesis. *Int J Cancer* **115**: 849–60.

Harris JF, Chambers AF, Hill RP, Ling V (1982). Metastatic variants are generated spontaneously at a high rate in mouse KHT tumor. *Proc Natl Acad Sci U S A* **79**: 5547–51.

Hazan RB, Phillips GR, Qiao RF, Norton L, Aaronson SA (2000). Exogenous expression of N-cadherin in breast cancer cells induces cell migration, invasion, and metastasis. *J Cell Biol* **148**: 779–90.

Ho-Tin-Noe B, Goerge T, Wagner DD (2009). Platelets: guardians of tumor vasculature. *Cancer Res* **69**: 5623–26.

Honn KV, Tang DG, Grossi I, Duniec ZM, Timar J, Renaud C et al. (1994). Tumor cell-derived 12(S)-hydroxyeicosatetraenoic acid induces microvascular endothelial cell retraction. *Cancer Res* **54**: 565–74.

Hugo H, Ackland ML, Blick T, Lawrence MG, Clements JA, Williams ED et al. (2007). Epithelial–mesenchymal and mesenchymal–epithelial transitions in carcinoma progression. *J Cell Physiol* **213**: 374–83.

Hunter KW, Crawford NP, Alsarraj J (2008). Mechanisms of metastasis. *Breast Cancer Res* **10(Suppl 1)**: S2.

Iravani S, Mao W, Fu L, Karl R, Yeatman T, Jove R et al. (1998). Elevated c-Src protein expression is an early event in colonic neoplasia. *Lab Invest* **78**: 365–71.

Joyce T, Cantarella D, Isella C, Medico E, Pintzas A (2009). A molecular signature for Epithelial to Mesenchymal transition in a human colon cancer cell system is revealed by large-scale microarray analysis. *Clin Exp Metastasis* **26**: 569–87.

Joyce JA, Pollard JW (2009). Microenvironmental regulation of metastasis. *Nat Rev Cancer* **9**: 239–52.

Juliano RL (2002). Signal transduction by cell adhesion receptors and the cytoskeleton: functions of integrins, cadherins, selectins, and immunoglobulin-superfamily members. *Annu Rev Pharmacol Toxicol* **42**: 283–323.

Kalluri R, Zeisberg M (2006). Fibroblasts in cancer. *Nat Rev Cancer* **6**: 392–401.
Kang Y, Siegel PM, Shu W, Drobnjak M, Kakonen SM, Cordon-Cardo C et al. (2003). A multigenic program mediating breast cancer metastasis to bone. *Cancer Cell* **3**: 537–49.
Kannagi R, Izawa M, Koike T, Miyazaki K, Kimura N (2004). Carbohydrate-mediated cell adhesion in cancer metastasis and angiogenesis. *Cancer Sci* **95**: 377–84.
Kaplan RN, Rafii S, Lyden D (2006). Preparing the "soil": the premetastatic niche. *Cancer Res* **66**: 11089–93.
Karkkainen MJ, Makinen T, Alitalo K (2002). Lymphatic endothelium: a new frontier of metastasis research. *Nat Cell Biol* **4**: E.
Kerbel R, Folkman J (2002). Clinical translation of angiogenesis inhibitors. *Nat Rev Cancer* **2**: 727–39.
Khalique L, Ayhan A, Whittaker JC, Singh N, Jacobs IJ, Gayther SA et al. (2009). The clonal evolution of metastases from primary serous epithelial ovarian cancers. *Int J Cancer* **124**: 1579–86.
Khatib AM, Auguste P, Fallavollita L, Wang N, Samani A, Kontogiannea M et al. (2005). Characterization of the host proinflammatory response to tumor cells during the initial stages of liver metastasis. *Am J Pathol* **167**: 749–59.
Kim YJ, Borsig L, Han HL, Varki NM, Varki A (1999). Distinct selectin ligands on colon carcinoma mucins can mediate pathological interactions among platelets, leukocytes, and endothelium. *Am J Pathol* **155**: 461–72.
Kim S, Iizuka K, Aguila HL, Weissman IL, Yokoyama WM (2000). In vivo natural killer cell activities revealed by natural killer cell-deficient mice. *Proc Natl Acad Sci U S A* **97**: 2731–36.
Kitadai Y, Sasaki T, Kuwai T, Nakamura T, Bucana CD, Fidler IJ (2006). Targeting the expression of platelet-derived growth factor receptor by reactive stroma inhibits growth and metastasis of human colon carcinoma. *Am J Pathol* **169**: 2054–65.
Klein CA (2009). Parallel progression of primary tumours and metastases. *Nat Rev Cancer* **9**: 302–12.
Kramer SA, Farnham R, Glenn JF, Paulson DF (1981). Comparative morphology of primary and secondary deposits of prostatic adenocarcinoma. *Cancer* **48**: 271–73.
Lamalice L, Le Boeuf F, Huot J (2007). Endothelial cell migration during angiogenesis. *Circ Res* **100**: 782–94.
Le NH, Franken P, Fodde R (2008). Tumour-stroma interactions in colorectal cancer: converging on beta-catenin activation and cancer stemness. *Br J Cancer* **98**: 1886–93.
Leon SA, Shapiro B, Sklaroff DM, Yaros MJ (1977). Free DNA in the serum of cancer patients and the effect of therapy. *Cancer Res* **37**: 646–50.
Leupold JH, Asangani I, Maurer GD, Lengyel E, Post S, Allgayer H (2007). Src induces urokinase receptor gene expression and invasion/intravasation via activator protein-1/p-c-Jun in colorectal cancer. *Mol Cancer Res* **5**: 485–96.
Li H, Fan X, Houghton J (2007). Tumor microenvironment: the role of the tumor stroma in cancer. *J Cell Biochem* **101**: 805–15.
Liao D, Johnson RS (2007). Hypoxia: a key regulator of angiogenesis in cancer. *Cancer Metastasis Rev* **26**: 281–90.
Lifsted T, Le Voyer T, Williams M, Muller W, Klein-Szanto A, Buetow KH et al. (1998). Identification of inbred mouse strains harboring genetic modifiers of mammary tumor age of onset and metastatic progression. *Int J Cancer* **77**: 640–44.
Litvinov SV, Balzar M, Winter MJ, Bakker HA, Briaire-de Bruijn IH, Prins F et al. (1997). Epithelial cell adhesion molecule (Ep-CAM) modulates cell-cell interactions mediated by classic cadherins. *J Cell Biol* **139**: 1337–48.
Lujambio A, Esteller M (2009). How epigenetics can explain human metastasis: a new role for microRNAs. *Cell Cycle* **8**: 377–82.
Lunt SJ, Chaudary N, Hill RP (2009). The tumor microenvironment and metastatic disease. *Clin Exp Metastasis* **26**: 19–34.
Luzzi KJ, MacDonald IC, Schmidt EE, Kerkvliet N, Morris VL, Chambers AF et al. (1998). Multistep nature of metastatic inefficiency: dormancy of solitary cells after successful extravasation and limited survival of early micrometastases. *Am J Pathol* **153**: 865–73.

Maetzel D, Denzel S, Mack B, Canis M, Went P, Benk M et al. (2009). Nuclear signalling by tumour-associated antigen EpCAM. *Nat Cell Biol* **11**: 162–71.

Malmberg KJ, Ljunggren HG (2006). Escape from immune- and nonimmune-mediated tumor surveillance. *Semin Cancer Biol* **16**: 16–31.

Mantovani A, Allavena P, Sica A, Balkwill F (2008). Cancer-related inflammation. *Nature* **454**: 436–44.

Massague J (2008). TGFbeta in Cancer. *Cell* **134**: 215–30.

Mehlen P, Puisieux A (2006). Metastasis: a question of life or death. *Nat Rev Cancer* **6**: 449–58.

Meijer J, Zeelenberg IS, Sipos B, Roos E (2006). The CXCR5 chemokine receptor is expressed by carcinoma cells and promotes growth of colon carcinoma in the liver. *Cancer Res* **66**: 9576–82.

Melendez-Zajgla J, Del Pozo L, Ceballos G, Maldonado V (2008). Tissue inhibitor of metalloproteinases-4. The road less traveled. *Mol Cancer* **7**: 85.

Miles FL, Pruitt FL, van Golen KL, Cooper CR (2008). Stepping out of the flow: capillary extravasation in cancer metastasis. *Clin Exp Metastasis* **25**: 305–24.

Minard ME, Ellis LM, Gallick GE (2006). Tiam1 regulates cell adhesion, migration and apoptosis in colon tumor cells. *Clin Exp Metastasis* **23**: 301–13.

Mizukami Y, Jo WS, Duerr EM, Gala M, Li J, Zhang X et al. (2005). Induction of interleukin-8 preserves the angiogenic response in HIF-1alpha-deficient colon cancer cells. *Nat Med* **11**: 992–97.

Mizukami Y, Kohgo Y, Chung DC (2007). Hypoxia inducible factor-1 independent pathways in tumor angiogenesis. *Clin Cancer Res* **13**: 5670–74.

Mook OR, Frederiks WM, Van Noorden CJ (2004). The role of gelatinases in colorectal cancer progression and metastasis. *Biochim Biophys Acta* **1705**: 69–89.

Morse M, Langer L, Starodub A, Hobeika A, Clay T, Lyerly HK (2007). Current immunotherapeutic strategies in colon cancer. *Surg Oncol Clin N Am* **16**: 873–900.

Mueller L, Goumas FA, Affeldt M, Sandtner S, Gehling UM, Brilloff S et al. (2007a). Stromal fibroblasts in colorectal liver metastases originate from resident fibroblasts and generate an inflammatory microenvironment. *Am J Pathol* **171**: 1608–18.

Mueller L, Goumas FA, Himpel S, Brilloff S, Rogiers X, Broering DC (2007b). Imatinib mesylate inhibits proliferation and modulates cytokine expression of human cancer-associated stromal fibroblasts from colorectal metastases. *Cancer Lett* **250**: 329–38.

Muller A, Homey B, Soto H, Ge N, Catron D, Buchanan ME et al. (2001). Involvement of chemokine receptors in breast cancer metastasis. *Nature* **410**: 50–56.

Murdoch C, Muthana M, Coffelt SB, Lewis CE (2008). The role of myeloid cells in the promotion of tumour angiogenesis. *Nat Rev Cancer* **8**: 618–31.

Nakagawa H, Liyanarachchi S, Davuluri RV, Auer H, Martin EW Jr., de la Chapelle A et al. (2004). Role of cancer-associated stromal fibroblasts in metastatic colon cancer to the liver and their expression profiles. *Oncogene* **23**: 7366–77.

Narita T, Kawakami-Kimura N, Kasai Y, Hosono J, Nakashio T, Matsuura N et al. (1996). Induction of E-selectin expression on vascular endothelium by digestive system cancer cells. *J Gastroenterol* **31**: 299–301.

Naumov GN, MacDonald IC, Weinmeister PM, Kerkvliet N, Nadkarni KV, Wilson SM et al. (2002). Persistence of solitary mammary carcinoma cells in a secondary site: a possible contributor to dormancy. *Cancer Res* **62**: 2162–68.

Nguyen DX, Bos PD, Massague J (2009). Metastasis: from dissemination to organ-specific colonization. *Nat Rev Cancer* **9**: 274–84.

Nicolson GL (1988). Cancer metastasis: tumor cell and host organ properties important in metastasis to specific secondary sites. *Biochim Biophys Acta* **948**: 175–224.

Nieswandt B, Hafner M, Echtenacher B, Mannel DN (1999). Lysis of tumor cells by natural killer cells in mice is impeded by platelets. *Cancer Res* **59**: 1295–300.

Olumi AF, Grossfeld GD, Hayward SW, Carroll PR, Tlsty TD, Cunha GR (1999). Carcinoma-associated fibroblasts direct tumor progression of initiated human prostatic epithelium. *Cancer Res* **59**: 5002–11.

Ostrand-Rosenberg S (2008). Immune surveillance: a balance between protumor and antitumor immunity. *Curr Opin Genet Dev* **18**: 11–18.

Owens LV, Xu L, Craven RJ, Dent GA, Weiner TM, Kornberg L et al. (1995). Overexpression of the focal adhesion kinase (p125FAK) in invasive human tumors. *Cancer Res* **55**: 2752–55.

Paget D (1889). The distribution of secondary growths in cancer of the breast. *Lancet* **1**: 571–73.

Palumbo JS, Talmage KE, Massari JV, La Jeunesse CM, Flick MJ, Kombrinck KW et al. (2007). Tumor cell-associated tissue factor and circulating hemostatic factors cooperate to increase metastatic potential through natural killer cell-dependent and-independent mechanisms. *Blood* **110**: 133–41.

Park YG, Zhao X, Lesueur F, Lowy DR, Lancaster M, Pharoah P et al. (2005). Sipa1 is a candidate for underlying the metastasis efficiency modifier locus Mtes1. *Nat Genet* **37**: 1055–62.

Pawelek JM, Chakraborty AK (2008). The cancer cell–leukocyte fusion theory of metastasis. *Adv Cancer Res* **101**: 397–444.

Pollard JW (2004). Tumour-educated macrophages promote tumour progression and metastasis. *Nat Rev Cancer* **4**: 71–78.

Polyak K, Weinberg RA (2009). Transitions between epithelial and mesenchymal states: acquisition of malignant and stem cell traits. *Nat Rev Cancer* **9**: 265–73.

Popovic ZV, Sandhoff R, Sijmonsma TP, Kaden S, Jennemann R, Kiss E et al. (2007). Sulfated glycosphingolipid as mediator of phagocytosis: SM4s enhances apoptotic cell clearance and modulates macrophage activity. *J Immunol* **179**: 6770–82.

Pyke C, Salo S, Ralfkiaer E, Romer J, Dano K, Tryggvason K (1995). Laminin-5 is a marker of invading cancer cells in some human carcinomas and is coexpressed with the receptor for urokinase plasminogen activator in budding cancer cells in colon adenocarcinomas. *Cancer Res* **55**: 4132–39.

Rabinovitz I, Mercurio AM (1997). The integrin alpha6beta4 functions in carcinoma cell migration on laminin-1 by mediating the formation and stabilization of actin-containing motility structures. *J Cell Biol* **139**: 1873–84.

Radinsky R (1995). Molecular mechanisms for organ-specific colon carcinoma metastasis. *Eur J Cancer* **31A**: 1091–95.

Radinsky R, Ellis LM (1996). Molecular determinants in the biology of liver metastasis. *Surg Oncol Clin N Am* **5**: 215–29.

Ramaswamy S, Ross KN, Lander ES, Golub TR (2003). A molecular signature of metastasis in primary solid tumors. *Nat Genet* **33**: 49–54.

Ribatti D, Mangialardi G, Vacca A (2006). Stephen Paget and the 'seed and soil' theory of metastatic dissemination. *Clin Exp Med* **6**: 145–49.

Rosenberg SA (2001). Progress in human tumour immunology and immunotherapy. *Nature* **411**: 380–84.

Samak R, Israel L (1982). [Extraction and identification of circulating immune complexes from the serum of cancer patient by affinity chromatography followed by high pressure steric exclusion chromatography. Demonstration of their effect on the mitogenesis of normal lymphocytes]. *Ann Med Interne (Paris)* **133**: 362–66.

Smyth MJ, Swann J, Kelly JM, Cretney E, Yokoyama WM, Diefenbach A et al. (2004). NKG2D recognition and perforin effector function mediate effective cytokine immunotherapy of cancer. *J Exp Med* **200**: 1325–35.

Solinas G, Garlanda MF, Mantovani A, Allavena P (2010). Inflammation-mediated promotion of invasion and metastasis. *Cancer Metastasis Rev* DOI 10.1007/s10555-010-9227-2

Stein U, Walther W, Arlt F, Schwabe H, Smith J, Fichtner I et al. (2009). MACC1, a newly identified key regulator of HGF-MET signaling, predicts colon cancer metastasis. *Nat Med* **15**: 59–67.

Subramaniam V, Gardner H, Jothy S (2007). Soluble CD44 secretion contributes to the acquisition of aggressive tumor phenotype in human colon cancer cells. *Exp Mol Pathol* **83**: 341–46.

Sundar SS, Ganesan TS (2007). Role of lymphangiogenesis in cancer. *J Clin Oncol* **25**: 4298–307.

Sundlisaeter E, Dicko A, Sakariassen PO, Sondenaa K, Enger PO, Bjerkvig R (2007). Lymphangiogenesis in colorectal cancer–prognostic and therapeutic aspects. *Int J Cancer* **121**: 1401–9.

Suzuki M, Mose ES, Montel V, Tarin D (2006). Dormant cancer cells retrieved from metastasis-free organs regain tumorigenic and metastatic potency. *Am J Pathol* **169**: 673–81.

Takeda K, Smyth MJ, Cretney E, Hayakawa Y, Yamaguchi N, Yagita H et al. (2001). Involvement of tumor necrosis factor-related apoptosis-inducing ligand in NK cell-mediated and IFN-gamma-dependent suppression of subcutaneous tumor growth. *Cell Immunol* **214**: 194–200.

Talmadge JE, Donkor M, Scholar E (2007). Inflammatory cell infiltration of tumors: Jekyll or Hyde. *Cancer Metastasis Rev* **26**: 373–400.

Taylor J, Hickson J, Lotan T, Yamada DS, Rinker-Schaeffer C (2008). Using metastasis suppressor proteins to dissect interactions among cancer cells and their microenvironment. *Cancer Metastasis Rev* **27**: 67–73.

Thiery JP, Sleeman JP (2006). Complex networks orchestrate epithelial-mesenchymal transitions. *Nat Rev Mol Cell Biol* **7**: 131–42.

Tischoff I, Tannapfel A (2008). [Epigenetic alterations in colorectal carcinomas and precancerous lesions]. *Z Gastroenterol* **46**: 1202–6.

Trainer DL, Kline T, Hensler G, Greig R, Poste G (1988). Clonal analysis of the malignant properties of B16 melanoma cells treated with the DNA hypomethylating agent 5-azacytidine. *Clin Exp Metastasis* **6**: 185–200.

Tremblay PL, Auger FA, Huot J (2006). Regulation of transendothelial migration of colon cancer cells by E-selectin-mediated activation of p38 and ERK MAP kinases. *Oncogene* **25**: 6563–73.

Tremblay PL, Huot J, Auger FA (2008). Mechanisms by which E-selectin regulates diapedesis of colon cancer cells under flow conditions. *Cancer Res* **68**: 5167–76.

Vernon AE, Bakewell SJ, Chodosh LA (2007). Deciphering the molecular basis of breast cancer metastasis with mouse models. *Rev Endocr Metab Disord* **8**: 199–213.

Walzog B, Gaehtgens P (2000). Adhesion molecules: the path to a new understanding of acute inflammation. *News Physiol Sci* **15**: 107–13.

Wang Y, Klijn JG, Zhang Y, Sieuwerts AM, Look MP, Yang F et al. (2005). Gene-expression profiles to predict distant metastasis of lymph-node-negative primary breast cancer. *Lancet* **365**: 671–79.

Weiss L (1990). Metastatic inefficiency. *Adv Cancer Res* **54**: 159–211.

Weiss L, Nannmark U, Johansson BR, Bagge U (1992). Lethal deformation of cancer cells in the microcirculation: a potential rate regulator of hematogenous metastasis. *Int J Cancer* **50**: 103–7.

Wong CW, Lee A, Shientag L, Yu J, Dong Y, Kao G et al. (2001). Apoptosis: an early event in metastatic inefficiency. *Cancer Res* **61**: 333–38.

Wyckoff JB, Jones JG, Condeelis JS, Segall JE (2000). A critical step in metastasis: in vivo analysis of intravasation at the primary tumor. *Cancer Res* **60**: 2504–11.

Yang H, Crawford N, Lukes L, Finney R, Lancaster M, Hunter KW (2005). Metastasis predictive signature profiles pre-exist in normal tissues. *Clin Exp Metastasis* **22**: 593–603.

Yang X, Pursell B, Lu S, Chang TK, Mercurio AM (2009). Regulation of {beta}4-integrin expression by epigenetic modifications in the mammary gland and during the epithelial-to-mesenchymal transition. *J Cell Sci* **122**: 2473–80.

Yang J, Weinberg RA (2008). Epithelial-mesenchymal transition: at the crossroads of development and tumor metastasis. *Dev Cell* **14**: 818–29.

Yates CC, Shepard CR, Stolz DB, Wells A (2007). Co-culturing human prostate carcinoma cells with hepatocytes leads to increased expression of E-cadherin. *Br J Cancer* **96**: 1246–52.

Zeelenberg IS, Ruuls-Van Stalle L, Roos E (2003). The chemokine receptor CXCR4 is required for outgrowth of colon carcinoma micrometastases. *Cancer Res* **63**: 3833–39.

Zeisberg EM, Potenta S, Xie L, Zeisberg M, Kalluri R (2007). Discovery of endothelial to mesenchymal transition as a source for carcinoma-associated fibroblasts. *Cancer Res* **67**: 10123–28.

Zeng Q, Chen S, You Z, Yang F, Carey TE, Saims D et al. (2002). Hepatocyte growth factor inhibits anoikis in head and neck squamous cell carcinoma cells by activation of ERK and Akt signaling independent of NFkappa B. *J Biol Chem* **277**: 25203–8.

Zvibel I, Halpern Z, Papa M (1998). Extracellular matrix modulates expression of growth factors and growth-factor receptors in liver-colonizing colon-cancer cell lines. *Int J Cancer* **77**: 295–301.

Chapter 2
PHYSIOPATHOLOGY OF COLORECTAL METASTASIS

Cristiano Ferrario[1] and Mark Basik[2,3]
[1] Department of Oncology, McGill University, Montreal, QC, Canada,
e-mail: cristianoferrario@gmail.com
[2] Department of Oncology, McGill University, Montreal, QC, Canada
[3] Segal Cancer Center, Jewish General Hospital, Montreal, QC, Canada,
e-mail: mark.basik@mcgill.ca

Abstract: Colorectal metastatic disease is ultimately responsible for almost all of the mortality resulting from colorectal cancer. The spread of colorectal cancer to 'vital' target organs such as the liver and the lung compromises normal physiology and usually leads to organ failure and death. Colorectal cancer also spreads to other, less 'vital' organs such as bone and the peritoneum, whose diminished function may lead to significant morbidity during the course of the disease. In this chapter, we will discuss mechanisms and patterns of spread of colorectal cancer to metastatic sites, how these metastases affect normal organ physiology, and what factors affect the progression of metastatic disease in different sites.

Key words: Liver metastasis · Chemokines and chemokine receptors · Tumour dormancy · Circulating tumour cells · Iatrogenic factors

2.1 Mechanisms of Metastatic Spread

2.1.1 Circulatory Spread

As described in Chapter 1 in this book, the development of metastatic disease in colorectal cancer, as in all cancers, is a complex and highly selective process, depending on the interaction between host factors and specific characteristics of cancer cells. A 'traditional' view of the physiopathology of this process sees it as a gradual progression starting from local extension of the primary tumour, followed by invasion of the lymphatic system in its local terminals, spread of cancer cells to the regional lymph nodes (LN), and eventually a widespread hematogenic progression, leading to microscopic cancer involvement of distant organs (micrometastases), then growing to macroscopic clinically detectable lesions. However, growing evidence supports the possibility that invasion into blood vessels can also occur early in the natural history of cancer development. Indeed, it is not uncommon in clinical practice to observe cases of colorectal cancers (CRCs) with no apparent involvement of regional lymph nodes, and which still go on to develop liver metastases. Indeed, the 5-year survival of Dukes stage B colon cancer (confined to the colonic wall, without evidence of lymph node metastases) is 85–90%, meaning that about 10–15% of patients do develop distant metastatic disease as a consequence of direct invasion into blood vessels, while apparently skipping lymph nodes close to the colonic wall.

The final destination of both lymphatic and hematogenous spread for the colon is the liver. The lymphatic drainage of the upper part of the rectum is also the liver through the portal venous circulation, whereas the lower part of the rectum is drained 'systemically', through lymphatics and veins associated with the iliac vessels. We will examine in closer detail the two major mechanisms of metastatic spread, lymphatic and hematogenous.

2.1.1.1 Lymphatic Spread

To categorize CRCs according to their prognosis, either the Dukes or the Tumor-Node-Metastases (TNM) 'staging' systems are generally used by oncologists. In both systems, the presence of lymph node metastases is the most important prognostic factor after curative surgery for CRC, and is also of critical importance for selecting patients for adjuvant treatments, which are usually recommended for patients with node-positive disease (Dukes C or stage III TNM) rather than node-negative (Dukes A/B or stage I/II TNM)

The development of lymph node metastases is a general characteristic of carcinomas, and lymphatic tumour cell dissemination is a relatively early and common event in CRC, usually preceding hematogenic tumour cell dissemination (Weitz et al., 1999). As other tumour types, it remains controversial as to whether tumour cells actually further metastasize from regional lymph nodes to other organs, or if the presence of lymphatic metastases simply reflects a more aggressive intrinsic tumour phenotype, and that lymphatic metastases are not themselves the source of distant metastases (Das and Skobe, 2008).

The process of cancer cell invasion into lymphatic vessels is different from their entry into blood vessels (hematogenous intravasation), and relatively easier, as malignant cells do not have to traverse inter-endothelial tight junctions, pericytes, nor an intact basement membrane (Saharinen et al., 2004). For this reason, it is traditionally considered a more passive process, whereby cancer cells 'shed' by the primary tumour can gain access to pre-existing lymphatics, and be drained to the regional lymph nodes, that function as intermediate way stations (Sleeman, 2000).

Neoplastic cells enter lymphatic vessels draining the site where the primary tumour grows, and are then transported to the subcapsular sinus of a regional node, through the afferent lymphatic vessels. This does not necessarily translate into a neoplastic colonization, which would require cells to survive and proliferate in the nodal 'filter'. Indeed, the presence of isolated tumour cells (<0.2 mm) in a lymph node has no known prognostic relevance (Bilchik and Nora, 2002). Cancer cells can remain localized in a lymph node station for a variable amount of time. If they survive and start proliferating, they initially create micrometastases (between 0.2 and 2 mm) (Fig. 2.1). In Dukes A/B colon cancers, lymph node micrometastases correlate with a higher risk of distant metastases, and with a lower 5-year overall survival (van Schaik et al., 2009). In draining nodes, cancer cells are filtered and concentrated in a restricted space, and in time their aggregation can favour their survival. Micrometastases can evolve to larger nodal metastases (>2 mm, defining Dukes C), and in some cases the excessive tumour growth leads to rupture of the lymph node capsule and extracapsular extension of neoplastic cells. At the same time, the neoplastic clone can also spread, usually in a relatively ordered fashion, from each node to the adjacent ones. Nevertheless, in approximately 11% of CRC patients, 'skip' lymph node metastases are found, in which distant nodes are involved by cancer colonization, while those closer to the primary tumour are negative, possibly as a consequence of circulation in unknown lymphatic channels (Yamamo et al., 1998).

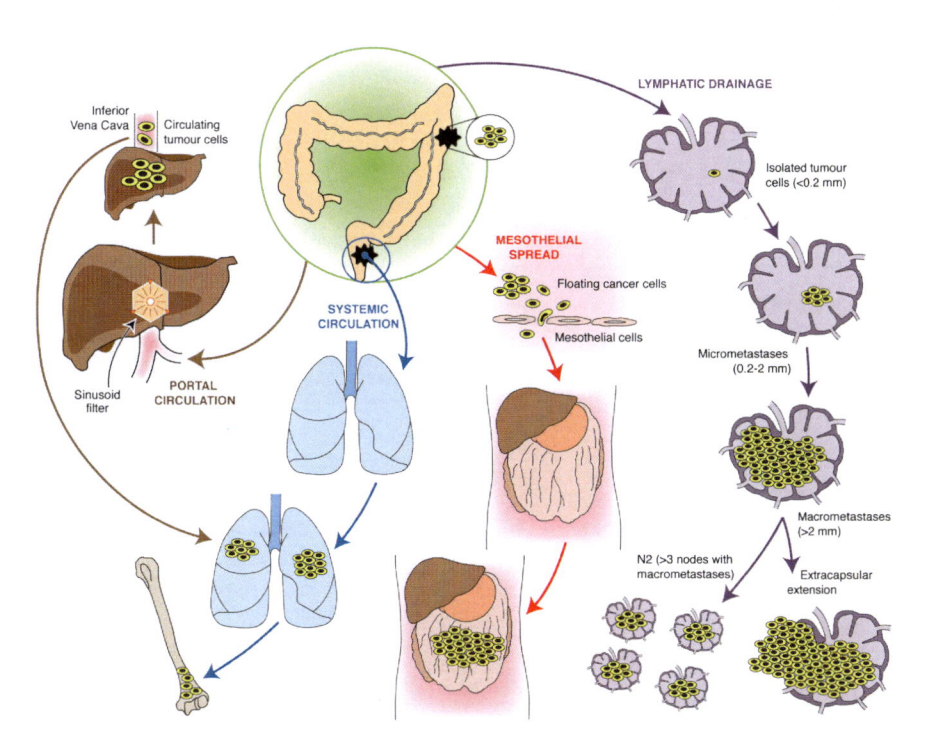

Fig. 2.1 The metastatic spread of colorectal cancer. Colon and rectal cancers metastasize using four paths: via the portal circulation to the liver and eventually to the systemic circulation; mesothelial spread to the peritoneal surfaces including the omentum; lymphatic spread with progressive local nodal growth; and, only for rectal cancer, spread directly into the systemic circulation

The traditional view of lymphatic spread as a passive process has been challenged by more recent findings on the biology of tumour-associated lymphangiogenesis, which will be discussed in further depth in Chapter 9. Immunohistochemical studies revealed the presence of many peri-tumoural lymphatic vessels associated with primary human CRCs (Omachi et al., 2007), while intra-tumoural lymphatics are scarce and typically distorted and compressed (Liang et al., 2006), probably as a consequence of high intra-tumour interstitial pressure. Both intra- and peri-tumoural lymphatics have a higher proliferative index than lymphatics in normal tissues, supporting the notion of lymphangiogenesis in CRC. Significant contradictions still exist across studies on lymphangiogenesis, with disagreement on the prognostic role of lymphatic vessel density (LVD). Most studies favour a prognostic role for peri-tumoural, but not intra-tumoural LVD and lymphovascular invasion (Longatto-Filho et al., 2008). The inconsistency of such findings suggests that mechanisms other than lymphangiogenesis may contribute to tumour cell infiltration and spread via the lymphatic system.

Members of the vascular endothelial growth factor (VEGF) family, VEGF-C and VEGF-D, also produced by tumour-associated macrophages (TAMs), were studied for their role in lymphangiogenesis (see Table 2.1). High expression of VEGF-C and -D is found at the deep invasive margin in approximately half of resected CRCs (Furodi et al., 2002; Onogawa et al., 2004). The expression of VEGF-C at the invasive margin, as opposed to its expression in the central or superficial parts of the tumour, correlates with LN metastases and higher risk of death. In vitro studies show that VEGF-C increases the contraction frequency and pump flow of collecting lymphatics, through activation of VEGF-Receptor 3 (VEGFR3) (Breslin et al., 2007). Finally, tumour-derived VEGF-C has been implicated in cell-cell interactions, stimulating proliferation and chemotaxis of lymphatic endothelial cells. A different concept has been proposed by others, whereby lymphatic endothelial cells can secrete chemotactic agents (chemokines) attracting metastasizing cells. For example, the expression of chemokine receptor type 7 (CCR7) in CRC cells in archival specimens significantly correlates with LN metastasis and patient survival (Günther et al., 2005). In spite of these findings, it remains possible that the initial drainage of cancer cells to regional lymph nodes is indeed a relatively non-specific event.

However, once lymph node metastases are established in the first draining nodes, further colonization and substitution of other lymph nodes, especially the more distant ones, can be facilitated by a specific 'tropism' of cancer cells. As in distant metastases, cancer cells can use specific receptors to preferentially migrate to lymph nodes in a chemotactic fashion. In a recent study (Kawada et al., 2007), colon cancer cell lines transfected with the chemokine receptor CXCR3 were compared in an in vivo xenograft model to controls without CXCR3 expression. Interestingly, both cell lines disseminated to lymph nodes at a similar frequency at 2 weeks, suggesting an initially CXCR3-independent mode of spread. However, the CXCR3$^+$ clone had disseminated more to other lymph nodes at 4 weeks. At 6 weeks, metastases to distant lymph nodes were present in 59% versus 14% of CXCR3-positive and CXCR3-negative cell lines, respectively. In this model, liver

Table 2.1 Molecular factors involved in cell-cell interaction and relevant to the development of metastasis from colorectal cancer

Cancer cell		Interacting with		Effects
		Paired molecule	Cell type or tissue	
Chemokine receptors	CCR6	CCL20	Liver	Migration to liver
	CCR7	CCL19, CCL21	Lymphatic endothelial cells (ECs)	Favoring lymph node metastasis
	CXCR2	CXCL1	Liver	Migration to liver, engraftment of metastasis
	CXCR3	CXCL-4, -9, -10, -11	Lymph nodes & lung	Chemotaxis & spread to nodes (including distant nodes) and lungs
	CXCR4	SDF1/CXCL12	Sites of distant metastasis	Migration to premetastatic niche
Other receptors	Ob-Rb receptors	Leptin	Blood	Promoting invasiveness
	Tissue Factor	Coagulation factors VIIa, X	Blood	Protective microthrombi; activation of anti-apoptotic pathways
	Toll-like receptor-4 (TLR4)	Saturated fatty acids	Blood	Evasion of immune surveillance from macrophages
	Heparan-sulphate glycosaminoglycans	E- and P-selectins	Blood ECs	Adhesion for extravasation into distant organs
	Integrins ($\alpha v\beta 3$, $\alpha v\beta 6$)	Fibrinogen	Platelets	Aggregation with platelets, protection from shear forces and NKs
		VCAM-1, PECAM-1, ICAM-1	Mesothelium & hepatic sinusoid ECs	Peritoneal spread, adhesion and migration in the hepatic microvasculature
Secreted factors	VEGF	VEGFR2	Blood ECs	Vessel permeability, facilitating extravasation
	VEGF, Placental Growth Factor	VEGFR1	Bone marrow-derived progenitor cells	Mobilization of HPCs to create pre-metastatic niche
	VEGF-C & -D	VEGFR3	Lymphatic ECs	Lymphatic vessel contraction, favoring nodal metastasis
	Fas ligand	Fas receptor	Hepatocytes & liver ECs	Apoptosis of hepatic ECs & hepatocytes, extravasation & infiltration

metastases are unaffected by CXCR3 expression. The expression of CXCR3 in CRC cells correlates with lymph node metastases and poorer prognosis in human samples as well.

2.1.1.2 Hematogenous Spread

Hematogenous dissemination, starting with 'intravasation' of malignant cells into newly-formed tumour-associated vessels, is probably facilitated by the irregular endothelial lining formed during cancer neo-angiogenesis (please see Chapter 9, in this book). For cancers originating in the colon, migrating tumour cells drain from the venules of the primary tumour into the portal vein, so that the first 'filter' they encounter is the hepatic capillary (sinusoid), before they can enter the systemic circulation. On the other hand, because of its peculiar venous drainage, rectal cancer can either metastasize through the portal system when arising from the more cranial portion of the rectum, or through the inferior vena cava when arising from its caudal portion.

The mere entry of tumour cells into the circulation is not enough to give rise to clinically detectable metastases (Dukes D, or TNM stage IV), as intravasation is followed by many other rate-limiting steps making this a very inefficient process. From experimental models, it is calculated that approximately one million cells per gram of tumour are released into the bloodstream each day (Chang et al., 2000). Modern techniques can isolate circulating tumour cells (CTCs) even from small blood samples of cancer patients. CTCs are found in CRC patients, in a higher proportion in more advanced stages of disease: in 20.7% of patients with stage II disease, in 24.1% with stage III, and in 60.7% with stage IV ($p=$ 0.005) (Sastre et al., 2008). In patients with metastatic disease, a higher load of CTCs correlates with shorter progression-free survival and overall survival (Cohen et al., 2009), suggesting that the presence of CTCs in the blood reflects overall tumour burden and activity. In the case of breast cancer, the half-life of CTCs has been estimated to be as short as a few hours (Meng et al., 2004). Even if CTCs can be found in CRC patients regardless of tumour stage, their 'clearance' within 24 h after excision of the primary tumour is greater in lower stages (Dukes A and B) (Patel et al., 2002).

Several mechanisms are responsible of the clearance of CTCs. In the circulation, tumour cells encounter significant physical stresses, both from shear forces, and from mechanical constriction in small-diameter vessels (Fig. 2.2). Cancer cells drained from the portal circulation will meet the first filter of hepatic sinusoids that can be activated to secrete nitric oxide by mechanical contact with tumour cells, causing apoptosis of arrested tumour cells. The expression of glycoprotein DARC (Duffy blood group receptor) on endothelial cells can also contribute to the clearance of CTCs (Bandyopadhyay et al., 2006). DARC interacts with the CD82 antigen expressed on CTCs, causing them to undergo senescence. Finally, the immune system, particularly natural killer (NK) cells, can also actively attack CTCs, causing their death (Gassmann and Haier, 2008).

An efficient mechanism for CTCs to escape all these surveillance mechanisms consists in their aggregation with platelets and the resulting formation of tumour emboli (Guo and Giancotti, 2004). Cancer cells express Tissue Factor (TF, see

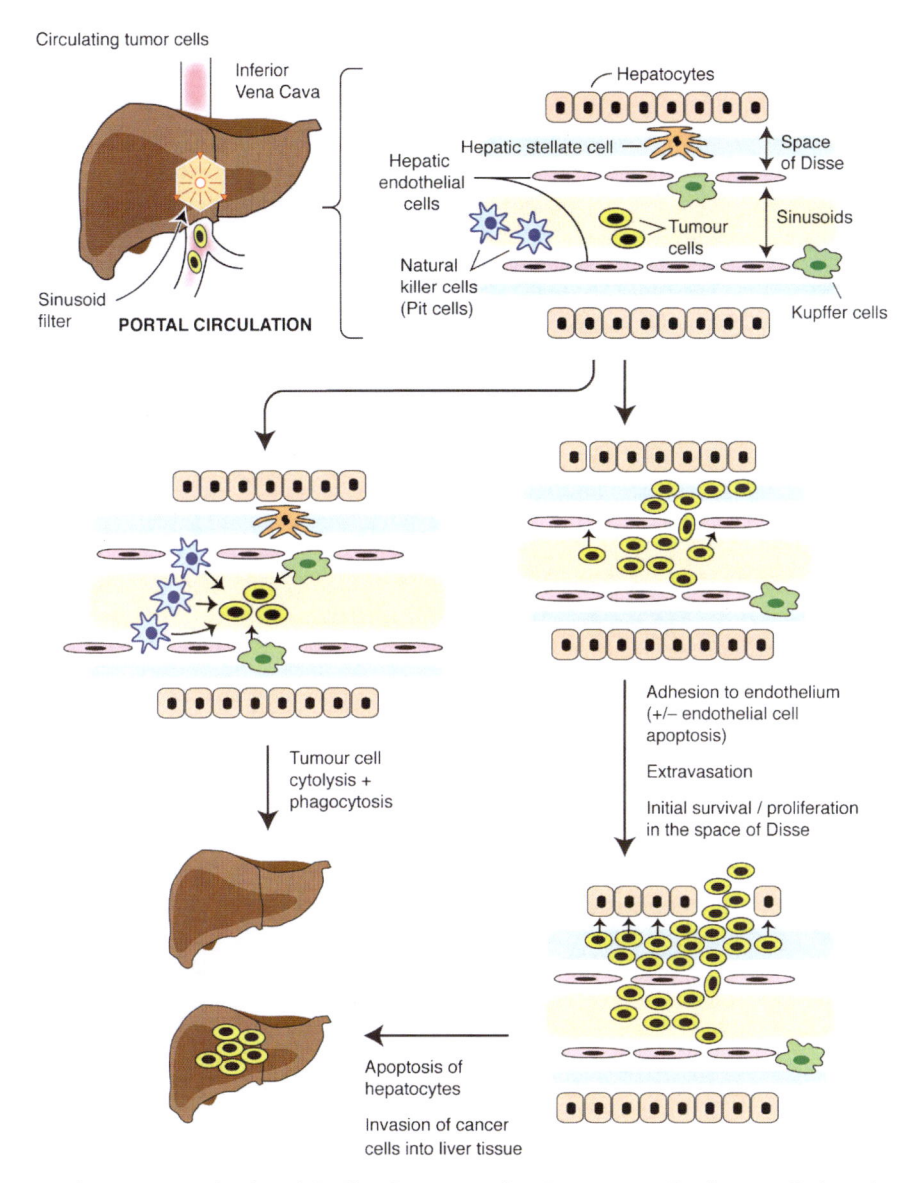

Fig. 2.2 The colonization of the liver by metastatic colon cancer cells. Cancer cells from the portal circulation remain trapped in the hepatic sinusoids, where they encounter the 'hepatic sinusoidal immune system': natural killer cells, Kupffer cells and hepatic endothelial cells. Natural killer and Kupffer cells that can move along the sinusoids normally aggregate around tumour cells, causing their cytolysis and phagocytosis. Alternatively, cancer cells that can evade and survive this immune surveillance, adhere to the liver microcirculation to extravasate, and may cause apoptosis of endothelial cells and hepatocytes, facilitating their invasion into the liver parenchyma. Initially, surviving cancer cells can be confined to the space of Disse and to Glisson's capsule, rich in extracellular matrix. In later stages, matrix proteins derived from liver-associated fibroblasts (stellate cells) will provide a substrate for cancer cell migration and further liver infiltration

Section 2.3.1.1 further below), a receptor for coagulation factors VIIa and X, that serves an important role in the formation of tumour cell-associated micro-thrombi (Im et al., 2004). Also, the expression and activation of integrin $\alpha v\beta 3$ on cancer cells, as well as on platelets, may contribute to the formation of such tumour emboli. Platelets can protect tumour cells from shear forces, and can hide them from NK immune and endothelial cells. Moreover, both platelets and fibrinogen were shown to increase metastatic potential by reducing the capacity of NK cells to clear newly established micrometastases (Palumbo et al., 2005). Interestingly, a high platelet count is associated with decreased survival in colorectal cancer, as in other tumour types (Jurasz et al., 2004).

Clusters of CTCs may arrest in small capillaries. Some cells that are capable of surviving can initially grow in the capillaries themselves, eventually causing vessel disruption (Al-Mehdi et al., 2000) and infiltration of the surrounding parenchyma in a relatively 'aspecific' way. Otherwise, single cells or small clusters of CTCs can extravasate through a more specific interaction with the vessel wall, in a way similar to leukocytes. Cancer cells can bind directly to endothelial cells, through the endothelial receptors E- and P-selectins (Kim et al., 1998). Extravasation is also facilitated by the production of VEGF from tumour cells that increase vascular permeability, disrupting endothelial intercellular junctions. The activation of Src kinases by VEGF in endothelial cells can mediate this process (Criscuoli et al., 2005).

Recently, it was found that primary cancers mobilize VEGF-Receptor 1-positive (VEGFR1$^+$) hematopoietic progenitor cells (HPCs) from the bone marrow (BM) to home to metastatic target organs, analogously to the recruitment of BM-derived cells to the primary tumour (Kaplan et al., 2005). The production of VEGF and Placental Growth Factor from the primary tumour directs VEGFR1$^+$ HPCs to preferentially localize to areas expressing increased levels of fibronectin. These HPCs can colonize distant organs even before the arrival of malignant cancer cells, creating a 'pre-metastatic niche', in association with the stromal cells of the target organ. The pre-metastatic niche is thought to create a favourable microenvironment for cancer cells, and in some cancer models, it was found to secrete stromal cell-derived factor-1 (SDF-1), a cytokine that facilitates the chemoattraction of malignant cells expressing the cognate receptor chemokine C-X-C motif receptor 4 (CXCR4) (Kaplan et al., 2005; Muller et al., 2001) (Table 2.1). In orthotopically-implanted CRC mice xenografts, mRNA levels of the cytokine chemokine ligand 1 (CXCL1) are increased in the pre-metastatic liver (before the development of metastasis) as compared to non-tumour-bearing mice (Yamamoto et al., 2008). The expression of the cognate receptor CXCR2 is detected predominantly on tumour cells in orthotopic tumours compared with ectopic tumours. Interestingly, the administration of TSU68, an inhibitor of VEGFR 2, platelet-derived growth factor receptor β (PDGFRβ) and fibroblast growth factor receptor 1 (FGFR 1), reduces the expression of chemokine ligand 1 (CXCL1) in the pre-metastatic liver, and results in a significant reduction of CRC liver metastasis compared to control.

The hematogenous spread is a very complex process, responsible for the development of distant visceral metastasis that accounts for most CRC-related deaths.

Recent discoveries, like the premetastatic niche, confirm the complexity of this process, 'orchestrated' by specific biological signaling at several sequential steps. It is plausible that a better elucidation of the molecules and mechanisms regulating each step will lead to the development of more adequate targeted therapeutic strategies.

2.1.2 Local Spread

Although the peritoneum, the lining of the abdominal cavity and of most intra-abdominal organs, has been thought of as a natural barrier to the trans-mural infiltration of cancer cells, peritoneal metastases are present in <10% of patients at diagnosis (synchronous metastases), but in 20–50% of patients with recurrent disease (metachronous metastases) (Koppe et al., 2006). Peritoneal carcinomatosis, in most cases, is believed to be the consequence of an alternative trans-coelomic spread in the peritoneal cavity, relatively distinct from lymphatic and hematogenous routes of dissemination. Such intra-peritoneal spread can develop in two ways (Sugarbaker, 1996): first, pre-operatively, as a result of full-thickness invasion of the bowel wall by the cancer (pT3-4), or by spontaneous bowel perforation; second, intra-operative spread can be favoured when in-transit tumour cells or emboli escape from dissected blood and lymph vessels or the bowel lumen.

The 'natural' development of peritoneal metastases involves the shedding of tumour cells from the invaded intestinal serosa, peritoneal transport usually by gravity towards the pelvis or, along the paracolic gutters to the sub-diaphragmatic spaces, and mesothelial adhesion mediated by adhesion molecules such as vascular cell adhesion molecule 1 (VCAM-1), platelet endothelial cell adhesion molecule 1 (PECAM-1), CXCR4, CD44, mucin 16 (MUC16) and intercellular adhesion molecule 1 (ICAM-1) (Ceelen and Bracke, 2009). Once mesothelial adhesion is achieved, invasion into the sub-mesothelial cells occurs probably at areas of peritoneal discontinuity, highlighting again the protective nature of the peritoneal lining. The omentum, the peritoneal fold attached to the transverse colon, is particularly susceptible to peritoneal metastases in part due to the presence of immunocompetent cell aggregates within it and its discontinuous mesothelial cell lining.

The possibility that any procedure or manipulation on a cancer might favour its dissemination has been a reason of concern for years. The presence of malignant cells on the surface of surgical tools or the gloves of the surgeon could potentially contribute to developments of metastatic implants in the abdominal cavity. Intra-operative contamination of the peritoneal cavity may explain why in up to 25% of patients with recurrent CRC to the peritoneal cavity is reported as the only site of relapse. Also in the case of patients with an intra-operative diagnosis of peritoneal carcinomatosis, only 23% are also found to have liver/lung metastases (Sadeghi et al., 2000). Therefore, it is likely that in some cases, peritoneal carcinomatosis may not necessarily be a hallmark of generalized disease.

The development of peritoneal metastases may be predicted by the detection of isolated tumour cells by immunocytology on peritoneal lavage of operated patients. The frequency of such cells depends on the assay being utilized, but varies between

18 and 25% when measured prior to surgical resection (Ceelen and Bracke, 2009). The presence of these cells serves as a marker for minimal residual disease, carrying a significant prognostic impact especially for more advanced stages (Schott et al., 1998). The incidence of positive peritoneal cytology is associated with the depth of tumour penetration, while other tumour characteristics (site of tumour, size, nodal status, differentiation, vascular or neural invasion) are not associated with this finding. Importantly, a positive cytology significantly correlates with a significantly higher rate of local or intra-peritoneal recurrence than in patients with a negative cytology (22.8% versus 8%) (Kanellos et al., 2003). Moreover, the presence of ascites is associated with a poor survival (Chu et al., 1989).

During surgery, the handling of the tumour can also result in spillage of tumour cells: free-floating tumour cells are found in peritoneal lavages performed at the time of surgery. In one study, the rate of tumour-positive cytology in peritoneal lavages increased from 13 to 21% after surgery for early stages of CRC (Varona et al., 2005).

2.1.3 Tumour Dormancy

Although most cancers are clinically diagnosed as limited to loco-regional disease, distant metastases can be detected months/years later, indicating that cancer cells had already spread in the form of distant 'micrometastases' at the time of the initial diagnosis. Deposits of single isolated tumour cells or avascular micrometastases maintain stable microscopic dimensions (tumour dormancy) until either the cancer cells or the microenvironment develops genetic/biological changes initiating a new phase of growth. The phase of tumour dormancy is difficult to investigate, but a few hypotheses have been generated to explain the basis of this phenomenon. It is possible that microscopically disseminated cancer cells enter the G0 phase of the cell cycle, especially when the switch from dormancy to the development of macroscopic metastases takes several years to occur. Alternatively, in a continuous cycle, a balance between cellular division and cell death could account for the stability of micrometastases. In this latter case, cell lysis can be a consequence of an unfavourable microenvironment, or of a lack of adequate blood supply. Similarly to the formation of the primary tumour, a pro-angiogenic switch is believed to take place also in the distant sites of metastases, with a change in the balance between anti- and pro-angiogenetic factors that allows neovascularization in the distant site of metastasis and growth to clinically detectable secondary lesions (Holmgren et al., 1995).

A recent clinical trial tested the impact of adjuvant administration of the anti-VEGF humanized antibody bevacizumab for 1 year in patients with operated colon cancer (Wolmark et al., 2009). In patients receiving bevacizumab, a significantly lower risk of relapse was observed only in the first year, coincident with bevacizumab treatment, suggesting that micrometastases already present are not eradicated by treatment with bevacizumab, but that the inhibition of the VEGF pathway during the year of treatment can prevent the angiogenic switch in the micrometastases, maintaining the state of tumour dormancy.

2.2 Sites of Metastasis and Consequences of Spread

CRC can metastasize to many organs with preferential targeting of the liver. It has always been evident that certain tumours preferentially metastatize to specific organs, while other organs (such as muscle) are rarely, if ever, sites of metastasis, leading Paget to first formulate the 'seed and soil' theory (Paget, 1889). A selective receptor-ligand interaction can account for an organ-specific extravasation in some cases. The best-studied ligand/receptor pair is the tumour cell receptor CXCR4 and its ligand SDF-1 (CXCL12), which is released into the bloodstream by those organs that are more commonly 'targets' of metastasis (Balkwill, 2004). The CXCR4 receptor is over-expressed in a variety of human cancers (Kakinuma and Hwang, 2006). In CRC cell lines over-expressing CXCR4, SDF-1 stimulates migration and invasion, and the over-expression of CXCR4 in CRC samples correlates with the presence of lymphatic and hematological metastases (Schimanski et al., 2005). The expression of the CXCR4 receptor was studied in primary CRC samples, and a higher expression was found to correlate with lymph node involvement at diagnosis. Moreover, high versus low expression of CXCR4 in primary tumour cells significantly predicts for tumour relapse after surgery in multivariate analysis. Interestingly, CXCR4 expression in liver metastases is higher than in matched primary tumours, supporting the theory that a higher expression of SDF-1 in the liver may selectively attract cells with increased levels of CXCR4 (Kim et al., 2005).

An alternative view of the mechanism of selection of the 'soil' by CTCs proposes a passive role of the microenvironment in the homing of cancer cells, based upon intravital imaging of hematogenous metastases (Chambers et al., 2002). This would imply that the predominant sites of metastases merely reflect the first pass of cancer cells in the circulation, and their entrapment in local capillaries. Tissue tropism would then be due to the ability of a small fraction of the cancer cells lodged in various tissues to survive, invade and grow in a particular tissue, possibly because of specific mutations in different subclones (Nguyen and Massague, 2007). A specific microenvironment could then offer growth factors particularly appropriate for that subclone, expressing a relevant cohort of genes.

Even if dissemination and homing were to depend on prevailing circulatory patterns, with passive entrapment in first-pass capillaries, the survival of tumour cells and their invasion and growth in the distant sites appear to be the real rate-limiting steps, where active adhesion and invasion of cancer cells likely depend on specific mechanisms, at present poorly defined.

2.2.1 Liver

Liver metastases are the major cause of death in CRC patients, and they are found in 10–25% of patients at diagnosis (synchronous metastases). Nevertheless, 20–50% of patients with no detectable metastasis at the time of resection of the primary tumour will develop liver metastases later on, in most cases within 5 years from diagnosis, with a peak in the first 2 years (Bird et al., 2006).

The liver is supplied by both the systemic and the portal circulation, the latter one thought to contribute to the particular tropism of colorectal cancer cells to the liver. In most other cancers (breast, lung, melanoma, gastric etc.) liver metastases are usually considered a hallmark of incurable disseminated disease. On the contrary, some cases of CRC with liver metastases that can be completely surgically resected appear to be 'curable'. In these cases, it is likely that the micrometastases from the primary tumour were 'filtered' by the liver capillaries in the first place, probably in a similar way as lymph node metastases in other cancer types, before gaining access to the systemic circulation. In a mouse model, intraportal injection of an adequate number of CRC cells led to development of liver metastases in up to 89% of animals. In 63% of the animals developing liver metastases, tumour cells also disseminated to the bone marrow (Thalheimer et al., 2009), suggesting that the risk of dissemination to the liver is higher than to the bone marrow, probably as a result of the specific lympho-venous drainage of CRCs.

2.2.1.1 Steps in Liver Invasion

CRC cells approach the liver parenchyma through the finer branches of the portal vein, and they can remain trapped either in these branches of the portal veins, or in the tortuous hepatic sinusoids, whose diameter is much smaller than that of CRC cells. Already at this stage, CRC cells encounter the 'hepatic sinusoidal immune system' (Vekemans and Braet, 2005), composed of: hepatic-specific NKs (pit cells) (Wisse et al., 1997), liver-specific macrophage Kupffer cells (KCs) (Naito et al., 2004) and hepatic endothelial cells (HECs) (Enomoto et al., 2004) (Fig. 2.3). NKs and KCs that can move along the sinusoids would normally aggregate around these tumour cells, causing their cytolysis and subsequent phagocytosis (Braet et al., 2007). In in vivo models, about 95% of CRC cells are eliminated in the liver sinusoids, by this synergistic action between KCs and NKs (Timmers et al., 2004), involving the production of interferon gamma (IFN-γ) and nitric oxide (NO).

Unfortunately, despite the presence of such an efficient filter-system, only very few tumour cells are needed to escape from the hepatic sinusoids, settle in the liver parenchyma and reactivate proliferation, eventually leading to the spreading of new tumour cells elsewhere in the liver ('secondary metastases'). For those CRC cells that can evade and survive sinusoidal immune surveillance, the specific adhesion to the liver microcirculation involves the binding of malignant cells to endothelial E-selectin in the phase of extravasation (Gout et al., 2008). Readers are referred to Chapters 1 and 7, in this book, for further information. Extravasation may also be facilitated by the expression of Fas ligand (FasL), a pro-apoptotic factor, by CRC cells, which may lead to apoptosis in Fas-expressing hepatic endothelial cells. The gaps created in such a way allow for cell-cell interactions between the tumour cells and the hepatocytes (Timmers et al., 2004), and again the expression of Fas on hepatocytes was proposed to render them susceptible to FasL-induced apoptosis, thus facilitating CRC cells invasion into the liver tissue (Vekemans et al., 2004).

Initially, cancer cells surviving in the liver are confined to the space of Disse and to Glisson's capsule, and metastasis initiates from these regions, rich in

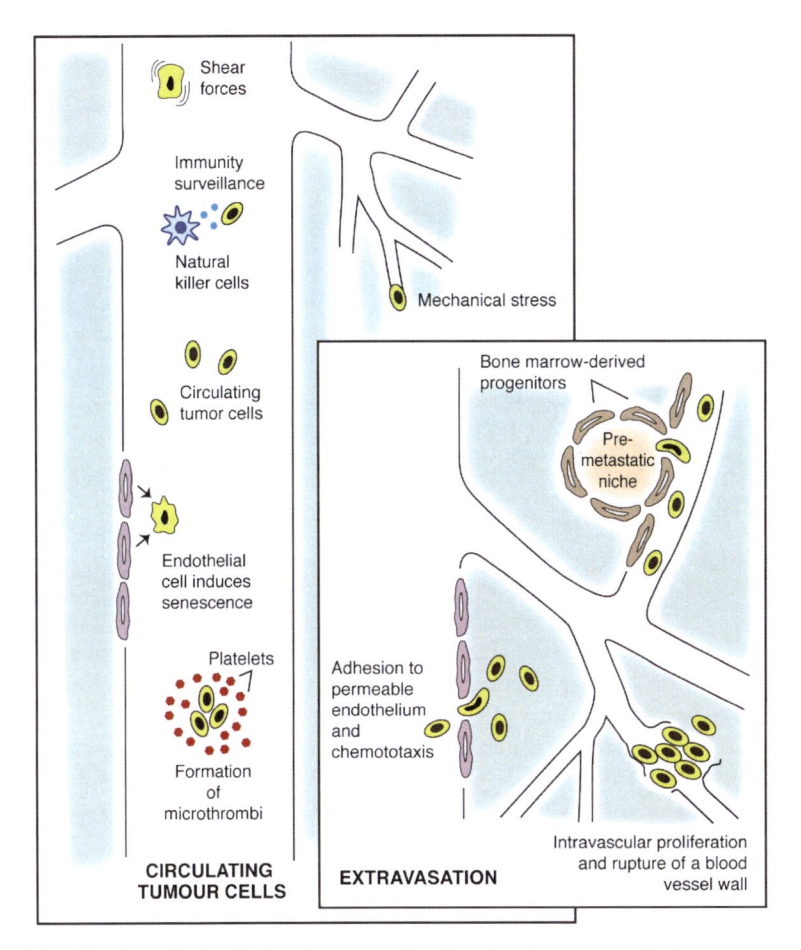

Fig. 2.3 The fate of circulating tumour cells. Circulating tumour cells have to overcome several hurdles, including shear forces, entrapment in small vessels, immune surveillance, and endothelium-induced senescence. Aggregation into microthrombi may facilitate their survival, enabling extravasation, i.e. exiting from the blood stream. The extravasation process can take place by chemotaxis, or by intravascular proliferation and rupture of the blood vessel wall. Colonization of target organs is facilitated by mobilization of bone marrow-derived progenitor cells that create a pre-metastatic niche, before the arrival of circulating tumour cells

extracellular matrix. In later stages, matrix proteins derived from liver-associated fibroblasts (stellate cells) are believed to provide a substrate for CRC cell migration and liver infiltration, while later on still, matrix proteins surrounding tumour nodules are used as a barrier preventing direct contact of cancer cells with KCs and NKs (Griffini et al., 1996).

Besides being directly supplied by the portal circulation, the liver is also thought to offer a particularly favourable microenvironment for the growth of CRC cells. It has been shown that the ability of tumour cells to metastasize in vivo to certain organs correlates with the ability of the cells to survive on extracellular matrix (ECM) derived from that organ (Doerr et al., 1989). For example, four out of four analyzed CRC cell lines grow better with ECM extracted from hepatocytes than with ECM from fibroblasts (Zvibel et al., 1998). Interestingly, the hepatocyte-derived ECM selectively enhances the clonal growth of the two cell lines with strong metastatic potential to the liver, but not of the two weakly metastatic ones. The heparin proteoglycans found in the ECM are thought to mediate this effect, as they modulate the expression of autocrine growth factors and growth factor receptors in tumour cells. The ECM of the normal liver is mainly found in the space of Disse, secreted by hepatocytes and endothelial cells. It consists mostly of type I and IV collagens, fibronectin, and the cell surface hepatocyte-specific proteoglycan, a part of the syndecan family (more often syndecan-2 or fibroglycan (Pierce et al., 1992)).

Moreover, cancer-associated fibroblasts (CAFs) extracted from liver metastases of CRC were found to produce growth factors that stimulate the growth of CRC cell lines, better than fibroblasts from uninvolved liver or normal skin (Nakagawa et al., 2004). Such growth factors include: PDGF, VEGF, FGF, CTCGF, transforming growth factor (TGF-β2) and cytokines (IL-6, MCP-1).

Finally, certain specific characteristics of CRC cells can mediate the particular tropism to the liver. A screening for genes whose expression correlates with CRC liver metastases led to the identification of phosphatase of regenerating liver-3 (PRL-3), a tyrosine phosphatase normally involved in angiogenesis (Saha et al., 2001), and more recently found to contribute to Src activation (Liang et al., 2007). The downregulation of PRL-3 in CRC cell lines has no impact on proliferation, but reduces cell motility and hepatic colonization in vivo. The overexpression of PRL-3 in human samples of CRC also significantly correlates both with liver and lung metastases (Kato et al., 2004).

Like other tumour types, CRC cancer cells can express membrane receptors physiologically involved in guiding the chemotaxis and migration of white blood cells into specific compartments, such as the aforementioned CXCR4 receptor. The aberrant expression of such receptors in CTCs can contribute to their 'targeting' of specific organs (Muller et al., 2001). Another example in CRC is the chemokine receptor chemokine type receptor 6 (CCR6), for which the only known ligand is CCL20 (or MIP-3α) (Schutyser et al., 2003), mainly expressed in mucosa-associated lymphoid tissues and in the liver. The CCL20-CCR6 pair drives migration of a subgroup of CD4+ T lymphocytes to the liver in normal conditions (Varona et al., 2005). Normal colon epithelial cells also express CCR6 (Yang et al., 2005), as do all CRC, but at very variable levels. Overall, CCR6 staining is significantly stronger in tumour cells, compared to adjacent normal mucosa. Interestingly, higher CCR6 expression is an independent predictor of synchronous liver metastases (Ghadjar et al., 2006), suggesting that CCR6 expression in CRC cells facilitates chemo-attraction by CCL20 expressed in the periportal area. Hepatic metastases show a lower expression of CCR6 than matched primary tumours, which is compatible with a CCL20-induced down-regulation (because of ligand-induced internalization and degradation of the receptor), as it happens for intra-hepatic T cells. Interestingly, CRC patients that develop liver metastases express significantly higher levels of

CCL20 in their normal liver tissues, compared with CRC patients without liver metastases (Rubie et al., 2006). This observation could be explained by a capacity of more aggressive tumours to up-regulate chemokine ligand 20 (CCL20) in the liver. In any case, it could represent a 'host-specific' factor, for which patients with a constitutively higher expression of CCL20 in the liver could be at higher risk for developing liver metastases independently of the biological aggressivity of their cancer. For example, CCL20 expression in the intestinal follicle-associated epithelium is highly inducible in response to inflammatory stimuli (Williams, 2006). In the liver, a decreased function of Kupffer cells can increase the inflammatory response to toxic agents, with an increased CCL20 expression, together with E-selectin and other cytokines (Kumagai et al., 2007).

The integrin family is composed of cell surface glycopotein adhesion receptors (please see Chapter 7 by Arabzadeh and Beauchemin, in this book). Recent in vivo experiments demonstrate a critical role in early stages of CRC liver metastasis for αv-integrins, being involved in tumour cell arrest, adhesion and migration within the hepatic microvasculature. Indeed, functional blocking of specific integrins significantly impairs these early stages of metastases development (Enns et al., 2005). Patients with high expression of the integrin $\alpha v \beta 6$ have higher risk of liver metastases than patients who are $\alpha v \beta 6$-negative (17% versus only 3%; $p<0.01$) (Yang et al., 2008).

2.2.1.2 Development of Liver Failure

The involvement of the liver can start with a limited number of discrete secondary nodules. With the exception of those patients where liver metastases can be radically resected, the disease usually evolves into multiple nodular implants, eventually causing significant hepatomegaly. Central necrosis is often found in the metastatic nodules, as they outgrow their blood supply. Liver metastases can grow to replace up to 80% of existing hepatic parenchyma, causing the liver to weigh several kilograms. It is often surprising how much liver can be replaced by cancer metastases without any clinical signs of liver failure.

Eventually, in the case of massive (>80%) or critical involvement (causing obstruction of major bile ducts), clinical signs of hepatic failure will develop, leading to the terminal phase of hepatic coma. Jaundice is an almost invariable finding, often together with pruritus, related to elevation of plasma bile acids and their deposition in skin and peripheral tissues. Hypo-albuminemia is also a consequence of impaired hepatic function and can slowly develop over the course of months, before the terminal phase. It predisposes to peripheral edema, and ascites formation. With severely impaired hepatic function, patients are also highly susceptible to failure of multiple organ systems, such as respiratory failure with pneumonia and sepsis, combined with renal failure. A coagulopathy develops, due to impaired hepatic synthesis of coagulation factors II, VII, IX and X. These patients develop a risk of bleeding that may lead to massive hemorrhage, or widespread petechiae. Hepatic encephalopathy is related to hyperammonemia, which impairs neuronal function, causes abnormal neurotransmission in the central nervous system, and induces generalized brain edema (Mousseau and Butterworth, 1994). The hepatorenal syndrome is another complication of hepatic failure, whereby acute renal failure develops in the absence of any other specific cause. It is associated with a drop in urine output and rise in blood urea and creatinine concentrations. The development of this syndrome seems to involve decreased renal perfusion (Van Roey and Moore, 1996).

In summary, the interplay of the complex factors regulating the seeding, survival and growth of metastatic CRC cells in the liver may eventually result in the overt manifestation of multiple liver metastases, which then almost always lead to liver failure and death.

2.2.2 Lungs

About 10–25% of patients with CRC develop pulmonary metastases, but only 2–4% have metastasis confined just to the lungs. Metastases typically appear as smooth, well-circumscribed and peripherally-located nodules, with a hypodense and rounded appearance on computer tomography (CT) scans. Most patients with lung metastases from CRC are asymptomatic. Symptoms are only reported in 10–20% of cases and reflect proximity to central airways: cough and hemoptysis are the most frequent complaints. Dyspnea is rarely observed.

Lung metastases from CRC are generally thought to be non-life-threatening, being much less likely than liver metastases to become poorly controllable by current treatments (including surgery), so that respiratory failure is a relatively rare cause of death in CRC patients, even in CRC patients with lung metastases.

Risk factors for the specific development of lung metastases in CRC have been reported. The site of the primary tumour (colon versus rectum) does not have an influence on the biology and prognosis of lung metastases, but rectal cancers can more frequently give rise to pulmonary metastases because of the rectum's dual venous drainage (caval and portal).

The mechanisms underlying the formation of lung metastasis are less understood than in the case of liver metastasis. It is thought that lung metastases may be enabled by the activation of CXCR3 in CRC cells. In one in vivo model (Cambien et al., 2009), activation of CXCR3 on CRC cells favours implantation and growth within lung tissues, without any effect on liver metastases. Interestingly, higher levels of both CXCR3 and its ligands are found in lung as compared to liver metastases.

2.2.3 Peritoneum

As mentioned above, peritoneal metastases develop in a minority of patients with CRC. Although these tumour deposits may be clinically silent when small, their growth may eventually lead to clinical symptoms due to small bowel obstruction and palpable masses in the abdomen and the abdominal wall. Unlike other forms of bowel obstruction, malignant small bowel obstruction does not usually resolve conservatively, but often requires surgical intervention due to intractable obstruction of the small bowel, not infrequently at multiple sites. At surgery, tumour deposits often have infiltrated the small bowel mesentery, leading to kinking of small bowel loops. When small bowel obstruction is due to pelvic peritoneal tumour deposits, it usually cannot be relieved by surgical resection of the obstructed loop of bowel, but requires intestinal bypass for symptom relief. Thus, although usually silent, peritoneal metastases may require complex surgical interventions for palliative relief of intestinal occlusive symptoms.

2.2.4 Bone and Bone Marrow

Bone metastases are a rare event in the early natural history of the disease, and they are usually a hallmark of very widespread disease, with a typical appearance several months after the clinical detection of metastases in other sites. Indeed, the overall incidence of bone metastases in CRC patients (6–10%) correlates with the number of previous treatments received, and they are more frequently found in patients with lung metastases (Sundermeyer et al., 2005). Bones are the only sites of disease in only 17% of patients with metastatic CRC (Kanthan et al., 1999). A recent study using sensitive tumour imaging techniques (PET scanning) reported that osseous metastases almost never occur without metastatic lesions to other organs (Roth et al., 2009). Resistant lung metastases were found to be a better predictor of the development of bone metastasis than liver metastases. Patients with primary rectal tumours are more likely to develop bone metastases (16% versus 8.6%, $p = 0.001$) than those with colon primary tumours. Bone metastases can disrupt the normal architecture of a bone, cause severe pain, and in some cases lead to pathological fractures.

When cancer cells enter the systemic circulation, they may not immediately home to those sites where eventually clinical metastases will develop, but rather first disseminate to other microenvironments, such as the lymph nodes and the bone marrow. It has been proposed that the bone marrow microenvironment may select subclones of cancer cells that subsequently will develop or improve their ability to migrate to distant sites. In particular, the bone marrow could provide a uniquely supportive stromal environment that is functioning physiologically to maintain the haematopoietic stem cell. So far, little experimental evidence has been reported to support such a hypothesis.

Little data is available on the frequency of bone marrow micrometastases in CRC patients (Weitz et al., 1999), but this does not appear to be a very early event, being less common than significant lymph node involvement in resected patients. As opposed to other tumour types, the clinical relevance of bone marrow micrometastases is yet to be validated in CRC patients: in 96 patients undergoing a curative resection with bone marrow (BM) aspiration at the time of surgery, 33% showed immunocytology-positive cells in the BM, but this finding did not correlate with 4-year survival (Schott et al., 1998). In another study on 47 patients undergoing surgical resection of liver metastases, 55% of them were also found to bear BM involvement by cytokeratin-positive cells, but this did not correlate with a higher risk of subsequent extrahepatic recurrence (Schoppmeyer et al., 2006).

2.2.5 Brain Metastasis

Brain metastases from CRC are rare in comparison to other cancer types (incidence 2–3%) (Mongan et al., 2009) but their incidence may be expected to increase as a result of recent improvements in overall survival of patients with metastatic disease. In a series of 39 cases with symptomatic brain metastases from CRC, the cerebellum was the most common area of brain involvement. As with bone metastases, concomitant widespread disease is usually present in patients diagnosed with brain metastases.

As in other solid cancers, it is likely that a particular tumour expression signature will be found to identify tumours at higher risk of specific organ metastases. These will require independent validation before clinical application is warranted. For the time being, expression of the CXCR4 receptor in primary colorectal cancer cells was found to be high in patients eventually developing brain metastases.

2.3 Factors Contributing to Metastatic Spread

The prognosis of a cancer is closely related to the risk of developing unresectable disease, usually meaning distant metastases. In clinical practice, the prognosis of resected cancers is estimated on the basis of tumour-related factors, such as clinical stage, grading, or other pathology findings. Nevertheless, this system is far from perfect. It is not uncommon to see patients relapsing with widespread disease after surgery for a node-negative tumour, or other cases of locally advanced cancers (node-positive, or pT4) that may be cured after resection of the primary tumour. These observations highlight both our need of a deeper understanding of the biology of each cancer, independently of its stage, and the remarkable lack of evidence regarding prognostic factors beyond those related to tumour characteristics. Here, we will focus on selected factors that not only predict for, but may functionally or physiologically contribute to the development of metastatic disease in CRC.

2.3.1 Tumour Factors

2.3.1.1 Tissue Factor

Tissue factor (TF, also known as thromboplastin) is a glycoprotein transmembrane receptor. Upon binding of the coagulation factors X and VIIa (FVIIa), TF is responsible for initiating proteolytic events that lead to the generation of thrombin, the primary trigger for the extrinsic coagulation cascade, together with fibrin deposition (Bach, 1988). TF is found on the surface of various cells, but it can be upregulated up to a 1,000-fold higher in tumour cells with metastatic potential than in non-metastatic cells (Mueller et al., 1992). The expression of TF is detected in 57% of colorectal cancers, and it is an independent risk factor for the development of liver metastases in this population (Seto et al., 2000). FVIIa binding to

TF causes the intracellular activation of extracellular signal-regulated kinase (ERK) mitogen-activated (MAP) kinases and phosphatidyl-inositol-3 (PI-3) kinase, with an anti-apoptotic effect, and upregulation of growth factors and genes regulating cell organization and motility (Versteeg et al., 2004a). Moreover, FVIIa and TF induce cell survival through inhibition of anoikis (Versteeg et al., 2004b), a special form of apoptosis that occurs when cells detach from the extracellular matrix and thus lack adhesion signalling. It appears that FVIIa/TF signalling can replace adhesion signalling in metastatic cells, leading to aberrant cell survival and ability to travel through the bloodstream. The TF receptor has also been proposed to function as an adhesion molecule, mediating metastatic cell adhesion to the endothelium, prior to extravasation (Ott et al., 1998).

Finally, besides its downstream intracellular effect, TF can support the development of metastatic disease independently of its cytoplasmic domain, through cooperation with circulating hemostatic factors, including distal components of the coagulation cascade. In an in vivo sarcoma model, tumour TF favoured the early survival of micrometastases, both through fibrinogen-dependent inhibition of NK cell functions, and through a prothrombin-dependent, NK-independent mechanism (Palumbo et al., 2007).

2.3.1.2 EGFR

The epidermal growth factor (EGF) family, crucial to the growth of epithelial tumours, is composed of four Erb-B/HER receptors (Erb-B1, -B2, -B3 and -B4) and several ligands (EGF, TGFα, heparin-binding EGF-like growth factor/HB-EGF, amphiregulin, epiregulin) that bind to EGF-receptors, leading to their homo- or hetero-dimerization (Citri and Yarden, 2006).

The Erb-B1 receptor (or epidermal growth factor receptor, EGFR) is believed to be particular relevant to the biology of CRC and was proven to be a valid therapeutic target: EGFR-targeting antibodies are widely used in clinical practice for the treatment of this disease (de Castro-Caroeno et al., 2008). Beyond its putative role in carcinogenesis and growth of the primary tumour, EGFR is believed to actively contribute to the generation of CRC metastases. Highly metastatic CRC cells express >5-fold the number of EGFR mRNA transcripts compared to cells with low metastatic potential. After injection into nude mice, only cells with high expression of EGFR produce a high incidence of liver metastasis (Radinsky et al., 1995). Some discrepancy exists in published literature regarding EGFR status in clinical samples. Concordance in the expression of total EGFR in primary CRC and matched liver/lung metastases ranges between 50 and 94% of the cases (Scartozzi et al., 2004; Italiano et al., 2005).

Interestingly, in vivo models suggest that the development of liver metastases can depend on a tissue-specific functional activation of EGFR detected as increased expression of phospho-EGFR (p-EGFR). Increased p-EGFR is observed both peripherally and centrally in liver metastases growing in nude mice, as opposed to primary tumours growing orthotopically, where little or no immunoreactivity for p-EGFR is found (Parker et al., 1998). These findings reflect a preferential activation of EGFR in liver metastases, as the overall expression of EGFR (independently of its functional state) is similar in primary tumours implanted orthotopically or ectopically and in liver metastases, suggesting a higher expression of active ligands for EGFR in the hepatic microenvironment. In addition, amphiregulin, HB-EGF and heregulins are heparin-binding growth factors. When CRC cell lines are grown in vitro on hepatocyte-derived ECM, amphiregulin stimulates the growth of the highly metastatic cell line KM12SM, while inhibiting the growth of the weakly liver-colonizing KM12 cell line (Ciardello et al., 1991). Taken together, the above reports suggest a specific role for EGFR signaling in the formation and growth of liver metastases in colorectal cancer, further shown by the clinical success of molecules such as cetuximab (an anti-EGFR antibody) that target this pathway in this disease.

2.3.2 Host Factors

2.3.2.1 Immunity

It has been reported that the subgroup of CRC patients carrying a germline mutation in DNA repair genes forming part of the mismatch repair system (MMR) have a better prognosis, with minimal or no impact from adjuvant chemotherapy (Smyrk et al., 2001; Ribic et al., 2003). This different prognosis may be dependent on a peculiar tumour biology, but host factors may also play a role: a characteristic 'Crohn-like' inflammatory stromal reaction has been proposed to mediate this lower incidence of distant metastasis, as its presence also predicts for a better prognosis (Buckowitz et al., 2005). Preliminary data suggest that this inflammatory response correlates with a high density of tumour-infiltrating cytotoxic ($CD8^+$) lymphocytes that could indicate a cytotoxic anti-tumoural immune response. A better immune response in the host could theoretically have a dramatic impact in reducing the risk of developing metastatic disease. Nevertheless, little clinical evidence is available on the impact of immunity on CRC prognosis. In preclinical studies, splenectomy associates with a higher incidence and load of liver metastases in mouse models of CRC (Higashijima et al., 2009). A vaccine targeting the intestinal cancer mucosa antigen guanylyl cyclase C (GCC) was studied in an in vivo model of CRC lung metastases. This vaccine induces anti-tumour $CD8^+$ T-cell immunity and antitumour activity opposing the development of distant metastases (Snook et al., 2009).

The efficacy of the anti-tumour immune response can be altered by many conditions. The possible impact of stress and other psychological conditions has often been evoked. In another in vivo model using intraportal vein injection of CRC cells, social isolation of host mice is associated with a higher number and burden of liver metastases, as compared to the group-housed mice (Wu et al., 2000). Interestingly, social isolation seems to enhance tumour metastasis in part because of an immunosuppressive effect, as it is associated with a weaker proliferative response of splenocytes to various stimuli, suppression of splenic NK activity and macrophage-mediated cytotoxicity.

2.3.2.2 Diet, Exercise and Liver Disease

Several epidemiological studies have reported that diet and other lifestyle factors, such as physical activity, impact the risk of developing CRC (Martínez, 2005), but their impact on the risk of recurrence (meaning on the development of metastases after an initial diagnosis of localized CRC) was only more recently assessed. Obesity is associated with increased prevalence of metastases at diagnosis of prostate cancer (Gong et al., 2007). A prospective observational study on more than 1,000 patients operated for stage III CRC found a significantly higher risk of cancer relapse and cancer-related death for patients following a 'Western'-type of diet, characterized by high intakes of meat, fat, refined grains, desserts, as compared to patients on a more 'prudent' diet, with more fruits, vegetables, poultry, fish (hazard ratio for disease-free survival up to 3.25 for the groups with the largest differences in dietary patterns; 95% CI, 1.75–4.63) (Meyerhardt et al., 2007). The mechanisms underlying such an association are not clear. Indeed, in the same patient population, neither body mass index and obesity nor weight change after surgery seemed to be associated with an increased risk of CRC recurrence after surgery (Meyerhardt et al., 2008). On the contrary, maintaining good physical activity during follow-up after surgery did appear to reduce the risk of cancer recurrence in this patient population (hazard ratio 0.51, 95% CI 0.26–0.97) (Meyerhardt et al., 2006).

In in vivo models, obesity, hyperlipidemia and glucose intolerance were shown to increase circulating pro-inflammatory cytokines and pro-angiogenic factors, and to promote tumour growth and metastasis (Kimura and Sumiyoshi, 2007), so that obese animals develop higher metastatic tumour burden in the liver than lean controls (Earl et al., 2009). The adipocyte-produced peptide leptin that plays a key role in regulation of food intake, body weight and fat mass, was studied in vitro, and shown to promote invasiveness of CRC cells expressing the corresponding Ob-Rb receptors (Attoub et al., 2000). Moreover, leptin stimulates angiogenesis in in vivo models in a dose-dependent manner (Anagnostoulis et al., 2008), with a mitogenic effect on vascular endothelial cells (Park et al., 2001). Together with an increase in serum leptin, high levels of fatty acids can contribute to the development of CRC metastases in obese patients. In particular, saturated fatty acids, whose circulating levels are often increased in visceral fat obesity, serve as a naturally occurring ligand for Toll-like receptor-4 (TLR4) complex (Lee et al., 2001). TLR4 is the innate receptor for intestinal endotoxin (lipopolysaccharide) and is expressed in tumour cells, where it can mediate a pro-neoplastic effect due to evasion of immune surveillance and induction of tumour tolerance in tumour-infiltrating macrophages (Shi et al., 2006). In a similar way, endotoxin and circulating fatty acids are thought to contribute to liver injury, in both alcoholic and non-alcoholic steatohepatitis, as TLR4 is also expressed in the liver, and it induces cytokine expression and activates pro-inflammatory pathways. In steatotic livers, the expression of TLR4 is higher than in the normal liver from lean animals (Earl et al., 2009).

In an interesting murine model of high fat diet-induced liver disease, starting from hepatic steatosis to development of primary liver dysplasia, splenic injection of CRC cells results in an increased number of metastatic lesions in steatotic livers

(VanSaun et al., 2009). These in vivo observations could simply be due to the effects of high circulating levels of leptin, endotoxin and fatty acids both on cancer cells and in the liver. Nevertheless, it is also plausible that liver steatosis itself provides a permissive microenvironment for the growth of CRC cells with metastatic potential to the liver. For example, microcirculatory disturbances are worsened in fatty livers, which may induce prolonged hypoxia (Ijaz et al., 2003). Hypoxia is one of the most potent stimulators of tumour growth (Harris, 2002), and prolonged hypoxia after liver ischemia/reperfusion plays an important role in stimulating the growth of subclinical CRC liver micrometastases (van der Bilt et al., 2007). Indeed, another in vivo model was used to show that liver ischemia/reperfusion resulted in the stimulation of the growth of previously established liver metastases. In this model as well, a heavier load of liver metastases is observed in older mice and in mice with a higher degree of liver steatosis (van der Bilt et al., 2008). Overall, these findings suggest that the development of liver metastasis can be favoured by a more 'permissive' liver microenvironment. This mainly depends on concomitant host conditions (as in the case of underlying inflammation and associated hypoxia), but in some cases it can also be influenced by medical procedures (for example, inducing liver hypoxia).

2.3.3 Iatrogenic Factors

A major operation is followed by a pronounced state of immunosuppression for up to 3 weeks (Mels et al., 2001), and it is theoretically possible that this state can also affect KCs and NKs in the liver, normally devoted to the eradication of CRC cells drained and retained in the liver vasculature. Furthermore, with the inflammatory reaction that inevitably follows surgical trauma, several cytokines are released locally and into the systemic circulation, including interleukin 1 (IL-1β), IL-6, tumour necrosis factor alpha (TNFα) and VEGF. Not only can these mediators directly stimulate the growth and invasion of malignant cells, but they can also alter the integrity of blood vessels, up-regulate adhesion molecules on liver endothelial cells, and increase vessel permeability, thus favouring the adhesion and extravasation of CTCs.

Indeed, it has been reported that surgical trauma enhances the outgrowth of metastases (Coffey et al., 2003). In animal studies, surgery itself enhances the locoregional growth of the tumour. Intraperitoneal injection of cancer cells in rats results in a 2.5-fold increase in peritoneal tumour load, if the injection is performed after a thoracotomy (Raa et al., 2005). Importantly, a more invasive surgery is associated with a higher tumour load, when comparing laparoscopy (less invasive, closed surgery) to laparotomy (more invasive, open surgery) in animal models (Mutter et al., 1999). In another interesting animal model, surgical trauma significantly increased the adhesion of injected CRC cells in the liver, favoring the outgrowth of metastases. Interestingly, if tumour cells were pre-incubated before their injection with an anti-α2 integrin antibody, their capacity of adhesion re-normalized to baseline levels (van der Bij et al., 2008).

Relatively little evidence on this topic is available in humans. In a clinical trial (Lacy et al., 2002), 219 patient candidates for resection of colon cancer were randomized between an open colectomy and a less-invasive laparoscopy-assisted colectomy. Surprisingly, a lower risk of tumour relapse (HR 0.39, 95% CI 0.19–0.82) and lower disease-specific mortality (HR 0.38, 95% CI 0.16–0.91) was found for patients treated with laparoscopy. However, these results were not confirmed in other studies, and a recent multi-study Cochrane review of randomized controlled trials on more than 3,000 patients, found no difference in tumour recurrence after laparoscopic or open surgery (Kuhry et al., 2008).

Another example of iatrogenic local spread of cancer is that of biopsies. Liver surgeons usually recommend against biopsy of CRC liver metastases, because of concerns about the risk of local dissemination. In two retrospective analysis on 133 patients undergoing surgery for CRC liver metastases after a pre-operative liver biopsy, 16–19% had evidence of dissemination related to the biopsy (needle-track deposits), independently of the type of biopsy (Rodgers et al., 2003). In another provocative retrospective analysis, the 4-year survival rate after liver resection was 32.5% in patients undergoing liver biopsy, compared with 46.7% in patients without biopsy ($p=0.008$) (Jones et al., 2005). Despite the retrospective nature of these findings, a liver biopsy is probably contra-indicated in patients with potentially resectable disease.

Finally, with the increasing number of patients undergoing resection of CRC liver metastases, a particular concern has been raised regarding the possibility that both the inevitable ischemia/reperfusion during surgery, and the molecular changes associated with the subsequent liver regeneration process may influence the kinetics of tumour growth and contribute to recurrence (Cristophi et al., 2008). During hepatic resection, the blood flow to the liver is transiently reduced, to prevent excessive blood loss. In a standardized murine model of temporary partial liver clamping, pre-established micrometastases are stimulated by ischemia/reperfusion (van der Bilt et al., 2007). This effect is attributable to a microcirculatory failure, lasting up to 5 days, followed by the development of necrotic areas after 24 h, surrounded by a massive inflammatory infiltrate. This is accompanied by profound and prolonged peri-necrotic hypoxia, that causes stabilization of hypoxia-inducible factor (HIF)-1α, and massive peri-necrotic outgrowth of pre-established micrometastases.

After portal vein embolization for liver resection, the hepatic parenchyma regenerates, but the growth rate of liver metastases exceeds that of normal liver by almost eight times (Elias et al., 1999). The degree of liver resection seems to influence the degree of tumour growth stimulation (Slooter et al., 1995), and this effect occurs predominantly in the late phase of liver regeneration, rather than in the early phase (Harun et al., 2007). A variety of growth factors, cytokines and pro-angiogenic factors increase after resection of a significant fraction of functional liver parenchyma, in order to stimulate the passage of hepatocytes from phase G0 to G1. The paracrine effect of these factors is likely to play a key role in stimulating un-resected cancer cells. Indeed, if tumour dormancy of undetected micrometastases depends on the balance between apoptosis and proliferation and between pro- and anti-angiogenic factors, the production of cytokines and pro-angiogenic factors that normally accompanies liver regeneration could alter the microenvironment also of distant microscopic tumour deposits, and cause their reactivation. For example, the expression of hepatocyte growth factor (HGF) increases 6–8 h after partial liver resection (Huh et al., 2004). Similarly, angiogenic growth factors such as VEGF and a number of the EGFR ligands are also upregulated during liver regeneration (EGF, TGFα, amphiregulin, HB-EGF).

Other changes in the liver microenvironment after resection can also influence the phenotype of established metastases. For example, liver resection causes a significant increase of CXCR2 on the surface of tumour cells, the receptor for the chemokine CXCL1/macrophage-inflammatory protein-2 (MIP-2). Pre-clinical data show that the chemokine MIP-2 promotes angiogenesis in vivo, stimulates growth of CRC liver metastasis (Kollmar et al., 2006), and engraftment of CRC metastasis at extrahepatic sites, but with no effect on the growth of already established metastases (Kollmar et al., 2008).

Despite all of this preclinical evidence, there is no doubt that in about a quarter to a third of patients with isolated liver metastases from CRC, short- to medium-term survival can be achieved by liver resection, suggesting that complete eradication of tumour metastases in the liver is achievable in selected cases. However, the above factors help to explain the reappearance of 'new' liver metastases after apparently complete metastatic tumour resection, through the reactivation of dormant tumour cells invisible to radiologic and clinical examination of the liver.

2.4 Conclusion

The physiopathology of colorectal metastasis is a complex process, which through multiple pathways leads to the demise of the CRC patient. Many tumour, host and treatment-related factors interplay to lead to the deposition and growth of metastatic tumour deposits. The liver is the most common site of significant metastatic spread, while metastasis to the lung, peritoneal cavity and bone are less frequent sites. The molecular factors involved in tissue tropism are slowly being elucidated and may become targets for early therapeutic intervention in the near future.

Abbreviations and Acronyms

BM	Bone marrow
CAFs	Cancer-associated fibroblasts
CCL20	Chemokine ligand 20
CCR7	Chemokine receptor type 7
CRC	Colorectal cancer
CTCs	Circulating tumour cells
DARC	Duffy blood group receptor
ECM	Extracellular matrix
EGF	Epidermal growth factor

EGFR	Epidermal growth factor receptor
ERK	Extracellular signal-regulated kinase
FGF	Fibroblast growth factor
GCC	Guanylyl cyclase C
HECs	Hepatic endothelial cells
HGF	Hepatocyte growth factor
HR	Hormone receptor
ICAM-1	Intercellular adhesion molecule-1
IL-1	Interleukin-1
IFN-γ	Interferon gamma
KCs	Kupffer cells
LN	Lymph nodes
LVD	Lymphatic vessel density
MAP Kinase	Mitogen-activated protein kinase
MIP-2	Macrophage-inflammatory protein-2
NKs	Natural killer cells
NO	Nitric oxide
PDGFRβ	Platelet-derived growth factor receptor β
PECAM-1	Platelet endothelial cell adhesion molecule-1
(PI-3) Kinase	phosphatidyl-inositol-3 kinase
PRL-3	Phosphatase of regenerating liver-3
SDF-1	Stromal cell-derived factor 1
TF	Tissue Factor
TLR	Toll-like receptor
TNFα	Tumour necrosis factor α
TNM	Tumour-node-metastases
VCAM-1	Vascular adhesion molecule-1
VEGF	Vascular endothelial growth factor
VEGFR	VEGF receptor

References

Al-Mehdi AB, Tozawa K, Fisher AB, Shientag L, Lee A, Muschel RJ (2000). Intravascular origin of metastasis from the proliferation of endothelium-attached tumor cells: a new model for metastasis. *Nat Med* **6**: 100–02.

Anagnostoulis S, Karayiannakis AJ, Lambropoulou M, Efthimiadou A, Polychronidis A, Simopoulos C (2008). Human leptin induces angiogenesis in vivo. *Cytokine* **42**: 353–57.

Attoub S, Noe V, Pirola L, Bruyneel E, Chastre E, Mareel M (2000). Leptin promotes invasiveness of kidney and colonic epithelial cells via phosphoinositide 3-kinase-, rho-, and rac-dependent signaling pathways. *FASEB J* **14**: 2329–38.

Bach RR (1988). Initiation of coagulation by tissue factor. *CRC Crit Rev Biochem* **23**: 339–68.

Balkwill F (2004). Cancer and the chemokine network. *Nat Rev Cancer* **4**: 540–50.

Bandyopadhyay S, Zhan R, Chaudhuri A, Watabe M, Pai SK, Hirota S et al. (2006). Interaction of KAI1 on tumor cells with DARC on vascular endothelium leads to metastasis suppression. *Nat Med* **12**: 933–38.

Bilchik AJ, Nora DT (2002). Lymphatic mapping of nodal micrometastasis in colon cancer: putting the cart before the horse? *Ann Surg Oncol* **9**: 529–31.

Bird NC, Mangnall D, Majeed AW (2006). Biology of colorectal liver metastases: a review. *J Surg Oncol* **94**: 68–80.

Braet F, Nagatsuma K, Saito M, Soon L, Wisse E, Matsuura T (2007). The hepatic sinusoidal endothelial lining and colorectal liver metastases. *World J Gastroenterol* **13**: 821–25.

Breslin JW, Gaudreault N, Watson KD, Reynoso R, Yuan SY, Wu MH (2007). Vascular endothelial growth factor-C stimulates the lymphatic pump by a VEGF receptor-3-dependent mechanism. *Am J Physiol Heart Circ Physiol* **293H**: 709–18.

Buckowitz A, Knaebel HP, Benner A, Bläker H, Gebert J, Kienle P et al. (2005). Microsatellite instability in colorectal cancer is associated with local lymphocyte infiltration and low frequency of distant metastases. *Br J Cancer* **92**: 1746–53.

Cambien B, Karimdjee BF, Richard-Fiardo P, Bziouech H, Barthel R, Millet MA et al. (2009). Organ-specific inhibition of metastatic colon carcinoma by CXCR3 antagonism. *Br J Cancer* **100**: 1755–64.

Ceelen WP, Bracke ME (2009). Peritoneal minimal residual disease in colorectal cancer: mechanisms, prevention, and treatment. *Lancet Oncol* **10**: 72–79.

Chambers AF, Groom AC, MacDonald IC (2002). Dissemination and growth of cancer cells in metastatic sites. *Nature Rev Cancer* **2**: 563–72.

Chang YS, di Tomaso E, McDonald DM, Jones R, Jain RK, Munn LL (2000). Mosaic blood vessels in tumors: frequency of cancer cells in contact with flowing blood. *Proc Natl Acad Sci USA* **97**: 14608–13.

Chu DZ, Lang NP, Thompson C, Osteen PK, Westbrook KC (1989). Peritoneal carcinomatosis in nongynecologic malignancy. A prospective study of prognostic factors. *Cancer* **63**: 364–67.

Ciardello F, Kim N, Saeki T, Dono R, Persico MG, Plowman GD et al. (1991). Differential expression of epidermal growth factor-related proteins in human colorectal tumors. *Proc Natl Acad Sci USA* **88**: 7792–96.

Citri A, Yarden Y (2006). EGF-ERBB signalling: towards the system level. *Nat Rev Mol Cell Biol* **7**: 505–16.

Coffey JC, Wang JH, Smith MJ, Bouchier-Hayes D, Cotter TG, Redmond HP (2003). Excisional surgery for cancer cure: therapy at a cost. *Lancet Oncol* **4**: 760–68.

Cohen SJ, Punt CJA, Iannotti N, Saidman BH, Sabbath KD, Gabrail NY et al. (2009). Prognostic significance of circulating tumor cells in patients with metastatic colorectal cancer. *Ann Oncol* **20**: 1223–29.

Criscuoli ML, Nguyen M, Eliceiri BP (2005). Tumor metastasis but not tumor growth is dependent on Src-mediated vascular permeability. *Blood* **105**: 1508–14.

Cristophi C, Harun N, Fifis T (2008). Liver regeneration and tumor stimulation – a review of cytokine and angiogenic factors. *J Gastrointest Surg* **12**: 966–80.

Das S, Skobe M (2008). Lymphatic vessel activation in cancer. *Ann NY Acad Sci* **1131**: 235–41.

de Castro-Caroeño J, Belda-Iniesta C, Casado Sáenz E, Hernández Agudo E, Feliu Batlle J, González Barón M (2008). EGFR and colon cancer: a clinical view. *Clin Transl Oncol* **10**: 6–13.

Doerr R, Zvibel I, Chiuten D, D'Olimpio J, Reid LM (1989). Clonal growth of tumors on tissue-specific biomatrices and correlation with organ-site specificity of metastases. *Cancer Res* **49**: 384–92.

Earl TM, Nicoud IB, Pierce JM, Wright JP, Majoras NE, Rubin JE (2009). Silencing of TLR4 decreases liver tumor burden in a murine model of colorectal metastasis and hepatic steatosis. *Ann Surg Oncol* **16**: 1043–50.

Elias D, De Baere T, Roche A, Mducreux M, Leclere J, Lasser P (1999). During liver regeneration following right portal embolization the growth rate of liver metastases is more rapid than that of the liver parenchyma. *Br J Surg* **86**: 784–88.

Enns A, Korb T, Schlüter K, Gassmann P, Spiegel HU, Senninger N et al. (2005). Alphavbeta5-integrins mediate early steps of metastasis formation. *Eur J Cancer* **41**: 1065–72.

Enomoto K, Nishikawa Y, Omori Y, Tokairin T, Yoshida M, Ohi N et al. (2004). Cell biology and pathology of liver sinusoidal endothelial cells. *Med Electron Microsc* **37**: 208–15.

Furudoi A, Tanaka S, Haruma K, Kitadai Y, Yoshihara M, Chayama K, Shimamoto F (2002). Clinical significance of vascular endothelial growth factor C expression and angiogenesis at the deepest invasive site of advanced colorectal carcinoma. *Oncology* **62**: 157–66.

Gassmann P, Haier J (2008). The tumor cell-host organ interface in the early onset of metastatic organ colonisation. *Clin Exp Metastasis* **25**: 171–81.

Ghadjar P, Coupland SE, Na IK, Noutsias M, Letsch A, Stroux A et al. (2006). Chemokine receptor CCR6 expression level and liver metastases in colorectal cancer. *J Clin Oncol* **24**: 1910–16.

Gong Z, Agalliu I, Lin DW, Stanford JL, Kristal AR (2007). Obesity is associated with increased risks of prostate cancer metastasis and death after initial cancer diagnosis in middle-aged men. *Cancer* **109**: 1192–202.

Gout S, Tremblay PL, Huot J (2008). Selectins and selectin ligands in extravasation of cancer cells and organ selectivity of metastasis. *Clin Exp Metastasis* **25**: 335–44.

Griffini P, Smorenburg SM, Vogels IM, Tigchelaar W, Van Noorden CJ (1996). Kupffer cells and pit cells are not effective in the defense against experimentally induced colon carcinoma metastasis in rat liver. *Clin Exp Metastasis* **14**: 367–80.

Guo W, Giancotti FG (2004). Integrin signalling during tumour progression. *Nat Rev Mol Cell Biol* **5**: 816–26.

Günther K, Leier J, Henning G, Dimmler A, Weissbach R, Hohenberger W, Förster R (2005). Prediction of lymph node metastasis in colorectal carcinoma by expression of chemokine receptor CCR7. *Int J Cancer* **116**: 726–33.

Harris AL (2002). Hypoxia-a key regulatory factor in tumour growth. *Nat Rev Cancer* **2**: 38–47.

Harun N, Nikfarjam M, Muralidharan V, Christophi C (2007). Liver regeneration stimulates tumour metastases. *J Surg Res* **138**: 284–90.

Higashijima J, Shimada M, Chikakiyo M, Miyatani T, Yoshikawa K, Nishioka M et al. (2009). Effect of splenectomy on antitumor immune system in mice. *Anticancer Res* **29**: 385–93.

Holmgren L, O'Reilly MS, Folkman J (1995). Dormancy of micrometastases: balanced proliferation and apoptosis in the presence of angiogenesis suppression. *Nature Med* **1**: 149–53.

Huh CG, Factor VM, Sánchez A, Uchida K, Conner EA, Thorgeirsson SS (2004). Hepatocyte growth factor/c-met signaling pathway is required for efficient liver regeneration and repair. *Proc Natl Acad Sci USA* **101**: 4477–82.

Ijaz S, Yang W, Winslet MC, Seifalian AM (2003). Impairment of hepatic microcirculation in fatty liver. *Microcirculation* **10**: 447–56.

Im JH, Fu W, Wang H, Bhatia SK, Hammer DA, Kowalska MA, Muschel RJ (2004). Coagulation facilitates tumor cell spreading in the pulmonary vasculature during early metastatic colony formation. *Cancer Res* **64**: 8613–19.

Italiano A, Saint-Paul MC, Caroli-Bosc FX, François E, Bourgeon A, Benchimol D et al. (2005). Epidermal growth factor receptor (EGFR) status in primary colorectal tumors correlates with EGFR expression in related metastatic sites: biological and clinical implications. *Ann Oncol* **16**: 1503–07.

Jones OM, Rees M, John TG, Bygrave S, Plant G (2005). Biopsy of resectable colorectal liver metastases causes tumour dissemination and adversely affects survival after liver resection. *Br J Surg* **92**: 1165–68.

Jurasz P, Alonso-Escolano D, Radomski MW (2004). Platelet-cancer interactions: mechanisms and pharmacology of tumour cell-induced platelet aggregation. *Br J Pharmacol* **143**: 819–26.

Kakinuma T, Hwang ST (2006). Chemokines, chemokine receptors, and cancer metastasis. *J Leukoc Biol* **79**: 639–51.

Kanellos I, Demetriades H, Zintzaras E, Mandrali A, Mantzoros I, Betsis D (2003). Incidence and prognostic value of positive peritoneal cytology in colorectal cancer. *Dis Colon Rectum* **46**: 535–39.

Kanthan R, Loewy J, Kanthan SC (1999). Skeletal metastases in colorectal carcinomas: a Saskatchewa profile. *Dis Colon Rectum* **42**: 1592–97.

Kaplan RN, Riba RD, Zacharoulis S, Bramley AH, Vincent L, Costa C et al. (2005). VEGFR1-positive haematopoietic bone marrow progenitors initiate the pre-metastatic niche. *Nature* **438**: 820–27.

Kato H, Semba S, Miskad UA, Seo Y, Kasuga M, Yokozaki H (2004). High expression of PRL-3 promotes cancer cell motility and liver metastasis in human colorectal cancer. *Clin Cancer Res* **10**: 7318–28.

Kawada K, Hosogi H, Sonoshita M, Sakashita H, Manabe T, Shimahara Y et al. (2007). Chemokine receptor CXCR3 promotes colon cancer metastasis to lymph nodes. *Oncogene* **26**: 4679–88.

Kim YJ, Borsig L, Varki NM, Varki A (1998). P-selectin deficiency attenuates tumor growth and metastasis. *Proc Natl Acad Sci USA* **95**: 9325–30.

Kim J, Takeuchi H, Lam ST, Turner RR, Wang HJ, Kuo C et al. (2005). Chemokine receptor CXCR4 expression in colorectal cancer patients increases the risk of recurrence and for poor survival. *J Clin Oncol* **23**: 2744–53.

Kimura Y, Sumiyoshi M (2007). High-fat, high-sucrose, and high-cholesterol diets accelerate tumor growth and metastasis. *Nutr Cancer* **59**: 207–16.

Kollmar O, Junker B, Rupertus K, Scheuer C, Menger MD, Schilling MK (2008). Liver resection-associated macrophage inflammatory protein-2 stimulates engraftment but not growth of colorectal metastasis at extrahepatic sites. *J Surg Res* **145**: 295–302.

Kollmar O, Scheuer C, Menger MD, Schilling MK (2006). Macrophage inflammatory protein-2 promotes angiogenesis, cell migration, and tumor growth in hepatic metastasis. *Ann Surg Oncol* **13**: 263–75.

Koppe MJ, Boerman OC, Oyen WJG, Bleichrodt RP (2006). Peritoneal carcinomatosis of colorectal origin. *Ann Surg* **243**: 212–22.

Kuhry E, Schwenk W, Gaupset R, Romild U, Bonjer HJ (2008). Long-term outcome of laparoscopic surgery for colorectal cancer: a cochrane systematic review of randomised controlled trials. *Cancer Treat Rev* **34**: 498–504.

Kumagai K, Kiyosawa N, Ito K, Yamoto T, Teranishi M, Nakayama H, Manabe S (2007). Influence of Kupffer cell inactivation on cycloheximide-induced hepatic injury. *Toxicology* **241**: 106–18.

Lacy AM, García-Valdecasas JC, Delgado S, Castells A, Taurá P, Piqué JM, Visa J (2002). Laparoscopy-assisted colectomy versus open colectomy for treatment of non-metastatic colon cancer: a randomised trial. *Lancet* **359**: 2224–29.

Lee JY, Sohn KH, Rhee SH, Hwang D (2001). Saturated fatty acids, but not unsaturated fatty acids, induce the expression of cyclooxygenase-2 mediated through Toll-like receptor 4. *J Biol Chem* **276**: 16683–89.

Liang P, Hong JW, Ubukata H, Liu HR, Watanabe Y, Katano M (2006). Increased density and diameter of lymphatic microvessels correlate with lymph node metastasis in early stage invasive colorectal carcinoma. *Virchows Arch* **448**: 570–75.

Liang F, Liang J, Wang WQ, Sun JP, Udho E, Zhang ZY (2007). PRL3 promotes cell invasion and proliferation by down-regulation of Csk leading to Src activation. *J Biol Chem* **282**: 5413–19.

Longatto-Filho A, Pinheiro C, Ferreira L, Scapulatempo C, Alves VA, Baltazar F, Schmitt F (2008). Peritumoural, but not intratumoural, lymphatic vessel density and invasion correlate with colorectal carcinoma poor-outcome markers. *Virchows Arch* **452**: 133–38.

Martínez ME (2005). Primary prevention of colorectal cancer: lifestyle, nutrition, exercise. *Recent Results Cancer Res* **166**: 177–211.

Mels AK, Statius Muller MG, van Leeuwen PA, von Blomberg BM, Scheper RJ, Cuesta MA et al. (2001). Immune-stimulating effects of low-dose perioperative recombinant granulocyte-macrophage colony-stimulating factor in patients operated on for primary colorectal carcinoma. *Br J Surg* **88**: 539–44.

Meng S, Tripathy D, Frenkel EP, Shete S, Naftalis EZ, Huth JF et al. (2004). Circulating tumor cells in patients with breast cancer dormancy. *Clin Cancer Res* **10**: 8152–62.

Meyerhardt JA, Heseltine D, Niedzwiecki D, Hollis D, Saltz LB, Mayer RJ et al. (2006). Impact of physical activity on cancer recurrence and survival in patients with stage III colon cancer: findings from CALGB 89803. *J Clin Oncol* **24**: 3535–41.

Meyerhardt JA, Niedzwiecki D, Hollis D, Saltz LB, Hu FB, Mayer RJ et al. (2007). Association of dietary patterns with cancer recurrence and survival in patients with stage III colon cancer. *J Am Med Assoc* **298**: 754–64.

Meyerhardt JA, Niedzwiecki D, Hollis D, Saltz LB, Mayer RJ, Nelson H et al. (2008). Impact of body mass index and weight change after treatment on cancer recurrence and survival in patients with stage III colon cancer: findings from Cancer and Leukemia Group B 89803. *J Clin Oncol* **26**: 4109–15.

Mongan JP, Fadul CE, Cole BF, Zaki BI, Suriawinata AA, Ripple GH et al. (2009). Brain metastases from colorectal cancer: risk factors, incidence and the possible role of chemokines. *Clin Colorectal Cancer* **8**: 100–05.

Mousseau DD, Butterworth RF (1994). Current theories on the pathogenesis of hepatic encephalopathy. *Proc Soc Exp Biol Med* **206**: 329–44.

Mueller BM, Reisfeld RA, Edgington TS, Ruf W (1992). Expression of tissue factor by melanoma cells promotes efficient hematogenous metastasis. *Proc Natl Acad Sci USA* **89**: 11832–36.

Mutter D, Hajri A, Tassetti V, Solis-Caxaj C, Aprahamian M, Marescaux J (1999). Increased tumor growth and spread after laparoscopy vs laparotomy: influence of tumor manipulation in a rat model. *Surg Endosc* **13**: 365–70.

Müller A, Homey B, Soto H, Ge N, Catron D, Buchanan ME et al. (2001). Involvement of chemokine receptors in breast cancer metastasis. *Nature* **410**: 50–56.

Naito M, Hasegawa G, Ebe Y, Yammoto T (2004). Differentiation and function of Kupffer cells. *Med Electron Microsc* **37**: 16–28.

Nakagawa H, Liyanarachchic S, Davuluri RV, Auer H, Martin EW Jr, de la Chapelle A, Frankel WL (2004). Role of cancer-associated stromal fibroblasts in metastatic colon cancer to the liver and their expression profiles. *Oncogene* **23**: 7366–77.

Nguyen DX, Massague J (2007). Genetic determinants of cancer metastasis. *Nature Rev Genet* **8**: 341–52.

Omachi T, Kawai Y, Mizuno R, Nomiyama T, Miyagawa S, Ohhashi T, Nakayama J (2007). Immunohistochemical demonstration of proliferating lymphatic vessels in colorectal carcinoma and its clinico-pathological significance. *Cancer Lett* **246**: 167–72.

Onogawa S, Kitadai Y, Tanaka S, Kuwai T, Kimura S, Chayama K (2004). Expression of VEGF-C and VEGF-D at the invasive edge correlates with lymph node metastasis and prognosis of patients with colorectal carcinoma. *Cancer Sci* **95**: 32–39.

Ott I, Fischer E, Miyagi Y, Mueller BM, Ruf W (1998). A role for tissue factor in cell adhesion and migration mediated by interaction with actin-binding protein 280. *J Cell Biol* **140**: 1241–53.

Paget S (1889). The distribution of secondary growths in cancer of the breast. *Lancet* **1**: 571–73.

Palumbo JS, Talmage KE, Massari JV, La Jeunesse CM, Flick MJ, Kombrinck KW et al. (2005). Platelets and fibrin(ogen) increase metastatic potential by impeding natural killer cell-mediated elimination of tumor cells. *Blood* **105**: 178–85.

Palumbo JS, Talmage KE, Massari JV, La Jeunesse CM, Flick MJ, Kombrinck KW et al. (2007). Tumor cell-associated tissue factor and circulating hemostatic factors cooperate to increase metastatic potential through natural killer cell-dependent and –independent mechanisms. *Blood* **110**: 133–41.

Park HY, Kwon HM, Lim HJ, Hong BK, Lee JY, Park BE et al. (2001). Potential role of leptin in angiogenesis: leptin induces endothelial cell proliferation and expression of matrix metalloproteinases in vivo and in vitro. *Exp Mol Med* **33**: 95–102.

Parker C, Roseman BJ, Bucana CD, Tsan R, Radinsky R (1998). Preferential activation of the epidermal growth factor receptor in human colon carcinoma liver metastases in nude mice. *J Histochem Cytochem* **46**: 595–602.

Patel H, Le Marer N, Wharton RQ, Khan ZA, Araia R, Glover C et al. (2002). Clearance of circulating tumor cells after excision of primary colorectal cancer. *Ann Surg* **235**: 226–31.

Pierce A, Lyron M, Hampson IN, Cowling GJ, Gallagher JT (1992). Molecular cloning of the major cell surface heparan sulfate proteoglycan from rat liver. *J Biol Chem* **267**: 3894–900.

Raa ST, Oosterling SJ, van der Kaaij NP, van den Tol MP, Beelen RH, Meijer S et al. (2005). Surgery promotes implantation of disseminated tumor cells, but does not increase growth of tumor cell clusters. *J Surg Oncol* **92**: 124–29.

Radinsky R, Risin S, Fan D, Dong Z, Bielenberg D, Bucana CD, Fidler IJ (1995). Level and function of epidermal growth factor receptor predict the metastatic potential of human colon carcinoma cells. *Clin Cancer Res* **1**: 19–31.

Ribic CM, Sargent DJ, Moore MJ, Thibodeau SN, French AJ, Goldberg RM et al. (2003). Tumor microsatellite-instability status as a predictor of benefit from fluorouracil-based adjuvant chemotherapy for colon cancer. *N Engl J Med* **349**: 247–57.

Rodgers MS, Collinson R, Desai S, Stubbs RS, McCall JL (2003). Risk of dissemination with biopsy of colorectal liver metastases. *Dis Colon Rectum* **46**: 454–58.

Roth ES, Fetzer DT, Barron BJ, Joseph UA, Gayed IW, Wan DQ (2009). Does colon cancer ever metastasize to bone first? A temporal analysis of colorectal cancer progression. *BMC Cancer* **9**: 274.

Rubie C, Oliveira V, Kempf K, Wagner M, Tilton B, Rau B et al. (2006). Involvement of chemokine receptor CCR6 in colorectal cancer metastasis. *Tumor Biol* **27**: 166–74.

Sadeghi B, Arvieux C, Glehen O, Beaujard AC, Rivoire M, Baulieux J et al. (2000). Peritoneal carcinomatosis from non-gynecologic malignancies. *Cancer* **88**: 358–63.

Saha S, Bardelli A, Buckhaults P, Velculescu VE, Rago C, St Croix B et al. (2001). A phosphatase associated with metastasis of colorectal cancer. *Science* **294**: 1343–46.

Saharinen P, Tammela T, Karkkainen MJ, Alitalo K (2004). Lymphatic vasculature: development, molecular regulation and role in tumor metastasis and inflammation. *Trends Immunol* **25**: 387–95.

Sastre J, Maestro ML, Puente J, Veganzones S, Alfonso R, Rafael S et al. (2008). Circulating tumor cells in colorectal cancer: correlation with clinical and pathological variables. *Ann Oncol* **19**: 935–38.

Scartozzi M, Bearzi I, Berardi R, Mandolesi A, Fabris G, Cascinu S (2004). Epidermal growth factor receptor (EGFR) status in primary colorectal tumors does not correlate with EGFR expression in related metastatic sites: implications for treatment with EGFR-targeted antibodies. *J Clin Oncol* **22**: 4772–78.

Schimanski CC, Schwald S, Simiantonaki N (2005). Effect of chemokine receptors CXCR4 and CCR7 on the metastatic behavior of human colorectal cancer. *Clin Cancer Res* **11**: 1743–50.

Schoppmeyer K, Frühauf N, Oldhafer K, Seeber S, Kasimir-Bauer S (2006). Tumor cell dissemination in colon cancer does not predict extrahepatic recurrence in patients undergoing surgery for hepatic metastases. *Oncol Rep* **15**: 449–54.

Schott A, Vogel I, Krueger U, Kalthoff H, Schreiber HW, Schmiegel W et al. (1998). Isolated tumor cells are frequently detectable in the peritoneal cavity of gastric and colorectal cancer patients and serve as a new prognostic marker. *Ann Surg* **227**: 372–79.

Schutyser E, Struyf S, Van Damme J (2003). The CC chemokine CCL20 and its receptor CCR6. *Cytokine Growth Factor Rev* **14**: 409–26.

Seto S, Onodera H, Kaido T, Yoshikawa A, Ishigami S, Arii S, Imamura M (2000). Tissue factor expression in human colorectal carcinoma: correlation with hepatic metastasis and impact on prognosis. *Cancer* **88**: 295–301.

Shi H, Kokoeva MV, Inouye K, Tzameli I, Yin H, Flier JS (2006). TLR4 links innate immunity and fatty acid-induced insulin resistance. *J Clin Invest* **116**: 3015–25.

Sleeman JP (2000). The lymph node as a bridgehead in the metastatic dissemination of tumors. *Recent Results Cancer Res* **157**: 55–81.

Slooter GD, Marquet RL, Jeekel J, Ijzermans JN (1995). Tumour growth stimulation after partial hepatectomy can be reduced by treatment with tumour necrosis factor alpha. *Br J Surg* **82**: 129–32.

Smyrk TC, Watson P, Kaul K, Lynch HT (2001). Tumor-infiltrating lymphocytes are a marker for microsatellite instability in colorectal carcinoma. *Cancer* **91**: 2417–22.

Snook AE, Li P, Stafford BJ (2009). Lineage-specific T-cell responses to cancer mucosa antigen oppose systemic metastases without inflammatory disease. *Cancer Res* **69**: 3537–44.

Sugarbaker PH (1996). Observations concerning cancer spread within the peritoneal cavity and concepts supporting an ordered pathophysiology. *Cancer Treat Res* **82**: 79–100.

Sundermeyer ML, Merepol NJ, Rogatko A, Wang H, Cohen SJ (2005). Changing patterns of bone and brain metastases in patients with colorectal cancer. *Clin Colorectal Cancer* **5**: 108–13.

Thalheimer A, Otto C, Bueter M, Illert B, Gattenlohner S, Gasser M et al. (2009). The intraportal injection model: a practical animal model for hepatic metastases and tumor cell dissemination in human colon cancer. *BMC Cancer* **9**: 29.

Timmers M, Vekemans K, Vermijlen D, Asosingh K, Kuppen P, Bouwens L et al. (2004). Interactions between rat colon carcinoma cells and Kupffer cells during the onset of hepatic metastasis. *Int J Cancer* **112**: 793–802.

van der Bilt JD, Kranenburg O, Borren A, van Hillegersberg R, Borel Rinkes IH (2008). Ageing and hepatic steatosis exacerbate ischemia/reperfusion-accelerated outgrowth of colorectal micrometastases. *Ann Surg Oncol* **15**: 1392–98.

van der Bij GJ, Oosterling SJ, Bögels M, Bhoelan F, Fluitsma DM, Beelen RH et al. (2008). Blocking α2 integrins on rat CC531 s colon carcinoma cells prevents operation-induced augmentation of liver metastases outgrowth. *Hepatology* **47**: 532–43.

van der Bilt JD, Soeters ME, Duyverman AM, Nijkamp MW, Witteveen PO, van Diest PJ et al. (2007). Perinecrotic hypoxia contributes to ischemia/reperfusion-accelerated outgrowth of colorectal micrometastases. *Am J Pathol* **170**: 1379–88.

Van Roey G, Moore K (1996). The hepatorenal syndrome. *Pediatr Nephrol* **10**: 100–07.

VanSaun MN, Lee IK, Washington MK, Matrisian L, Gorden DL (2009). High fat diet induced hepatic steatosis establishes a permissive microenvironment for colorectal metastases and promotes primary dysplasia in a murine model. *Am J Pathol* **175**: 355–64.

van Schaik PM, Hermans E, van der Linden JC, Pruijt JRM, Ernst MF, Bosscha K (2009). Micro-metastases in stages I and II colon cancer are a predictor of the development of distant metastases and worse disease-free survival. *Eur J Surg Oncol* **35**: 492–96.

Varona R, Cadenas V, Gómez L, Martínez-A C, Márquez G (2005). CCR6 regulates CD4+ T-cell-mediated acute graft-versus-host disease responses. *Blood* **106**: 18–26.

Vekemans K, Braet F (2005). Structural and functional aspects of the liver and liver sinusoidal cells in relation to colon carcinoma metastasis. *World J Gastroenterol* **11**: 5095–102.

Vekemans K, Braet F, Wisse E (2004). DiO-labeled CC351 s colon carcinoma cells traverse the hepatic sinusoidal endothelium via the Fas/FasL pathway. *J Gastrointest Surg* **8**: 371–72, author reply 372.

Versteeg HH, Spek CA, Peppelenbosch MP, Richel DJ (2004a). Tissue factor and cancer metastasis: the role of intracellular and extracellular signaling pathways. *Mol Med* **10**: 6–11.

Versteeg HH, Spek CA, Richel DJ, Peppelenbosch MP (2004b). Coagulation factors VIIa and Xa inhibit apoptosis and anoikis. *Oncogene* **23**: 410–17.

Weitz J, Kienle P, Magener A, Koch M, Schrödel A, Willeke F et al. (1999). Detection of disseminated colorectal cancer cells in lymph nodes, blood and bone marrow. *Clin Cancer Res* **5**: 1830–36.

Williams IR (2006). CCR6 and CCL20: partners in intestinal immunity and lymphorganogenesis. *Ann NY Acad Sci* **1072**: 52–61.

Wisse E, Luo D, Vermijlen D, Kanellopoulou C, De Zanger R, Braet F (1997). On the function of pit cells, the liver-specific natural killer cells. *Semin Liver Dis* **17**: 265–86.

Wolmark N, Yothers G, O'Connell JO, Sharif S, Atkins JN, Seay TE et al. (2009). A phase III trial comparing mFOLFOX6 to mFOLFOX6 plus bevacizumab in stage II or III carcinoma of the colon: results of NSABP protocol C-08. *J Clin Oncol* **27**: 18 s.

Wu W, Yamaura T, Murakami K, Murata J, Matsumoto K, Watanabe H, Saiki I (2000). Social isolation stress enhanced liver metastasis of murine colon 26-L5 carcinoma cells by suppressing immune response in mice. *Life Sci* **66**: 1827–38.

Yamamo Y, Takahashi K, Yasuno M, Sakoma T, Mori T (1998). Clinicopathological characteristics of skipping lymph node metastases in patients with colorectal cancer. *Jap J Clin Oncol* **28**: 6378–82.

Yamamoto M, Kikuchi H, Ohta M, Kawabata T, Hiramatsu Y, Kondo K et al. (2008). TSU68 prevents liver metastasis of colon cancer xenografts by modulating the premetastatic niche. *Cancer Res* **68**: 9754–62.

Yang CC, Ogawa H, Dwinell MB, McCole DF, Eckmann L, Kagnoff MF (2005). Chemokine receptor CCR6 transduces signals that activate p130 Cas and alter cAMP-stimulated ion transport in human intestinal epithelial cells. *Am J Physiol Cell Physiol* **288**: C321–C28.

Yang GY, Xu KS, Pan ZQ, Zhang ZY, Mi YT, Wang JS et al. (2008). Integrin alpha v beta 6 mediates the potential for colon cancer cells to colonize in and metastasize to the liver. *Cancer Sci* **99**: 879–87.

Zvibel I, Brill S, Halpern Z, Papa M (1998). Hepatocyte extracellular matrix modulates expression of growth factors and growth factors receptors in human colon cancer cells. *Exp Cell Res* **245**: 123–31.

Chapter 3

THE GENETICS OF COLORECTAL CANCER

Andrew M. Kaz[1] and William M. Grady[2]
[1] Fred Hutchinson Cancer Research Center, Seattle, WA, USA
[2] Fred Hutchinson Cancer Research Center, Seattle, WA, USA
e-mail: wgrady@fhcrc.org

Abstract: Colorectal cancer arises as the result of the accumulation of genetic alterations (including gene mutations and amplification) and epigenetic modifications (such as aberrant DNA methylation and chromatin modifications) that transform normal colonic epithelial cells into adenocarcinoma cells. Loss of genomic stability and the resulting genetic changes appears to be a crucial molecular and pathogenic step that occurs early in the tumourigenic process and permits a sufficient number of alterations in tumour suppressor genes and oncogenes to accumulate in a clone of cells to result in their eventual transformation into cancer. Substantial progress has been made recently concerning potential causes of chromosomal instability in colorectal cancer and in determining the effects of the various forms of genomic instability on the biological and clinical behavior of colon tumours. Furthermore, progress has been made in terms of understanding the specific signalling pathways that are frequently deregulated in colorectal cancers. Although the discovery of genes involved in colorectal cancer metastasis remains a challenge, advancements in our understanding of the molecular genetics of this process have occurred, both with traditional familial/linkage studies and also utilizing state-of-the-art genome-wide searches. The evaluation of the cause and role of the genetic events involved in colorectal cancer formation has the potential to yield more effective prevention and treatment strategies for this disease.

Key words: Mutations · Genetics · Tumour suppressor genes · Oncogenes · Signalling pathways · Gene

3.1 Introduction

Colorectal cancer develops due to the progressive accumulation of genetic and epigenetic alterations that lead to the transformation of normal colorectal epithelium to colorectal adenocarcinoma. The loss of genomic stability is a critical molecular and pathophysiologic step in this process and serves to create a permissive environment for mutations in tumour suppressor genes and oncogenes. Alterations in these genes, which include *APC, CTNNB1, KRAS, BRAF, SMAD4, TP53, PIK3CA,* and *TGFBR2,* appear to promote colorectal tumourigenesis by perturbing signalling pathways, including the wingless/Wnt (WNT), phosphatidyl inositol 3 kinase (PI3K) and transforming growth factor β (TGF-β) signalling pathways, or by affecting genes that regulate central behaviors of cells such as DNA repair, proliferation, etc.

The process of colorectal carcinogenesis usually follows a succession of histologic changes called the adenoma-to-carcinoma sequence. The steps in this pathway are believed to unfold over a 10- to 15-year period and involve simultaneous histological and molecular changes. The ultimate consequence of these genetic alterations on the cell is the acquisition of key biological characteristics that are central to the malignant phenotype, including insensitivity to anti-growth signals, the ability to evade apoptosis, limitless replicative potential, and the ability to invade and metastasize (Hanahan and Weinberg, 2000). Previous analyses of the molecular genetics of colorectal cancer have made it clear that its development is a multi-step process that is characterized by genomic instability, i.e. the loss of the cell's ability to maintain its wild-type DNA coding sequence through the repair of DNA mutations, and epigenetic instability, which is the focus of Chapter 4 by Carmona and Esteller in this book. In a background of genomic and epigenetic instability, genetic and epigenetic alterations accumulate and collaborate to drive the initiation and progression of colorectal cancer (Fearon and Vogelstein, 1990; Kinzler and Vogelstein, 1996; Lengauer et al., 1998).

Colorectal neoplasms appear to be most frequently initiated by alterations that affect the Wingless/Wnt signalling pathway. The newly initiated neoplasm then progresses as the result of the accumulation of sequential genetic or epigenetic events that either activate oncogenes or inactivate tumour suppressor genes that are involved in other signalling pathways, including the RAS-RAF-mitogen-activated protein kinase (MAPK) pathway, TGF-β pathway, and the PI3K-v-akt murine thymoma viral oncogene homolog (AKT) pathway (Bardelli et al., 2003; Parsons et al., 2005). The identification of these abnormalities has provided potential targets for the development of new therapies for the prevention and/or treatment of colorectal tumours throughout their progression from normal epithelium to adenocarcinoma.

3.2 The Adenoma-to-Carcinoma Sequence

The evolution of normal epithelial cells to adenocarcinoma by and large follows a predictable progression of histological and concurrent genetic changes (Fig. 3.1). These genetic mutations provide cells with a growth advantage and lead to the clonal

3 The Genetics of Colorectal Cancer

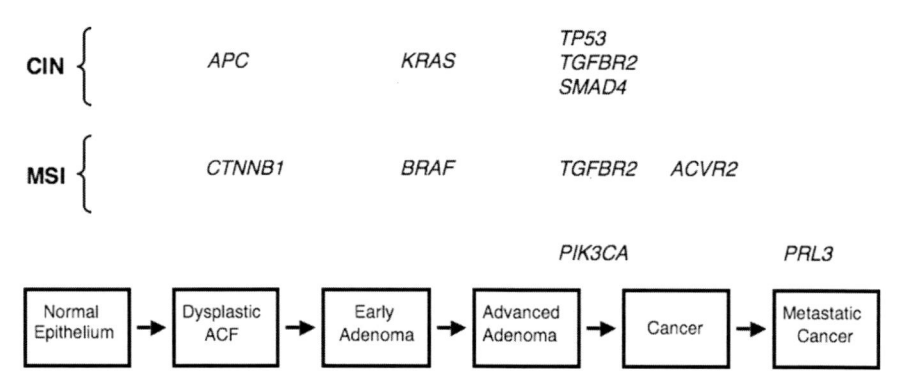

```
         APC            KRAS         TP53
CIN {                                TGFBR2
                                     SMAD4

         CTNNB1         BRAF         TGFBR2    ACVR2
MSI {
                                     PIK3CA              PRL3
```

Normal Epithelium → Dysplastic ACF → Early Adenoma → Advanced Adenoma → Cancer → Metastatic Cancer

Fig. 3.1 Schematic diagram of the adenoma-to-carcinoma progression sequence. Each histological step in the process is depicted as a *box*. Above the histologic sequence is a list of the genes that are commonly altered at that step in the progression sequence in the setting of two recognized forms of genomic instability that occur in colorectal cancer, chromosomal instability (CIN) and microsatellite instability (MSI). The genes are listed above the histologic steps in which they presumably occur during the adenoma-to-cancer sequence

expansion of the altered cells. Until recently, it was believed that only conventional tubular and tubulovillous adenomatous polyps had the potential to undergo malignant transformation; however, it now also appears that some colorectal cancers can evolve from a subset of polyps called sessile serrated adenomas, which arise in unique molecular as well as histologic events (Goldstein, 2006; Jass, 2004). These serrated adenomas appear to have the potential to transform into adenocarcinomas through a hyperplastic polyp → serrated adenoma → adenocarcinoma progression sequence (Goldstein, 2006; Kambara et al., 2004). Serrated polyps that arise in the right colon commonly display a form of genomic instability termed microsatellite instability as well as epigenetic instability characterized by aberrant cytosine-phosphate-guanine (CpG) island DNA methylation, whereas those that arise in the left colon are typically microsatellite stable and frequently carry mutations in *KRAS* (Jass, 2004; Noffsinger, 2009).

3.3 Mechanisms of Genomic Instability

3.3.1 Overview

Genomic instability, which is the loss of the ability of the cell to maintain the fidelity of its DNA, is a fundamental aspect of colorectal tumourigenesis (Little et al., 2008). At least three forms of genomic instability have been identified in colorectal cancer: (1) microsatellite instability (MSI), (2) chromosome instability (i.e. aneusomy, gains and losses of chromosomal regions) (CIN), and (3) chromosomal translocations (Grady, 2004). The etiology of CIN has been identified in only a small subset of colorectal cancers. In contrast, MSI is known to result from inactivating mutations or from the aberrant methylation of genes in the DNA Mismatch Repair (MMR) family, which repairs DNA base-pair mismatches that arise during DNA replication. The timing of the loss of genomic stability, either chromosomal instability (CIN) or microsatellite instability (MSI), during the initiation and progression of colorectal cancer appears to be after adenoma formation, but before progression to frank malignancy. In fact, both CIN and MSI can be detected in colorectal adenomas (Aaltonen et al., 1994; Bomme et al., 1998; Grady et al., 1998; Jacoby et al., 1995; Rooney et al., 1999; Shih et al., 2001; Wong et al., 1999). Despite the accumulation of data demonstrating the presence of genomic instability in early colorectal tumours, the causative role of genomic instability in cancer remains a source of considerable controversy (Grady, 2004; Lengauer et al., 1998). Nonetheless, genomic instability provides an attractive target for anti-cancer therapies because it is nearly ubiquitous in colorectal cancer and is a unique characteristic of cancer cells that is absent in normal epithelial cells (Goel et al., 2007; Ostwald et al., 2009). The feasibility of targeting genomic instability for anti-cancer treatments has been shown using in vitro systems (Chen et al., 2000).

3.3.2 Chromosome Instability

Chromosomal instability is the most common type of genomic instability observed in colorectal cancer, occurring in approximately 85% of colorectal tumours. However, despite the high frequency of CIN in colorectal cancer and the fact that aneuploidy has long been appreciated as a hallmark of cancer our understanding of the mechanisms of CIN is still rudimentary. It is open to debate whether aneuploidy is simply a condition that occurs non-specifically during tumour formation, which tumour cells can tolerate because of independence from the normal mechanisms that control cell growth and death, or whether it represents an active process of chromosomal instability that is itself an important element in a tumour's development. The recognition that colorectal cancers display recurrent and tumour-specific chromosome abnormalities implies that this process is not random or merely accessory, but more likely that chromosomal instability plays a direct role in tumour progression by increasing clonal diversity (Grady, 2004; Hermsen et al., 2002; Maley et al., 2006).

A significant challenge in understanding chromosomal instability relates to the complexity of the mechanisms that regulate and maintain CIN. In *Saccharomyces cerevisiae*, more than 100 genes have been shown to cause a CIN phenotype when mutated (Jin et al., 1998; Kolodner et al., 2002). These genes regulate a variety of cellular processes, including chromosome condensation, sister-chromatid cohesion, kinetochore structure and function, microtubule formation, and cell-cycle checkpoint regulation. Yet, despite this complexity, progress has been made in identifying a genetic etiology for aneuploidy and presumably CIN in a subset of colorectal cancers. Over the past decade, mutations or amplification of genes known to cause experimental forms of CIN have been identified in cancer, including *BUB1, ATM, ATR, BRCA1, BRCA2, STK15, PLK1,* and *CDC4* (Bischoff et al., 1998; Cahill et al.,

1998; Rajagopalan et al., 2002; Rotman and Shiloh, 1998; Smith et al., 1998; Zhang et al., 1998; Zhou et al., 1998). Using a broader methodology, Wang et al. employed computational analyses to identify over 1,000 possible genes that could lead to genomic instability based on their homology to genes in yeast and *Drosophila melanogaster*. This group identified somatic mutations in a subset of these genes in cancers, but the role of these genes in causing CIN has not yet been determined (Wang et al., 2004b). In another comprehensive approach, Barber et al. screened 102 human homologues of 96 yeast CIN genes and identified mutations in five genes, most of which regulate sister chromatid cohesion. Functional analysis of these mutations revealed they could lead to chromosomal instability. The most notable genes identified were *murein formation gene cluster E 11* (*MRE11*) and cell division cycle 4 (*CDC4*), which have been shown in independent studies to regulate genomic instability, as noted below (Barber et al., 2008).

Some potential candidate genes that mediate CIN have been confirmed in multiple subsets of colorectal cancers. For example, somatic mutations in *hCDC4*, also known as *F-box/WD repeat-containing protein 7* (*Fbw7*) or *Archipelago*, were found in 11.5% of human colorectal cancers (N=22/190) and in 6.9% of colon adenomas (Rajagopalan et al., 2004). CDC4 is an evolutionarily conserved E3 ubiquitin ligase that regulates the G1→S checkpoint. The functional consequence of *CDC4* inactivation was demonstrated by disrupting both alleles through homologous recombination in the karyotypically stable colorectal cancer cell lines HCT116 and DLD1. This resulted in nuclear atypia, an increased frequency of multipolar spindles, and chromosome instability. Notably, this effect was dependent on an increase in cyclin E, which is a substrate of CDC4 (Rajagopalan et al., 2004; Rajagopalan and Lengauer, 2004). Others have shown that the inhibition of cyclin E degradation in mice leads to tumours that display genomic instability, and that Fbxw7/hCDC4 cooperates with p53 to suppress tumour formation (Loeb et al., 2005; Perez-Losada et al., 2005). It appears that Cdc4 is regulated by p53 and is one of the downstream effectors of p53-mediated regulation of genomic stability, particularly in the setting of genomic stress. Notably, Cdc4 may affect genomic stability not only through its regulation of cyclin E, but also via Notch and/or Jun (Perez-Losada et al., 2005). Together, these data support the concept of a genetic basis for CIN and the premise that deregulation of mechanisms that mediate DNA integrity lead to an assortment of outcomes that ultimately induce CIN.

3.3.3 DNA Mismatch Repair Inactivation and Microsatellite Instability

Genomic instability results from the inactivation or inhibition of the normal cellular mechanisms used to maintain DNA fidelity. Defects in two of these mechanisms, the Mismatch Repair (MMR) and Base Excision Repair (BER) systems, have been identified in independent subsets of colorectal cancer. The MMR system consists of a complex of proteins that attaches to double-stranded DNA and recognizes and repairs base pair mismatches that occur during DNA replication

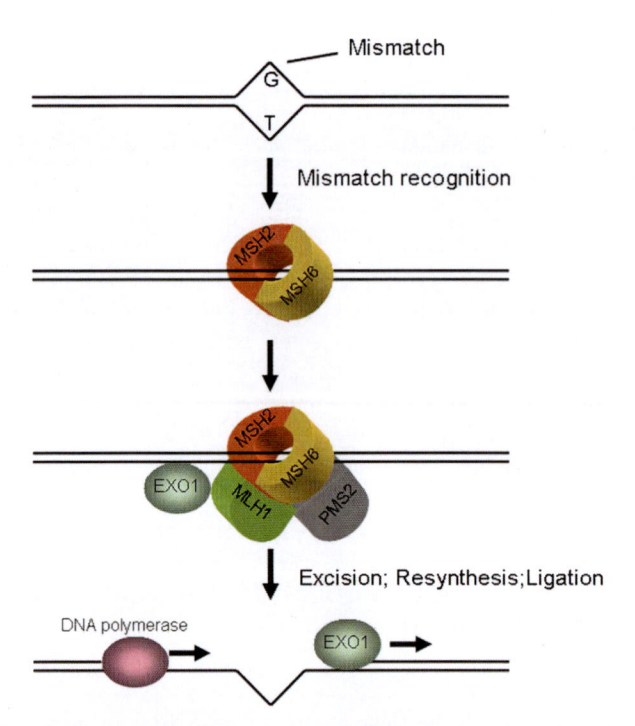

Fig. 3.2 **Depiction of the mismatch repair (MMR) system**, which plays an important role in recognizing and repairing DNA mismatches that occur during DNA replication, homologous recombination, and various forms of DNA damage. MSH (MutS homologues) proteins form heterodimers with each other to perform specific MMR functions. For example, MSH2-MSH6 heterodimers (shown in figure) bind to single base-pair mismatches. Following the recognition of the sequence error, another heterodimer such as MLH1-PMS2 (MutL homologue 1 and post-meiotic segregation 2) along with the EXO1 exonuclease are recruited to the complex to complete the repair of the DNA. Ultimately, the mismatch is digested by EXO1 and the gap filled in by DNA polymerases

(Fig. 3.2). Inactivation of the MMR system occurs in 1–2% of colorectal cancers due to germline mutations in MMR system genes, including *mutL homolog 1*, (*MLH1*), *mutS homolog 2/6* (*MSH2* and *MSH6*), and *postmeiotic segregation increased 2* (*PMS2*), and is the etiology of the colorectal cancer family syndrome Lynch Syndrome (also known as Hereditary Nonpolyposis Colon Cancer; HNPCC) (Hampel et al., 2005; Lynch and de la Chapelle, 1999). In addition to Lynch Syndrome-related colon cancers, 15% of sporadic colorectal cancers have an inactivated MMR system due to the aberrant methylation of the *MLH1* gene promoter (Kane et al., 1997).

Microsatellite instability (MSI) occurs as a consequence of MMR inactivation and is recognized by frameshift mutations in microsatellite repeats located throughout the genome. Since many colorectal cancers demonstrate frameshift mutations at a small percentage of microsatellite repeats, the designation of a colorectal adenocarcinoma as 'microsatellite unstable' depends on the detection of greater than 30%

unstable loci from a panel of 5–10 loci previously selected at a National Cancer Institute consensus conference (Boland et al., 1998).

A thorough investigation of the MMR proteins has revealed that recognition of the base-base mismatches and insertion/deletion loops is performed by a heterodimer of either MSH2 and MSH6 or MSH2 and MSH3. Of interest, the MSH2-MSH3 heterodimer preferentially recognizes insertion/deletion loops and thus cannot compensate for loss of MSH6. Consequently, cancers arising due to a loss of MSH6 function display microsatellite instability predominantly in mononucleotide repeats and may exhibit an attenuated form of MSI called 'MSI-low'. MSI-low cancers are recognized clinically as possessing 10–29% unstable loci in the NCI consensus panel noted above (Jiricny, 1998). The MLH1, PMS1, and PMS2 proteins appear to operate primarily by repairing the base-base mismatches and insertion/deletion loops. A heterodimer of MLH1-PMS2 operates as a 'molecular matchmaker' and is involved in repairing mismatches in conjunction with DNA-polymerase ∂, and the replication factors proliferating cell nuclear antigen (PCNA), replication protein A (RPA), and replication factor C (RFC) as well as the $5' \rightarrow 3'$ exo/endonucleases EXO1 and FEN1 and other unidentified $3' \rightarrow 5'$ exonucleases and helicases (Jiricny, 1998; Kolodner et al., 1999).

The microsatellite instability that results from loss of MMR activity predominantly affects mono-, di-, and tri-nucleotide tracts. However, cell lines derived from these tumours also demonstrate up to a 1,000-fold increased mutation rate at expressed gene sequences, particularly at short sequence repeats (Eshleman et al., 1995). Genes that possess such 'microsatellite-like' repeats in their coding regions appear to be the targets relevant to carcinogenesis. This pathway to tumour formation appears to be distinct from that seen in colorectal cancers that are microsatellite stable (MSS) (Yamamoto et al., 1998). This pathway more commonly involves genes such as the TGF-β receptor type II tumour suppressor (*TGFBR2*), the activin receptor type II (*ACVR2*), and Bcl-2–associated X protein (*BAX*) than does the MSS pathway (Hempen et al., 2003; Markowitz et al., 1995). Importantly, MSI and the subsequent target gene mutations appear to occur throughout the adenoma-to-carcinoma progression at distinct phases of tumour progression (Grady et al., 1998). Overall, MSI appears to permit the accumulation of mutations in vulnerable genes that promote tumourigenesis, and these mutations ultimately contribute to the generation of colorectal cancer.

The relationship between the MSI pathway and other genetic pathways found in colorectal cancer is incompletely understood. One notable association is between mutant *V-raf murine sarcoma viral oncogene homolog B1* (*BRAF*) and sporadic MSI colorectal cancer (Deng et al., 2004). *BRAF* (*V600E*) mutations associate with sporadic MSI tumours that carry aberrantly methylated *MLH1*, but not MSI colorectal cancers arising in the setting of the Lynch Syndrome (Deng et al., 2004; Domingo et al., 2004). Alterations in the Wnt/Wingless pathway can be observed in tumours irrespective of MSI status (Huang et al., 1996). Mutations in adenomatous polyposis coli (*APC*) and β-catenin encoding gene (*CTNNB1*) can be found in 21 and 43% of MSI tumours, respectively (Konishi et al., 1996; Miyaki et al., 1999). In addition, the incidence of *KRAS* mutations appears to be as high as 22–31% in

MSI tumours, which is similar to the incidence observed in MSS colorectal cancers (Fujiwara et al., 1998; Olschwang et al., 1993). Mutations in tumor protein 53 (*TP53*) are less frequent in MSI cancers than in MSS cancers. The *TP53* mutation incidence in MSI colorectal cancers ranges between 0 and 40%, whereas the incidence in MSS tumours is between 31 and 67% (Eshleman et al., 1998; Fujiwara et al., 1998; Konishi et al., 1996; Olschwang et al., 1997). Of interest, monoallelic and biallelic *BAX* mutations and the aberrant methylation of *p14*^{ARF} are found frequently in MSI colorectal cancers and may serve to replace the role of mutant *TP53* in colorectal carcinogenesis (Mori et al., 2001; Shen et al., 2003). Thus, the microsatellite-mutator pathway appears to be initiated through changes in the Wnt/Wingless pathway and shares some alterations with the MSS colorectal cancer pathway. However, other events, such as mutations in *TP53* and *TGFBR2*, occur at different frequencies in the MSI versus the MSS pathway.

The impact of microsatellite instability on the clinical behaviour of colorectal cancers has been intensely investigated to date, but it is still unclear whether this molecular feature can be used to more accurately predict the behaviour of colorectal cancers. Several retrospective studies have shown mixed results regarding the effect of MSI on prognosis. Watanabe et al. found that in stage III colorectal cancer (CRC) patients, 18q LOH correlated with a reduction in 5-year survival from 74 to 50%. They also demonstrated that *TGFBR2 BAT-RII* mutations correlated with improved 5-year survival in tumours with MSI versus those without this mutation, from 74 to 46% respectively (Watanabe et al., 2001). In addition, a systematic review of MSI in colorectal cancer revealed a combined hazard ratio (HR) estimate for overall survival associated with MSI of 0.65 (95% CI, 0.59–0.71) (Popat et al., 2005).

3.3.4 Base Excision Repair Defects/MYH

Inactivation of a second 'DNA caretaker' mechanism, the Base Excision Repair (BER) system, is found in a subset of colorectal cancer cell lines and is the cause of an autosomal recessive form of adenomatous polyposis called the 'MYH-associated adenomatous polyposis (MAP) syndrome'(Chow et al., 2004). Germline mutations in *MYH*, which encodes a protein involved in base excision repair, is the cause of adenomatous polyposis in up to 5–10% of individuals who have an adenomatous polyposis syndrome. *MYH* germline mutations were discovered as a cause of adenomatous polyposis when investigators identified an excessive number of somatic G:C→A:T mutations in neoplasms of people with adenomatous polyposis but who had no detectable germline mutations in *APC* (Al-Tassan et al., 2002; Sampson et al., 2003; Sieber et al., 2003). This type of mutation is frequently a consequence of oxidative DNA damage that yields 8-oxo-7, 8-dihydro2′deoxyguanosine (8-oxodG), one of the most stable and deleterious products of oxidative DNA damage (Chow et al., 2004; Olinski et al., 1992). The BER system is responsible for repairing this form of DNA damage, which led investigators to assess candidate genes involved in this repair process, including *8-oxoguanine DNA glycosylase (OGG1), methylenetetrahydrofolate dehydrogenase (NADP*$^+$

dependent) *1* (*MTHF1*), and *MutY human homologue* (*MYH*), as potential genetic causes of adenomatous polyposis. Only *MYH* was affected by mutations in this screen.

The most common *MYH* germline mutations are Tyr165Cys and Gly382Asp, which account for 82% of the mutant alleles detected to date (Sieber et al., 2003). Despite the role of germline *MYH* mutations in the MYH Associated Polyposis (MAP) colorectal cancer family syndrome, somatic *MYH* mutations are uncommon in sporadic colorectal cancer. A study of 1,042 unselected colorectal cancer patients in Finland revealed no somatic *MYH* mutations (Chow et al., 2004; Halford et al., 2003). Of interest, the tumours arising in the setting of biallelic *MYH* germline mutations do not demonstrate differences in the frequency of *TP53, SMAD4,* or *TGFBR2* mutations but do show an absence of MSI or CIN, suggesting they follow a unique molecular pathway compared to sporadic colorectal cancer (Lipton et al., 2003). The discovery of *MYH* germline mutations in individuals with a hereditary colorectal cancer syndrome provides additional evidence for the importance of genomic instability in cancer development.

3.4 Common Deregulated Signalling Pathways

3.4.1 *The Wingless/Wnt Signalling Pathway*

3.4.1.1 APC

The role of genetic alterations in colorectal cancer formation was initially highlighted by the colorectal cancer family syndrome 'Familial Adenomatous Polyposis' (FAP). FAP is a hereditary colorectal cancer predisposition syndrome that is characterized by the development of hundreds to thousands of intestinal adenomatous polyps. The gene responsible for this syndrome, adenomatous polyposis coli (*APC*), was identified as the result of the discovery of an interstitial deletion on chromosome 5q in a patient affected with FAP as well as from classical linkage analyses of families affected by FAP (Groden et al., 1991; Herrera et al., 1986; Nishisho et al., 1991). The *APC* gene contains 15 exons and encodes a 310 kDa protein that possesses multiple functional domains that mediate oligomerization as well as binding to a variety of intracellular proteins, including β-catenin, γ-catenin, glycogen synthase kinase (GSK)-3β, axin, tubulin, End binding protein 1 (EB1), and homologue of Discs Large (hDLG) (Kinzler and Vogelstein, 1996). Germline mutations in *APC* result in FAP or one of its variants, Gardner's syndrome, attenuated FAP, and Turcott's syndrome (Foulkes, 1995; Soravia et al., 1998; Spirio et al., 1992).

APC is mutated in up to 70% of all sporadic colorectal adenocarcinomas. These mutations are detectable in the earliest stages of colorectal cancer, preceding other mutations (Chung, 2000; Miyaki et al., 1999; Miyoshi et al., 1992; Powell et al., 1992; Vogelstein et al., 1988). In fact, aberrant crypt foci, presumptive precursor lesions to colorectal cancer, have been found to harbour *APC* mutations (Jen et al., 1994b). The mutations observed in sporadic colorectal cancer occur most frequently in the 5′ end of exon 15 between amino acid residues 1280 and 1500 (Miyaki et al., 1994). The vast majority of *APC* mutations (>90%) result in premature stop codons and truncated gene products (Powell et al., 1993). These mutations are often accompanied by chromosomal deletion of the residual wild-type allele, but biallelic inactivation of *APC* can also occur by second somatic mutations and possibly by aberrant DNA methylation in the promoter region of the gene (Sakamoto et al., 2001; Spirio et al., 1998).

The fundamental tumourigenic effect of these *APC* mutations results from increased activation of Wingless/Wnt signalling (Fig. 3.3). Normally, GSK-3β forms a complex with APC, β-catenin, and axin and phosphorylates these proteins. The phosphorylation of β-catenin by GSK-3β targets it for ubiquitin-mediated proteasomal degradation. Truncating *APC* mutations prevent this process from occurring and cause an increase in the amount of cytoplasmic β-catenin, which can then translocate to the nucleus and interact with other transcription factors, such as T-cell factor/lymphoid enhancing factor (TCF/Lef) and C-terminal-binding protein 1 (CtBP1) to drive the genes involved with proliferation, etc. (Jin et al., 2008; Phelps et al., 2009). Consistent with the concept that increased Wnt-β-catenin pathway activity is a central tumour-promoting effect of *APC* mutations, oncogenic mutations in

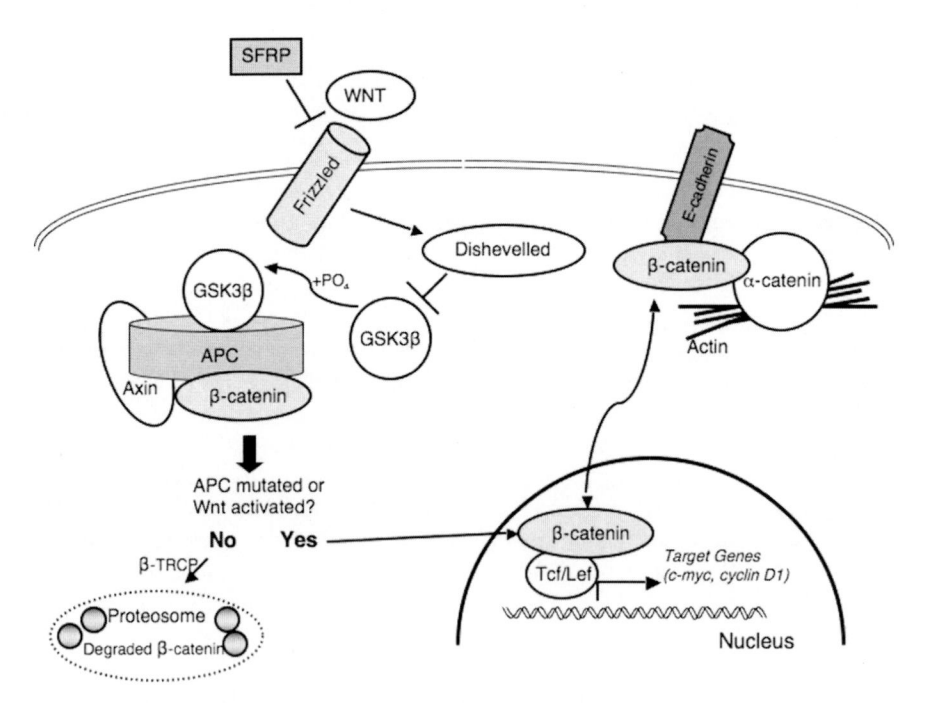

Fig. 3.3 Summary of key interactions in the Wnt signalling pathway, depicting the consequences of *APC* mutations on activation of the pathway. Binding of Wnt-1 to the frizzled receptor activates dishevelled, which inhibits GSK3-β phosphorylation of β-catenin, preventing its proteosomal degradation. Also shown are the interactions of APC with the actin cytoskeleton and the relationship of β-catenin with the E-cadherin cell adhesion structure and Tcf transcription factor

CTNNB1 have been observed in some colorectal cancers, as has methylation of secreted frizzled-related protein 2 and 4 (*SFRP2* and *SFRP4*), members of a family of secreted Wnt antagonists called secretory frizzled related proteins (Kitaeva et al., 1997; Sparks et al., 1998; Suzuki et al., 2004).

The clinical effects of *APC* mutations are best understood in the context of FAP, in which the location of the mutation associates with the phenotype and the occurrence of extra-intestinal tumours, such as desmoid tumours (Caspari et al., 1995; Gardner et al., 1997; Olschwang et al., 1993; Spirio et al., 1993). Polymorphisms in the *APC* gene, including *I1307K* and *E1317Q*, that associate with a slightly increased risk of colorectal have also been identified. *APC I1307K* occurs exclusively in people of Ashkenazi Jewish descent and results in a two-fold increased risk of colorectal adenomas and adenocarcinomas compared to the general population (Laken et al., 1997; Lothe et al., 1998). The *I1307K* polymorphism results from a transition from T to A at nucleotide 3920 in the *APC* gene and appears to produce a region of hypermutability that leads to inactivating mutations in the gene.

3.4.1.2 β-Catenin (*CTNNB1*)

β-catenin is a member of the APC/β-catenin/T cell factor-lymphoid enhancer factor (TCF/Lef) pathway that plays an important role in the majority of colorectal cancers. β-catenin is a homologue of *Armadillo*, and its expression is increased by activation of the Wnt signalling pathway (Aberle et al., 1994; Hulsken et al., 1994; Moon et al., 1997). Mutations in *CTNNB1* often render β-catenin insensitive to APC/β-catenin/GSK-3β-mediated degradation (Morin et al., 1997; Rubinfeld et al., 1997). One of the functions of β-catenin is to regulate transcription of a variety of genes through binding of transcription factors, including TCF/Lef-1, forkhead box, sub-group O (FOXO), CtBP1, Jun, etc. (Gan et al., 2008; Jin et al., 2008; Phelps et al., 2009). Accordingly, cancers with *APC* or *CTNNB1* mutations have increased β-catenin/Tcf-mediated transcription, which leads to the inappropriate expression of genes such as *CCND1* (the gene for cyclin D1) and v-myc myelocytomatosis viral oncogene homolog (*MYC*) (He et al., 1998; Shtutman et al., 1999). With regards to the specific nature of the *CTNNB1* mutations, these mutations are often missense mutations in the highly conserved aspartic acid 32 and presumably impair the ability of GSK-3β to phosphorylate β-catenin (Park et al., 1999). Mutations that abolish β-catenin binding with E-cadherin have also been identified and have been shown to impair cell adhesion (Kawanishi et al., 1995).

Like *APC* mutations, *CTNNB1* mutations play an essential role in early colorectal tumour formation. Mouse models with conditional *Ctnnb1* alleles that lead to the stabilization of β-catenin in the intestinal tract result in a phenotype similar to mice that have germline mutations in *Apc*, providing functional evidence that *CTNNB1* mutations in humans contribute to the formation of adenomas (Harada et al., 1999). Of interest, however, is the fact that the incidence of *CTNNB1* mutations decreases from 12.5% in benign adenomas to 1.4% in invasive cancers, suggesting that *CTNNB1* mutations do not favour the progression of adenomas to adenocarcinomas (Samowitz et al., 1999).

3.4.2 K-RAS, B-RAF and RAS-RAF-MAPK Signalling Pathway

3.4.2.1 K-RAS

One of the most prominent proto-oncogenes in colorectal carcinogenesis is *KRAS*, a member of the *RAS* family of genes. The *RAS* oncogenes, which include *HRAS*, *NRAS*, and *KRAS*, were initially discovered as the transforming genes of the Harvey and Kirsten murine sarcoma viruses (Ha-MSV, Ki-MSV) (Harvey, 1964; Kirsten and Mayer, 1967). *KRAS* is the most commonly mutated *RAS* family member in colorectal cancer, although *NRAS* mutations are also observed in a small percentage of colon cancers (Fearon, 1995).

The *RAS* family of genes encodes a highly conserved family of 21 kDa proteins that are involved in signal transduction. A chief function of the Ras proteins is to couple growth factors to the Raf-mitogen-activated protein (MAP) kinase signal transduction pathway, which leads to the nuclear expression of early response genes (Bokoch and Der, 1993). The protein encoded by *KRAS* has three domains that mediate the following processes: (1) binding to guanosine triphosphate or diphosphate (GTP/GDP), (2) attachment to the inner surface of the plasma membrane after post-translational modification (isoprenylation) of the carboxy terminus, and (3) interaction with cellular targets.

KRAS mutations can be detected in 37–41% of colorectal cancers. In fact, the most common mutations observed in human cancers involve *KRAS* codons 12, 13, and 61, which correspond to areas in the GTP/GDP binding domains in the KRAS protein, although they can also occur in codons 117 and 146 (Crook et al., 2009). These mutations lead to an increased fraction of KRAS in the activated state, which in turn leads to activation of the RAS-RAF-MAPK signalling pathway, promoting cell proliferation and increased survival as well as other pro-tumourigenic effects (Fang and Richardson, 2005; Janda et al., 2002; Scheele et al., 1995). The *KRAS* mutations appear to occur after *APC* mutations in the temporal progression of adenoma to cancer and appear to cooperate with mutant *APC* to deregulate Wnt signalling (Phelps et al., 2009; Vogelstein et al., 1988). Of interest, though, *KRAS* mutations are not mandatory for the malignant conversion of adenomas to adenocarcinomas. Furthermore, from the aspect of clinical management of colorectal cancer, mutant *KRAS* has been found to predict resistance to the anti-epidermal growth factor receptor (EGFR) monoclonal antibodies cetuximab and panitumumab, and is being used as a biomarker to direct the care of patients with metastatic colorectal cancer (Allegra et al., 2009).

3.4.2.2 B-RAF

BRAF, a gene that encodes a protein kinase that is activated by KRAS, is mutated in 27–31% of MSI and 5% of MSS colorectal cancers (Lubomierski et al., 2005; Rajagopalan et al., 2002). *BRAF* mutations can be identified in aberrant crypt foci, adenomas, and adenocarcinomas (Beach et al., 2005). Eighty percent of the mutations are *V600E* mutations, which occur almost exclusively in MSI cancers and lead to activation of the ERK and NFκB pathways (Ikenoue et al., 2004). *BRAF* and *KRAS* mutations appear to be mutually exclusive, suggesting that mutations in either gene affect tumour formation by activating the RAS-RAF-MAPK pathway. *BRAF* mutations occur rarely in MSI colorectal cancers that develop in the setting of the Lynch Syndrome, and are closely associated with CpG island methylator phenotype (CIMP) colorectal cancers, suggesting that there may be two distinct molecular pathways for the formation of sporadic MSI colorectal cancers (Deng et al., 2004; Domingo et al., 2004; Samowitz et al., 2005; Wang et al., 2003).

3.4.3 p53 (TP53)

The p53 protein, which forms a stable complex with the SV40 large T antigen, was ultimately shown to be a tumour suppressor gene in a variety of cancer types (Ochiai and Hirohashi, 1997). Early studies of this gene demonstrated that *TP53* is located at 17p13.1 and is mutated in 50% of primary human tumours, including tumours of the gastrointestinal tract (Iacopetta et al., 2006; Somasundaram, 2000). p53 is a transactivation factor involved in maintaining genomic stability through the control of cell cycle progression and induction of apoptosis in response to genotoxic stress (Somasundaram, 2000). The protein encoded by *TP53* has been structurally divided into four domains: (1) an acidic amino-terminal domain (codons 1–43) required for transcriptional activation; (2) a central sequence-specific DNA-binding domain (codons 100–300); (3) a tetramerization domain (codons 324–355); and (4) a C-terminal regulatory domain (codons 363–393), rich in basic amino acids and believed to regulate the core DNA-binding domain (Somasundaram, 2000). The spectrum of mutations in *TP53* seen in colorectal cancer appears similar to that seen in other tumours, with clustering at four hot spots in highly conserved regions (domains II-V). *TP53* is mutated in approximately 30–50% of colorectal adenocarcinomas and the mutations localize primarily to exons 5–8 (Iacopetta et al., 2006; Vogelstein et al., 1988; 1989). One-third of these mutations result in loss of the p53 transactivation function (Iacopetta et al., 2006). *TP53* mutations have not been observed in colorectal adenomas, but rather appear to be late events in the adenoma-to-carcinoma sequence that may mediate the transition from adenoma to carcinoma (Vogelstein et al., 1988). Mutation of *TP53* coupled with loss of heterozygosity (LOH) of the wild-type allele was found to coincide with the appearance of carcinoma in an adenoma, providing additional evidence for its role in the transition from benign adenoma to adenocarcinoma (Baker et al., 1990; Boland et al., 1995; Kikuchi-Yanoshita et al., 1992; Ohue et al., 1994). Mutant *TP53* is also more common in distal colon cancer and rectal cancer (30–40% of tumours) compared to proximal colon cancer (approximately 20%), perhaps secondary to the increased frequency of MSI cancers in the proximal colon, which have a low frequency of *TP53* mutations (Iacopetta et al., 2006).

p53 normally serves to regulate cell growth and division in the context of genotoxic stress. It is expressed at very low levels in the cell until it is activated by poorly-understood mechanisms as a result of genotoxic stress (i.e. DNA damage due to gamma irradiation, ultraviolet irradiation, or chemotherapeutic agents) (Lane, 1993). Its activation results in the transcription of genes that directly regulate cell cycle progression and apoptosis, including $p21^{WAF1/CIP1}$, *GADD45*, *MDM2*, *14-3-3-σ*, *BAX*, *B99*, *TSP1*, *KILLER/DR5*, *FAS/APO1*, *CYCLIN G*, and others (Somasundaram, 2000). Expression of many of these genes effectively halts DNA replication and induces DNA repair (el-Deiry et al., 1994; 1993; Lin et al., 1992; Smith et al., 1994). This function of p53 to identify DNA damage and stimulate cell cycle arrest and DNA repair or apoptosis explains p53's label 'guardian of the genome' (Dameron et al., 1994; Lane, 1993; Levine, 1997). Mouse models have demonstrated that the biological role of mutant *TP53* depends on the location of the mutation and that the effect may predominantly be on apoptosis or on genomic stability (Iwakuma et al., 2004). To date, the role of mutant *TP53* as a predictive or prognostic biomarker remains controversial and has not proven robust enough for clinical use despite its clear effects on the molecular behaviour of colorectal cancers (Midgley et al., 2009; Walther et al., 2009).

3.4.4 The Phosphatidyl Inositol 3-Kinase (PI3K) Pathway

The phosphatidyl inositol 3-kinases are a family of lipid kinases that regulate the activity of other kinases, such as AKT and p70S6K, and ultimately affect cell proliferation, apoptosis and cell motility, which are hallmark biological functions that are commonly deregulated in cancer (Vivanco and Sawyers, 2002). Recently, large-scale mutational analyses of members of the PI3K signalling pathway have identified mutations that activate this pathway in a large proportion of colorectal cancers (Parsons et al., 2005; Samuels et al., 2004). In one study, gain-of-function mutations in *PIK3CA*, the p110α catalytic subunit of PI3K, were found in 32% of colorectal cancers (Samuels et al., 2004). Analysis of 76 colorectal adenomas and 199 colorectal cancers detected these *PIK3CA* mutations only in advanced adenomas or colorectal cancers, suggesting that these defects influence the transition of adenomas to adenocarcinomas (Samuels et al., 2004).

In addition to mutations in *PIK3CA*, mutations in other members of the PI3K pathway have been detected in a series of 180 colorectal cancers, including mitogen activated protein-kinase kinase-4 (*MKK4/JNKK1*), myosin light-chain kinase-2 (*MYLK2*), phosphoinositide-dependent protein kinase-1 (*PDK1*), p21-activated kinase 4 (*PAK4*), v-akt murine thymoma viral oncogene homologue-2 kinase (*AKT2*) and several others (Parsons et al., 2005). Furthermore, inactivating mutations in phosphatase and tensin homolog deleted on chromosome 10 (*PTEN*) a lipid dual-specificity phosphatase, and in *PIK3R1*, the p85α regulatory subunit of PI3K, have been demonstrated in 5 and 2% of colorectal cancers, respectively (Philp et al., 2001; Vivanco and Sawyers, 2002). MSI colorectal cancers have a higher frequency of *PTEN* mutations (30%) than CIN tumours (9%) as the result of microsatellite repeat mutation hotspots in exons five and eight (53% of all mutations), which has been predicted to lead to an increased susceptibility to therapies targeting the PI3K pathway (Danielsen et al., 2008; Vilar et al., 2009). Remarkably, mutations that affect the PI3K pathway can be detected in nearly 40% of colorectal cancers, and these mutations are nearly mutually exclusive, suggesting that they exert comparable tumourigenic effects through the activation of the PI3K pathway (Parsons et al., 2005).

3.4.5 TGF-β Signalling Pathways

Transforming growth factor β (TGF-β) is a multi-functional cytokine that can induce growth inhibition, apoptosis and differentiation in intestinal epithelial cells (Fynan and Reiss, 1993; Markowitz and Roberts, 1996). The TGF-β pathway is deregulated in approximately 75% of colorectal cancer cell lines and is one of the most common pathways affected by mutations, suggesting it is an important tumour suppressor pathway in colorectal cancer (Chittenden et al., 2008; Grady et al., 1999). Evidence of TGF-β's role in colorectal cancer formation came first from studies that demonstrated colorectal cancer cell lines were resistant to the normal growth inhibitory effects of TGF-β (Hoosein et al., 1989).

TGF-β mediates its effects on cells through the heteromeric TGF-β receptor complex that consists of type I (TGFBR1) and type II (TGFBR2) components (Fig. 3.4). TGFBR1 and TGFBR2 are serine-threonine kinases that phosphorylate

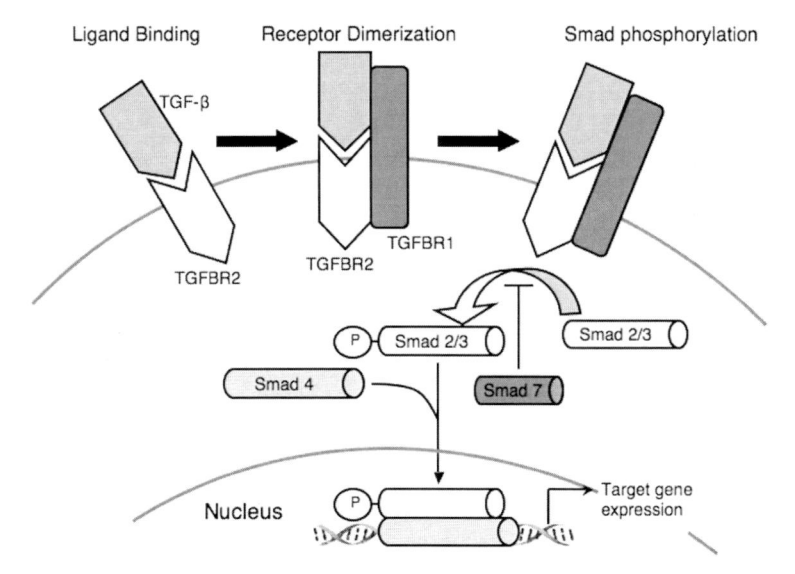

Fig. 3.4 Representation of the Transforming Growth Factor-β (TGF-β) signalling pathway, which is frequently deregulated in colorectal cancer. The pathway plays a critical role in the regulation of cell growth, differentiation, and development in a wide range of biological systems. In general, signalling is initiated by ligand-induced oligomerization of the TGFBR2 and TGFBR1 serine/threonine receptor kinases followed by phosphorylation of the cytoplasmic signalling molecules Smad2 and Smad3. Carboxy-terminal phosphorylation of Smads by activated receptors results in their association with the signalling transducer Smad4, and translocation to the nucleus. Activated Smads regulate diverse biological effects by binding to transcription factors, resulting in modulation of transcription

downstream signalling proteins upon activation (Massague, 1996). After becoming activated by TGF-β binding to TGFBR2, TGFBR1 propagates the signal from the receptor through the phosphorylation of downstream proteins, including the Smad proteins (Smad2 and Smad3) and non-Smad proteins (including PI3K, p38MAPK, and RhoA) (Markowitz and Roberts, 1996; Wakefield and Roberts, 2002). The Smad pathway is the most extensively characterized post-TGF-β-receptor pathway. For the majority of the non-Smad pathways, it is not apparent whether pathway activation is a direct or indirect effect of TGF-β receptor activation.

The downstream transcriptional targets of the TGF-β signalling pathway are involved in the regulation of a variety of cellular functions, including cell proliferation, extracellular matrix production, and immune surveillance. These functions are not only an integral part of tissue homeostasis, but also are logical targets for dysregulation in colorectal carcinogenesis. Elements involved in growth regulation that are clearly influenced in part by TGF-β include growth regulation proteins, such as MYC, cyclin D1, cyclin-dependent kinase (cdk4), p21, p27, p15, and Rb as well as proteins involved in differentiation, apoptosis, angiogenesis, and extracellular matrix remodelling (Alexandrow and Moses, 1995; Ewen et al., 1993; Fava et al., 1990; Geng and Weinberg, 1993; Grady, 2005; Hannon and Beach, 1994; Howe et al., 1991). It appears that certain effector proteins, such as p21 and cdk4, are regulated differentially depending on the degree of TGF-β signal pathway activation and/or on the interaction with other signalling pathways, creating another layer of regulatory control on TGF-β's effects on proliferation that could be disrupted in cancer cells (Gong et al., 2003; Rojas et al., 2009; Seoane et al., 2004; Wang et al., 2004a). With regards to the effects of TGF-β signalling pathway deregulation on other cell behaviours, the extracellular matrix proteins and regulators of extracellular matrix proteins (fibronectin, tenascin, and plasminogen activator inhibitor 1), apoptosis-associated proteins, and senescence-related proteins appear to be altered by TGF-β pathway mutations in colorectal cancers as well (Grady and Markowitz, 2008; Keeton et al., 1991; Zhao, 1999).

The disruption of the production of normal extracellular matrix may play a role in tumour invasion. In support of this concept, *TGFBR2* mutations in MSI colorectal adenomas are only detected in areas of high-grade dysplasia or in adenomas with concurrent adenocarcinoma, suggesting that TGFBR2 inactivation promotes the malignant transition of colorectal adenomas to adenocarcinomas (Grady et al., 1998). Furthermore, in vivo mouse models deficient in intestinal $Tgfbr2$ ($Fabp^{4xat-132}$ $Cre;Tgfbr2^{flx/flx}$ and $Villin-Cre;Tgfbr2^{flx/flx};Apc^{1638\ N/wt}$ mice) demonstrate a significant increase in adenocarcinomas compared to mice with an intact TGFBR2 (Biswas et al., 2004; Munoz et al., 2006; Trobridge et al., 2009).

3.4.5.1 *TGFBR2*

Functionally significant mutations in *TGFBR2* have been identified in up to 30% of colorectal cancers, and the mutational inactivation of TGFBR2 is the most common mechanism identified to date for inactivating the TGF-β signalling pathway in colorectal cancer (Grady et al., 1999; Markowitz et al., 1995). No alterations in

TGFBR1 or the type III TGF-β receptor (*TGFBR3*) have been observed in studies of TGF-β-resistant colorectal cancer cell lines, suggesting mutational inactivation of *TGFBR2* is a particularly favorable event that leads to tumour formation. Markowitz et al. have demonstrated that mutational inactivation of *TGFBR2* is an extremely common event in MSI colorectal cancers. *TGFBR2* has a microsatellite-like region in exon 3 that consists of a 10 base-pair polyadenine tract, making it particularly susceptible to errors in the setting of MSI (Markowitz et al., 1995; Myeroff et al., 1995; Parsons et al., 1995). In a series of 110 MSI colorectal cancers, 100 were found to carry *BAT-RII* mutations. In almost all of these cases, the mutations were biallelic, consistent with the tumour suppressor function of TGFBR2 (Parsons et al., 1995).

TGFBR2's task as a tumour suppressor gene in colorectal cancer has been further elucidated by studies in mouse models. Deletion of a conditional *Tgfbr2* allele in the colorectal epithelium promotes the growth of colorectal adenocarcinomas in the azoxymethane mouse model of colorectal cancer (Biswas et al., 2004). Of interest, *TGFBR2* mutation plays its role in tumour formation in the context of other gene mutations and acts to promote the progression of colon neoplasms (Munoz et al., 2006; Trobridge et al., 2009). Further support for *TGFBR2*'s role as a tumour suppressor gene in colorectal cancer comes from the demonstration of *TGFBR2* mutations in colorectal cancer cell lines that are microsatellite stable (MSS). *TGFBR2* mutations have been found in 15% ($n=3/14$) of TGF-β-resistant MSS colorectal cancer cell lines (Grady et al., 1999). In aggregate, the overall incidence of *TGFBR2* mutations in both MSS and MSI colorectal cancers appears to be 30% (Grady et al., 1999). Interestingly, in a study of colorectal cancer cell lines, the incidence of TGF-β resistance was found to be 55% despite the cell lines frequently having wild-type *TGFBR1* and *TGFBR2* (Grady et al., 1999). Presumably, these cancers have inactivated the TGF-β signalling pathway via genetic or epigenetic alterations in post-receptor pathway molecules, further underscoring the importance of the TGF-β signalling pathway in colorectal cancer formation.

3.4.5.2 The SMAD Genes

It has been determined that a deleted region on chromosome 18q that is shared among colorectal cancers is the locus of a number of tumour suppressor genes implicated in colorectal cancer formation, including *DCC*, *SMAD2*, and *SMAD4*, all of which have been shown to be mutated in colon cancer (Eppert et al., 1996; Fearon and Vogelstein, 1990; Nagatake et al., 1996). The Smad proteins serve as intracellular mediators that regulate TGF-β superfamily signalling. Numerous studies have identified three major classes of Smad proteins: (1) the receptor-regulated Smads (R-Smads: Smads1, 2, 3, and 5), which are direct targets of the TGF-β receptor family type I kinases; (2) the common Smads (Co-Smads: Smad4) which form heteromeric complexes with the R-Smads and propagate the TGF-β-mediated signal; and (3) the inhibitory Smads (I-Smads: Smad6 and Smad7) which antagonize TGF-β signalling.

In light of the known tumour suppressor effects of the TGF-β signalling pathway and the role the Smad proteins play in propagating this signal, it is not surprising that alterations in some of the *SMAD* genes have been discovered in colorectal cancer. Mutational inactivation of *SMAD2* and *SMAD4* has been observed in a high percentage of pancreatic cancers and in 5–16% of colorectal cancers (Eppert et al., 1996; Hahn et al., 1996; Riggins et al., 1996; Takagi et al., 1996). The effect of these mutations upon colorectal carcinogenesis is being investigated in a number of animal models. One murine model, a compound heterozygote $Smad4^{+/-}/Apc\Delta^{716}$, develops colorectal cancer (unlike the $Apc\Delta^{716}$ mouse, which only develops small intestinal adenomas) (Takaku et al., 1998). This mouse model suggests that *SMAD4* inactivation may play a role in the progression of colorectal cancers as opposed to their initiation. However, in other contexts, *SMAD4* mutations appear to initiate tumour formation. Mature $Smad4^{+/-}$ mice do not develop colorectal cancer, but instead develop gastric and intestinal juvenile polyps and invasive gastric cancer (Takaku et al., 1999; Xu et al., 2000). Furthermore, germline mutations in *SMAD4* have been found in approximately one third of individuals with Juvenile Polyposis (JPS), an autosomal dominant syndrome characterized by gastrointestinal hamartomatous polyps and an increased risk of gastrointestinal cancer, consistent with the concept that haploid insufficiency of *SMAD4* may contribute to tumour initiation (Friedl et al., 1999; Howe et al., 1998; Roth et al., 1999). Importantly, though, the polyps observed in JPS and the invasive cancers in the $Smad4^{+/-}$ mouse have been shown to have allelic loss of *SMAD4*, supporting the concept that biallelic inactivation of *SMAD4* is required for cancer formation (Woodford-Richens et al., 2000; Xu et al., 2000). Taken together, these studies suggest that *SMAD4* is a tumour suppressor gene in colorectal cancer and is one of the targets of 18q LOH. However, given the frequency of 18q LOH versus detected *SMAD4* mutations or deletions, there are likely other tumour suppressor loci on 18q21.

The 18q21 region, which also contains the *SMAD7* gene, was further evaluated in a recent genome-wide association study of colorectal cancer cases (Pittman et al., 2009). While it has been shown that *SMAD7* single nucleotide polymorphisms (SNPs) influence colorectal cancer risk (Broderick et al., 2007; Tenesa et al., 2008), the underlying basis for this risk had not been previously defined. Pittman et al. sequenced the 17-kb 18q21 region and evaluated all variants in 2,532 CRC cases and 2,607 normal controls and found that a novel C to G SNP at 44,703,563 bp was maximally associated with CRC risk. They proposed that this novel SNP is a functional alteration leading to CRC predisposition through differential *SMAD7* expression and, therefore, abnormal TGF-β signalling (Pittman et al., 2009).

Although the *SMAD2* gene is also located at 18q21, mutations in *SMAD2* have been found in only 0–5% of cancers (Eppert et al., 1996; Riggins et al., 1996; Takenoshita et al., 1998). The other *SMAD* genes are not frequently altered in colorectal cancer, despite the fact that *SMAD3* and *SMAD6* are located on chromosome 15q21–22, which is a frequent site of allelic loss in colorectal cancer (Arai et al., 1998; Park et al., 2000; Riggins et al., 1996). In conclusion, *SMAD* mutations appear to play a role in tumour formation in a subset of colorectal cancers, but are not as widespread as mutations in *TGFBR2*. This raises the possibility that there are non-Smad TGF-β signalling pathways that play an essential role in the tumour suppressor activity of *TGFBR2*.

The effect of 18q LOH, and thus presumably inactivation of *SMAD2* and/or *SMAD4*, on the clinical behavior of colon carcinomas has been subjected to intense scrutiny with inconclusive results to date. Assessment of LOH of 18q using microsatellite markers in stage II colon cancer has found either no correlation with the clinical behavior of the cancer or an association with more aggressive cancer behavior (Carethers et al., 1998; Jen et al., 1994a; Laurent-Puig et al., 1992; Martinez-Lopez et al., 1998; Zhou et al., 2002). The reason for the discrepancy is unclear, but may relate to different microsatellite loci that were used in the different studies and thus the specific region of 18q that was assessed by each group. Adding to this confusion, *SMAD4* diploidy and *TGFBR2 BAT-RII* mutations associate with improved survival after adjuvant chemotherapy, but Smad4 expression correlates inversely with prognosis (Alazzouzi et al., 2005; Alhopuro et al., 2005; Boulay et al., 2002; Watanabe et al., 2001). Thus, the effect of alterations in the Smad proteins on the clinical behavior of cancer is unclear at this time.

3.4.5.3 *TGF-β Superfamily Receptors*: *ACVR2 and BMPR1A*

The TGF-β superfamily not only includes TGF-β1, TGF-β2, and TGF-β3, but also the BMPs (Bone Morphogenetic Proteins), activin, nodal, GDFs (Growth and Differentiation Factors) and inhibin. Germline mutations in *SMAD4* and *BMPR1A*, a type I receptor for the Bone Morphogenetic Proteins (BMPs), in families with Juvenile Polyposis (JPS) have implicated inactivation of BMP signalling in this subset of hereditary colorectal cancers. Nonsense and missense germline mutations in *BMPR1A* have been identified in JPS families, including 44–47delTGTT, 715C>T, 812G>A and 961delC affecting exons 1, 7, and 8 respectively (Howe et al., 2001). Alterations in *SMAD4* account for 5–62% of cases and published mutations to date include deletions (1244–1247delAGAC), missense mutations and frameshift mutations in exons 5, 6, 8, 9, 10 and 11(Friedl et al., 2002). The 1244–1247delAGAC mutation has been identified in multiple unrelated families and appears to be a mutation hot spot in the gene (Howe et al., 2002).

The BMPs are a group of at least 15 disulfide-linked dimeric proteins and include BMP-2, BMP-4 and BMP-7 (OP-1). They have a broad range of biological functions, including the regulation of morphogenesis in various tissues and organs during development as well as the regulation of growth, differentiation, chemotaxis and apoptosis in monocytes, epithelial cells, mesenchymal cells and neuronal cells (Kawabata et al., 1998). As with the TGF-β receptor, the Smad pathway is the best-understood post-BMP receptor pathway. The R-Smads, Smads1 and 5 partner with Smad4 (Co-Smad) to transduce BMP-mediated signals from the BMP receptors (Kawabata et al., 1998). Thus, the identification of both *BMPR1A* and *SMAD4* germline mutations in JPS families strongly implicates BMP signalling disruption in the pathogenesis of this syndrome.

Activin is a secreted dimeric ligand, composed of either Activin βA and/or Activin βB, that activates intracellular signalling pathways that include the

SMAD2/3-SMAD4 pathway via a heteromeric receptor which is composed of a type I receptor (ACVRL1, ACTRIA, or ACTRIB) and a type II receptor (ACVR2 or ACVR2B) (de Caestecker, 2004). Mutations in *ACVR2* have been found to occur in 58–90% of MSI colorectal cancers as the result of a polyadenine tract in the coding region of the gene (Deacu et al., 2004; Mori et al., 2001). The identification of mutations that affect activin, TGF-β and BMP signalling implicates at least three members of the TGF-β family as members of tumour suppressor pathways in colorectal cancer.

3.5 Genome-Wide Analyses of Colorectal Cancer Genes

In general, the oncogenes and tumour suppressor genes related to the initiation and progression of colorectal cancer described in the aforementioned sections have been discovered by linkage analyses in cancer-prone families, by the evaluation of chromosomal abnormalities in tumours, or by sequence analysis of candidate genes (Parsons et al., 2005). Now, with the relatively recent development and refinement of genome-wide sequencing and bioinformatics technologies, it is possible to evaluate the entire cancer cell genome in an inclusive and unbiased fashion. Sjöblom et al. recently examined a large number of breast and colon cancer genes by focusing on protein-coding sequences termed the consensus coding sequences (CCDS) which contain the full-length protein-coding genes that are identical among the RefSeq and Ensembl reference databases (Sjoblom et al., 2006). Their analysis of over 13,000 genes in 11 colon and 11 breast cancers revealed each tumour possessed an average of approximately 90 mutant genes that would be predicted to potentially play a role in tumour formation. Utilizing a set of criteria to focus attention upon the most likely contributors to the neoplastic process (i.e. excluding those genes exhibiting silent genetic changes, changes that were present in normal controls and known polymorphisms) they identified 189 genes (an average of 11 per tumour) that were mutated at a statistically significant frequency in colorectal cancers and that were predicted to affect multiple cellular processes, including motility, transport, adhesion, transcription and invasion. A key validation of this data relied upon re-identification of genes previously shown to be somatically mutated in human cancers, such as *APC*. All of the consensus coding sequences for genes previously shown to be mutated in >10% of either breast or colorectal cancers were found to be candidate cancer genes in this study, including *TP53, APC, KRAS, SMAD4*, and *FBXW7* (*CDC4*) (Sjoblom et al., 2006).

In another study, large-scale sequencing analyses were used to evaluate protein tyrosine kinases (PTKs) and phosphatases (PTPs), proteins critical to intracellular signalling pathways including cell growth, apoptosis and invasion. Only a handful of tyrosine phosphatases have previously been directly implicated in cancer. Wang et al. utilized bioinformatics analyses and Hidden Markov Models to identify all 87 known PTPs plus seven putative PTPs (Wang et al., 2004c). The 1,375 coding exons of all of the PTPs were analyzed in 18 colorectal cancers using PCR and DNA sequencing and compared to matched normal tissue. In this manner, they were able to identify six PTP genes containing somatic mutations (*PTPRF, PTPRG, PTPRT, PTPN3, PTPN13, PTPN14*); when an additional 157 colorectal cancers were examined, 77 mutations were found in the six genes, overall affecting 26% of the colorectal tumours. In 16 samples, both alleles of the tyrosine phosphatase gene were mutated; the majority of the tumours with *PTP* gene mutations also carried mutations in *BRAF* or *KRAS* (Wang et al., 2004c). The results of this study therefore suggest a role for protein tyrosine phosphatases in colorectal carcinogenesis. Thus, these genome-wide sequencing studies have identified novel genes involved in colorectal cancer and have begun to define the number of mutations typically acquired by colorectal cancers during their formation.

3.6 Metastasis Genes

One of the fundamental challenges in cancer biology is the identification of genes that contribute to the metastatic and lethal cancer phenotype. Intense investigation in this area has led to the identification of promising candidate genes that may influence the metastatic potential of the primary colorectal cancer. Metastasis-associated phosphatase of regenerating liver-3 (PRL3), a phosphatase, was found over-expressed in 12 of 12 colorectal cancer liver metastases, but not in matched colorectal cancer primaries from the same patients (Saha et al., 2001). Moreover, in 3 of 12 cases, PRL3 over-expression was accompanied by marked *PRL3* gene amplification, suggesting that PRL3 over-expression is a primary genetic event selected for during metastasis. Osteopontin is a protein that also appears to have potential to predict the metastatic potential of colorectal cancer. Osteopontin was identified through expression array studies and is 15-fold over-expressed in primary colorectal cancers and 27-fold over-expressed in liver metastases (Yeatman and Chambers, 2003). Osteopontin is a phosphoglycoprotein that can bind to several integrins as well as CD44 and has been shown to contribute to the malignant phenotype in breast cancer (Furger et al., 2001; Yeatman and Chambers, 2003). To date, neither PRL3 nor osteopontin has been shown to have the ability to predict the metastatic potential of colorectal cancer in a prospective clinical trial.

Using cancer-focused oligonucleotide microarrays, Slaby et al. analyzed gene expression profiles of 20 CRC samples and identified three genes (*HSP110, HYOU1* and *TCTP*) that were significantly up-regulated in primary tumours of patients who developed lymph node metastasis (Slaby et al., 2009). In an independent group of 30 patients, they validated the differences in HSP110 expression by real-time PCR, demonstrating significant up-regulation of HSP110 expression in colorectal tumours compared to adjacent non-tumoural tissue ($p<0.0003$).

Expression array analyses have been used to establish a pattern of 115 genes that discriminates stage-matched metastatic from non-metastatic primary colorectal tumours (Fritzmann et al., 2009). Among these, the TGF-β inhibitor BAMBI was highly expressed in approximately half of metastatic primary tumours and

Table 3.1 Genes mutated in colorectal cancer: the following table lists the genes previously noted to play a role in the process of colorectal carcinogenesis. Listed next to each gene is the pathway affected by the gene (or its function), the type and frequency of the gene alteration, and whether or not germline mutations have been described

Gene	Affected pathway/function	Alteration identified in colorectal cancer	Frequency of mutant genes in colorectal cancers (approximate)	Germline mutations in cancer family syndromes	Comments/additional references
APC	Wingless/Wnt pathway	Mutation	70%	Yes	Germline mutation is cause of Familial Adenomatous Polyposis (FAP)
CTNNB1	"	Mutation	2%	No	More common in MSI cancers
AXIN2	"	Mutation	Uncommon	Yes	Cause of attenuated polyposis (Lammi et al., 2004; Liu et al., 2000)
SFRP1	"	Methylation	90%	No	(Suzuki et al., 2004)
SFRP2	"	Methylation	85%	No	(Suzuki et al., 2004)
KRAS	Ras-Raf pathway	Mutation	40%	No	
BRAF	"	Mutation	30% MSI/5% MSS CRCs	No	V600E is mutation hotspot in BRAF
PIK3CA	PI3K signaling pathway	Mutation	30%	No	
PIK3R1	"	Mutation	5%	No	
PTEN	"	Mutation	Uncommon in MSS cancers, 10% in MSI cancers	Yes	Germline mutation is cause of Cowden's syndrome

(continued)

3 The Genetics of Colorectal Cancer

Table 3.1 (continued)

Gene	Affected pathway/function	Alteration identified in colorectal cancer	Frequency of mutant genes in colorectal cancers (approximate)	Germline mutations in cancer family syndromes	Comments/additional references
TP53		Mutation	>50%	Yes	Germline mutations cause Li-Fraumeni syndrome, which may be cause of some cases of early onset CRC (Wong et al., 2006)
p14ARF		Methylation	20%	No	
STK11 (LKB1)		Mutation	Uncommon	Yes	Cause of Peutz-Jeghers Syndrome (PJS)
TGFBR2	TGF-β signaling pathway	Mutation	25–30%	Yes[a]	Mutations more common in MSI CRCs
TGFBR1	"	Polymorphism	Rare somatic mutations	Yes	TGFBR1*A polymorphism associated with cancer risk (Pasche et al., 2005)
SMAD4	TGF-β and BMP signaling pathway	Mutation	16%	Yes	Germline mutation is cause of Juvenile Polyposis Syndrome (JPS)

(continued)

Table 3.1 (continued)

Gene	Affected pathway/function	Alteration identified in colorectal cancer	Frequency of mutant genes in colorectal cancers (approximate)	Germline mutations in cancer family syndromes	Comments/additional references
SMAD2	TGF-β signaling pathway	Mutation	2%	No	
ACVR2	Activin/TGF-β signaling pathway	Mutation	60–90% of MSI CRCs	No	More common in MSI cancers
BMPR1A	BMP signaling pathway	Mutation	–	Yes	Mutation is uncommon in sporadic CRCs
MYH	Base excision repair	Mutation	Rare somatic mutations	Yes	Cause of 5–10% of adenomatous polyposis cases
MLH1	Mismatch Repair (MMR)	Methylation	10% of sporadic cases	Yes	Most common gene affected in Lynch Syndrome (HNPCC)
MSH2	"	Mutation	Uncommon	Yes	Cause of Lynch Syndrome (HNPCC)
MSH6	"	Mutation	Rare somatic mutations	Yes	"
PMS2	"	Mutation	Rare somatic mutations	Yes	"

[a]*TGFBR2* germline mutation is a cause of Marfan-like syndrome and does not cause a cancer family syndrome (Mizuguchi et al., 2004). CRC=colorectal cancer

metastases but not in nonmetastatic tumours. BAMBI is a target of canonical Wnt signalling that involves the beta-catenin coactivator BCL9–2. This group observed an inverse correlation between the level of BAMBI expression and metastasis-free survival time of patients. In mice, over-expression of BAMBI caused colon cancer cells to form tumours that metastasized more frequently to the liver and lymph nodes than control cancer cells (Fritzmann et al., 2009). Thus, through a variety of experimental approaches, genes that may play a role in the metastatic behaviour of colorectal cancer are being identified (Table 3.1). These genes are candidates for validation studies in model systems and other cohorts of patients with colorectal cancer.

3.7 Conclusions

Investigation of the molecular pathogenesis of colorectal cancer has yielded many insights into the genetic mechanisms driving the tumourigenesis process and to the identification of many potential therapeutic targets. Key insights from the assessment of the molecular genetics and epigenetics of colorectal cancer include the multistep nature of carcinogenesis, the central role of tumour suppressor pathways, the role of DNA repair genes and genomic stability in cancer formation, and the role of the Wingless/Wnt, RAS-RAF-MAPK, PI3K, and TGF-β signalling pathways in tumour formation. Even with these insights, the molecular origin of the metastatic phenotype that directly accounts for cancer lethality remains unknown. In addition, the translation of molecular genetics to new diagnostic and prognostic assays and therapeutic modalities remains promising and is beginning to have a major impact on the clinical management of colorectal cancer. With additional forthcoming research, this field of inquiry promises to yield important answers to these and other pertinent questions.

Abbreviations and Acronyms

ACVR2	Activin receptor type II
BAX	Bcl-2–associated X protein
BER	Base Excision Repair
BMPs	Bone Morphogenetic Proteins
BRAF	V-raf murine sarcoma viral oncogene homolog B1
CCDS	Consensus coding sequences
CDC4	Cell division cycle 4
Cdk4	Cyclin-dependent kinase 4
CIMP	CpG island methylator phenotype
CIN	Microsatellite instability
CpG	Cytosine-phosphate-guanine
CRC	Colorectal cancer
CtBP1	C-terminal-binding protein 1
CTNNB1	β-catenin encoding gene
EB1	End binding protein

FAP	Familial adenomatous polyposis
Fbw7	F-box/WD repeat-containing protein 7
FOXO	Forkhead box, sub-group O
EGFR	Epidermal growth factor receptor
GDFs	Growth and differentiation factors
GSK-3β	Glycogen synthase kinase-3β
hDLG	Homologue of Discs Large
HNPCC	Hereditary nonpolyposis colon cancer
HR	Hazard ratio
JPS	Juvenile polyposis
LOH	Loss of heterozygosity
MAP	MYH-Associated adenomatous polyposis syndrome
MAPK	Mitogen-activated protein kinase
MKK4/JNKK1	Mitogen activated protein-kinase kinase-4
MSH	Muts homolog, colon cancer, nonpolyposis type 1 (*E. coli*)
MLH1	MutL homolog 1, colon cancer, nonpolyposis type 2 (MLH1)
MMR	DNA Mismatch Repair
MRE11	Murein formation gene cluster E
MSI	Microsatellite instability
MSS	Microsatellite stable
MTHF1	Methylenetetrahydrofolate dehydrogenase (NADP+ dependent) 1
MYC	v-myc myelocytomatosis viral oncogene homolog
MYH	MutY human homologue
MYLK2	Myosin light-chain kinase-2
OGG1	8-Oxoguanine DNA glycosylase
PAK4	p21-activated kinase 4
PCNA	Proliferating cell nuclear antigen
PDK1	Phosphoinositide-dependent protein kinase-1
PI3K/AKT	Phosphatidyl inositol 3 kinase/v-akt murine thymoma viral oncogene homologue 1
PMS2	Postmeiotic segregation increased 2
PRL-3	Metastasis-associated phosphatase of regenerating liver-3
PTEN	Phosphatase and tensin homolog deleted on chromosome 10
PTK	Protein tyrosine kinase
PTP	Phosphatase
RFC	Replication factor C
RPA	Replication protein A
SNP	Single nucleotide polymorphisms
SFRP	Secreted frizzled-related protein
TCF/Lef	T-cell factor/lymphoid enhancing factor
TGFβ	Transforming growth factor β
TGFBR2	TGF-β receptor type II
TP53	Tumor protein 53
WNT	Wingless/Wnt

References

Aaltonen L, Peltomaki P, Mecklin J-P, Jarvinen H, Jass J, Green J et al. (1994). Replication errors in benign and malignant tumors from hereditary nonpolyposis colorectal cancer patients. *Cancer Res* **54**: 1645–48.

Aberle H, Butz S, Stappert J, Weissig H, Kemler R, Hoschuetzky H (1994). Assembly of the cadherin-catenin complex in vitro with recombinant proteins. *J Cell Sci* **107**: 3655–63.

Al-Tassan N, Chmiel NH, Maynard J, Fleming N, Livingston AL, Williams GT et al. (2002). Inherited variants of MYH associated with somatic G:C–>T:A mutations in colorectal tumors. *Nat Genet* **30**: 227–32.

Alazzouzi H, Alhopuro P, Salovaara R, Sammalkorpi H, Jarvinen H, Mecklin JP et al. (2005). SMAD4 as a prognostic marker in colorectal cancer. *Clin Cancer Res* **11**: 2606–11.

Alexandrow MG, Moses HL (1995). Transforming growth factor beta and cell cycle regulation. *Cancer Res* **55**: 1452–57.

Alhopuro P, Alazzouzi H, Sammalkorpi H, Davalos V, Salovaara R, Hemminki A et al. (2005). SMAD4 levels and response to 5-fluorouracil in colorectal cancer. *Clin Cancer Res* **11**: 6311–16.

Allegra CJ, Jessup JM, Somerfield MR, Hamilton SR, Hammond EH, Hayes DF et al. (2009). American Society of Clinical Oncology provisional clinical opinion: testing for KRAS gene mutations in patients with metastatic colorectal carcinoma to predict response to anti-epidermal growth factor receptor monoclonal antibody therapy. *J Clin Oncol* **27**: 2091–96.

Arai T, Akiyama Y, Okabe S, Ando M, Endo M, Yuasa Y (1998). Genomic structure of the human Smad3 gene and its infrequent alterations in colorectal cancers. *Cancer Lett* **122**: 157–63.

Baker SJ, Preisinger AC, Jessup JM, Paraskeva C, Markowitz S, Willson JK et al. (1990). p53 gene mutations occur in combination with 17p allelic deletions as late events in colorectal tumorigenesis. *Cancer Res* **50**: 7717–22.

Barber TD, McManus K, Yuen KW, Reis M, Parmigiani G, Shen D et al. (2008). Chromatid cohesion defects may underlie chromosome instability in human colorectal cancers. *Proc Natl Acad Sci USA* **105**: 3443–48.

Bardelli A, Parsons DW, Silliman N, Ptak J, Szabo S, Saha S et al. (2003). Mutational analysis of the tyrosine kinome in colorectal cancers. *Science* **300**: 949.

Beach R, Chan AO, Wu TT, White JA, Morris JS, Lunagomez S et al. (2005). BRAF mutations in aberrant crypt foci and hyperplastic polyposis. *Am J Pathol* **166**: 1069–75.

Bischoff JR, Anderson L, Zhu Y, Mossie K, Ng L, Souza B et al. (1998). A homologue of Drosophila aurora kinase is oncogenic and amplified in human colorectal cancers. *EMBO J* **17**: 3052–65.

Biswas S, Chytil A, Washington K, Romero-Gallo J, Gorska AE, Wirth PS et al. (2004). Transforming Growth Factor β Receptor Type II Inactivation Promotes the Establishment and Progression of Colon Cancer. *Cancer Res* **64**: 4687–92.

Bokoch GM, Der CJ (1993). Emerging concepts in the Ras superfamily of GTP-binding proteins. *FASEB J* **7**: 750–59.

Boland CR, Sato J, Appelman HD, Bresalier RS, Feinberg AP (1995). Microallelotyping defines the sequence and tempo of allelic losses at tumour suppressor gene loci during colorectal cancer progression. *Nat Med* **1**: 902–09.

Boland C, Thibodeau S, Hamilton S, Sidransky D, Eshleman J, Burt R et al. (1998). National Cancer Institute workshop on microsatellite instability for cancer detection and familial predispostion:development of international criteria for the determination of microsatellite instability in colorectal cancer. *Cancer Res* **58**: 5248–57.

Bomme L, Bardi G, Pandis N, Fenger C, Kronborg O, Heim S (1998). Cytogenetic analysis of colorectal adenomas: karyotypic comparisons of synchronous tumors. *Cancer Genet Cytogenet* **106**: 66–71.

Boulay JL, Mild G, Lowy A, Reuter J, Lagrange M, Terracciano L et al. (2002). SMAD4 is a predictive marker for 5-fluorouracil-based chemotherapy in patients with colorectal cancer. *Br J Cancer* **87**: 630–34.

Broderick P, Carvajal-Carmona L, Pittman AM, Webb E, Howarth K, Rowan A et al. (2007). A genome-wide association study shows that common alleles of SMAD7 influence colorectal cancer risk. *Nat Genet* **39**: 1315–17.

Cahill D, Lengauer C, Yu J, Riggins G, Willson J, Markowitz S et al. (1998). Mutations of mitotic checkpoint genes in human cancers. *Nature* **392**: 300–03.

Carethers JM, Hawn MT, Greenson JK, Hitchcock CL, Boland CR (1998). Prognostic significance of allelic lost at chromosome 18q21 for stage II colorectal cancer [see comments]. *Gastroenterology* **114**: 1188–95.

Caspari R, Olschwang S, Friedl W, Mandl M, Boisson C, Boker T et al. (1995). Familial adenomatous polyposis: desmoid tumours and lack of ophthalmic lesions (CHRPE) associated with APC mutations beyond codon 1444. *Hum Mol Genet* **4**: 337–40.

Chen WD, Eshleman JR, Aminoshariae MR, Ma AH, Veloso N, Markowitz SD et al. (2000). Cytotoxicity and mutagenicity of frameshift-inducing agent ICR191 in mismatch repair-deficient colon cancer cells. *J Natl Cancer Inst* **92**: 480–85.

Chittenden TW, Howe EA, Culhane AC, Sultana R, Taylor JM, Holmes C et al. (2008). Functional classification analysis of somatically mutated genes in human breast and colorectal cancers. *Genomics* **91**: 508–11.

Chow E, Thirlwell C, Macrae F, Lipton L (2004). Colorectal cancer and inherited mutations in base-excision repair. *Lancet Oncol* **5**: 600–06.

Chung D (2000). The genetic basis of colorectal cancer:insights into critical pathways of tumorigenesis. *Gastroenterology* **119**: 854–65.

Crook S, Seth R, Jackson D, Ilyas M (2009). Concomitant mutations and splice variants in KRAS and BRAF demonstrate complex perturbation of the Ras/Raf signalling pathway in Colorectal Cancer. *Gut* **58**: 1234–41.

Dameron KM, Volpert OV, Tainsky MA, Bouck N (1994). Control of angiogenesis in fibroblasts by p53 regulation of thrombospondin-1. *Science* **265**: 1582–84.

Danielsen SA, Lind GE, Bjornslett M, Meling GI, Rognum TO, Heim S et al. (2008). Novel mutations of the suppressor gene PTEN in colorectal carcinomas stratified by microsatellite instability- and TP53 mutation- status. *Hum Mutat* **29**: E252–E62.

Deacu E, Mori Y, Sato F, Yin J, Olaru A, Sterian A et al. (2004). Activin type II receptor restoration in ACVR2-deficient colon cancer cells induces transforming growth factor-beta response pathway genes. *Cancer Res* **64**: 7690–96.

de Caestecker M (2004). The transforming growth factor-beta superfamily of receptors. *Cytokine Growth Factor Rev* **15**: 1–11.

Deng G, Bell I, Crawley S, Gum J, Terdiman JP, Allen BA et al. (2004). BRAF mutation is frequently present in sporadic colorectal cancer with methylated hMLH1, but not in hereditary nonpolyposis colorectal cancer. *Clin Cancer Res* **10**: 191–95.

Domingo E, Laiho P, Ollikainen M, Pinto M, Wang L, French AJ et al. (2004). BRAF screening as a low-cost effective strategy for simplifying HNPCC genetic testing. *J Med Genet* **41**: 664–68.

el-Deiry WS, Harper JW, O'Connor PM, Velculescu VE, Canman CE, Jackman J et al. (1994). WAF1/CIP1 is induced in p53-mediated G1 arrest and apoptosis. *Cancer Res* **54**: 1169–74.

el-Deiry WS, Tokino T, Velculescu VE, Levy DB, Parsons R, Trent JM et al. (1993). WAF1, a potential mediator of p53 tumor suppression. *Cell* **75**: 817–25.

Eppert K, Scherer S, Ozcelik H, Pirone R, Hoodless P, Kim H et al. (1996). MADR2 maps to 18q21 and encodes a TGFß-regulated MAD-related protein that is functionally mutated in colorectal cancer. *Cell* **86**: 543–52.

Eshleman J, Casey G, Kochera M, Sedwick W, Swinler S, Veigl M et al. (1998). Chromosome number and structure both are markedly stable in RER colorectal cancers and are not destabilized by mutation of p53. *Oncogene* **17**: 719–25.

Eshleman J, Lang E, Bowerfind G, Parsons R, Vogelstein B, Willson J et al. (1995). Increased mutation rate at the *hprt* locus accompanies microsatellite instability in colon cancer. *Oncogene* **10**: 33–37.

Ewen ME, Sluss HK, Whitehouse LL, Livingston DM (1993). TGF beta inhibition of Cdk4 synthesis is linked to cell cycle arrest. *Cell* **74**: 1009–20.

Fang JY, Richardson BC (2005). The MAPK signalling pathways and colorectal cancer. *Lancet Oncol* **6**: 322–27.

Fava RA, Casey TT, Wilcox J, Pelton RW, Moses HL, Nanney LB (1990). Synthesis of transforming growth factor-beta 1 by megakaryocytes and its localization to megakaryocyte and platelet alpha-granules. *Blood* **76**: 1946–55.

Fearon E (1995). Molecular Genetics of Colorectal Cancer. *Ann N Y Acad Sci* **768**: 101–10.

Fearon E, Vogelstein B (1990). A genetic model for colorectal tumorigenesis. *Cell* **61**: 759–67.

Foulkes WD (1995). A tale of four syndromes: familial adenomatous polyposis, Gardner syndrome, attenuated APC and Turcot syndrome. *QJM* **88**: 853–63.

Friedl W, Kruse R, Uhlhaas S, Stolte M, Schartmann B, Keller KM et al. (1999). Frequent 4-bp deletion in exon 9 of the SMAD4/MADH4 gene in familial juvenile polyposis patients. *Genes Chromos Cancer* **25**: 403–06.

Friedl W, Uhlhaas S, Schulmann K, Stolte M, Loff S, Back W et al. (2002). Juvenile polyposis: massive gastric polyposis is more common in MADH4 mutation carriers than in BMPR1A mutation carriers. *Hum Genet* **111**: 108–11.

Fritzmann J, Morkel M, Besser D, Budczies J, Kosel F, Brembeck FH et al. (2009). A colorectal cancer expression profile that includes transforming growth factor beta inhibitor BAMBI predicts metastatic potential. *Gastroenterolology* **137**: 165–75.

Fujiwara T, Stolker JM, Watanabe T, Rashid A, Longo P, Eshleman JR et al. (1998). Accumulated clonal genetic alterations in familial and sporadic colorectal carcinomas with widespread instability in microsatellite sequences. *Am J Pathol* **153**: 1063–78.

Furger KA, Menon RK, Tuckl AB, Bramwelll VH, Chambers AF (2001). The functional and clinical roles of osteopontin in cancer and metastasis. *Curr Mol Med* **1**: 621–32.

Fynan TM, Reiss M (1993). Resistance to inhibition of cell growth by transforming growth factor-beta and its role in oncogenesis. *Crit Rev Oncog* **4**: 493–540.

Gan XQ, Wang JY, Xi Y, Wu ZL, Li YP, Li L (2008). Nuclear Dvl, c-Jun, beta-catenin, and TCF form a complex leading to stabilization of beta-catenin-TCF interaction. *J Cell Biol* **180**: 1087–100.

Gardner RJ, Kool D, Edkins E, Walpole IR, Macrae FA, Nasioulas S et al. (1997). The clinical correlates of a 3' truncating mutation (codons 1982–1983) in the adenomatous polyposis coli gene. *Gastroenterology* **113**: 326–31.

Geng Y, Weinberg RA (1993). Transforming growth factor beta effects on expression of G1 cyclins and cyclin-dependent protein kinases. *Proc Natl Acad Sci USA* **90**: 10315–19.

Goel A, Nagasaka T, Arnold CN, Inoue T, Hamilton C, Niedzwiecki D et al. (2007). The CpG island methylator phenotype and chromosomal instability are inversely correlated in sporadic colorectal cancer. *Gastroenterology* **132**: 127–38.

Goldstein NS (2006). Serrated pathway and APC (conventional)-type colorectal polyps: molecular-morphologic correlations, genetic pathways, and implications for classification. *Am J Clin Pathol* **125**: 146–53.

Gong J, Ammanamanchi S, Ko TC, Brattain MG (2003). Transforming growth factor beta 1 increases the stability of p21/WAF1/CIP1 protein and inhibits CDK2 kinase activity in human colon carcinoma FET cells. *Cancer Res* **63**: 3340–46.

Grady WM (2004). Genomic instability and colon cancer. *Cancer Metast Rev* **23**: 11–27.

Grady WM (2005). Epigenetic events in the colorectum and in colon cancer. *Biochem Soc Trans* **33**: 684–88.

Grady WM, Markowitz SD (2008). TGF-ß signaling pathway and tumor suppression. In: Derynck R, Miyazono K (eds) *The TGF-ß Family*, 1st edn. Cold Spring Harbor Laboratory Press: Cold Spring Harbor, pp 889–938.

Grady WM, Myeroff LL, Swinler SE, Rajput A, Thiagalingam S, Lutterbaugh JD et al. (1999). Mutational inactivation of transforming growth factor-beta receptor type II in microsatellite stable colon cancers. *Cancer Res* **59**: 320–24.

Grady W, Rajput A, Myeroff L, Liu D, Kwon K-H, Willis J et al. (1998). Mutation of the type II transforming growth factor-ß receptor is coincident with the transformation of human colon adenomas to malignant carcinomas. *Cancer Res* **58**: 3101–04.

Groden J, Thliveris A, Samowitz W, Carlson M, Gelbert L, Albertsen H et al. (1991). Identification and characterization of the familial adenomatous polyposis coli gene. *Cell* **66**: 589–600.

Hahn S, Schutte M, Shamsul Hoque A, Moskaluk C, da Costa L, Rozenblum E et al. (1996). *DPC4*, a candidate tumor supressor gene at human chromosome 18q21.1. *Science* **271**: 350–53.

Halford SE, Rowan AJ, Lipton L, Sieber OM, Pack K, Thomas HJ et al. (2003). Germline mutations but not somatic changes at the MYH locus contribute to the pathogenesis of unselected colorectal cancers. *Am J Pathol* **162**: 1545–48.

Hampel H, Frankel WL, Martin E, Arnold M, Khanduja K, Kuebler P et al. (2005). Screening for the Lynch syndrome (hereditary nonpolyposis colorectal cancer). *N Engl J Med* **352**: 1851–60.

Hanahan D, Weinberg RA (2000). The hallmarks of cancer. *Cell* **100**: 57–70.

Hannon G, Beach D (1994). p15^{INK4B} is a potential effector of TGF-ß-induced cell cycle arrest. *Nature* **371**: 257–61.

Harada N, Tamai Y, Ishikawa T, Sauer B, Takaku K, Oshima M et al. (1999). Intestinal polyposis in mice with a dominant stable mutation of the beta-catenin gene. *EMBO J* **18**: 5931–42.

Harvey J (1964). An unidentified virus which causes the rapid production of tumors in mice. *Nature* **204**: 1104–1105.

He TC, Sparks AB, Rago C, Hermeking H, Zawel L, da Costa LT et al. (1998). Identification of c-MYC as a target of the APC pathway [see comments]. *Science* **281**: 1509–12.

Hempen PM, Zhang L, Bansal RK, Iacobuzio-Donahue CA, Murphy KM, Maitra A et al. (2003). Evidence of selection for clones having genetic inactivation of the activin A type II receptor (ACVR2) gene in gastrointestinal cancers. *Cancer Res* **63**: 994–99.

Hermsen M, Postma C, Baak J, Weiss M, Rapallo A, Sciutto A et al. (2002). Colorectal adenoma to carcinoma progression follows multiple pathways of chromosomal instability. *Gastroenterology* **123**: 1109–19.

Herrera L, Kakati S, Gibas L, Pietrzak E, Sandberg AA (1986). Gardner syndrome in a man with an interstitial deletion of 5q. *Am J Med Genet* **25**: 473–76.

Hoosein N, McKnight M, Levine A, Mulder K, Childress K, Brattain D et al. (1989). Differential sensitivity of subclasses of human colon carcinoma cell lines to the growth inhibitory effects of transforming growth factor-ß1. *Exp Cell Res* **181**: 442–53.

Howe JR, Bair JL, Sayed MG, Anderson ME, Mitros FA, Petersen GM et al. (2001). Germline mutations of the gene encoding bone morphogenetic protein receptor 1A in juvenile polyposis. *Nat Genet* **28**: 184–87.

Howe PH, Draetta G, Leof EB (1991). Transforming growth factor beta 1 inhibition of p34cdc2 phosphorylation and histone H1 kinase activity is associated with G1/S-phase growth arrest. *Mol Cell Biol* **11**: 1185–94.

Howe JR, Roth S, Ringold JC, Summers RW, Jarvinen HJ, Sistonen P et al. (1998). Mutations in the SMAD4/DPC4 gene in juvenile polyposis [see comments]. *Science* **280**: 1086–88.

Howe JR, Shellnut J, Wagner B, Ringold JC, Sayed MG, Ahmed AF et al. (2002). Common deletion of SMAD4 in juvenile polyposis is a mutational hotspot. *Am J Hum Genet* **70**: 1357–62.

Huang J, Papadopoulos N, McKinley A, Farrington S, Curtis L, Wyllie A et al. (1996). APC mutations in colorectal tumors with mismatch repair deficiency. *Proc Natl Acad Sci USA* **93**: 9049–54.

Hulsken J, Birchmeier W, Behrens J (1994). E-cadherin and APC compete for the interaction with beta-catenin and the cytoskeleton. *J Cell Biol* **127**: 2061–69.

Iacopetta B, Russo A, Bazan V, Dardanoni G, Gebbia N, Soussi T et al. (2006). Functional categories of TP53 mutation in colorectal cancer: results of an International Collaborative Study. *Ann Oncol* **17**: 842–47.

Ikenoue T, Hikiba Y, Kanai F, Aragaki J, Tanaka Y, Imamura J et al. (2004). Different effects of point mutations within the B-Raf glycine-rich loop in colorectal tumors on mitogen-activated protein/extracellular signal-regulated kinase kinase/extracellular signal-regulated kinase and nuclear factor kappaB pathway and cellular transformation. *Cancer Res* **64**: 3428–35.

Iwakuma T, Parant JM, Fasulo M, Zwart E, Jacks T, de Vries A et al. (2004). Mutation at p53 serine 389 does not rescue the embryonic lethality in mdm2 or mdm4 null mice. *Oncogene* **23**: 7644–50.

Jacoby R, Marshall D, Kailas S, Schlack S, Harms B, Love R (1995). Genetic instability associated with adenoma to carcinoma progression in hereditary nonpolyposis colon cancer. *Gastroenterology* **109**: 73–82.

Janda E, Lehmann K, Killisch I, Jechlinger M, Herzig M, Downward J et al. (2002). Ras and TGF[beta] cooperatively regulate epithelial cell plasticity and metastasis: dissection of Ras signaling pathways. *J Cell Biol* **156**: 299–313.

Jass JR (2004). Hyperplastic polyps and colorectal cancer: is there a link? *Clin Gastroenterol Hepatol* **2**: 1–8.

Jen J, Kim H, Piantadosi S, Liu ZF, Levitt RC, Sistonen P et al. (1994a). Allelic loss of chromosome 18q and prognosis in colorectal cancer [see comments]. *N Engl J Med* **331**: 213–21.

Jen J, Powell SM, Papadopoulos N, Smith KJ, Hamilton SR, Vogelstein B et al. (1994b). Molecular determinants of dysplasia in colorectal lesions. *Cancer Res* **54**: 5523–26.

Jin T, George Fantus I, Sun J (2008). Wnt and beyond Wnt: multiple mechanisms control the transcriptional property of beta-catenin. *Cell Signal* **20**: 1697–704.

Jin D, Spencer F, Jeang K (1998). Human T cell leukemia virus type 1 oncoprotein Tax targets the human mitotic checkpoint protein MAD1. *Cell* **93**: 81–91.

Jiricny J (1998). Replication errors: cha(lle)nging the genome. *EMBO J* **17**: 6427–36.

Kambara T, Simms LA, Whitehall VL, Spring KJ, Wynter CV, Walsh MD et al. (2004). BRAF mutation is associated with DNA methylation in serrated polyps and cancers of the colorectum. *Gut* **53**: 1137–44.

Kane M, Loda M, Gaida G, Lipman J, Mishra R, Goldman H et al. (1997). Methylation of the *hMLH1* promoter correlates with lack of expression of hMLH1 in sporadic colon tumors and mismatch repair-defective human tumor cell lines. *Cancer Res* **57**: 808–11.

Kawabata M, Imamura T, Miyazono K (1998). Signal transduction by bone morphogenetic proteins. *Cytokine Growth Factor Rev* **9**: 49–61.

Kawanishi J, Kato J, Sasaki K, Fujii S, Watanabe N, Niitsu Y (1995). Loss of E-cadherin-dependent cell-cell adhesion due to mutation of the beta-catenin gene in a human cancer cell line, HSC-39. *Mol Cell Biol* **15**: 1175–81.

Keeton MR, Curriden SA, van Zonneveld AJ, Loskutoff DJ (1991). Identification of regulatory sequences in the type 1 plasminogen activator inhibitor gene responsive to transforming growth factor beta. *J Biol Chem* **266**: 23048–52.

Kikuchi-Yanoshita R, Konishi M, Ito S, Seki M, Tanaka K, Maeda Y et al. (1992). Genetic changes of both p53 alleles associated with the conversion from colorectal adenoma to early carcinoma in familial adenomatous polyposis and non-familial adenomatous polyposis patients. *Cancer Res* **52**: 3965–71.

Kinzler KW, Vogelstein B (1996). Lessons from Hereditary Colorectal Cancer. *Cell* **87**: 159–70.

Kirsten W, Mayer L (1967). Morphologic responses to a murine erythroblastosis virus. *J Nat Cancer Inst* **39**: 311–35.

Kitaeva M, Grogan L, Williams J, Dimond E, Nakahara K, Hausner P et al. (1997). Mutations in ß-catenin are uncommon in colorectal cancer occurring in occasional replication error-positive tumors. *Cancer Res* **57**: 4478–81.

Kolodner RD, Putnam CD, Myung K (2002). Maintenance of genome stability in Saccharomyces cerevisiae. *Science* **297**: 552–57.

Kolodner R, Tytell J, Schmeits J, Kane M, Gupta R, Weger J et al. (1999). Germ-line *msh6* mutations in colorectal cancer families. *Cancer Res* **59**: 5068–74.

Konishi M, Kikuchi-Yanoshita R, Tanaka K, Muraoka M, Onda A, Okumura Y et al. (1996). Molecular nature of colon tumors in hereditary nonpolyposis colon cancer, familial polyposis, and sporadic colon cancer. *Gastroenterology* **111**: 307–17.

Laken SJ, Petersen GM, Gruber SB, Oddoux C, Ostrer H, Giardiello FM et al. (1997). Familial colorectal cancer in Ashkenazim due to a hypermutable tract in APC. *Nat Genet* **17**: 79–83.

Lammi L, Arte S, Somer M, Jarvinen H, Lahermo P, Thesleff I et al. (2004). Mutations in AXIN2 cause familial tooth agenesis and predispose to colorectal cancer. *Am J Hum Genet* **74**: 1043–50.

Lane DP (1993). Cancer. A death in the life of p53 [news; comment]. *Nature* **362**: 786–7.

Laurent-Puig P, Olschwang S, Delattre O, Remvikos Y, Asselain B, Melot T et al. (1992). Survival and acquired genetic alterations in colorectal cancer [see comments]. *Gastroenterology* **102**: 1136–41.

Lengauer C, Kinzler K, Vogelstein B (1998). Genetic instabilities in human cancers. *Nature* **396**: 643–49.

Levine AJ (1997). p53, the cellular gatekeeper for growth and division. *Cell* **88**: 323–31.

Lin D, Shields MT, Ullrich SJ, Appella E, Mercer WE (1992). Growth arrest induced by wild-type p53 protein blocks cells prior to or near the restriction point in late G1 phase. *Proc Natl Acad Sci USA* **89**: 9210–14.

Lipton L, Halford SE, Johnson V, Novelli MR, Jones A, Cummings C et al. (2003). Carcinogenesis in MYH-associated polyposis follows a distinct genetic pathway. *Cancer Res* **63**: 7595–99.

Little MP, Vineis P, Li G (2008). A stochastic carcinogenesis model incorporating multiple types of genomic instability fitted to colon cancer data. *J Theor Biol* **254**: 229–38.

Liu W, Dong X, Mai M, Seelan RS, Taniguchi K, Krishnadath KK et al. (2000). Mutations in AXIN2 cause colorectal cancer with defective mismatch repair by activating beta-catenin/TCF signalling. *Nat Genet* **26**: 146–7.

Loeb KR, Kostner H, Firpo E, Norwood T, D Tsuchiya T, Clurman BE et al. (2005). A mouse model for cyclin E-dependent genetic instability and tumorigenesis. *Cancer Cell* **8**: 35–47.

Lothe RA, Hektoen M, Johnsen H, Meling GI, Andersen TI, Rognum TO et al. (1998). The APC gene I1307K variant is rare in Norwegian patients with familial and sporadic colorectal or breast cancer. *Cancer Res* **58**: 2923–4.

Lubomierski N, Plotz G, Wormek M, Engels K, Kriener S, Trojan J et al. (2005). BRAF mutations in colorectal carcinoma suggest two entities of microsatellite-unstable tumors. *Cancer* **104**: 952–61.

Lynch HT, de la Chapelle A (1999). Genetic susceptibility to non-polyposis colorectal cancer. *J Med Genet* **36**: 801–18.

Maley CC, Galipeau PC, Finley JC, Wongsurawat VJ, Li X, Sanchez CA et al. (2006). Genetic clonal diversity predicts progression to esophageal adenocarcinoma. *Nat Genet* **38**: 468–73.

Markowitz S, Roberts A (1996). Tumor supressor activity of the TGF-ß pathway in human cancers. *Cytokine Growth Factor Rev* **7**: 93–102.

Markowitz S, Wang J, Myeroff L, Parsons R, Sun L, Lutterbaugh J et al. (1995). Inactivation of the type II TGF-ß receptor in colon cancer cells with microsatellite instability. *Science* **268**: 1336–38.

Martinez-Lopez E, Abad A, Font A, Monzo M, Ojanguren I, Pifarre A et al. (1998). Allelic loss on chromosome 18q as a prognostic marker in stage II colorectal cancer [see comments]. *Gastroenterology* **114**: 1180–87.

Massague J (1996). TGF-ß signaling: receptors, transducers, and mad proteins. *Cell* **85**: 947–50.

Midgley RS, Yanagisawa Y, Kerr DJ (2009). Evolution of nonsurgical therapy for colorectal cancer. *Nat Clin Pract Gastroenterol Hepatol* **6**: 108–20.

Miyaki M, Iijima T, Kimura J, Yasuno M, Mori T, Hayashi Y et al. (1999). Frequent mutation of beta-catenin and APC genes in primary colorectal tumors from patients with hereditary nonpolyposis colorectal cancer. *Cancer Res* **59**: 4506–09.

Miyaki M, Konishi M, Kikuchi-Yanoshita R, Enomoto M, Igari T, Tanaka K et al. (1994). Characteristics of somatic mutation of the adenomatous polyposis coli gene in colorectal tumors. *Cancer Res* **54**: 3011–20.

Miyoshi Y, Nagase H, Ando H, Horii A, Ichii S, Nakatsuru S et al. (1992). Somatic mutations of the APC gene in colorectal tumors: mutation cluster region in the APC gene. *Hum Mol Genet* **1**: 229–33.

Mizuguchi T, Collod-Beroud G, Akiyama T, Abifadel M, Harada N, Morisaki T et al. (2004). Heterozygous TGFBR2 mutations in Marfan syndrome. *Nat Genet* **36**: 855–60.

Moon RT, Brown JD, Yang-Snyder JA, Miller JR (1997). Structurally related receptors and antagonists compete for secreted Wnt ligands. *Cell* **88**: 725–28.

Mori Y, Yin J, Rashid A, Leggett BA, Young J, Simms L et al. (2001). Instabilotyping: comprehensive identification of frameshift mutations caused by coding region microsatellite instability. *Cancer Res* **61**: 6046–49.

Morin PJ, Sparks AB, Korinek V, Barker N, Clevers H, Vogelstein B et al. (1997). Activation of beta-catenin-Tcf signaling in colon cancer by mutations in beta-catenin or APC [see comments]. *Science* **275**: 1787–90.

Munoz N, Upton M, Rojas A, Washington M, Lin L, Chytil A et al. (2006). Transforming growth factor beta receptor type II inactivation induces transformation of intestinal neoplasms initiated by Apc mutation. *Cancer Res* **66**: 9837–44.

Myeroff L, Parsons R, Kim S-J, Hedrick L, Cho K, Orth K et al. (1995). A transforming growth factor ß receptor type II gene mutation common in colon and gastric but rare in endometrial cancers with microsatellite instability. *Cancer Res* **55**: 5545–47.

Nagatake M, Takagi Y, Osada H, Uchida K, Mitsudomi T, Saji S et al. (1996). Somatic in vivo alterations of the DPC4 gene at 18q21 in human lung cancers. *Cancer Res* **56**: 2718–20.

Nishisho I, Nakamura Y, Miyoshi Y, Miki Y, Ando H, Horii A et al. (1991). Mutations of chromosome 5q21 genes in FAP and colorectal cancer patients. *Science* **253**: 665–69.

Noffsinger AE (2009). Serrated polyps and colorectal cancer: new pathway to malignancy. *Annu Rev Pathol* **4**: 343–64.

Ochiai A, Hirohashi S (1997). Multiple genetic alterations in gastric cancer. In: Sugimura T, Sasako M (eds.) *Gastric Cancer*. Oxford University Press: New York, pp. 87–99.

Ohue M, Tomita N, Monden T, Fujita M, Fukunaga M, Takami K et al. (1994). A frequent alteration of p53 gene in carcinoma in adenoma of colon. *Cancer Res* **54**: 4798–804.

Olinski R, Zastawny T, Budzbon J, Skokowski J, Zegarski W, Dizdaroglu M (1992). DNA base modifications in chromatin of human cancerous tissues. *FEBS Lett* **309**: 193–98.

Olschwang S, Hamelin R, Laurent-Puig P, Thuille B, De Rycke Y, Li YJ et al. (1997). Alternative genetic pathways in colorectal carcinogenesis. *Proc Natl Acad Sci USA* **94**: 12122–27.

Olschwang S, Tiret A, Laurent-Puig P, Muleris M, Parc R, Thomas G (1993). Restriction of ocular fundus lesions to a specific subgroup of APC mutations in adenomatous polyposis coli patients. *Cell* **75**: 959–68.

Ostwald C, Linnebacher M, Weirich V, Prall F (2009). Chromosomally and microsatellite stable colorectal carcinomas without the CpG island methylator phenotype in a molecular classification. *Int J Oncol* **35**: 321–27.

Park WS, Oh RR, Park JY, Lee SH, Shin MS, Kim YS et al. (1999). Frequent somatic mutations of the beta-catenin gene in intestinal-type gastric cancer. *Cancer Res* **59**: 4257–60.

Park WS, Park JY, Oh RR, Yoo NJ, Lee SH, Shin MS et al. (2000). A distinct tumor suppressor gene locus on chromosome 15q21.1 in sporadic form of colorectal cancer. *Cancer Res* **60**: 70–73.

Parsons R, Myeroff LL, Liu B, Willson JK, Markowitz SD, Kinzler KW et al. (1995). Microsatellite instability and mutations of the transforming growth factor beta type II receptor gene in colorectal cancer. *Cancer Res* **55**: 5548–50.

Parsons DW, Wang TL, Samuels Y, Bardelli A, Cummins JM, DeLong L et al. (2005). Colorectal cancer: mutations in a signalling pathway. *Nature* **436**: 792.

Pasche B, Knobloch TJ, Bian Y, Liu J, Phukan S, Rosman D et al. (2005). Somatic acquisition and signaling of TGFBR1*6A in cancer. *J Am Med Assoc* **294**: 1634–46.

Perez-Losada J, Mao JH, Balmain A (2005). Control of genomic instability and epithelial tumor development by the p53-Fbxw7/Cdc4 pathway. *Cancer Res* **65**: 6488–92.

Phelps RA, Chidester S, Dehghanizadeh S, Phelps J, Sandoval IT, Rai K et al. (2009). A two-step model for colon adenoma initiation and progression caused by APC loss. *Cell* **137**: 623–34.

Philp AJ, Campbell IG, Leet C, Vincan E, Rockman SP, Whitehead RH et al. (2001). The phosphatidylinositol 3'-kinase p85alpha gene is an oncogene in human ovarian and colon tumors. *Cancer Res* **61**: 7426–29.

Pittman AM, Naranjo S, Webb E, Broderick P, Lips EH, van Wezel T et al. (2009). The colorectal cancer risk at 18q21 is caused by a novel variant altering SMAD7 expression. *Genome Res* **19**: 987–93.

Popat S, Hubner R, Houlston RS (2005). Systematic review of microsatellite instability and colorectal cancer prognosis. *J Clin Oncol* **23**: 609–18.

Powell SM, Petersen GM, Krush AJ, Booker S, Jen J, Giardiello FM et al. (1993). Molecular diagnosis of familial adenomatous polyposis [see comments]. *N Engl J Med* **329**: 1982–87.

Powell SM, Zilz N, Beazer-Barclay Y, Bryan TM, Hamilton SR, Thibodeau SN et al. (1992). APC mutations occur early during colorectal tumorigenesis. *Nature* **359**: 235–37.

Rajagopalan H, Bardelli A, Lengauer C, Kinzler KW, Vogelstein B, Velculescu VE (2002). Tumorigenesis: RAF/RAS oncogenes and mismatch-repair status. *Nature* **418**: 934.

Rajagopalan H, Jallepalli PV, Rago C, Velculescu VE, Kinzler KW, Vogelstein B et al. (2004). Inactivation of hCDC4 can cause chromosomal instability. *Nature* **428**: 77–81.

Rajagopalan H, Lengauer C (2004). hCDC4 and genetic instability in cancer. *Cell Cycle* **3**: 693–4.

Riggins G, Thiagalingam S, Rozenblum E, Weinstein C, Kern S, Hamilton S et al. (1996). Mad-related genes in the human. *Nat Genet* **13**: 347–49.

Rojas A, Padidam M, Cress D, Grady WM (2009). TGF-ß receptor levels regulated the specificity of signaling pathway activation and biological effects of TGF-ß. *Biochim Biophys Acta-Mol Cell Res* **1793**: 1165–73.

Rooney P, Murray G, Stevenson D, Haites N, Cassidy J, McLeod H (1999). Comparative genomic hybridization and chromosomal instability in solid tumors. *Br J Cancer* **80**: 862–73.

Roth S, Sistonen P, Salovaara R, Hemminki A, Loukola A, Johansson M et al. (1999). SMAD genes in juvenile polyposis. *Genes Chromos Cancer* **26**: 54–61.

Rotman G, Shiloh Y (1998). ATM:from gene to function. *Human Mol Gen* **7**: 1555–63.

Rubinfeld B, Albert I, Porfiri E, Munemitsu S, Polakis P (1997). Loss of beta-catenin regulation by the APC tumor suppressor protein correlates with loss of structure due to common somatic mutations of the gene. *Cancer Res* **57**: 4624–30.

Saha S, Bardelli A, Buckhaults P, Velculescu VE, Rago C, Croix BS et al. (2001). A phosphatase associated with metastasis of colorectal cancer. *Science* **294**: 1343–46.

Sakamoto Y, Kitazawa R, Maeda S, Kitazawa S (2001). Methylation of CpG loci in 5'-flanking region alters steady-state expression of adenomatous polyposis coli gene in colon cancer cell lines. *J Cell Biochem* **80**: 415–23.

Samowitz WS, Albertsen H, Herrick J, Levin TR, Sweeney C, Murtaugh MA et al. (2005). Evaluation of a large, population-based sample supports a CpG island methylator phenotype in colon cancer. *Gastroenterology* **129**: 837–45.

Samowitz WS, Powers MD, Spirio LN, Nollet F, van Roy F, Slattery ML (1999). Beta-catenin mutations are more frequent in small colorectal adenomas than in larger adenomas and invasive carcinomas. *Cancer Res* **59**: 1442–44.

Sampson JR, Dolwani S, Jones S, Eccles D, Ellis A, Evans DG et al. (2003). Autosomal recessive colorectal adenomatous polyposis due to inherited mutations of MYH. *Lancet* **362**: 39–41.

Samuels Y, Wang Z, Bardelli A, Silliman N, Ptak J, Szabo S et al. (2004). High frequency of mutations of the PIK3CA gene in human cancers. *Science* **304**: 554.

Scheele JS, Rhee JM, Boss GR (1995). Determination of absolute amounts of GDP and GTP bound to Ras in mammalian cells: comparison of parental and Ras-overproducing NIH 3T3 fibroblasts. *Proc Natl Acad Sci USA* **92**: 1097–100.

Seoane J, Le HV, Shen L, Anderson SA, Massague J (2004). Integration of Smad and forkhead pathways in the control of neuroepithelial and glioblastoma cell proliferation. *Cell* **117**: 211–23.

Shen L, Kondo Y, Hamilton SR, Rashid A, Issa JP (2003). P14 methylation in human colon cancer is associated with microsatellite instability and wild-type p53. *Gastroenterology* **124**: 626–33.

Shih IM, Zhou W, Goodman SN, Lengauer C, Kinzler KW, Vogelstein B (2001). Evidence that genetic instability occurs at an early stage of colorectal tumorigenesis. *Cancer Res* **61**: 818–22.

Shtutman M, Zhurinsky J, Simcha I, Albanese C, D'Amico M, Pestell R et al. (1999). The cyclin D1 gene is a target of the beta-catenin/LEF-1 pathway. *Proc Natl Acad Sci USA* **96**: 5522–27.

Sieber OM, Lipton L, Crabtree M, Heinimann K, Fidalgo P, Phillips RK et al. (2003). Multiple colorectal adenomas, classic adenomatous polyposis, and germ-line mutations in MYH. *N Engl J Med* **348**: 791–99.

Sjoblom T, Jones S, Wood LD, Parsons DW, Lin J, Barber TD et al. (2006). The consensus coding sequences of human breast and colorectal cancers. *Science* **314**: 268–74.

Slaby O, Sobkova K, Svoboda M, Garajova I, Fabian P, Hrstka R et al. (2009). Significant overexpression of Hsp110 gene during colorectal cancer progression. *Oncol Rep* **21**: 1235–41.

Smith ML, Chen IT, Zhan Q, Bae I, Chen CY, Gilmer TM et al. (1994). Interaction of the p53-regulated protein Gadd45 with proliferating cell nuclear antigen [see comments]. *Science* **266**: 1376–80.

Smith AJ, Matthews JB, Hall RC (1998). Transforming growth factor-beta1 (TGF-beta1) in dentine matrix. Ligand activation and receptor expression. *Eur J Oral Sci* **106**(**Suppl 1**): 179–84.

Somasundaram K (2000). Tumor suppressor p53: regulation and function. *Front Biosci* **5**: D424–D37.

Soravia C, Berk T, Madlensky L, Mitri A, Cheng H, Gallinger S et al. (1998). Genotype-phenotype correlations in attenuated adenomatous polyposis coli. *Am J Hum Genet* **62**: 1290–301.

Sparks AB, Morin PJ, Vogelstein B, Kinzler KW (1998). Mutational analysis of the APC/beta-catenin/Tcf pathway in colorectal cancer. *Cancer Res* **58**: 1130–34.

Spirio L, Olschwang S, Groden J, Robertson M, Samowitz W, Joslyn G et al. (1993). Alleles of the APC gene: an attenuated form of familial polyposis. *Cell* **75**: 951–57.

Spirio L, Otterud B, Stauffer D, Lynch H, Lynch P, Watson P et al. (1992). Linkage of a variant or attenuated form of adenomatous polyposis coli to the adenomatous polyposis coli (APC) locus. *Am J Hum Genet* **51**: 92–100.

Spirio LN, Samowitz W, Robertson J, Robertson M, Burt RW, Leppert M et al. (1998). Alleles of APC modulate the frequency and classes of mutations that lead to colon polyps. *Nat Genet* **20**: 385–88.

Suzuki H, Watkins DN, Jair KW, Schuebel KE, Markowitz SD, Dong Chen W et al. (2004). Epigenetic inactivation of SFRP genes allows constitutive WNT signaling in colorectal cancer. *Nat Genet* **36**: 417–22.

Takagi Y, Kohmura H, Futamura M, Kida H, Tanemura H, Shimokawa K et al. (1996). Somatic alterations of the DPC4 gene in human colorectal cancers in vivo. *Gastroenterology* **111**: 1369–72.

Takaku K, Miyoshi H, Matsunaga A, Oshima M, Sasaki N, Taketo MM (1999). Gastric and duodenal polyps in Smad4 (Dpc4) knockout mice. *Cancer Res* **59**: 6113–17.

Takaku K, Oshima M, Miyoshi H, Matsui M, Seldin M, Taketo M (1998). Intestinal tumorigenesis in compound mutant mice of both *Dpc4* (*Smad4*) and *Apc* genes. *Cell* **92**: 645–56.

Takenoshita S, Tani M, Mogi A, Nagashima M, Nagamachi Y, Bennett WP et al. (1998). Mutation analysis of the Smad2 gene in human colon cancers using genomic DNA and intron primers. *Carcinogenesis* **19**: 803–07.

Tenesa A, Farrington SM, Prendergast JG, Porteous ME, Walker M, Haq N et al. (2008). Genome-wide association scan identifies a colorectal cancer susceptibility locus on 11q23 and replicates risk loci at 8q24 and 18q21. *Nat Genet* **40**: 631–37.

Trobridge P, Knoblaugh S, Washington MK, Munoz NM, Tsuchiya KD, Rojas A et al. (2009). TGF-ss receptor inactivation and mutant Kras induce intestinal neoplasms in mice via a ss-catenin independent pathway. *Gastroenterology* **136**: 1680–88.

Vilar E, Mukherjee B, Kuick R, Raskin L, Misek DE, Taylor JM et al. (2009). Gene expression patterns in mismatch repair-deficient colorectal cancers highlight the potential therapeutic role of inhibitors of the phosphatidylinositol 3-kinase-AKT-mammalian target of rapamycin pathway. *Clin Cancer Res* **15**: 2829–39.

Vivanco I, Sawyers CL (2002). The phosphatidylinositol 3-Kinase AKT pathway in human cancer. *Nat Rev Cancer* **2**: 489–501.

Vogelstein B, Fearon ER, Hamilton SR, Kern SE, Preisinger AC, Leppert M et al. (1988). Genetic alterations during colorectal-tumor development. *N Engl J Med* **319**: 525–32.

Vogelstein B, Fearon ER, Kern SE, Hamilton SR, Preisinger AC, Nakamura Y et al. (1989). Allelotype of colorectal carcinomas. *Science* **244**: 207–11.

Wakefield LM, Roberts AB (2002). TGF-beta signaling: positive and negative effects on tumorigenesis. *Curr Opin Genet Dev* **12**: 22–29.

Walther A, Johnstone E, Swanton C, Midgley R, Tomlinson I, Kerr D (2009). Genetic prognostic and predictive markers in colorectal cancer. *Nat Rev Cancer* **9**: 489–99.

Wang Z, Cummins JM, Shen D, Cahill DP, Jallepalli PV, Wang TL et al. (2004b). Three classes of genes mutated in colorectal cancers with chromosomal instability. *Cancer Res* **64**: 2998–3001.

Wang L, Cunningham JM, Winters JL, Guenther JC, French AJ, Boardman LA et al. (2003). BRAF mutations in colon cancer are not likely attributable to defective DNA mismatch repair. *Cancer Res* **63**: 5209–12.

Wang J, Sergina N, Ko TC, Gong J, Brattain MG (2004a). Autocrine and exogenous transforming growth factor beta control cell cycle inhibition through pathways with different sensitivity. *J Biol Chem* **279**: 40237–44.

Wang Z, Shen D, Parsons DW, Bardelli A, Sager J, Szabo S et al. (2004c). Mutational analysis of the tyrosine phosphatome in colorectal cancers. *Science* **304**: 1164–66.

Watanabe T, Wu TT, Catalano PJ, Ueki T, Satriano R, Haller DG et al. (2001). Molecular predictors of survival after adjuvant chemotherapy for colon cancer. *N Engl J Med* **344**: 1196–206.

Wong DJ, Foster SA, Galloway DA, Reid BJ (1999). Progressive region-specific de novo methylation of the p16 CpG island in primary human mammary epithelial cell strains during escape from M(0) growth arrest. *Mol Cell Biol* **19**: 5642–51.

Wong P, Verselis SJ, Garber JE, Schneider K, DiGianni L, Stockwell DH et al. (2006). Prevalence of early onset colorectal cancer in 397 patients with classic Li-Fraumeni syndrome. *Gastroenterology* **130**: 73–79.

Woodford-Richens K, Williamson J, Bevan S, Young J, Leggett B, Frayling I et al. (2000). Allelic loss at SMAD4 in polyps from juvenile polyposis patients and use of fluorescence in situ hybridization to demonstrate clonal origin of the epithelium. *Cancer Res* **60**: 2477–82.

Xu X, Brodie SG, Yang X, Im YH, Parks WT, Chen L et al. (2000). Haploid loss of the tumor suppressor Smad4/Dpc4 initiates gastric polyposis and cancer in mice. *Oncogene* **19**: 1868–74.

Yamamoto H, Sawai H, Weber T, Rodriguez-Bigas M, Perucho M (1998). Somatic frameshift mutations in DNA mismatch repair and proapoptosis genes in hereditary nonpolyposis colorectal cancer. *Cancer Res* **58**: 997–1003.

Yeatman TJ, Chambers AF (2003). Osteopontin and colon cancer progression. *Clin Exp Metast* **20**: 85–90.

Zhang H, Tombline G, Weber B (1998). BRCA1, BRCA2, and DNA damage reponse: collision or collusion. *Cell* **92**: 433–36.

Zhao Y (1999). Transforming growth factor-beta (TGF-beta) type I and type II receptors are both required for TGF-beta-mediated extracellular matrix production in lung fibroblasts. *Mol Cell Endocrinol* **150**: 91–97.

Zhou W, Goodman SN, Galizia G, Lieto E, Ferraraccio F, Pignatelli C et al. (2002). Counting alleles to predict recurrence of early-stage colorectal cancers. *Lancet* **359**: 219–25.

Zhou H, Kuang J, Zhong L, Kuo W-l, Gray J, Sahin A et al. (1998). Tumour amplified kinase STK15/BTAK induces centrosome amplification, aneuploidy and transformation. *Nat Genet* **20**: 189–93.

Chapter 4

EPIGENETICS OF COLORECTAL CANCER

F. Javier Carmona[1] and Manel Esteller[2]

[1] Cancer Epigenetics and Biology Program (PEBC), Bellvitge Institute for Biomedical Research (IDIBELL), 08907 L'Hospitalet, Barcelona, Catalonia, Spain

[2] Cancer Epigenetics and Biology Program (PEBC), Bellvitge Institute for Biomedical Research (IDIBELL), 08907 L'Hospitalet, Barcelona, Catalonia, Spain, e-mail: mesteller@iconcologia.net

Abstract: Epigenetic research is increasingly gaining prominence as it provides new insights in explaining human diseases, as well as new diagnostic and prognostic tools. Colorectal cancer is a prime model for cancer epigenetics, as aberrant DNA methylation processes characterize all stages of the disease. This chapter recapitulates the contribution of epigenetics to colorectal cancer research, emphasizing its connection to human cancer metastasis.

Key words: Epigenetics · DNA methylation · Histones · MicroRNAs · Metastasis

4.1 Introduction

'Epigenetics' is a term used to describe mitotically and meiotically heritable states of gene activity that are not due to changes in DNA sequence. Epigenetic events are important in all aspects of biology. Research carried out within the past decade has shown that these processes have a key role in carcinogenesis and tumour progression.

Epigenetic modifications are stable marks, resulting from covalent chemical alterations on chromatin. These changes determine gene expression and can be inherited throughout mitotic divisions without affecting the primary DNA sequence. In contrast to genetic information, which is homogeneous in an organism regardless of cell type, epigenetic modifications are characteristic of different cell types or differentiation states and play a key role in defining the transcriptome, which ultimately determines the identity of each cell type (Fisher, 2002). Epigenetic information is stored by covalent modifications of two classes of biomolecules: DNA and histones. Epigenetic mechanisms also involve positioning of histone variants, ATP-dependent nucleosome remodelling and non-coding RNAs. This chapter will explore the roles of these various forms of epigenetic modifications and their relationship with colorectal cancer (CRC).

So far, the most widely studied epigenetic modification in humans is the cytosine methylation of DNA within the dinucleotide cytosine phosphate guanine (CpG). Approximately 3–6% of all cytosine residues are methylated in a normal human genome. The chemical reaction is carried out by DNA methyltransferases (DNMTs) and consists on the addition of a methyl group on the 5′ position of the cytosine pyrimidinic ring. There are two major DNMTs: DNMT1, which is responsible for the maintenance of methylation patterns and DNMT3B that carries out de novo methylation in association with DNA replication processes.

The distribution of the CpG dinucleotides in the genome is not random. Indeed, they tend to cluster in CpG islands: CpG-rich regions located at the 5′ end region whether or not the gene is being transcribed (Bird, 2002). The promoter and first exon of approximately 60% of human genes are usually unmethylated in normal cells.

Histone marks also exhibit a wide range of possible combinations that, in coordination with DNA methylation events, regulate chromatin architecture and modulate gene transcription. Covalent modifications of histone proteins can orchestrate conformational changes of chromatin, converting densely compacted and inactive (hetero-) chromatin to active open (eu-) chromatin. There are at least eight distinct types of modifications found within histones, including acetylation, methylation, phosphorylation and ubiquitination. Specific antibodies and mass spectrometry have identified over 60 different residues on histones where modifications can take place (Berger, 2007; Kouzarides, 2007; Martin and Zhang, 2005; Shilatifard, 2006). Increased complexity comes partly from the fact that methylation at lysines and arginines may take up to three forms: mono-, di-, or trimethylation of lysines and mono- or dimethylation (asymmetric or symmetric) of arginines (Kouzarides, 2007).

An additional layer of intricacy arises from the dynamic cross-talk that occurs between different histone marks while recruiting protein complexes, as well as those between histone modifications and DNA methylation signatures, which directly affect chromatin conformation (Esteller, 2007a).

MicroRNAs (miRNAs) are a new class of non-coding regulatory RNAs that have recently been described. They are small non-coding RNAs of about 22 nucleotides in length that regulate gene expression in a number of eukaryotic organisms (He and Hannon, 2004). miRNAs play key roles in all cellular processes, as they control the expression of genes involved in proliferation, differentiation, apoptosis and development. Moreover, recent studies report altered miRNA expression patterns in cancer (Lu et al., 2005; Melo et al., 2009). Some of these are down-regulated while others are overexpressed, suggesting that they play different roles as either tumour suppressor genes or oncogenes, respectively (Lu et al., 2005; Melo et al., 2009). Furthermore, miRNA expression has been linked with epigenetic regulation through DNA methylation (Lujambio et al., 2007; Saito and Jones, 2006), and a specific miRNA DNA methylation profile has been linked to metastatic development (Lujambio et al., 2008).

Concerted epigenetic phenomena are natural and essential for many biological functions, but if they occur improperly, there can have major adverse health effects. Epigenetic alterations have been identified in almost all types of human cancer, and may be involved in all stages of tumour development and progression (Esteller, 2008). For this reason, epigenetics have been promoted to front rank becoming a field of intense biomedical research.

Despite the intense investigation carried out in this field over the past decades, it is only recently that we have witnessed a dramatic increase in information about the roles of these alterations in disease. Major contributions to this knowledge have come from the development of genome-wide approaches for studying histone modifications on a genomic scale. These methods combine Chromatin Immunoprecipitation (ChIP) with high-throughput techniques including DNA microarrays and high-throughput sequencing (ChIP-ChIP and ChIP-Seq, respectively). In the field of DNA methylation, genome-wide techniques have also been developed that enable researchers to interrogate the methylation status of specific regions of the genome or identify the entire spectrum of genes silenced by epigenetic mechanisms during cancer development (Bibikova et al., 2006; Suzuki et al., 2002).

Colorectal cancer is now increasingly cited as a prime example of a disease in which epigenetic changes influence tumourigenesis. Numerous studies have reported a wide range of epigenetic lesions that affect the initial stages of tumour development and lead to malignant carcinoma. Several DNA methylation defects, abnormal histone marks as well as aberrant miRNA expression are known to coincide with CRC progression (Fig. 4.1), and they are still the subject of intense

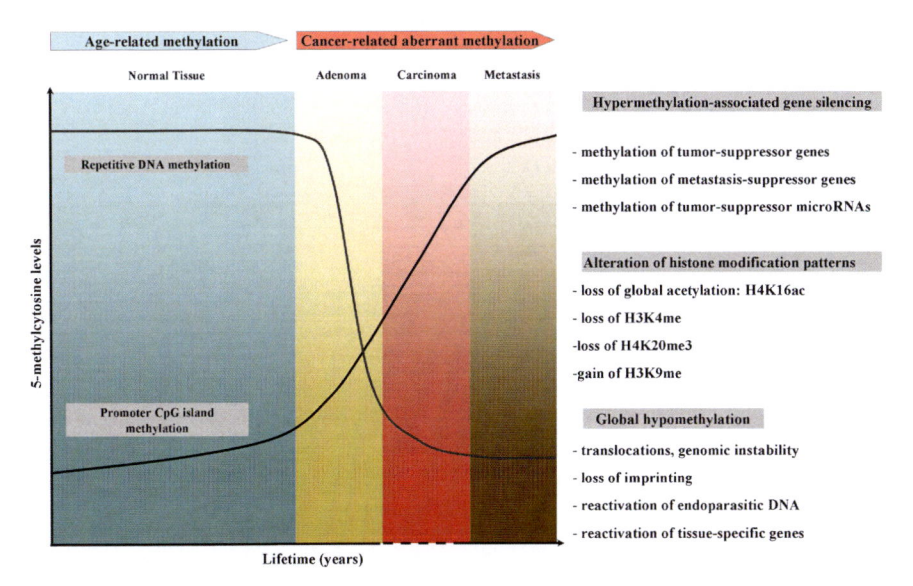

Fig. 4.1 Epigenetic defects occurring during colorectal cancer progression. In conjunction with phenotypic cellular changes and the accumulation of genetic defects, there is a progressive loss of total DNA methylation content that leads to genetic instability, an increased frequency of hypermethylated CpG islands that inactivates tumour suppressor genes, and an increased histone modification imbalance as the disease develops

investigation as key events in the carcinogenic sequence (Grady, 2005). Epigenetics offer new opportunities for the clinical management of the disease due to the plasticity of the epigenetic changes and the potential to revert them. Currently, CRC epigenetics is a burgeoning field and constitutes a remarkable model for comprehending how epigenetics and genetics interact to trigger malignancy.

4.2 DNA Methylation Defects in Colorectal Cancer

In colorectal neoplasias, aberrant DNA methylation arises very early in tumour (Kondo and Issa, 2004). Consequently, research over the past few years has accumulated evidence that epigenetic changes such as promoter hypermethylation and loss of imprinting (LOI) can occur in histologically normal epithelium. These normal epithelia give rise to a polyclonal cell population from which neoplastic clones can develop (Ehrlich, 2002).

The mechanisms underlying these alterations are still under investigation and have not yet been fully clarified. It is generally accepted that, compared with normal tissue, cancer cells undergo a process of global hypomethylation accompanied by regional hypermethylation of specific gene-associated CpG islands that are normally unmethylated (Fig. 4.1). DNA methylation defects in relation to cancer were first reported in 1983 (Feinberg and Vogelstein, 1983). From that moment on, several milestones were met in succession: hypermethylation of tumour suppressor genes (Greger et al., 1989), the development of a mouse model for cancer epigenetics (Christofori et al., 1995), the association of specific DNA methylation profiles with tumour types (Costello et al., 2000; Esteller et al., 2001), the arrival of the first epigenetic drug-based therapy (Issa and Kantarjian, 2005) and the onset of epigenomics (Esteller, 2007a).

Bearing in mind all the above, identification of DNA methylation signatures in CRC and other types of cancer should be helpful, not only for detecting potential markers for diagnosis, chemo-prediction and prognosis, but also in the depiction of the pathways of progression.

4.2.1 Hypomethylation of DNA

In spite of the advances in epigenetic research in cancer, the role of DNA hypomethylation in colorectal neoplasia remains unclear. However, there are some well-defined aspects of the loss of 5-methylcytosine (5mC) content in colorectal tumourigenesis as compared to the paired normal mucosa.

Thus, DNA hypomethylation in colorectal carcinomas was the first epigenetic event to be described in human cancer. It is considered to be an early event in hyperproliferative lesions of the colon (Feinberg and Vogelstein, 1983). For instance, the genomic 5mC content has been measured at different stages in tumour development and its decay has been frequently detected in pre-neoplastic lesions (Gama-Sosa et al., 1983). This strongly suggests that demethylation may have a function in tumour initiation, rather than in progression since the extent of global hypomethylation does not appear to increase significantly with tumour progression (Bariol et al., 2003). In this regard, in *Dnmt1* hypomorph mice, DNA hypomethylation was sufficient to induce T-cell lymphomas (Gaudet et al., 2003) and was also directly involved in gains and losses of whole chromosomes and mitotic dysfunction, generating genetic instability in colon cancer cell lines (Lengauer et al., 1997). However, this does not exclude the possibility that punctual hypomethylation events may facilitate tumoural progression. The decrease of genomic methylation in the context of hyperplastic polyps and carcinomas compared with their normal counterpart may reflect an increase in the proliferative potential of these lesions, as 5mC content inversely correlated with proliferative potential as measured by PCNA immunostaining (Bariol et al., 2003). This evidence confers a causal role in cancer initiation on global genomic hypomethylation.

Hypomethylation events generally affect repetitive DNA sequences, ranging from highly repeated, interspersed DNA sequences (long terminal repeats (LTRs), retrotransposons, retrovirus) in diverse types of cancers to moderate-copy repeats and satellite DNA (Sat-alpha). In normal tissue, methylation of these sequences is understood as a defence mechanism of the cell to keep these elements silent. However, many of these are reactivated in vivo by tumour-associated DNA demethylation (Wolffe and Matzke, 1999). The up-regulation of their transcription programs is generally associated with genomic instability: *LINE-1* (long interspersed nuclear element 1) and even more *Alu* repeats have been reported to mediate cancer-associated gene insertions, as occurs when the *APC* gene is disrupted by *LINE-1* insertion in CRC (Miki et al., 1992; Rothberg et al., 1997). In particular, tumoural hypomethylation of *LINE-1* was recently identified in a cohort study as an independent indicator associated with shorter survival among colon cancer patients (Ogino et al., 2008). It has been demonstrated that transcription reactivation of latent viruses or retroviruses, specially the human endogeneous retrovirus K (*HERV-K*) family and many solitary regulatory elements derived with transcription-inducing capacity (Casau et al., 1999; Leib-Mosch et al., 1993) and more rarely, hypomethylation, can also induce expression of single-copy genes, which, in some cases, can contribute to different stages of tumour progression, as will be discussed further.

The majority of the protein-coding genes undergoing hypomethylation-associated activation does not show any apparent relation to carcinogenesis and could be considered bystander alterations with no relevant functional role. Irizarry and colleagues used a genome-wide approach to address a comprehensive analysis of the normal and cancer cell methylome. This platform did not examine the repetitive sequences, consequently, the enrichment in DNA hypomethylation was not due to repetitive DNA (Irizarry et al., 2009). The screening was performed on colon tumours and normal mucosa from the same subjects and was validated through bisulfite pyrosequencing. With this approach, cancer-related genes previously reported in various types of cancer were identified. Furthermore, the study also pointed out comparable amounts of hypermethylation and hypomethylation with differences in the distribution of these alterations; hypomethylation

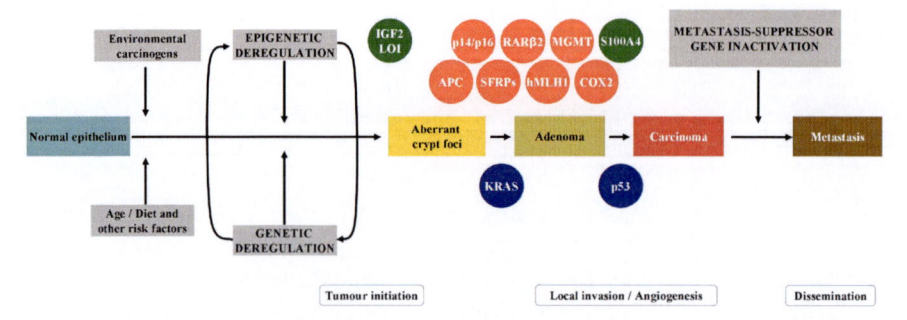

Fig. 4.2 The epigenetic contribution to the malignant phenotype. During CRC progression, interplay between genetic and epigenetic deregulation contributes to the enhancement of malignant properties. Yet, in a pre-malignant lesion, LOI of *IGF2* is also observed in surrounding normal mucosa. Tumour suppressor gene hypermethylation cooperates with genetic mutations to emphasize the cancerous phenotype, compromising all major cellular pathways, including cell cycle regulation (*p14/p16*), Wnt pathway (*APC*), DNA repair (*hMLH1*), apoptosis (*SFRP1*) and inflammation (*COX2*) among others. In metastasis formation, hypermethylation of metastasis suppressor genes confers invasive abilities on tumoural cells in order for them to colonize and establish themselves in other organs

was not associated with a CpG island in 34% of cases (Irizarry et al., 2009). This is consistent with previous findings that reported decreases in 5mC levels in the core of the gene rather than in the promoter. Such is the case for the third exon of *MYC* in CRC when compared with the corresponding normal tissue (Sharrard et al., 1992), the second intron of *S100A4*, where hypomethylation correlated with an enhancement of gene expression in colon adenocarcinoma cells (Fig. 4.2) (Nakamura and Takenaga, 1998), and some other examples displaying cancer-associated hypomethylation (Baylin, 2005; Esteller, 2006; Feltus et al., 2006; Wynter et al., 2006; Xu et al., 2004). Nevertheless, few studies have addressed the functional consequences of these events thereby playing down the relation between hypomethylation and transcriptional reactivation. Hence, no specific profiles have been identified regarding the reactivation of these sequences. These investigations aim to spot consistent biomarkers for diagnosis and prognosis, as has been done with B-melanoma antigens (*BAGE*) loci, melanoma-associated antigen (*MAGE-A1*) and *MAGEA3*, *S100A4* and ubiquitin carboxy terminal esterase L1 (*UCHL1*), among others, whose hypomethylation is linked with CRC development and progression through their effect on altered pathways (Grunau et al., 2008; Kim et al., 2006; Mizukami et al., 2008; Nakamura and Takenaga, 1998). These markers enrich the record of currently analyzed epigenetic alterations and could be taken into account alongside other biomarkers to develop reliable diagnostic tests.

Another interesting group of genes that are frequent targets of altered DNA methylation and expression patterns in cancer are imprinted genes. These genes exhibit a parent-of-origin-determined expression whose maintenance is crucial for normal development, and display the methylated status of their promoter region in normal tissue (Malik et al., 2000). LOI has been reported to occur at the genomic insulin-like growth factor (*IGF2*) and mouse mesoderm-specific transcript (*MEST*) loci in lung cancer, at *TP73* in gastric cancer, and at GTP-binding RAS-like 3 (*DIRAS3*) and GTP-binding RAS-like *NOEY2* in breast cancer, being *IGF2* the best studied in relation to CRC development (Kang et al., 2000; Lee et al., 1999; Ogawa et al., 1993; Pedersen et al., 1999; Yu et al., 1999). Normal imprinting of *IGF2* is thought to occur through differential methylation between parental alleles at particular regions called differential methylation regions (DMRs). As a result of aberrant DMR hypomethylation, LOI of *IGF2* locus results in overexpression of IGF2, a mitogenic factor that promotes cell survival (Cui et al., 2002; Nakagawa et al., 2001). This alteration was first identified in Wilm's tumours as the most common modification (Malik et al., 2000) and was later detected in many other tumour types, including CRC (Cui et al., 1998; Rainier et al., 1993). In this particular cancer, LOI is of special relevance since so far, it is the only alteration that has been associated with both cancer and normal tissue, and it is correlated with a five-fold greater frequency of colorectal neoplasia (Cui et al., 2003; Woodson et al., 2004). Furthermore, LOI of *IGF2* was also assessed in peripheral blood lymphocytes (PBLs), whereby strong associations were found between LOI in PBLs and LOI in the colon, independently of the area examined, suggesting that some field effect may predispose a shift to malignancy. In Feinberg's model of the *epigenetic progenitor origin of human cancer* (Feinberg et al., 2006), LOI of *IGF2* is the first step towards the development of a commonly recognized neoplasia, by which the epigenetic disruption of progenitor cells would smooth the way to initiating further epigenetic and genetic mutations (Fig. 4.2). Nonetheless, prospective studies are needed to clarify the relevance of this alteration in tumourigenesis.

Another subject of current research seeks associations between hypo- and hypermethylation events, but none has yet been found. Therefore, results obtained so far suggest that tumour-associated DNA hypomethylation contributes to carcinogenesis and tumour progression by mechanisms and pathways that are independent of those followed by aberrant DNA hypermethylation (Ehrlich, 2002).

In summary, hypomethylation of repetitive DNA sequences has been shown to play a significant role in the development of cancer by inducing karyotypic instability and, indirectly, affecting the expression of genes. On the other hand, the single-copy gene hypomethylation events and their transcriptional consequences have been little studied in comparison to the investigation into repression-linked hypermethylation of tumour-suppressor genes in cancer. Then again, as described above, a number of studies have evaluated the correlation between decreases in DNA methylation levels and tumour-grade progression and stage, as well as with other prognostic factors (De Smet et al., 1996; Hawkins and Ward, 2001; Hernandez-Blazquez et al., 2000; Narayan et al., 1998; Paz et al., 2002). Therefore, as we gain insight into the contribution of DNA hypomethylation in cancer and metastasis, new weapons will become available that will allow clinicians to better fight and defeat this malignancy.

4.3 Inactivation of Tumour Suppressor Genes by CpG Island Hypermethylation

Promoter CpG island hypermethylation is considered a common hallmark of all human cancers (Esteller, 2007a) since its association with aberrant transcriptional silencing involves inactivation of tumour suppressor genes, in addition to mutations (Herman and Baylin, 2003). In fact, the number of cancer-related genes affected by epigenetic inactivation equals or surpasses the number of those inactivated by mutation (Jones and Baylin, 2002).

The first tumour suppressor gene found to be regulated by promoter methylation was *RB1* (a negative cell-cycle regulator) (Ohtani-Fujita et al., 1993). Subsequently, other tumour suppressors involved in almost all cellular pathways were found to be inactivated in cancer by promoter hypermethylation, including *VHL* (associated with von Hippel-Lindau disease) (Herman et al., 1994), cyclin D kinase (*CDKN2A*) and *CDKN2B* (Herman et al., 1996; Merlo et al., 1995; Otterson et al., 1995), homologue to MutL *E. coli* (*hMLH1*) (Herman et al., 1998) and breast cancer susceptibility gene 1 (*BRCA1*) (Esteller et al., 2000b).

Different strategies have been used to identify new genes undergoing methylation-associated inactivation in cancer cells, including transcriptional (Suzuki et al., 2002; Yamashita et al., 2002), genomic (Costello et al., 2000), and candidate gene (Esteller et al., 2001) approaches. An interesting study published by our group reported new epigenetically silenced tumour suppressor genes, using the colon cancer cell line HCT-116 and its counterpart in which two major DNMTs (1 and 3b) had been silenced (Paz et al., 2003). Using two molecular screenings for different methylated loci, a new set of genes with methylation-associated silencing in colon cancer was unmasked. These included genes with potentially important roles in tumourigenesis, such as the cadherin member *FAT*, the homeobox genes *LMX-1* and *DUX-4*, and other genes whose role in transformation has not been characterized, such as the calcium channel alpha1I or the thromboxane A2 receptor (Paz et al., 2003). These approaches aimed to study methylation changes at a global genomic level such as differential methylation hybridization (DMH) that uses a CpG island microarray enriched in single-copy genes (Huang et al., 1999) and amplification of inter-methylated sites (AIMS), a PCR-based assay for identifying anonymous sequences exhibiting differential methylation (Frigola et al., 2002). Another fruitful strategy in the search for new methylated genes in human cancer combined methylated DNA immunoprecipitation (MeDIP) technology with comprehensive gene promoter arrays (Weber et al., 2005). This approach resulted in the identification of new hypermethylated genes (*RASGRF2, HOXD1* and *BHLHB9*) in human colorectal tumourigenesis (Jacinto et al., 2007), thus covering most of the disrupted pathways of cancer cells (Hanahan and Weinberg, 2000). In addition, it helped to identify the hypermethylation of the identified candidate genes as early events in the pathway towards full-blown colorectal tumours. New array-based technologies are increasing the record of genes exhibiting aberrant methylation associated with cancer (Calvanese et al., 2008) and a refined analysis of the data obtained will add more names to the already expanding list.

The publication of several specific CpG island hypermethylation profiles of human cancer revealed that methylation is targeted to specific pathways involved in cell immortalization and transformation (Costello et al., 2000; Esteller et al., 2001). This could imply either that methylation targets specific pathways or that subclonal populations exhibiting more advantageous features conferred by specific methylation patterns are selected for spreading. In carcinogenesis, genes common to all cancers become inactive through promoter methylation, in addition to those affected in particular types of cancer. Such is the case for *p16INK4A*, *p14ARF*, *MGMT*, *APC* and *hMLH1* methylation profiles in gastrointestinal tumours – the most hypermethylated tumour types – whereas breast cancer matches for *p16INK4A* but also shows *BRCA1* and *DAPK* hypermethylation (Esteller, 2007b; Esteller et al., 2001). Future research will define specific methylation profiles through the comparison of healthy and tumoural samples, different tumour types and tumoural stages and outcomes, in a genome-wide manner, shedding light on the processes that lead to malignancy (Table 4.1) (Esteller, 2007a).

Unlike genetic mutations, epigenetic alterations do not permanently inactivate genes. Instead, the genes are kept in a dormant state, but due to the dynamism of epigenetic processes this status can be reverted, as occurs when epigenetic drugs are used. What influence the environment has on switching between different epigenetic conditions is highly relevant. This was thoroughly demonstrated in a study of monozygotic twins which showed that epigenetic differences arise during their lifetime due to their distinct lifestyles, diet, carcinogen exposure etc., thereby explaining differences in the penetrance of disease (Fraga et al., 2005a). The influence of environmental factors on the epigenome of the cells is another expanding field of research. Particularly with respect to colon cancer, many groups have investigated the influence of folate deficiency, alcohol intake and other dietary habits on the acquisition of methylation patterns that subsequently lead to CRC predisposition (Giovannucci, 2002; Kim, 2004; 2005; van Engeland et al., 2003). Another related issue is the gain of methylation at certain genes linked to age. Ahuja *et al.* have shown that aberrant CpG island methylation occurs in histologically normal colon epithelium in an age-dependent manner, and that half the genes involved in this age-related methylation are the same as those involved in colon carcinogenesis (Ahuja et al., 1998). Similarly, abnormal DNA methylation of specific loci acknowledged in the aberrant crypt foci has been considered to be the earliest precursor lesion for colon adenocarcinoma (Chan et al., 2002a, b; Li et al., 2003; Ramirez et al., 2008; Rashid et al., 2001). Epigenetic changes have also been characterized in normal mucosa surrounding colorectal neoplastic lesions, including *hMLH1*, *MGMT*, *p16INK4a* and *E-Cadherin* methylation (Fig. 4.2) (Ramirez et al., 2008). Overall, it seems that environmental factors play an important role in the configuration and alteration of normal epigenetic patterns. This evidence further demonstrates how the initiation of epigenetic events can induce additional genetic and epigenetic alterations leading to tumour development.

Table 4.1 Genes undergoing promoter hypermethylation-associated silencing in colorectal cancer

Gene	Function	Frecuency (%)	Stage	References
APC	Signal transduction, beta-catenin regulation, apoptosis, cell migration	10–50	Increasing methylation with tumoural progression	Esteller et al. (2000c)
BMP3	Cell differentiation	>80	Increasing methylation with tumoural progression	Loh et al. (2008)
CDH13	Cell signaling, cell adhesion	30–70	Aberrant crypt foci	Hibi et al. (2005)
p16^{INK4A}	Cell-cycle regulation, apoptosis	15–30	Aberrant crypt foci	Merlo et al. (1995) and Gonzalez-Zulueta et al. (1995)
CHFR	Mitotic stress checkpoint	30–40	Transition to adenoma	Toyota et al. (2003) and Corn et al. (2003)
COX-2	Inflammatory response, cell proliferation	~80	Transition to carcinoma	Lee et al. (2004)
CRBP1	retinoic acid metabolic process	–	–	Esteller et al. (2002)
DAPK	Apoptosis, signal transduction	30–50	Increasing methylation with tumoural progression	Lee et al. (2004)
DKK1	Wnt signaling pathway	10–20	Transition to carcinoma	Gonzalez-Sancho et al. (2005)
ER	Growth and differentiation	~80	Transition to adenoma	Issa et al. (1994)
GSTP1	Apoptosis	5–10	Transition to carcinoma	Esteller et al. (2001) and Lee et al. (2004)
LKB1	Cell signalling, cell polarity	5–10	Transition to carcinoma	Esteller et al. (2000a)
MAL	Cell differentiation, apoptosis	60–80	Aberrant crypt foci and benign lesions	Lind et al. (2008)
MGMT	Repair of DNA guanosine methyl adduct	30–40	Transition to adenoma	Lee et al. (2004)
hMLH1	Mismatch repair	10–20	Transition to carcinoma	Kim et al. (2003)
NELL1	Cell growth, cell differentiation, cell adhesion	–	–	Mori et al. (2006)
PAX6	Cell differentiation	–	–	Toyota et al. (1999)

(continued)

Table 4.1 (continued)

Gene	Function	Frecuency (%)	Stage	References
$p14^{ARF}$	Cell cycle regulation	10–30	Transition to adenoma	Esteller et al. (2000d)
$RAR\beta2$	Apoptosis, cell proliferation, signal transduction	–	–	Spurling et al. (2008)
RASSF1A	DNA repair, cell cycle regulation	> 50	Transition to carcinoma	Lee et al. (2004)
RASGRF2	Cell signaling	30–50	Transition to adenoma	Jacinto et al. (2007)
SOCS1	Cell signaling, cell polarity	5–10	–	Hibi et al. (2005)
SFRP1	Wnt signaling pathway	5–10	Transition to carcinoma	Caldwell et al. (2004)
THBS1	Angiogenesis, response to hypoxia, MAPK signalling	10–20	Transition to carcinoma	Kim et al. (2005)
TIMP3	Matrix remodelling, tissue invasion	10–30	Transition to carcinoma	Lee et al. (2004)
TPEF	Cell signaling	~80	Aberrant crypt foci and benign lesions	Sabbioni et al. (2003)
WT1	Cell cycle regulation	50–70	–	Hiltunen et al. (1997)

In conclusion, CRC is a heterogeneous disease. Different molecular signatures are found, depending on variables such as age, sex, type of precursor lesion and affected region. An extensive panel of tumour suppressor genes that become silenced in association with promoter hypermethylation in cancer has been described (Table 4.1). Moreover, the search for methylation profiles and specific markers are contributing to solving the puzzle of the cancer cell hypermethylome, providing the scientific community with new, reliable tools that will enable a refined diagnosis and prognosis of cancer patients (Esteller, 2008).

4.4 Epigenetic Regulation of microRNA in Cancer

It was not until very recently that research on miRNAs has emerged as a promising field. Yet in 2005, Lu et al. observed a general miRNA imbalance in most, if not all types of cancer assessed (Lu et al., 2005). Some miRNAs are down-regulated – generally tumour suppressor miRNAs- whilst others are over-expressed – oncomiRNAs – contributing to the malignant phenotype. Since miRNAs play regulatory roles in all cellular processes, a precise assessment of changes in miRNA expression can provide new clues about basic mechanisms of cancer.

Altered miRNA expression in cancer can be a consequence of several mechanisms including chromosomal abnormalities (Hayashita et al., 2005), epigenetic changes (Lujambio et al., 2007; Saito and Jones, 2006) and genetic mutations causing defects in the miRNA processing machinery (Melo et al., 2009). Regarding epigenetic regulation of miRNAs, it was demonstrated that single-stranded RNAs could also be subject of regulation by DNA methylation (Lujambio et al., 2007; Saito and Jones, 2006). Again, the conjunction of epigenetic tools and miRNA expression profiling led to the discovery of two tumour suppressor miRNAs. Indeed, *miR-127* and *miR-124a*, which negatively regulate the expression of oncogenes *BCL6* and *CDK6* respectively, were identified and feature methylation-associated silencing in the HCT-116 colon cancer cell line and primary tumours (Lujambio et al., 2007; Saito and Jones, 2006). This research was followed by the identification of other miRNAs regulated by epigenetic mechanisms, such as *miR-9-1* (Lehmann et al., 2008), *miR-193a*, *miR-137* (Kozaki et al., 2008) and *miR-342* (Grady et al., 2008), which also undergo aberrant methylation in cancer. Approximately 50% of miRNAs described are embedded in CpG islands, and therefore are prone to aberrant regulation through DNA methylation processes (Weber et al., 2007). Many publications have highlighted that epigenetic deregulation of miRNAs in cancer is a widespread phenomenon, as shown for *miR-9-1, miR-193a, miR-137, miR-342, miR-203* among others (Bueno et al., 2008; Grady et al., 2008; Kozaki et al., 2008; Lehmann et al., 2008).

Interestingly, a recent study reported truncating genetic mutations in TAR RNA-binding protein 2 (*TARBP2*), a component of the miRNA processing machinery, as an important cause for miRNA down-regulation in cancer (Melo et al., 2009). The presence of *TARBP2* mutations causes a defect in the processing of miRNAs and provokes a destabilization in the DICER1 protein, enhancing the tumoural phenotype and explaining the observed defects in the expression of mature miRNAs in tumours with microsatellite instability (Melo et al., 2009). Cells with a TRBP deficiency showed a 90% reduction in the efficiency of endogenous processing of miRNAs, most of them with tumour suppressor capacities. The re-introduction of TRBP in the deficient cells was accompanied by the down-regulation of their target oncoproteins. Conversely, the tumoural phenotype was enhanced upon *TARBP2* interference in TRBP wild-type cells due to an impairment of pre-miRNA processing. Parallel results were obtained after assessing *TARBP2* disruption in human primary tumours with microsatellite instability, emphasizing the importance of miRNA disparity in relation to cancer (Melo et al., 2009).

4.5 microRNAS as Metastasis Switches

A new role for miRNAs in metastasis has recently emerged. As occurs in early stages of tumour development, some miRNAs act as oncogenes and are over-expressed, whereas tumour suppressor miRNAs are down-regulated. microRNAs also play a leading role in metastasis development. Through their ability to affect the expression of protein-coding genes, these non-coding RNAs have the power to alter cellular processes such as those involved in cancer development and progression.

Several lines of evidence support the existence of miRNAs with metastasis promoter and suppressor capacities. On the one hand, it has been found that *miR-10b* and *miR-155* are regulated as part of a metastatic gene expression program conducted by the *TWIST1* transcription factor (Kong et al., 2008; Ma et al., 2007). On the other hand, a miRNA hypermethylation profile was found to predict the presence of lymph node metastases in various types of tumours (Lujambio et al., 2008). These findings showed increased activity upon treatment with demethylating agents, and were able to inhibit motility, tumour growth and metastasis formation through down-regulation of their oncogenic targets (Lujambio et al., 2008). Additionally, several other metastasis-promoting miRNAs have been characterized, including *miR-373* and *miR-372* through their effect in CD44 metastasis-suppressor inactivation (Voorhoeve et al., 2006); and *miR-21* that was found to enhance the metastatic phenotype in colon cancer and other cancer models (Asangani et al., 2008).

In contrast to this, miRNAs can also have opposite roles and act as inhibitors of various steps involved in metastasis. *MiR-335* and *miR-206* were the first metastasis-suppressor miRNAs described in breast cancer. They were significantly repressed in metastatic foci, and their re-introduction was found to inhibit cell adhesion, migration and invasion, resulting in a reduction of the metastatic phenotype (Tavazoie et al., 2008). Similarly, *miR-29c* reduces metastasis formation through the inhibition of extracellular matrix degrading proteins (Sengupta et al., 2008), and the same occurs with the *miR-146* family and the inhibition of nuclear kappa factor light chain-enhancer of activated B cells (NF-κβ) pathway resulting in a reduction of metastatic potential as observed in a breast cancer model (Bhaumik et al., 2008).

In conclusion, research based on miRNAs biology is proving to be a promising area of investigation in the fight against cancer. Firstly, it provides new important insights into tumour and metastasis biology; secondly, it is a source of biomarkers that can be used to predict the occurrence of metastasis; and finally, it may help in identifying targets for the clinical management of different types of cancer.

4.6 Histone Modification Defects in Colon Cancer

Epigenetic alterations in cancer cells do not only involve DNA methylation defects. They occur in a wider context of epigenetic deregulation that also involves aberrant histone modifications.

There is growing evidence that histone modifications play a role in pre-marking genes prone to CpG cancer-related hypermethylation. The timing of gene silencing was first investigated (Mutskov and Felsenfeld, 2004). Through an elegant manner, it was found that global histone acetylation levels, which are normally correlated with an active transcription state, decreased in conjunction with another activation mark, the loss of di- and trimethylation of lysine 4 at histone 3 (H3K4 me2/me3). This occurs before the gain of permanent repressive modifications such as methylation of lysine 9 at histone 3 (H3K9me) and CpG island promoter hypermethylation. Moreover, once the repressive status is acquired, it is positively fed back to ensure the silent condition and to propagate it to neighbouring chromatin domains (Mutskov and Felsenfeld, 2004). These experiments were performed in non-transformed animal cell lines, but the mechanism could be extended to what takes place in normal and tumoural human cells, although this has yet to be confirmed. However, some recent reports have shown the presence of pre-existing epigenetic repressive programs by which genes undergoing de novo CpG island methylation would be marked by EZH2-containing Polycomb (PcG) complex with lysine 27 trimethylation in histone 3 (H3K27me3) early on in development. This suggests that this particular histone modification may be specifically associated with methylated CpG island genes in colon cancer cell lines (Ohm et al., 2007; Schlesinger et al., 2007; Widschwendter et al., 2007). The presence of this particular mark was detected in embryonic and normal tissue cells, but was only involved in the recruitment of DNA methylation machinery when transformation occurred (Widschwendter et al., 2007). Consistent with these observations, Baylin's group found that PcG complexes and histone methyltransferases conferred both active and repressive (H3K27me and H3K4me, respectively) marks on some genes. By acquiring this bivalent state, genes were kept at low transcription rates which were then permanently silenced through the recruitment of DNA methyltransferases as transformation followed. This prevented anti-proliferative genes from being expressed by hypermethylation of their promoters, and contributed to the abnormal clonal expansion of cells exhibiting advantageous methylation patterns (Ohm et al., 2007). Therefore, the PcG-marked genes found in these studies represent a template for aberrant stable methylation in cancer. Overall, it seems that transcriptional repression by PcG complexes is a necessary precursor to DNA methylation.

Finally, our laboratory has also contributed to the description of altered histone modification patterns in cancer progression (Fig. 4.1). Genome-wide methods such as HPCE and mass spectrometry were employed to detect altered patterns of histone marks. Specifically, loss of lysine 16 acetylation and lysine 20 trimethylation in histone 4 was described as an early event, even occurring in benign lesions. It was found to accumulate up to the most malignant stages, causing transcriptional repression of targeted sequences. This mechanism was studied in colon cancer, but also extends to other types of cancer, thereby constituting a common hallmark of human cancer (Fraga et al., 2005b). Another study assessed global levels of individual histone modifications in tissues obtained from prostate cancer patients and provided evidence that changes in bulk histone modifications of cancer cells predict clinical outcome (Seligson et al., 2005). Similar approaches have not so far been used with CRC, but would be very informative for predicting patient prognosis, responsiveness to treatment, survival, etc. as well as providing information about the molecular basis of this type of cancer.

The combined evidence suggests that histone modifications work synergistically with each other and are important for maintaining methylation patterns in normal and cancer cells. The study of histone modifications in relation to cancer is an expanding field that still has much to offer. Since they are implicated in a multitude of cellular processes, the elucidation of their roles in association with disease will be the focus of intense research in the coming years.

4.7 Epigenetic Contribution to Colorectal Cancer Metastasis

Seminal contributions have emerged from the *epigenetic factory* in relation to colorectal cancer metastasis.

DNA methylation defects affecting the metastatic spread of tumour cells have been reported for many candidate genes that underwent hypermethylation-associated silencing during tumour formation, and whose re-induction, both by DNA demethylating agents or transgene transfection, impaired the invasion of colon cancer cells and inhibited the formation of metastasis. Inactivation of these genes favoured all stages in the metastatic cascade.

Promoter hypermethylation of *RUNX3* was detected in colon cancer cell lines (Ku et al., 2004) and it was subsequently found that its anti-tumoural effect as an angiogenesis inhibitor, through inhibition of *VEGF*, was barred at early stages of cancer development. *RUNX3* gene transfer suppressed *VEGF* expression in human gastric cancer cells, which in turn correlated with a significantly impaired angiogenic potential of human gastric cancer cells and inhibited metastasis formation in animal models (Peng et al., 2006). Similar results have been reported for epigenetic inactivation of the metastasis suppressor *RECK* which enhances the invasion of human colon cancer cells (Cho et al., 2007). In addition, hypoxia is known to be a common condition in tumours, facilitating both tumour angiogenesis and metastasis by activating gene-expression programs that trigger invasion, proteolysis and tumour cell migration. Epigenetic deregulation of such processes is found in *uPA* and *uPAR* (urokinase-type plasminogen activator and receptor, respectively) in which hypomethylation-linked re-expression has been reported in a wide range of cancers with high invasive or metastatic potential (Pakneshan et al., 2005). Additionally, hypomethylation-associated over-expression of S100A4 in advanced stages is related to the aggressiveness of colorectal carcinoma (Cho et al., 2005). Moreover, Wendt and co-workers reported methylation-related inactivation of the *CXCL12* chemokine locus and associated metastasis development due to deregulation of apoptosis signalling (Wendt et al., 2006). Reactivation of *CXCL12* in stable gene transfectants showed that in vivo metastatic tumour formation was prevented (Wendt et al., 2006).

Other cases have been discovered in the course of metastasis development. For example, a high degree of methylation of *TPEF* (transmembrane protein containing epidermal growth factor and follistatin domain) has been reported in liver metastasis (Ebert et al., 2005). $p16^{INK4}$ and $p14^{ARF}$, two distinctive cell-cycle regulators, exhibit promoter hypermethylation that correlates with lymph node metastasis (Lee et al., 2006). Also, as mentioned before, a miRNA methylation signature was found, in which *miR-148a*, *miR-34b/c* and *miR-9* hypermethylation was significantly associated with the appearance of lymph node metastasis (Lujambio et al., 2008).

Hitherto, the importance of epigenetics in colorectal metastasis is becoming increasingly apparent as new technologies emerge, innovative experimental approaches are developed and comprehensive analyses are undertaken. Nevertheless, there is still a long road ahead that will require the combination of basic and translational research in order to extend our understanding of human cancer metastasis.

4.8 Epigenetic Biomarkers and Therapies

Unlike tumour suppressor genes inactivated by genetic alterations, genes silenced by epigenetic mechanisms are intact and responsive to reactivation by small molecules (Kopelovich et al., 2003). On one hand, the widespread DNA methylation observed in neoplasia has encouraged research on hypomethylating agents for the therapeutic management of cancer, as a mechanism of inducing tumour-cell differentiation, growth arrest, and re-expression of tumour-silencing agents inactivated by promoter hypermethylation. On the other hand, the stability of methylation events related to cancer has permitted the identification of a large panel of biomarkers used in clinical practice (Table 4.1) (Santini et al., 2001).

Two drugs, 5-azacytidine (5aza, Vidaza) and 5-aza-2'-deoxycytidine (5dC, Decitabine), are the standard bearers of epigenetic cancer therapy. Both have demonstrated their effectiveness in reducing DNA methylation levels by covalently trapping the methyltransferase machinery, leading to cellular differentiation and re-expression of several proteins. While 5aza incorporates primarily into RNA and exerts its function on rapidly dividing cells, 5dC slips into DNA, blocking its synthesis and producing a severe cytotoxic effect. Many examples in the literature show that in vitro pharmacological inhibition of methyltransferase results in the reactivation of gene expression for genes silenced either physiologically or pathologically, including *p16INK4A* and *MLH1*. Treatment with methylation inhibitor 5dAza notably extends the doubling time of neoplastic cell lines, but not of normal fibroblast cell lines (Bender et al., 1998; Lantry et al., 1999). In addition, blockade of cytosine methylation has been shown to prevent or reverse the onset of neoplasia in several animal models (Laird et al., 1995).

The use of 5aza in the treatment of haematological malignancies was approved by the US Food and Drug Administration (FDA) in 2004, and has already achieved important victories for patients, alone and in combination with other drugs such as histone deacetylase inhibitors (HDACs) (Gore and Hermes-DeSantis, 2008). However, these demethylating agents have not yet been shown to have significant response rates in the treatment of solid tumours (Yoo and Jones, 2006).

The second major layer of epigenetic therapy involves targeting histone deacetylases. Pharmacological HDACis of class I and II display a wide range of anti-tumour effects as inducers of growth arrest, differentiation, and cytotoxicity (Mariadason,

2008) and have turned out to be efficient chemopreventive agents. These agents are divided into four groups: short-chain fatty acids, hydroxamic acids, cyclic tetrapeptides and benzamides. Among these, trichostatin A (TSA) and suberoylanilide hydroxamic acid (SAHA) have been used experimentally for decades and have achieved growth inhibition and apoptosis in colon cancer cells (Bolden et al., 2006; Bordonaro et al., 1999; Mariadason et al., 2000). In addition, TSA was also approved by the FDA for the treatment of cutaneous T-cell lymphoma. Furthermore, synergy between 5dC and TSA has succeeded in reactivating methylated tumour suppressor genes (Cameron et al., 1999). Combining demethylating agents and HDACis provides a means of reducing the side effects associated with the former drugs.

Epigenetic research is leading investigators towards novel methods of treating cancer, and the therapies implemented are fulfilling expectations. However, there is much work still to be done. Shortening the translational bridge between the laboratory and the clinic will require close interactions between researchers, who understand the disease's biology and the mechanisms of action of the drugs under development and physicians, who are aware of patients' needs.

Abbreviations and Acronyms

APC	Adenomatous polyposis coli
BAGE	B-melanoma antigens
BRCA1	Breast cancer susceptibility gene 1
CDKN2A	Cyclin D kinase N2A
ChIP	Chromatin Immunoprecipitation
CRC	Colorectal cancer
CpG	Cytosine-phosphate-guanine
DIRAS	GTP-binding RAS-like 3
DNMTs	DNA methyltransferases
5mC	5-methylcytosine
HDACs	Histone deacetylases
HERV	Human endogenous retrovirus
IGF	Insulin like growth factor
LINE-1	Long interspersed nuclear element 1
LOI	Loss of imprinting
LTR	Long terminal repeat
MAGE	Melanoma-associated antigens
MeDIP	Methylated DNA immunoprecipitation
MEST	Mouse mesoderm-specific transcript
miRNA	microRNA
MeDIP	Methylated DNA immunoprecipitation
MEST	Mouse mesoderm-specific transcript
miRNA	microRNA
NF-kB	Nuclear factor kappa light chain enhancer of activated B cells

SAHA   Suberoylanilide hydroxamic acid
TARBP2   TAR RNA-binding protein 2
TPEF   Transmembrane protein containing epidermal growth factor and follistatin domain
TSA   Trichostatin
VHL   Von Hippel-Lindau

References

Ahuja N, Li Q, Mohan AL, Baylin SB, Issa JP (1998). Aging and DNA methylation in colorectal mucosa and cancer. *Cancer Res* **58**: 5489–94.

Asangani IA, Rasheed SA, Nikolova DA, Leupold JH, Colburn NH, Post S et al. (2008). MicroRNA-21 (miR-21) post-transcriptionally downregulates tumor suppressor Pdcd4 and stimulates invasion, intravasation and metastasis in colorectal cancer. *Oncogene* **27**: 2128–36.

Bariol C, Suter C, Cheong K, Ku SL, Meagher A, Hawkins N et al. (2003). The relationship between hypomethylation and CpG island methylation in colorectal neoplasia. *Am J Pathol* **162**: 1361–71.

Baylin SB (2005). DNA methylation and gene silencing in cancer. *Nat Clin Pract Oncol* **2** (Suppl 1): S4–S11.

Bender CM, Pao MM, Jones PA (1998). Inhibition of DNA methylation by 5-aza-2′-deoxycytidine suppresses the growth of human tumor cell lines. *Cancer Res* **58**: 95–101.

Berger SL (2007). The complex language of chromatin regulation during transcription. *Nature* **447**: 407–12.

Bhaumik D, Scott GK, Schokrpur S, Patil CK, Campisi J, Benz CC (2008). Expression of microRNA-146 suppresses NF-kappaB activity with reduction of metastatic potential in breast cancer cells. *Oncogene* **27**: 5643–47.

Bibikova M, Lin Z, Zhou L, Chudin E, Garcia EW, Wu B et al. (2006). High-throughput DNA methylation profiling using universal bead arrays. *Genome Res* **16**: 383–93.

Bird A (2002). DNA methylation patterns and epigenetic memory. *Genes Dev* **16**: 6–21.

Bolden JE, Peart MJ, Johnstone RW (2006). Anticancer activities of histone deacetylase inhibitors. *Nat Rev Drug Discov* **5**: 769–84.

Bordonaro M, Mariadason JM, Aslam F, Heerdt BG, Augenlicht LH (1999). Butyrate-induced apoptotic cascade in colonic carcinoma cells: modulation of the beta-catenin-Tcf pathway and concordance with effects of sulindac and trichostatin A but not curcumin. *Cell Growth Differ* **10**: 713–20.

Bueno MJ, Perez de Castro I, Gomez de Cedron M, Santos J, Calin GA, Cigudosa JC et al. (2008). Genetic and epigenetic silencing of microRNA-203 enhances ABL1 and BCR-ABL1 oncogene expression. *Cancer Cell* **13**: 496–506.

Caldwell GM, Jones C, Gensberg K, Jan S, Hardy RG, Byrd P et al. (2004). The Wnt antagonist sFRP1 in colorectal tumorigenesis. *Cancer Res* **64**: 883–88.

Calvanese V, Horrillo A, Hmadcha A, Suarez-Alvarez B, Fernandez AF, Lara E et al. (2008). Cancer genes hypermethylated in human embryonic stem cells. *PLoS One* **3**: e3294.

Cameron EE, Bachman KE, Myohanen S, Herman JG, Baylin SB (1999). Synergy of demethylation and histone deacetylase inhibition in the re-expression of genes silenced in cancer. *Nat Genet* **21**: 103–7.

Casau AE, Vaughan JE, Lozano G, Levine AJ (1999). Germ cell expression of an isolated human endogenous retroviral long terminal repeat of the HERV-K/HTDV family in transgenic mice. *J Virol* **73**: 9976–83.

Chan AO, Broaddus RR, Houlihan PS, Issa JP, Hamilton SR, Rashid A (2002a). CpG island methylation in aberrant crypt foci of the colorectum. *Am J Pathol* **160**: 1823–30.

Chan AO, Issa JP, Morris JS, Hamilton SR, Rashid A (2002b). Concordant CpG island methylation in hyperplastic polyposis. *Am J Pathol* **160**: 529–36.

Cho YG, Kim CJ, Nam SW, Yoon SH, Lee SH, Yoo NJ et al. (2005). Overexpression of S100A4 is closely associated with progression of colorectal cancer. *World J Gastroenterol* **11**: 4852–56.

Cho CY, Wang JH, Chang HC, Chang CK, Hung WC (2007). Epigenetic inactivation of the metastasis suppressor RECK enhances invasion of human colon cancer cells. *J Cell Physiol* **213**: 65–69.

Christofori G, Naik P, Hanahan D (1995). Deregulation of both imprinted and expressed alleles of the insulin-like growth factor 2 gene during beta-cell tumorigenesis. *Nat Genet* **10**: 196–201.

Corn PG, Summers MK, Fogt F, Virmani AK, Gazdar AF, Halazonetis TD et al. (2003). Frequent hypermethylation of the 5′ CpG island of the mitotic stress checkpoint gene Chfr in colorectal and non-small cell lung cancer. *Carcinogenesis* **24**: 47–51.

Costello JF, Fruhwald MC, Smiraglia DJ, Rush LJ, Robertson GP, Gao X et al. (2000). Aberrant CpG-island methylation has non-random and tumour-type-specific patterns. *Nat Genet* **24**: 132–38.

Cui H, Cruz-Correa M, Giardiello FM, Hutcheon DF, Kafonek DR, Brandenburg S et al. (2003). Loss of IGF2 imprinting: a potential marker of colorectal cancer risk. *Science* **299**: 1753–55.

Cui H, Horon IL, Ohlsson R, Hamilton SR, Feinberg AP (1998). Loss of imprinting in normal tissue of colorectal cancer patients with microsatellite instability. *Nat Med* **4**: 1276–80.

Cui H, Onyango P, Brandenburg S, Wu Y, Hsieh CL, Feinberg AP (2002). Loss of imprinting in colorectal cancer linked to hypomethylation of H19 and IGF2. *Cancer Res* **62**: 6442–46.

De Smet C, De Backer O, Faraoni I, Lurquin C, Brasseur F, Boon T (1996). The activation of human gene MAGE-1 in tumor cells is correlated with genome-wide demethylation. *Proc Natl Acad Sci USA* **93**: 7149–53.

Ebert MP, Mooney SH, Tonnes-Priddy L, Lograsso J, Hoffmann J, Chen J et al. (2005). Hypermethylation of the TPEF/HPP1 gene in primary and metastatic colorectal cancers. *Neoplasia* **7**: 771–78.

Ehrlich M (2002). DNA methylation in cancer: too much, but also too little. *Oncogene* **21**: 5400–13.

Esteller M (2006). CpG island methylation and histone modifications: biology and clinical significance. *Ernst Schering Res Found Workshop* **57**: 115–26.

Esteller M (2007a). Cancer epigenomics: DNA methylomes and histone-modification maps. *Nat Rev Genet* **8**: 286–98.

Esteller M (2007b). Epigenetic gene silencing in cancer: the DNA hypermethylome. *Hum Mol Genet* **16**(Spec No 1): R50–R59.

Esteller M (2008). Epigenetics in cancer. *N Engl J Med* **358**: 1148–59.

Esteller M, Avizienyte E, Corn PG, Lothe RA, Baylin SB, Aaltonen LA et al. (2000a). Epigenetic inactivation of LKB1 in primary tumors associated with the Peutz-Jeghers syndrome. *Oncogene* **19**: 164–68.

Esteller M, Corn PG, Baylin SB, Herman JG (2001). A gene hypermethylation profile of human cancer. *Cancer Res* **61**: 3225–29.

Esteller M, Guo M, Moreno V, Peinado MA, Capella G, Galm O et al. (2002). Hypermethylation-associated Inactivation of the Cellular Retinol-Binding-Protein 1 Gene in Human Cancer. *Cancer Res* **62**: 5902–5.

Esteller M, Silva JM, Dominguez G, Bonilla F, Matias-Guiu X, Lerma E et al. (2000b). Promoter hypermethylation and BRCA1 inactivation in sporadic breast and ovarian tumors. *J Natl Cancer Inst* **92**: 564–69.

Esteller M, Sparks A, Toyota M, Sanchez-Cespedes M, Capella G, Peinado MA et al. (2000c). Analysis of adenomatous polyposis coli promoter hypermethylation in human cancer. *Cancer Res* **60**: 4366–71.

Esteller M, Tortola S, Toyota M, Capella G, Peinado MA, Baylin SB et al. (2000d). Hypermethylation-associated inactivation of p14(ARF) is independent of p16(INK4a) methylation and p53 mutational status. *Cancer Res* **60**: 129–33.

Feinberg AP, Ohlsson R, Henikoff S (2006). The epigenetic progenitor origin of human cancer. *Nat Rev Genet* **7**: 21–33.

Feinberg AP, Vogelstein B (1983). Hypomethylation distinguishes genes of some human cancers from their normal counterparts. *Nature* **301**: 89–92.

Feltus FA, Lee EK, Costello JF, Plass C, Vertino PM (2006). DNA motifs associated with aberrant CpG island methylation. *Genomics* **87**: 572–79.

Fisher AG (2002). Cellular identity and lineage choice. *Nat Rev Immunol* **2**: 977–82.

Fraga MF, Ballestar E, Paz MF, Ropero S, Setien F, Ballestar ML et al. (2005a). Epigenetic differences arise during the lifetime of monozygotic twins. *Proc Natl Acad Sci USA* **102**: 10604–9.

Fraga MF, Ballestar E, Villar-Garea A, Boix-Chornet M, Espada J, Schotta G et al. (2005b). Loss of acetylation at Lys16 and trimethylation at Lys20 of histone H4 is a common hallmark of human cancer. *Nat Genet* **37**: 391–400.

Frigola J, Ribas M, Risques RA, Peinado MA (2002). Methylome profiling of cancer cells by amplification of inter-methylated sites (AIMS). *Nucl Acids Res* **30**: e28.

Gama-Sosa MA, Slagel VA, Trewyn RW, Oxenhandler R, Kuo KC, Gehrke CW et al. (1983). The 5-methylcytosine content of DNA from human tumors. *Nucl Acids Res* **11**: 6883–94.

Gaudet F, Hodgson JG, Eden A, Jackson-Grusby L, Dausman J, Gray JW et al. (2003). Induction of tumors in mice by genomic hypomethylation. *Science* **300**: 489–92.

Giovannucci E (2002). Epidemiologic studies of folate and colorectal neoplasia: a review. *J Nutr* **132**: 2350S–2355S.

Gonzalez-Sancho JM, Aguilera O, Garcia JM, Pendas-Franco N, Pena C, Cal S et al. (2005). The Wnt antagonist DICKKOPF-1 gene is a downstream target of beta-catenin/TCF and is downregulated in human colon cancer. *Oncogene* **24**: 1098–103.

Gonzalez-Zulueta M, Bender CM, Yang AS, Nguyen T, Beart RW, Van Tornout JM et al. (1995). Methylation of the 5′ CpG island of the p16/CDKN2 tumor suppressor gene in normal and transformed human tissues correlates with gene silencing. *Cancer Res* **55**: 4531–35.

Gore SD, Hermes-DeSantis ER (2008). Future directions in myelodysplastic syndrome: newer agents and the role of combination approaches. *Cancer Control* **15**(Suppl): 40–49.

Grady WM (2005). Epigenetic events in the colorectum and in colon cancer. *Biochem Soc Trans* **33**: 684–88.

Grady WM, Parkin RK, Mitchell PS, Lee JH, Kim YH, Tsuchiya KD et al. (2008). Epigenetic silencing of the intronic microRNA hsa-miR-342 and its host gene EVL in colorectal cancer. *Oncogene* **27**: 3880–88.

Greger V, Passarge E, Hopping W, Messmer E, Horsthemke B (1989). Epigenetic changes may contribute to the formation and spontaneous regression of retinoblastoma. *Hum Genet* **83**: 155–58.

Grunau C, Brun ME, Rivals I, Selves J, Hindermann W, Favre-Mercuret M et al. (2008). BAGE hypomethylation, a new epigenetic biomarker for colon cancer detection. *Cancer Epidemiol Biomarkers Prev* **17**: 1374–79.

Hanahan D, Weinberg RA (2000). The hallmarks of cancer. *Cell* **100**: 57–70.

Hawkins NJ, Ward RL (2001). Sporadic colorectal cancers with microsatellite instability and their possible origin in hyperplastic polyps and serrated adenomas. *J Natl Cancer Inst* **93**: 1307–13.

Hayashita Y, Osada H, Tatematsu Y, Yamada H, Yanagisawa K, Tomida S et al. (2005). A polycistronic microRNA cluster, miR-17-92, is overexpressed in human lung cancers and enhances cell proliferation. *Cancer Res* **65**: 9628–32.

He L, Hannon GJ (2004). MicroRNAs: small RNAs with a big role in gene regulation. *Nat Rev Genet* **5**: 522–31.

Herman JG, Baylin SB (2003). Gene silencing in cancer in association with promoter hypermethylation. *N Engl J Med* **349**: 2042–54.

Herman JG, Jen J, Merlo A, Baylin SB (1996). Hypermethylation-associated inactivation indicates a tumor suppressor role for p15INK4B. *Cancer Res* **56**: 722–27.

Herman JG, Latif F, Weng Y, Lerman MI, Zbar B, Liu S et al. (1994). Silencing of the VHL tumor-suppressor gene by DNA methylation in renal carcinoma. *Proc Natl Acad Sci USA* **91**: 9700–4.

Herman JG, Umar A, Polyak K, Graff JR, Ahuja N, Issa JP et al. (1998). Incidence and functional consequences of hMLH1 promoter hypermethylation in colorectal carcinoma. *Proc Natl Acad Sci USA* **95**: 6870–75.

Hernandez-Blazquez FJ, Habib M, Dumollard JM, Barthelemy C, Benchaib M, de Capoa A et al. (2000). Evaluation of global DNA hypomethylation in human colon cancer tissues by immunohistochemistry and image analysis. *Gut* **47**: 689–93.

Hibi K, Kodera Y, Ito K, Akiyama S, Nakao A (2005). Aberrant methylation of HLTF, SOCS-1, and CDH13 genes is shown in colorectal cancers without lymph node metastasis. *Dis Colon Rectum* **48**: 1282–86.

Hiltunen MO, Koistinaho J, Alhonen L, Myohanen S, Marin S, Kosma VM et al. (1997). Hypermethylation of the WT1 and calcitonin gene promoter regions at chromosome 11p in human colorectal cancer. *Br J Cancer* **76**: 1124–30.

Huang TH, Perry MR, Laux DE (1999). Methylation profiling of CpG islands in human breast cancer cells. *Hum Mol Genet* **8**: 459–70.

Irizarry RA, Ladd-Acosta C, Wen B, Wu Z, Montano C, Onyango P et al. (2009). The human colon cancer methylome shows similar hypo- and hypermethylation at conserved tissue-specific CpG island shores. *Nat Genet* **41**: 178–86.

Issa JP, Kantarjian H (2005). Azacitidine. *Nat Rev Drug Discov* (Suppl): S.

Issa JP, Ottaviano YL, Celano P, Hamilton SR, Davidson NE, Baylin SB (1994). Methylation of the oestrogen receptor CpG island links ageing and neoplasia in human colon. *Nat Genet* **7**: 536–40.

Jacinto FV, Ballestar E, Ropero S, Esteller M (2007). Discovery of epigenetically silenced genes by methylated DNA immunoprecipitation in colon cancer cells. *Cancer Res* **67**: 11481–86.

Jones PA, Baylin SB (2002). The fundamental role of epigenetic events in cancer. *Nat Rev Genet* **3**: 415–28.

Kang MJ, Park BJ, Byun DS, Park JI, Kim HJ, Park JH et al. (2000). Loss of imprinting and elevated expression of wild-type p73 in human gastric adenocarcinoma. *Clin Cancer Res* **6**: 1767–71.

Kim YI (2004). Folate and DNA methylation: a mechanistic link between folate deficiency and colorectal cancer? *Cancer Epidemiol Biomarkers Prev* **13**: 511–19.

Kim YI (2005). Nutritional epigenetics: impact of folate deficiency on DNA methylation and colon cancer susceptibility. *J Nutr* **135**: 2703–9.

Kim KH, Choi JS, Kim IJ, Ku JL, Park JG (2006). Promoter hypomethylation and reactivation of MAGE-A1 and MAGE-A3 genes in colorectal cancer cell lines and cancer tissues. *World J Gastroenterol* **12**: 5651–57.

Kim H, Kim YH, Kim SE, Kim NG, Noh SH, Kim H (2003). Concerted promoter hypermethylation of hMLH1, p16INK4A, and E-cadherin in gastric carcinomas with microsatellite instability. *J Pathol* **200**: 23–31.

Kim HC, Roh SA, Ga IH, Kim JS, Yu CS, Kim JC (2005). CpG island methylation as an early event during adenoma progression in carcinogenesis of sporadic colorectal cancer. *J Gastroenterol Hepatol* **20**: 1920–26.

Kondo Y, Issa JP (2004). Epigenetic changes in colorectal cancer. *Cancer Metastasis Rev* **23**: 29–39.

Kong W, Yang H, He L, Zhao JJ, Coppola D, Dalton WS et al. (2008). MicroRNA-155 is regulated by the transforming growth factor beta/Smad pathway and contributes to epithelial cell plasticity by targeting RhoA. *Mol Cell Biol* **28**: 6773–84.

Kopelovich L, Crowell JA, Fay JR (2003). The epigenome as a target for cancer chemoprevention. *J Natl Cancer Inst* **95**: 1747–57.

Kouzarides T (2007). Chromatin modifications and their function. *Cell* **128**: 693–705.

Kozaki K, Imoto I, Mogi S, Omura K, Inazawa J (2008). Exploration of tumor-suppressive microRNAs silenced by DNA hypermethylation in oral cancer. *Cancer Res* **68**: 2094–105.

Ku JL, Kang SB, Shin YK, Kang HC, Hong SH, Kim IJ et al. (2004). Promoter hypermethylation downregulates RUNX3 gene expression in colorectal cancer cell lines. *Oncogene* **23**: 6736–42.

Laird PW, Jackson-Grusby L, Fazeli A, Dickinson SL, Jung WE, Li E et al. (1995). Suppression of intestinal neoplasia by DNA hypomethylation. *Cell* **81**: 197–205.

Lantry LE, Zhang Z, Crist KA, Wang Y, Kelloff GJ, Lubet RA et al. (1999). 5-Aza-2'-deoxycytidine is chemopreventive in a 4-(methyl-nitrosamino)-1-(3-pyridyl)-1-butanone-induced primary mouse lung tumor model. *Carcinogenesis* **20**: 343–46.

Lee MP, DeBaun MR, Mitsuya K, Galonek HL, Brandenburg S, Oshimura M et al. (1999). Loss of imprinting of a paternally expressed transcript, with antisense orientation to KVLQT1, occurs frequently in Beckwith-Wiedemann syndrome and is independent of insulin-like growth factor II imprinting. *Proc Natl Acad Sci USA* **96**: 5203–8.

Lee S, Hwang KS, Lee HJ, Kim JS, Kang GH (2004). Aberrant CpG island hypermethylation of multiple genes in colorectal neoplasia. *Lab Invest* **84**: 884–93.

Lee M, Sup Han W, Kyoung Kim O, Hee Sung S, Sun Cho M, Lee SN et al. (2006). Prognostic value of p16INK4a and p14ARF gene hypermethylation in human colon cancer. *Pathol Res Pract* **202**: 415–24.

Lehmann U, Hasemeier B, Christgen M, Muller M, Romermann D, Langer F et al. (2008). Epigenetic inactivation of microRNA gene hsa-mir-9-1 in human breast cancer. *J Pathol* **214**: 17–24.

Leib-Mosch C, Haltmeier M, Werner T, Geigl EM, Brack-Werner R, Francke U et al. (1993). Genomic distribution and transcription of solitary HERV-K LTRs. *Genomics* **18**: 261–69.

Lengauer C, Kinzler KW, Vogelstein B (1997). DNA methylation and genetic instability in colorectal cancer cells. *Proc Natl Acad Sci USA* **94**: 2545–50.

Li H, Myeroff L, Smiraglia D, Romero MF, Pretlow TP, Kasturi L et al. (2003). SLC5A8, a sodium transporter, is a tumor suppressor gene silenced by methylation in human colon aberrant crypt foci and cancers. *Proc Natl Acad Sci USA* **100**: 8412–17.

Lind GE, Ahlquist T, Kolberg M, Berg M, Eknaes M, Alonso MA et al. (2008). Hypermethylated MAL gene – a silent marker of early colon tumorigenesis. *J Transl Med* **6**: 13.

Loh K, Chia JA, Greco S, Cozzi SJ, Buttenshaw RL, Bond CE et al. (2008). Bone morphogenic protein 3 inactivation is an early and frequent event in colorectal cancer development. *Genes Chromosomes Cancer* **47**: 449–60.

Lu J, Getz G, Miska EA, Alvarez-Saavedra E, Lamb J, Peck D et al. (2005). MicroRNA expression profiles classify human cancers. *Nature* **435**: 834–38.

Lujambio A, Calin GA, Villanueva A, Ropero S, Sanchez-Cespedes M, Blanco D et al. (2008). A microRNA DNA methylation signature for human cancer metastasis. *Proc Natl Acad Sci USA* **105**: 13556–61.

Lujambio A, Ropero S, Ballestar E, Fraga MF, Cerrato C, Setien F et al. (2007). Genetic unmasking of an epigenetically silenced microRNA in human cancer cells. *Cancer Res* **67**: 1424–29.

Ma L, Teruya-Feldstein J, Weinberg RA (2007). Tumour invasion and metastasis initiated by microRNA-10b in breast cancer. *Nature* **449**: 682–88.

Malik K, Salpekar A, Hancock A, Moorwood K, Jackson S, Charles A et al. (2000). Identification of differential methylation of the WT1 antisense regulatory region and relaxation of imprinting in Wilms' tumor. *Cancer Res* **60**: 2356–60.

Mariadason JM (2008). HDACs and HDAC inhibitors in colon cancer. *Epigenetics* **3**: 28–37.

Mariadason JM, Corner GA, Augenlicht LH (2000). Genetic reprogramming in pathways of colonic cell maturation induced by short chain fatty acids: comparison with trichostatin A, sulindac, and curcumin and implications for chemoprevention of colon cancer. *Cancer Res* **60**: 4561–72.

Martin C, Zhang Y (2005). The diverse functions of histone lysine methylation. *Nat Rev Mol Cell Biol* **6**: 838–49.

Melo SA, Ropero S, Moutinho C, Aaltonen LA, Yamamoto H, Calin GA et al. (2009). A TARBP2 mutation in human cancer impairs microRNA processing and DICER1 function. *Nat Genet* **41**: 365–70.

Merlo A, Herman JG, Mao L, Lee DJ, Gabrielson E, Burger PC et al. (1995). 5′ CpG island methylation is associated with transcriptional silencing of the tumour suppressor p16/CDKN2/MTS1 in human cancers. *Nat Med* **1**: 686–92.

Miki Y, Nishisho I, Horii A, Miyoshi Y, Utsunomiya J, Kinzler KW et al. (1992). Disruption of the APC gene by a retrotransposal insertion of L1 sequence in a colon cancer. *Cancer Res* **52**: 643–45.

Mizukami H, Shirahata A, Goto T, Sakata M, Saito M, Ishibashi K et al. (2008). PGP9.5 methylation as a marker for metastatic colorectal cancer. *Anticancer Res* **28**: 2697–700.

Mori Y, Cai K, Cheng Y, Wang S, Paun B, Hamilton JP et al. (2006). A genome-wide search identifies epigenetic silencing of somatostatin, tachykinin-1, and 5 other genes in colon cancer. *Gastroenterology* **131**: 797–808.

Mutskov V, Felsenfeld G (2004). Silencing of transgene transcription precedes methylation of promoter DNA and histone H3 lysine 9. *EMBO J* **23**: 138–49.

Nakagawa H, Chadwick RB, Peltomaki P, Plass C, Nakamura Y, de La Chapelle A (2001). Loss of imprinting of the insulin-like growth factor II gene occurs by biallelic methylation in a core region of H19-associated CTCF-binding sites in colorectal cancer. *Proc Natl Acad Sci USA* **98**: 591–96.

Nakamura N, Takenaga K (1998). Hypomethylation of the metastasis-associated S100A4 gene correlates with gene activation in human colon adenocarcinoma cell lines. *Clin Exp Metastasis* **16**: 471–79.

Narayan A, Ji W, Zhang XY, Marrogi A, Graff JR, Baylin SB et al. (1998). Hypomethylation of pericentromeric DNA in breast adenocarcinomas. *Int J Cancer* **77**: 833–38.

Ogawa O, Eccles MR, Szeto J, McNoe LA, Yun K, Maw MA et al. (1993). Relaxation of insulin-like growth factor II gene imprinting implicated in Wilms' tumour. *Nature* **362**: 749–51.

Ogino S, Nosho K, Kirkner GJ, Kawasaki T, Chan AT, Schernhammer ES et al. (2008). A cohort study of tumoral LINE-1 hypomethylation and prognosis in colon cancer. *J Natl Cancer Inst* **100**: 1734–38.

Ohm JE, McGarvey KM, Yu X, Cheng L, Schuebel KE, Cope L et al. (2007). A stem cell-like chromatin pattern may predispose tumor suppressor genes to DNA hypermethylation and heritable silencing. *Nat Genet* **39**: 237–42.

Ohtani-Fujita N, Fujita T, Aoike A, Osifchin NE, Robbins PD, Sakai T (1993). CpG methylation inactivates the promoter activity of the human retinoblastoma tumor-suppressor gene. *Oncogene* **8**: 1063–67.

Otterson GA, Khleif SN, Chen W, Coxon AB, Kaye FJ (1995). CDKN2 gene silencing in lung cancer by DNA hypermethylation and kinetics of p16INK4 protein induction by 5-aza 2′deoxycytidine. *Oncogene* **11**: 1211–16.

Pakneshan P, Szyf M, Rabbani SA (2005). Methylation and inhibition of expression of uPA by the RAS oncogene: divergence of growth control and invasion in breast cancer cells. *Carcinogenesis* **26**: 557–64.

Paz MF, Avila S, Fraga MF, Pollan M, Capella G, Peinado MA et al. (2002). Germ-line variants in methyl-group metabolism genes and susceptibility to DNA methylation in normal tissues and human primary tumors. *Cancer Res* **62**: 4519–24.

Paz MF, Wei S, Cigudosa JC, Rodriguez-Perales S, Peinado MA, Huang TH et al. (2003). Genetic unmasking of epigenetically silenced tumor suppressor genes in colon cancer cells deficient in DNA methyltransferases. *Hum Mol Genet* **12**: 2209–19.

Pedersen IS, Dervan PA, Broderick D, Harrison M, Miller N, Delany E et al. (1999). Frequent loss of imprinting of PEG1/MEST in invasive breast cancer. *Cancer Res* **59**: 5449–51.

Peng Z, Wei D, Wang L, Tang H, Zhang J, Le X et al. (2006). RUNX3 inhibits the expression of vascular endothelial growth factor and reduces the angiogenesis, growth, and metastasis of human gastric cancer. *Clin Cancer Res* **12**: 6386–94.

Rainier S, Johnson LA, Dobry CJ, Ping AJ, Grundy PE, Feinberg AP (1993). Relaxation of imprinted genes in human cancer. *Nature* **362**: 747–49.

Ramirez N, Bandres E, Navarro A, Pons A, Jansa S, Moreno I et al. (2008). Epigenetic events in normal colonic mucosa surrounding colorectal cancer lesions. *Eur J Cancer* **44**: 2689–95.

Rashid A, Shen L, Morris JS, Issa JP, Hamilton SR (2001). CpG island methylation in colorectal adenomas. *Am J Pathol* **159**: 1129–35.

Rothberg PG, Ponnuru S, Baker D, Bradley JF, Freeman AI, Cibis GW et al. (1997). A deletion polymorphism due to Alu-Alu recombination in intron 2 of the retinoblastoma gene: association with human gliomas. *Mol Carcinog* **19**: 69–73.

Sabbioni S, Miotto E, Veronese A, Sattin E, Gramantieri L, Bolondi L et al. (2003). Multigene methylation analysis of gastrointestinal tumors: TPEF emerges as a frequent tumor-specific aberrantly methylated marker that can be detected in peripheral blood. *Mol Diagn* **7**: 201–7.

Saito Y, Jones PA (2006). Epigenetic activation of tumor suppressor microRNAs in human cancer cells. *Cell Cycle* **5**: 2220–22.

Santini V, Kantarjian HM, Issa JP (2001). Changes in DNA methylation in neoplasia: pathophysiology and therapeutic implications. *Ann Intern Med* **134**: 573–86.

Schlesinger Y, Straussman R, Keshet I, Farkash S, Hecht M, Zimmerman J et al. (2007). Polycomb-mediated methylation on Lys27 of histone H3 pre-marks genes for de novo methylation in cancer. *Nat Genet* **39**: 232–36.

Seligson DB, Horvath S, Shi T, Yu H, Tze S, Grunstein M et al. (2005). Global histone modification patterns predict risk of prostate cancer recurrence. *Nature* **435**: 1262–66.

Sengupta S, den Boon JA, Chen IH, Newton MA, Stanhope SA, Cheng YJ et al. (2008). MicroRNA 29c is down-regulated in nasopharyngeal carcinomas, up-regulating mRNAs encoding extracellular matrix proteins. *Proc Natl Acad Sci USA* **105**: 5874–78.

Sharrard RM, Royds JA, Rogers S, Shorthouse AJ (1992). Patterns of methylation of the c-myc gene in human colorectal cancer progression. *Br J Cancer* **65**: 667–72.

Shilatifard A (2006). Chromatin modifications by methylation and ubiquitination: implications in the regulation of gene expression. *Annu Rev Biochem* **75**: 243–69.

Spurling CC, Suhl JA, Boucher N, Nelson CE, Rosenberg DW, Giardina C (2008). The short chain fatty acid butyrate induces promoter demethylation and reactivation of RARbeta2 in colon cancer cells. *Nutr Cancer* **60**: 692–702.

Suzuki H, Gabrielson E, Chen W, Anbazhagan R, van Engeland M, Weijenberg MP et al. (2002). A genomic screen for genes upregulated by demethylation and histone deacetylase inhibition in human colorectal cancer. *Nat Genet* **31**: 141–49.

Tavazoie SF, Alarcon C, Oskarsson T, Padua D, Wang Q, Bos PD et al. (2008). Endogenous human microRNAs that suppress breast cancer metastasis. *Nature* **451**: 147–52.

Toyota M, Ho C, Ahuja N, Jair KW, Li Q, Ohe-Toyota M et al. (1999). Identification of differentially methylated sequences in colorectal cancer by methylated CpG island amplification. *Cancer Res* **59**: 2307–12.

Toyota M, Sasaki Y, Satoh A, Ogi K, Kikuchi T, Suzuki H et al. (2003). Epigenetic inactivation of CHFR in human tumors. *Proc Natl Acad Sci USA* **100**: 7818–23.

van Engeland M, Weijenberg MP, Roemen GM, Brink M, de Bruine AP, Goldbohm RA et al. (2003). Effects of dietary folate and alcohol intake on promoter methylation in sporadic colorectal cancer: the Netherlands cohort study on diet and cancer. *Cancer Res* **63**: 3133–37.

Voorhoeve PM, le Sage C, Schrier M, Gillis AJ, Stoop H, Nagel R et al. (2006). A genetic screen implicates miRNA-372 and miRNA-373 as oncogenes in testicular germ cell tumors. *Cell* **124**: 1169–81.

Weber M, Davies JJ, Wittig D, Oakeley EJ, Haase M, Lam WL et al. (2005). Chromosome-wide and promoter-specific analyses identify sites of differential DNA methylation in normal and transformed human cells. *Nat Genet* **37**: 853–62.

Weber B, Stresemann C, Brueckner B, Lyko F (2007). Methylation of human microRNA genes in normal and neoplastic cells. *Cell Cycle* **6**: 1001–5.

Wendt MK, Johanesen PA, Kang-Decker N, Binion DG, Shah V, Dwinell MB (2006). Silencing of epithelial CXCL12 expression by DNA hypermethylation promotes colonic carcinoma metastasis. *Oncogene* **25**: 4986–97.

Widschwendter M, Fiegl H, Egle D, Mueller-Holzner E, Spizzo G, Marth C et al. (2007). Epigenetic stem cell signature in cancer. *Nat Genet* **39**: 157–58.

Wolffe AP, Matzke MA (1999). Epigenetics: regulation through repression. *Science* **286**: 481–86.

Woodson K, Flood A, Green L, Tangrea JA, Hanson J, Cash B et al. (2004). Loss of insulin-like growth factor-II imprinting and the presence of screen-detected colorectal adenomas in women. *J Natl Cancer Inst* **96**: 407–10.

Wynter CV, Kambara T, Walsh MD, Leggett BA, Young J, Jass JR (2006). DNA methylation patterns in adenomas from FAP, multiple adenoma and sporadic colorectal carcinoma patients. *Int J Cancer* **118**: 907–15.

Xu XL, Yu J, Zhang HY, Sun MH, Gu J, Du X et al. (2004). Methylation profile of the promoter CpG islands of 31 genes that may contribute to colorectal carcinogenesis. *World J Gastroenterol* **10**: 3441–54.

Yamashita K, Upadhyay S, Osada M, Hoque MO, Xiao Y, Mori M et al. (2002). Pharmacologic unmasking of epigenetically silenced tumor suppressor genes in esophageal squamous cell carcinoma. *Cancer Cell* **2**: 485–95.

Yoo CB, Jones PA (2006). Epigenetic therapy of cancer: past, present and future. *Nat Rev Drug Discov* **5**: 37–50.

Yu Y, Xu F, Peng H, Fang X, Zhao S, Li Y et al. (1999). NOEY2 (ARHI), an imprinted putative tumor suppressor gene in ovarian and breast carcinomas. *Proc Natl Acad Sci USA* **96**: 214–19.

Chapter 5

CANCER-INITIATING CELLS IN COLORECTAL CANCER

Antonija Kreso[1], Liane Gibson[2] and Catherine Adell O'Brien[2-4]

[1] Department of Molecular and Medical Genetics, University of Toronto, Toronto, ON, Canada
[2] Division of Cell and Molecular Biology, University Health Network, Toronto, ON, Canada
[3] Division of General Surgery, University Health Network, Toronto, ON, Canada
[4] Toronto General Hospital, Toronto, ON, Canada,
e-mail: cobrien@uhnresearch.ca

Abstract: Colorectal cancer is the second leading cause of death from cancer (men and women combined) in the US and Canada. The mainstay of treatment remains surgical resection and although new agents are constantly emerging to treat colorectal cancer, to date none of the agents have been successful at curing patients with advanced disease. In recent years, there has been an increasing interest in the notion that cancers are organized as a hierarchy with the cancer-initiating cell (C-IC or cancer stem cell) existing at the apex. The C-ICs only represent a subset of the total tumour cells, however, research indicates that they are responsible for both the initiation and maintenance of tumour growth. This chapter will focus on the current state of knowledge in the colorectal C-IC (CC-IC) field, commencing with a summary of the cell surface markers that have been utilized to isolate these cells. The identification of CC-ICs has also led to a number of questions being raised in the field including whether or not they play a role in chemoresistance and metastasis. Lastly, this chapter will also address the challenges that the CC-IC field faces and the approaches being utilized to better understand these cells and determine their clinical relevance.

Key words: Colon cancer metastasis · Colon cancer initiating cells (CC-ICs) · Chemotherapy

5.1 Introduction

It has long been appreciated that tumours are composed of cells that display morphological heterogeneity (Dick, 2008). In 1961, Southam et al. published a set of experiments where they autologously injected tumour cells into patients' thighs; in order to observe tumour growth, they required a minimum injection of 10^6 cells (Southam and Brunschwig, 1961). Interestingly, the number of tumour cells required to obtain growth was inversely correlated to the stage and grade of the original neoplasm, with more advanced and poorly differentiated tumours requiring fewer cells to seed a tumour in the thigh. These experiments clearly demonstrated that tumour cells are not only morphologically different, but that they also exhibit functional heterogeneity.

Two models were put forth to explain why tumour cells are functionally heterogeneous in their ability to initiate and maintain tumour growth (Fig. 5.1). The stochastic model stated that every cell within a tumour had the ability to sustain the

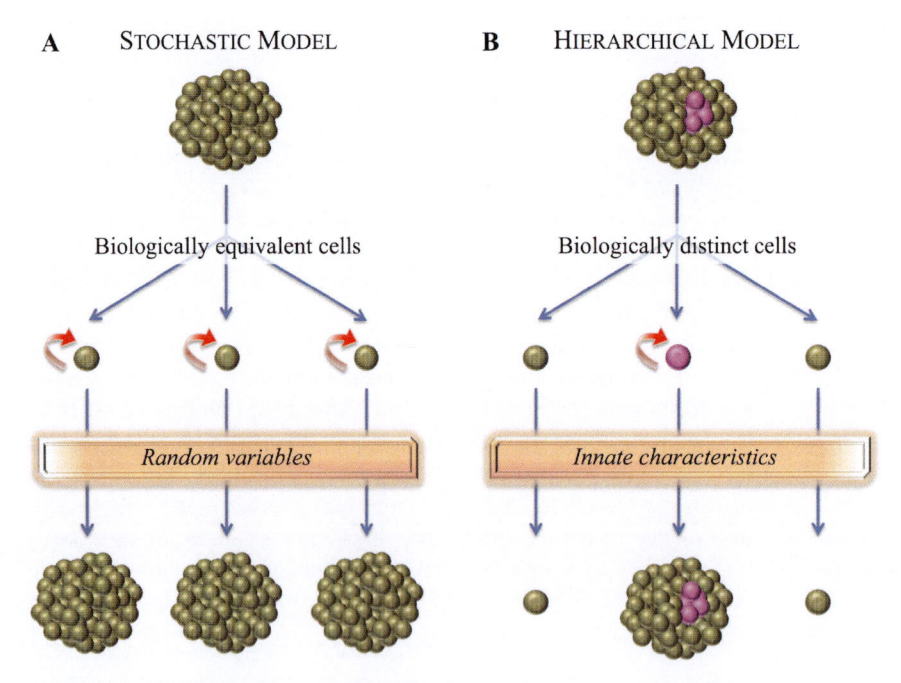

Fig. 5.1 Models to explain tumour heterogeneity. (**a**) The stochastic model predicts that the distinct ability of tumour cells to initiate tumours is governed by random variables, such as entry into the cell cycle, a low probability stochastic event. According to this model, it should not be possible to fractionate cells with differential tumour initiation properties. (**b**) The hierarchical or cancer stem cell model predicts that there is a subset of cancer cells that are responsible for establishing and maintaining tumour growth. According to this model, it should be possible to prospectively isolate these cancer stem cells, or cancer-initiating cells (C-ICs), based on the expression of specific cell surface markers

tumour and this was governed by entry into the cell cycle, a low probability stochastic event. According to this model, one would not be able to prospectively isolate the cell subset that is responsible for sustaining the tumour. In contrast, the cancer stem cell (CSC) model (also known as the hierarchical model) suggested that there is a subset of cancer cells that is responsible for establishing and maintaining tumour growth. According to this model, one should be able to prospectively isolate the CSC or cancer-initiating cell (C-IC) based on cell surface marker expression (Reya et al., 2001).

The initial evidence to support the CSC model stemmed from work published in 1994 by John Dick and colleagues (Bonnet and Dick, 1997; Lapidot et al., 1994). They isolated a subset of acute myelogenous leukemia (AML) cells, based on a specific cell surface phenotype ($CD34^+CD38^-$), that were solely capable of transferring the disease in immune deficient mouse models. The leukemia stem cells (LSCs) were defined by the ability to: (i) generate a xenograft that was histologically representative of the parent tumour from which they were derived; (ii) self-renew as demonstrated by serial passage in a xenograft assay; and (iii) give rise to daughter cells that possessed proliferative capacity but were unable to establish or maintain the AML clone upon serial passage (Clarke et al., 2006).

The principles of the CSC model were not tested in a solid tumour until a decade after the initial work in leukemia was published (Pardal et al., 2003). This was due in large part to the paucity of solid tumour xenograft models generated from single cell suspensions and the inability to sort the cells based on cell surface markers. The technical hurdles were surmounted in 2003 when Michael Clarke's group tested the CSC model in the context of breast cancer (Al-Hajj et al., 2003). They were able to prospectively isolate a subset of breast cancer cells ($CD44^+CD24^-$) that were solely responsible for sustaining the disease in an immune-compromised mouse model. The CSC subset could be serially passaged and the xenografts generated were histologically heterogeneous, resembling the parent tumour from which they were derived. These results demonstrated that the same CSC principles that had previously been shown to apply in an AML model could also be translated to a solid tumour. Since the initial publication in breast cancer, a plethora of papers have been published identifying C-ICs in numerous cancers including: brain (Singh et al., 2004), colon (O'Brien et al., 2007; Ricci-Vitiani et al., 2007), head and neck (Prince et al., 2007), pancreas (Hermann et al., 2007; Li et al., 2007), lung (Eramo et al., 2008), prostate (Collins et al., 2005; Patrawala et al., 2006), and sarcoma (Wu et al., 2007).

The application of the CSC model to solid tumours has led to many questions being raised with regards to the clinical and biological relevance of these cells. Increasing evidence has demonstrated that the C-ICs possess mechanisms to survive radiation therapy and many of the conventional chemotherapies (Fig. 5.2) (Eyler and Rich, 2008). This raises an important biological question of whether C-ICs represent the source of metastatic disease, which would render them the most relevant cells to study when developing new therapeutics (Wang, 2007). These questions remain unanswered; however, the expanding interest in C-ICs is in large part fueled by these possibilities. The aim of this chapter will be to review the current state of knowledge

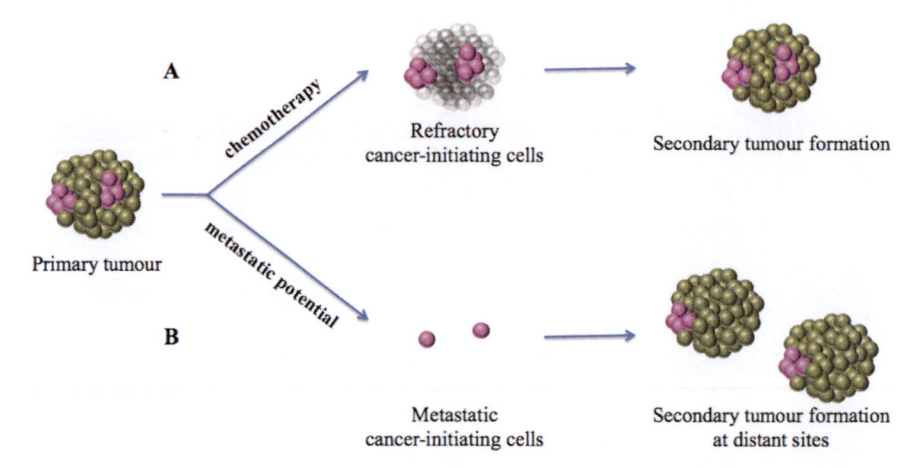

Fig. 5.2 Hypothetical models to account for the role of CC-ICs in tumour relapse and metastasis. (a) After chemotherapy, refractory CC-ICs survive which possess the ability to self-renew and proliferate extensively, allowing them to re-generate a new tumour. (b) CC-ICs are postulated to be responsible for the establishment of metastatic disease. Based on their ability to endure environmental stressors, it is thought that C-ICs may possess the inherent biological mechanisms that give them an advantage during the metastatic process

in the field of colon cancer-initiating cells (CC-ICs) with a particular focus on their role in the metastatic process.

5.2 The Cell Surface Phenotype of Colon Cancer-Initiating Cells

Proof of the CSC model is dependent on demonstrating functional heterogeneity amongst the cells of a given tumour. Of equal importance is the ability to prospectively identify the tumour-initiating fraction based on a specific cell surface phenotype. Over the past 5 years, a number of C-IC surface markers have been identified in a wide range of solid tumours (O'Brien et al., 2009). This chapter will focus on the markers that have been published in colorectal cancer including: CD133 (O'Brien et al., 2007; Ricci-Vitiani et al., 2007), CD44 (Dalerba et al., 2007), CD166 (Dalerba et al., 2007), and aldehyde dehydrogenase (ALDH) (see Table 5.1) (Huang et al., 2009).

CD133 was the first cell surface marker utilized to isolate the tumour-initiating cells in colon cancer (O'Brien et al., 2007; Ricci-Vitiani et al., 2007). It was originally identified as a cell surface antigen present on hematopoietic and neural stem cells (Miraglia et al., 1997; Uchida et al., 2000; Yin et al., 1997). It is a five transmembrane domain glycoprotein, which is postulated to play a role in cell polarity; however, much work is still required to clearly delineate its functional role (Mizrak et al., 2008). In 2003, Singh et al. were the first group to utilize CD133 expression to separate solid tumour C-ICs (Singh et al., 2004). In a non-obese diabetic/severe combined immune-deficient (NOD/SCID) murine xenograft

Table 5.1 Prospective isolation of colon cancer-initiating cells (CC-ICs)

References	CC-IC marker(s)	Injection site	Mouse strain	Minimum cell number for tumour engraftment	Range of marker expression in tumours (%)
O'Brien et al. (2007)	CD133+	Renal capsule	NOD/SCID	100	1.8–24.5
Ricci-Vitiani et al. (2007)	CD133+	Subcutaneous	SCID	3,000	0.7–6.1
Dalerba et al. (2007)	EpCAM^{high}CD44+	Subcutaneous	NOD/SCID	200–500	0.03–38
Dalerba et al. (2007)	EpCAM^{high}CD44+CD166[1]	Subcutaneous	NOD/SCID	1,000	3.3–35.6
Todaro et al. (2007)	CD133+	Subcutaneous	Nude	2,500–5,000	0.3–3
Haraguchi et al. (2008)	CD133−	Subcutaneous	NOD/SCID	10,000	0.3–82
Haraguchi et al. (2008)	CD44+	Subcutaneous	NOD/SCID	10,000	11.5–58.4
Haraguchi et al. (2008)	CD133+CD44+	Subcutaneous	NOD/SCID	10,000	0.2–50.5
Chu et al. (2009)	CD44^{high}	Subcutaneous	SCID/Bg	1,000	5–24
Chu et al. (2009)	CD44^{high}ALDH+	Subcutaneous	SCID/Bg	100	1.5–9
Huang et al. (2009)	ALDH[1]	Subcutaneous	NOD/SCID	25–100	3.5±1
Huang et al. (2009)	ALDH−CD44−	Subcutaneous	NOD/SCID	no data	1.3±0.6
Huang et al. (2009)	ALDH+CD133+	Subcutaneous	NOD/SCID	no data	0.9–0.2

model, orthotopic injection of as few as 100 CD133$^+$ brain cancer cells gave rise to a xenograft that was histologically similar to the parent tumour from which it was derived. In contrast, injection of up to 10^5 CD133$^-$ brain cancer cells did not give rise to a xenograft. Since the initial publication in brain tumours, CD133 has been found to mark the tumourigenic fraction in a range of solid tumours including: colon (O'Brien et al., 2007; Ricci-Vitiani et al., 2007), pancreas (Hermann et al., 2007), lung (Eramo et al., 2008), and prostate (Collins et al., 2005).

Two groups utilizing two different murine xenograft models initially published the identification of CD133 as a marker of CC-ICs. One group employed a NOD/SCID renal subcapsular xenograft model to demonstrate that CD133$^+$ human colon cancer cells were enriched in tumour-initiating capacity (O'Brien et al., 2007). In contrast, the CD133$^-$ colon cancer cells did not give rise to xenografts with one exception at the highest cell concentration (2×10^5 cells). Similar results were published by Ricci-Vitiani et al. using CD133 in a SCID mouse subcutaneous xenograft model. They demonstrated that 3,000 CD133$^+$ human colon cancer cells could initiate tumours, whereas 10^6 unfractionated cells did not initiate tumours (Ricci-Vitiani et al., 2007). Interestingly, the two groups demonstrated significant variation in the percentage of CD133$^+$ cells in the colon cancers studied: the range being 1.8–24.5% in one study (O'Brien et al., 2007) and 0.7–6.1% in the other (Ricci-Vitiani et al., 2007). Each of these studies represented a small sample size and therefore future work will be required to determine the range of CD133 expression in a larger sample size of human colon cancers.

It is important to recognize that the CD133$^+$ population of colon cancer cells is heterogeneous and not every CD133$^+$ cell represents a CC-IC; rather, CD133 enriches for tumour-initiating capacity (O'Brien et al., 2007). This is best illustrated by carrying out in vivo limiting dilution assays (LDAs), which enables one to calculate the CC-IC frequency in the unfractionated colon cancer cells, as well as in the CD133$^+$ subset. Utilizing LDA experiments, O'Brien et al. determined that the pooled CC-IC frequency for their cohort of 17 patients was approximately 1 in 56,000 unfractionated colon cancer cells (O'Brien et al., 2007). The CC-IC activity was significantly enriched in the CD133$^+$ subset, where one in 262 CD133$^+$ colon cancer cells was calculated by LDA to be a CC-IC. This represented a greater than 200 fold enrichment in CC-IC activity in the CD133$^+$ cells, as compared to the bulk colon cancer cells. It should be noted that this CC-IC frequency was derived from pooled LDAs carried out on the 17 colon cancers in the study. Ideally both unfractionated and fractionated LDAs should be completed for each individual tumour, thereby obtaining CC-IC frequencies and percent enrichment specific for each colon cancer.

The third publication on CC-ICs utilized an adhesion molecule, CD44, to identify the tumour-initiating fraction in human colon cancer (Dalerba et al., 2007; Nagano and Saya, 2004). Initially identified as a C-IC marker in breast cancer (Al-Hajj et al., 2003), CD44 has since been utilized to identify the tumourigenic fraction in a variety of solid tumours, including: colon (Dalerba et al., 2007), pancreas (Li et al., 2007), and head and neck (Prince et al., 2007). In colon cancer, Dalerba et al. identified that the combined expression of epithelial cell adhesion molecule (EpCAM) and CD44 in colorectal cancer cells enriched for tumour-initiating potential in a NOD/SCID subcutaneous xenograft model (Dalerba et al., 2007). They were able to obtain xenograft formation with the injection of, as few as, 200–500 EpCAM^{high}CD44$^+$ cells, whereas 10^4 EpCAM^{low}CD44$^-$ cells did not form xenografts. The tumours derived from the EpCAM^{high}/CD44$^+$ cells reproduced the morphological and histological heterogeneity of the parent tumours from which they were derived. The study consisted of a total of eight colorectal cancer specimens and the frequency of the EpCAM^{high}/CD44$^+$ population ranged from 0.8 to 38%. The authors detected CD133 expression on some of the colon cancers studied; they noted that CD44$^+$ cells typically co-expressed CD133, with the CD44$^+$ cells representing the smaller subset (Dalerba et al., 2007). The authors also studied CD44 in the context of another marker, CD166, a mesenchymal stem cell marker (Bruder et al., 1998). It has previously been published that a subset of colorectal cancers express CD166 and that increased CD166 expression levels have been associated with poor clinical outcome in colorectal cancer (Weichert et al., 2004). Utilizing two un-passaged primary colorectal cancer specimens and a xenografted sample, the authors demonstrated that the tumour-initiating capacity existed solely in the EpCAM$^+$CD44$^+$CD166$^+$ colon cancer cells; a subpopulation that ranged from 3.3 to 35.6% of the total tumour cells. As per all studies in this field, the sample size was small with six out of the eight samples tested being from high passage xenografts and only two of the samples being tested directly from the patient tumour. Since the Dalerba et al. study, another group has also identified the combined use of CD133 and CD44 as a useful tool to further purify the tumour-initiating fraction (Haraguchi et al., 2008). Interestingly, yet another study found that the CD44 alone provided better purification, as opposed to using it in combination with CD133 (Chu et al., 2009). It should be acknowledged that published studies in this area typically test a very small number of samples, with the last two aforementioned studies testing less than five colon cancer samples each. This is likely one of the main factors leading to the conflicting results.

Additional markers continue to be identified that can segregate CC-ICs and non-CC-ICs. For example, aldehyde dehydrogenase 1 (ALDH1), a detoxifying enzyme that oxidizes intracellular aldehydes, has been used to enrich for CC-ICs (Chu et al., 2009; Huang et al., 2009). Huang et al. showed that 100 ALDH1$^+$ primary human colon cancer cells could initiate xenografts in mice, and as few as 25 ALDH1$^+$ colon cancer xenograft-derived cells could be serially cultured in NOD/SCID mice (Huang et al., 2009). They also studied ALDH1 in the context of known CC-IC markers, CD44 and CD133. The percentage of cancer cells expressing only ALDH1 was 3.5±1.0%. In contrast, the cell subsets expressing either CD44 or CD133 were significantly larger being 19.5±6.9% and 24.8±6.0%, respectively. The proportion of colorectal cancer cells positive for both ALDH1 and CD44 was 1.3%±0.6%. The authors found that the use of CD44 in combination with ALDH1 did not provide any further enrichment of the tumour-initiating activity, as compared to the use of ALDH1 alone. Both the ALDH1$^+$ and the ALDH1$^+$CD44$^+$ cells displayed tumour-initiation rates of approximately 70%. The combination of CD133 with ALDH1 revealed a population that comprised 0.9±0.2% of the total cancer cells. Unlike the use of CD44, the combination of CD133 and ALDH1 did reveal enrichment in the tumour-initiating capacity. The ALDH1⁺ tumour-initiation rate was 58% when used alone. However, this was increased to 89% in the xenografts derived from the cancer cells expressing both CD133⁺ALDH1⁺. The authors also noted that the injection of CD44⁻ or CD133⁻ colon cancer cells did not give rise to xenograft formation; yet, the injection of ALDH⁺CD44⁻ or ALDH⁺CD133⁻ demonstrated tumour-initiation rates of 70 and 44%, respectively. The authors attributed this observation to the fact that the cells expressed ALDH1, which conferred the tumour-initiating capacity. The ALDH1⁺ fraction only constitutes a small proportion of the total CD44⁻ and CD133⁻ populations, therefore the authors hypothesized that these fractions typically did not form xenografts because the ALDH⁺CD44⁻ and ALDH⁺CD133⁻ cells are typically present in such low concentrations. Once again, the study consisted of a small sample size with the majority being highly passaged xenografts; nevertheless, it clearly demonstrates that this work is becoming increasingly complex with the addition of each potential CC-IC marker.

Future studies will be required to validate the combined use of CD133, CD44, CD166, and ALDH1 to further purify the CC-IC fraction. It is very possible that different subtypes of human colon cancers will have CC-ICs identified by distinct cell surface phenotypes; however, determining this will require larger scale studies looking at a variety of markers and multiple combinations thereof.

5.3 Colon Cancer-Initiating Cells and Chemoresistance

In recent years, there have been a number of studies published in a variety of solid tumour xenograft models demonstrating radiation and chemotherapeutic resistance of the C-IC subset (Bao et al., 2006; Li et al., 2008; Ma et al., 2008). Todaro et al. were the first to publish evidence that the CC-IC and non-CC-IC fractions of human colon cancers responded differently to conventional chemotherapeutic agents, such as 5-Fluorouracil (5-FU) and oxaliplatin (Todaro et al., 2007). Utilizing CD133 as the CC-IC marker, they demonstrated that CD133⁺ cells were relatively resistant to standard chemotherapeutic agents. In contrast, CD133⁻ cells derived from the same tumours were highly sensitive to both in vivo and in vitro treatment with 5-FU or oxaliplatin. The authors determined that one of the mechanisms by which the CD133⁺ cells protect themselves from conventional chemotherapies is through the autocrine production of interleukin-4 (IL-4). By treating mice with a neutralizing antibody against IL-4, they were able to render previously resistant CD133⁺ colon cancer cells sensitive to treatment with oxaliplatin and/or 5-FU, thereby leading to an overall decrease in the number of CD133⁺ cells (Todaro et al., 2007). Interestingly, the increased chemosensitivity in the cancer cells, following treatment with the IL-4 antibody, was associated with a reduction in pro-survival molecules, such as caspase 8 homolog FLICE inhibitory protein (cFLIP), B-cell lymphoma extra-large protein (Bcl-x_L), and phosphoprotein enriched in diabetes (PED) in the CD133⁺ fraction (Todaro et al., 2007).

Another study published by Dylla et al. looked at the response of CC-ICs (ESA$^+$CD44$^+$) to irinotecan or cyclophosphamide (CPA) treatment (Dylla et al., 2008). Human colon cancer cells were utilized to generate xenografts, which were subsequently treated for 2 weeks with irinotecan. Following treatment, the xenografts were harvested and it was determined that the percentage of tumour cells displaying the CC-IC phenotype was increased by 61% in the xenografts treated with irinotecan, as compared to untreated control xenografts. Furthermore, the xenografts were tested in a limiting dilution serial transplantation assay and only the cells displaying the CC-IC phenotype could generate tumours in both the irinotecan and control treated groups (Dylla et al., 2008). The authors demonstrated that not only was there an increase in CC-IC marker expression after exposure to irinotecan, but that this change was also functionally important because it was associated with an increase in the tumour-initiating capacity.

To investigate the relationship between CPA treatment and CC-ICs the authors used a different approach. Existing literature suggests that resistance to CPA results from high ALDH activity. Interestingly, when Dylla et al. studied colon cancer cells for ALDH1 expression, it was determined that the CC-IC fraction (ESA$^+$CD44$^+$) possessed the majority of the ALDH1 activity (Dylla et al., 2008). Moreover, the tumour-initiating potential was greater in the ESA$^+$CD44$^+$ALDH1$^+$ versus the ESA$^+$CD44$^+$ALDH1$^-$ colon cancer cells. Phenotypically the ALDH1$^+$ subpopulation of ESA$^+$CD44$^+$ cells was consistently higher after CPA treatment, as compared to the vehicle-treated controls (67±6.3% versus 56.8±6.8% respectively). Interestingly, the inhibition of ALDH1 activity either by short-hairpin RNA interference or chemical-mediated inhibition by diethylaminobenzaldehyde did not significantly inhibit xenograft growth. However, the decreased ALDH1 activity did render the cells sensitive to CPA treatment, resulting in a significant inhibitory effect on xenograft growth (Dylla et al., 2008). Interestingly, the inhibition of ALDH1 activity did not have any effect on the resistance of CC-ICs to irinotecan, indicating that the mechanism of resistance is drug-specific. This work was the first to demonstrate the complex mechanisms utilized by CC-ICs to protect themselves from the stressors in their environment and confer a survival advantage. One can assume that there are multiple survival mechanisms utilized by the CC-ICs; deciphering these mechanisms and developing methods to perturb them will require better purification and a deeper understanding of CC-IC biology.

5.4 The Role of Cancer-Initiating Cells in Metastases

There are striking similarities between the understanding of how cancer cells metastasize and the emerging functional definition of C-ICs. Interestingly, both the C-IC and fully metastatic cells represent rare clones within primary tumours (Chiang and Massague, 2008). In animal models, 0.01% or fewer cancer cells entering the circulation develop into metastases (Chambers et al., 2002; Luzzi et al., 1998). The low metastatic efficiency of cancer cells may be related to the extreme environmental stresses that these cells are exposed to upon entering the circulation, including: lack of oxygen or nutrients, a low pH, and reactive oxygen species (ROS) (Gupta and Massague, 2006). It has been postulated that only those cancer cells that acquire an aggressive phenotype capable of overcoming these environmental stressors will survive to give rise to a metastatic lesion. According to the CSC model, only C-ICs are capable of initiating and maintaining the tumour, which often leads to the assumption that C-ICs must be the cells responsible for metastatic dissemination. The relationship between C-ICs and metastasis, although theoretically plausible, requires experimental proof. This field remains at a very nascent stage; preliminary research suggests that the C-ICs may be the cells most responsible for metastases.

The first evidence that supported a potential role for C-ICs in metastasis was published in breast cancer, where it was determined that the majority of early disseminated cancer cells detected in the bone marrow of breast cancer patients have a putative breast cancer stem cell phenotype (Balic et al., 2006). This led researchers to question whether C-ICs in breast cancer have biological properties that facilitate their metastatic spread and enable them to colonize distant sites. In support of this hypothesis, Diehn et al. published work in breast cancer, as well as in other solid tumours, which indicated that C-ICs express increased levels of free radical scavenging systems and consequently have lower levels of ROS when compared to their non-tumour initiating counterparts (Diehn et al., 2009). To assess whether the lower levels of ROS detected in the CSC fraction was providing them with a survival advantage, the authors pharmacologically depleted glutathione (GSH); this in turn led to an increase in the ROS levels. GSH is a critical cellular antioxidant that has been implicated in both the chemotherapy and radiotherapy resistance of cancer cells. The depletion of GSH and the resulting increase in ROS levels in the C-IC subset significantly decreased their clonogenicity suggesting that the low ROS levels provide the C-ICs with a survival advantage. High ROS levels are one of the recognized barriers to a cancer cell's ability to successfully metastasize (Chiang and Massague, 2008). Therefore, it is interesting that C-ICs possess mechanisms to maintain lower ROS levels, which may function to protect these cells against environmental stressors and give them an advantage during the metastatic process.

More recently, Li and colleagues demonstrated that in brain cancer xenografts, the C-IC subset preferentially expresses hypoxia-inducible factor 2α (HIF2α) and multiple HIF-regulated genes, as compared to the non-tumour-initiating fraction (Li et al., 2009). Targeting HIF2α in the C-IC population inhibited self-renewal, proliferation, and attenuated xenograft growth in vivo. They also determined that HIF2α is required for vascular endothelial growth factor (VEGF) expression in the C-IC subset (Li et al., 2009). This result supports the notion that C-ICs can preferentially survive in hypoxic environments and furthermore it suggests that C-ICs possess the ability to establish the vascular niche for the tumour. In summary, evidence is emerging that C-ICs share a number of characteristics with the cells that are able to successfully metastasize. It is easy to assume that the C-ICs are therefore responsible for metastatic disease but the experimental evidence is very limited at this time and will require extensive work to conclusively answer this question.

To date, there have been no published papers looking at metastasis and the role of C-ICs in human colorectal cancer. However, a very elegant study was published by Hermann et al. that explored these questions in the context of pancreatic adenocarcinoma C-ICs (Hermann et al., 2007). First, they determined that CD133 marks only a small subset of pancreatic tumour cells and that only the CD133$^+$ cells are able to initiate tumours when injected into the pancreas of immuno-compromised mice (Hermann et al., 2007). Injection of 10^6 CD133$^-$ cells did not produce tumours, thereby confirming that in their system the C-IC activity existed only within the CD133$^+$ pancreatic cancer cells. In addition to primary pancreatic cancer tissue, they also studied two pancreatic cancer cell lines, L3.6pl and FG, which have high and low metastatic potential, respectively. Utilizing an orthotopic xenograft model, they demonstrated that both cell lines possessed a CD133$^+$ C-IC subset, however, only CD133$^+$ cells from the L3.6pl cell line possessed the ability to metastasize. The CD133$^+$ cells from the FG cell line could form a xenograft at the site of injection but lacked any metastatic capability (Hermann et al., 2007). The authors noted that only the L3.6pl cell line expressed the chemokine (C-X-C motif) receptor CXCR4 and questioned whether this might be playing a role in the ability of these CD133$^+$ cells to metastasize. Interestingly, CXCR4 and its ligand, stromal derived growth factor 1 (SDF-1) (also known as CXC chemokine ligand 12 [CXCL12]), play important roles in the survival of both breast and renal cancer cells at sites of metastasis (Muller et al., 2001; Staller et al., 2003; Zagzag et al., 2005). To determine whether CXCR4 is functionally important in pancreatic adenocarcinoma C-ICs and metastasis, the L3.6pl (high metastatic ability) CD133$^+$ cell population was fractionated based on CXCR4 expression. The CD133$^+$CXCR4$^+$ and CD133$^+$CXCR4$^-$ cell subsets were both capable of generating xenografts at the site of injection in NOD/SCID mice, demonstrating that the tumour-initiating capacity of the two cell subsets was equivalent. However, when they analyzed the blood from the xenograft-bearing mice they found that only the double positive cells (CD133$^+$CXCR4$^+$) could be detected in the circulation and this correlated with a metastatic phenotype in the mice. Furthermore, they inhibited CXCR4 pharmacologically, which resulted in abrogated metastasis in their murine xenograft model (Hermann et al., 2007). This work was the first to describe heterogeneity in the C-IC compartment, where a distinct subset of C-ICs was responsible for metastatic dissemination. One could hypothesize that there might be a subset of C-ICs that preferentially disseminates to a specific organ depending on the cell surface phenotype and micro-environmental niche that best support its survival. It is clear that there are currently more questions than answers as they relate to C-ICs and their role in metastasis. Understanding this relationship will provide insight into the mechanisms that cancer cells employ to survive hostile environments, as well as potentially providing insight into why tumours have well-defined patterns of metastasis (Paget, 1989).

5.5 Cancer-Initiating Cells as Biomarkers

The identification of C-IC markers has led to an intense interest in being able to utilize these cell surface phenotypes as prognostic indicators. The most logical method in which to approach this question is through the utilization of immunohistochemistry (IHC) techniques to quantitate the expression of the cell surface markers and correlate this information back to stage, grade, and disease-free survival. The numbers of publications in this field remain limited and although initial results have been very interesting, larger studies are required before clinically relevant biomarkers are validated (Choi et al., 2009; Ginestier et al., 2007; Horst et al., 2009a, 2008). The first study reviewed a series of 77 colorectal cancer patients, of whom 21 (27%) died of colorectal cancer within 5 years of diagnosis (Horst et al., 2008). They employed a semi-quantitative approach where tumours were scored as 0, <50%, or ≥50% $CD133^+$ cells. CD133 expression did not correlate with age, gender, or stage of the tumour. However, by multivariate analysis CD133 expression was demonstrated to be an independent marker for decreased patient survival: $CD133^{high}$ expression represented a relative risk of 2.45 as compared to the $CD133^{low}$ group (Horst et al., 2008).

More recently, Choi et al. studied the relationship between the expression of CC-IC phenotypic markers (CD133 and CD44) as they relate to colorectal cancer: stage, differentiation status, and outcomes (Choi et al., 2009). The retrospective study consisted of a consecutive series of 523 colorectal cancer cases with complete histopathological data. The authors concluded that CD133 and CD44 expression had no effect on overall survival by univariate or multivariate analysis. However, they did demonstrate that CD133 protein expression was higher in the more advanced stage colon cancers, whereas larger tumours (>5.5 cm) showed greater CD44 expression (Choi et al., 2009). These studies provide good examples of the ongoing controversy in the field of CC-IC research and demonstrate why no definite conclusions can be drawn based on the current published literature.

An important issue with the use of known C-IC markers for IHC studies is the understanding that the markers identified to date represent an enrichment of tumour-initiating activity. Further purification of the C-IC subset is required to better delineate the most relevant cells. An interesting approach to this problem is to combine C-IC markers with molecular markers of pathways postulated to have an essential role in the maintenance of the C-IC subset. This approach was employed by Horst et al. in a recent publication where they studied the co-expression of CD133 and nuclear β-catenin and correlated this to outcome data in colorectal cancer patients (Horst et al., 2009a). Previous work by this group had demonstrated that most colon cancers display a heterogeneous expression pattern of nuclear β-catenin, and increased expression was correlated with decreased survival (Horst et al., 2009b). Furthermore, there is data from other cancers that nuclear β-catenin may play an important role in maintaining C-ICs (Korkaya et al., 2009). The authors hypothesized that nuclear β-catenin, like CD133, may also mark the CC-IC subset. To test this, they studied the co-expression of the two markers in 162 stage IIa colon cancers. The combined evaluation proved to be very powerful in identifying patients with stage IIa disease that harbored an increased risk of recurrence. For the subset of patients whose tumours demonstrated the highest co-expression of CD133 and nuclear β-catenin, the 5-year survival rate was only 47±13%, a figure approaching the 5-year survival rates in stage IIIc patients (Horst et al., 2009a). However, the authors caution that these results remain preliminary and must be confirmed in larger studies. Future research using similar methods of combining CC-IC phenotypes with molecular markers from relevant pathways will hopefully lead to these biologically relevant marker combinations being employed as clinically useful prognostic indices.

A recent study by Ginestier et al. demonstrated that another marker, ALDH1, could prospectively identify the breast cancer cell subset capable of xenograft formation and serial transplantation (Ginestier et al., 2007). As mentioned previously in this chapter, ALDH1 has also been identified as a C-IC marker in colon cancer (Huang et al., 2009). Interestingly, apart from identifying ALDH1 as a C-IC marker in breast cancer, they also studied a series of 577 breast cancer patients and determined that expression of ALDH1 correlated with poor prognosis. The relative risk of death due to cancer was 1.76 for patients with ALDH1-positive tumours as compared to patients with ALDH1-low or -negative tumours (Ginestier et al., 2007). The potential value of ALDH1 as a prognostic marker in colon cancer remains to be studied.

5.6 Cancer-Initiating Cells and Clinical Trials

There is a keen interest to determine the clinical relevance of C-ICs and an essential aspect to answering this question requires incorporating the study of C-ICs into clinical trials. Li et al. were the first to study C-ICs in the context of a neo-adjuvant clinical trial for locally advanced breast cancer patients (Li et al., 2008). The authors compared the C-IC subset (CD44$^+$CD24$^-$) following conventional chemotherapy (docetaxol or doxorubicin and cyclophosphamide) alone or with the addition of lapatinib (an epidermal growth factor receptor/HER2 inhibitor). Tumour samples were obtained pre- and post-treatment and tested both phenotypically and functionally for C-IC activity. The functional testing included in vitro mammosphere formation efficiency (MFSE) and in vivo xenograft formation. The tumours treated with chemotherapy alone demonstrated an enrichment in cells displaying the C-IC CD44$^+$CD24$^-$ phenotype. In contrast, the patients that received chemotherapy with lapatinib did not display any enrichment in the C-IC phenotype (Li et al., 2008). It is important to appreciate that the phenotypic assessment is insufficient to draw any conclusions when used in isolation without functional correlation. The gold standard is to functionally assess tumourigenicity or self-renewal potential of the cancer cells by in vivo limiting dilution analysis. Li et al. were able to demonstrate that not only was there a phenotypic change in the profile of the tumours, but this also translated to a functional change because the tumours treated with lapatinib possessed decreased self-renewal capacity as measured by MFSE and xenograft formation, as compared to the tumours only treated with conventional chemotherapy (Li et al., 2008). The authors hypothesized that the observed phenotypic and functional C-IC changes may in part explain the survival benefit conferred by lapatinib. However, the trial was preliminary and larger trials will have to be carried out to confirm these findings. To dates no colorectal cancer clinical trials have been published that have incorporated the study of C-ICs. The principles applied by Li et al. provide an excellent framework for colorectal cancer, as well as other solid tumours. By sampling the tumours pre- and post-treatment, they were able to both phenotypically and functionally test the self-renewal capacity of the tumours, both aspects being essential when determining the clinical relevance of C-ICs.

The ability to carry out informative clinical trials will be essential because one of the main criticisms of the C-IC field is that the majority of the work is currently carried out in xenograft models. This has raised many issues about whether researchers are simply detecting the cancer cells that can engraft in immuno-compromised mouse models, leading many to question the clinical relevance of C-ICs in the context of human patients (Visvader and Lindeman, 2008). The longevity of the C-IC field will strongly depend on the ability to demonstrate that C-ICs are clinically relevant in the context of human patients as determined by large prospective randomized clinical trials.

5.7 Cell of Origin and C-ICs

The notion that human cancers are organized in a hierarchical manner with a C-IC at the apex in many ways recapitulates the organization of normal tissue architecture (Wang and Dick, 2005). This is probably best exemplified in highly regenerating normal tissues, such as the hematopoietic and intestinal systems (Tan et al., 2006). This has led to some confusion in the field partly due to the commonly utilized nomenclature of 'cancer stem cell', and partly due to the undeniable similarities between normal and cancer stem cells, namely the capacity for self-renewal (Jordan et al., 2006). However, it is important to emphasize that although the CSC model states that there is a stem-like cell that maintains the tumour, it does not suggest that the C-ICs are derived from normal stem cells. This question delves into the 'cell of origin' of cancer and represents a field of study unto itself. There is data in other organ systems, namely hematopoietic, that C-ICs can arise from normal stem cells or progenitors (Cozzio et al., 2003; Jamieson et al., 2004; Krivtsov et al., 2006). In the instance of solid tumours, there is much less known about the normal hierarchical structures of the tissues and therefore these questions remain to be answered (Barker et al., 2009; Zhu et al., 2009). The ability to combine these two fields of research will lead to a better understanding of how C-ICs develop.

To dates CC-ICs have not been identified in mouse models of colorectal tumourigenesis; however, a number of murine studies have been published that identify putative markers of normal intestinal stem cells. The markers identified include leucine-rich-repeat containing G-protein-coupled receptor 5 (Lgr5), Prominin 1

(Prom1, the mouse homolog of CD133), and Bmi-1 (Barker et al., 2007; Sangiorgi and Capecchi, 2008; Zhu et al., 2009). Interestingly, Lgr5 and Prom1 are co-expressed in a subset of intestinal cells at the base of crypts, however, there are also intestinal cells that only express one or the other (Barker et al., 2009; Zhu et al., 2009). Barker et al. identified Lgr5 as a stem cell marker in murine small and large intestine by genetically tracing the progeny of marked Lgr5$^+$ intestinal cells (Barker et al., 2007). They demonstrated that long-term clones derived from single Lgr5$^+$ marked cells were capable of repopulating all the cells within the crypt and villus, including: enterocytes, goblet cells, Paneth cells, and enteroendocrine cells (Barker et al., 2007). Zhu et al. carried out similar experiments whereby they utilized lineage-tracing experiments to identify Prom1$^+$ cells as putative murine intestinal stem cells (Zhu et al., 2009). The Prom1$^+$ cells possessed the hallmark stem cell characteristics of multi-lineage differentiation and self-renewal, and were capable of repopulating an entire intestinal crypt over several weeks (Zhu et al., 2009). Both groups attempted to determine whether their 'stem cell subset' was susceptible to malignant transformation and approached this question by utilizing methods to perturb β-catenin function. In both studies the perturbation of β-catenin in either the Lgr5$^+$ or Prom1$^+$ cells led to adenoma formation. All of the intestinal cells forming the adenomas were derived from the mutated stem cell; however, in both studies only a small percentage of the cells within the adenoma retained expression of Lgr5 or Prom1, 6.5 and 7%, respectively. This finding supports the notion that a hierarchical organization exists even within adenomas and this may in part reflect the cell of origin of intestinal tumours. Adding further complexity to the picture, Barker et al. also studied the effect of increasing nuclear β-catenin in the progenitor cells of the intestine (i.e. Lgr5 negative cells) (Barker et al., 2009). They observed numerous microadenomas; however, the generation of adenomas was a rare occurrence, as compared to the number of adenomas detected in the Lgr5$^+$ cells. This demonstrates the complexity of the system and implies that progenitor cells may also possess the capacity to generate tumours albeit at a lower frequency. These are seminal studies in the field of intestinal stem cell biology and represent the first papers to functionally delve into the question of cell of origin in intestinal neoplasia. It will be very interesting to apply this knowledge to the human intestinal system in order to develop a better understanding of the early stages of malignant transformation and to determine if human intestinal stem cells can be identified using the same cell surface markers.

5.8 Controversies in the Cancer Stem Cell Field

To fully understand the current state of C-IC research, it is also important to have an understanding of the controversies that exist within the field. As mentioned previously in this chapter, one of the main criticisms of the CSC model is that it relies very heavily on the xenograft assay (Rosen and Jordan, 2009). This has led critics of the research to question whether a cell subset is being selected, capable of surviving in immuno-compromised mice. One method by which researchers are trying to address this criticism is by identifying C-IC fractions in transgenic mouse models of cancer. These models allow for syngeneic transplantation of specific cell subsets and therefore eliminate the cross-species barriers to engraftment. The work published to date is mostly examining mouse models of leukemia; it is clear from the results that the LSC frequency differs depending on the transgenic model (Kennedy et al., 2007). As one would expect, some models have a very high LSC frequency where almost all cells in the tumour have the capacity to self-renew (Kelly et al., 2007). However, there are other mouse models that possess a hierarchical organization. For example, in a phosphatase and tensin homolog (*Pten*) deletion model of AML, only one out of every 6×10^5 leukemic cells was able to reconstitute the disease in syngeneic transplantation assays (Yilmaz et al., 2006). It would be very informative to carry out similar studies in the commonly studied mouse models of colon cancer such as the *Adenomatous polyposis coli/multiple intestinal neoplasis* (*Apc/Min*) mouse model. Initial work in human cancers suggests that C-IC frequencies also vary between tumours. Determining the extent of the variation and the clinical relevance will require functional testing in a large number of patients with a broad range of tumour subtypes.

Another major criticism of the field is that it is over-simplifying a complex genetic disease. The notion that one cell surface marker can enrich for the most relevant cell type in a broad range of cancers is conceptually difficult for some cancer researchers to accept. Among colon cancers there is a significant amount of genetic variability, therefore it is difficult to imagine that this would not be reflected in the engrafting phenotype. This field remains at a very nascent stage and current work is being carried out to study C-ICs in the context of genetic changes within a specific tumour. Related work is also being carried out to study the C-IC subset using reporter constructs, which will provide a means to functionally study these cells in the context of the molecular pathways driving them (Korkaya et al., 2009).

5.9 Conclusions

The study of C-ICs in solid tumours has expanded exponentially over the past 5 years following the initial publication by Michael Clarke's group (Al-Hajj et al., 2003). It has provided a different way to study tumour initiation and maintenance. As a result, it has also led to numerous questions and controversies (Hill, 2006; Jordan et al., 2006). The purpose of this chapter was to provide an overview of what is currently known about C-ICs in colorectal cancer with an emphasis on how this relates to the metastatic process. Preliminary evidence indicates that CC-ICs are both biologically and clinically relevant (Dylla et al., 2008; Horst et al., 2008; Todaro et al., 2007). Albeit preliminary, the research relating to their clinical relevance suggests that these are the cells capable of surviving conventional chemotherapy. Furthermore, C-ICs share many characteristics with the rare clones within a cancer that are capable of successfully metastasizing. This has led to the question of whether C-ICs are the cells responsible for establishing metastases. There is evidence in support of this notion, particularly in the case of pancreatic adenocarcinoma (Hermann et al., 2007); however, definitive proof is pending. This will require a better understanding of the biology of the CC-ICs and the mechanisms they exploit to preferentially survive under environmentally stressful conditions. Larger scale studies are also required to develop a more complete appreciation of the biological diversity that exists within the C-IC subset.

The interest in the cancer stem cell field is driven in large part by the potential clinical relevance. The question that remains to be answered is whether targeting these cells will prove to be relevant in the context of treating human cancers. Current research should be focused on improved purification of CC-ICs, as well as understanding the biology that makes them so unique. It is only through achieving a deeper understanding of CC-ICs that we will be able to devise therapeutics to target the aberrant biology that underlies these cells.

Acknowledgements We gratefully acknowledge the advice and expertise of Dr. John Dick and all the members of the Dick lab for their advice and expertise.

Abbreviations and Acronyms

ALDH	Aldehyde dehydrogenase
AML	Acute myelogenous leukemia
Apc/Min	Adenomatous polyposis coli/multiple intestinal neoplasia
C-IC	Cancer-initiating cell
CC-IC	Colorectal C-IC
CPA	Cyclophosphamide
CSC	Cancer stem cell
CXC	Chemokine C-X-C motif
CXCR	Chemokine C-X-C motif receptor
EpCAM	Epithelial cell adhesion molecule
HIF2α	Hypoxia-inducible factor 2α
IHC	Immunohistochemistry
IL-4	Interleukin-4
LDA	Limiting dilution assay
Lgr5	Leucine-rich-repeat containing G-protein-coupled receptor 5
LSC	Leukemia stem cell
MFSE	Mammosphere formation efficiency
NOD/SCID	Non-obese diabetic/severe combined immune-deficient
PED	Phosphoprotein enriched in diabetes
Prom	Prominin
Pten	Phosphatase tensin homolog
SDF-1	Stromal derived growth factor 1
VEGF	Vascular endothelial growth factor

References

Al-Hajj M, Wicha MS, Benito-Hernandez A, Morrison SJ, Clarke MF (2003). Prospective identification of tumorigenic breast cancer cells. *Proc Natl Acad Sci USA* **100**: 3983–88.

Balic M, Lin H, Young L, Hawes D, Giuliano A, McNamara G et al. (2006). Most early disseminated cancer cells detected in bone marrow of breast cancer patients have a putative breast cancer stem cell phenotype. *Clin Cancer Res* **12**: 5615–21.

Bao S, Wu Q, McLendon RE, Hao Y, Shi Q, Hjelmeland AB et al. (2006). Glioma stem cells promote radioresistance by preferential activation of the DNA damage response. *Nature* **444**: 756–60.

Barker N, Ridgway RA, van Es JH, van de Wetering M, Begthel H, van den Born M et al. (2009). Crypt stem cells as the cells-of-origin of intestinal cancer. *Nature* **457**: 608–11.

Barker N, van Es JH, Kuipers J, Kujala P, van den Born M, Cozijnsen M et al. (2007). Identification of stem cells in small intestine and colon by marker gene Lgr5. *Nature* **449**: 1003–07.

Bonnet D, Dick JE (1997). Human acute myeloid leukemia is organized as a hierarchy that originates from a primitive hematopoietic cell. *Nat Med* **3**: 730–37.

Bruder SP, Ricalton NS, Boynton RE, Connolly TJ, Jaiswal N, Zaia J et al. (1998). Mesenchymal stem cell surface antigen SB-10 corresponds to activated leukocyte cell adhesion molecule and is involved in osteogenic differentiation. *J Bone Miner Res* **13**: 655–63.

Chambers AF, Groom AC, MacDonald IC (2002). Dissemination and growth of cancer cells in metastatic sites. *Nat Rev Cancer* **2**: 563–72.

Chiang AC, Massague J (2008). Molecular basis of metastasis. *N Engl J Med* **359**: 2814–23.

Choi D, Lee HW, Hur KY, Kim JJ, Park GS, Jang SH et al. (2009). Cancer stem cell markers CD133 and CD24 correlate with invasiveness and differentiation in colorectal adenocarcinoma. *World J Gastroenterol* **15**: 2258–64.

Chu P, Clanton DJ, Snipas TS, Lee J, Mitchell E, Nguyen ML et al. (2009). Characterization of a subpopulation of colon cancer cells with stem cell-like properties. *Int J Cancer* **124**: 1312–21.

Clarke MF, Dick JE, Dirks PB, Eaves CJ, Jamieson CH, Jones DL et al. (2006). Cancer stem cells–perspectives on current status and future directions: AACR Workshop on cancer stem cells. *Cancer Res* **66**: 9339–44.

Collins AT, Berry PA, Hyde C, Stower MJ, Maitland NJ (2005). Prospective identification of tumorigenic prostate cancer stem cells. *Cancer Res* **65**: 10946–51.

Cozzio A, Passegue E, Ayton PM, Karsunky H, Cleary ML, Weissman IL (2003). Similar MLL-associated leukemias arising from self-renewing stem cells and short-lived myeloid progenitors. *Genes Dev* **17**: 3029–35.

Dalerba P, Dylla SJ, Park IK, Liu R, Wang X, Cho RW et al. (2007). Phenotypic characterization of human colorectal cancer stem cells. *Proc Natl Acad Sci USA* **104**: 10158–63.

Dick JE (2008). Stem cell concepts renew cancer research. *Blood* **112**: 4793–807.

Diehn M, Cho RW, Lobo NA, Kalisky T, Dorie MJ, Kulp AN et al. (2009). Association of reactive oxygen species levels and radioresistance in cancer stem cells. *Nature* **458**: 780–83.

Dylla SJ, Beviglia L, Park IK, Chartier C, Raval J, Ngan L et al. (2008). Colorectal cancer stem cells are enriched in xenogeneic tumors following chemotherapy. *PLoS ONE* **3**: e2428.

Eramo A, Lotti F, Sette G, Pilozzi E, Biffoni M, Di Virgilio A et al. (2008). Identification and expansion of the tumorigenic lung cancer stem cell population. *Cell Death Differ* **15**: 504–14.

Eyler CE, Rich JN (2008). Survival of the fittest: cancer stem cells in therapeutic resistance and angiogenesis. *J Clin Oncol* **26**: 2839–45.

Ginestier C, Hur MH, Charafe-Jauffret E, Monville F, Dutcher J, Brown M et al. (2007). ALDH1 is a marker of normal and malignant human mammary stem cells and a predictor of poor clinical outcome. *Cell Stem Cell* **1**: 555–67.

Gupta GP, Massague J (2006). Cancer metastasis: building a framework. *Cell* **127**: 679–95.

Haraguchi N, Ohkuma M, Sakashita H, Matsuzaki S, Tanaka F, Mimori K et al. (2008). CD133+CD44+ population efficiently enriches colon cancer initiating cells. *Ann Surg Oncol* **15**: 2927–33.

Hermann PC, Huber SL, Herrler T, Aicher A, Ellwart JW, Guba M et al. (2007). Distinct populations of cancer stem cells determine tumor growth and metastatic activity in human pancreatic cancer. *Cell Stem Cell* **1**: 313–23.

Hill RP (2006). Identifying cancer stem cells in solid tumors: case not proven. *Cancer Res* **66**: 1891–95. discussion 1890.

Horst D, Kriegl L, Engel J, Jung A, Kirchner T (2009a). CD133 and nuclear beta-catenin: the marker combination to detect high risk cases of low stage colorectal cancer. *Eur J Cancer* **45**(11): 2034–40.

Horst D, Kriegl L, Engel J, Kirchner T, Jung A (2008). CD133 expression is an independent prognostic marker for low survival in colorectal cancer. *Br J Cancer* **99**: 1285–89.

Horst D, Reu S, Kriegl L, Engel J, Kirchner T, Jung A (2009b). The intratumoral distribution of nuclear beta-catenin is a prognostic marker in colon cancer. *Cancer* **115**: 2063–70.

Huang EH, Hynes MJ, Zhang T, Ginestier C, Dontu G, Appelman H et al. (2009). Aldehyde dehydrogenase 1 is a marker for normal and malignant human colonic stem cells (SC) and tracks SC overpopulation during colon tumorigenesis. *Cancer Res* **69**: 3382–89.

Jamieson CH, Ailles LE, Dylla SJ, Muijtjens M, Jones C, Zehnder JL et al. (2004). Granulocyte-macrophage progenitors as candidate leukemic stem cells in blast-crisis CML. *N Engl J Med* **351**: 657–67.

Jordan CT, Guzman ML, Noble M (2006). Cancer stem cells. *N Engl J Med* **355**: 1253–61.

Kelly PN, Dakic A, Adams JM, Nutt SL, Strasser A (2007). Tumor growth need not be driven by rare cancer stem cells. *Science* **317**: 337.

Kennedy JA, Barabe F, Poeppl AG, Wang JC, Dick JE (2007). Comment on "Tumor growth need not be driven by rare cancer stem cells". *Science* **318**: 1722. author reply 1722.

Korkaya H, Paulson A, Charafe-Jauffret E, Ginestier C, Brown M, Dutcher J et al. (2009). Regulation of mammary stem/progenitor cells by PTEN/Akt/beta-catenin signaling. *PLoS Biol* **7**: e1000121.

Krivtsov AV, Twomey D, Feng Z, Stubbs MC, Wang Y, Faber J et al. (2006). Transformation from committed progenitor to leukaemia stem cell initiated by MLL-AF9. *Nature* **442**: 818–22.

Lapidot T, Sirard C, Vormoor J, Murdoch B, Hoang T, Caceres-Cortes J et al. (1994). A cell initiating human acute myeloid leukaemia after transplantation into SCID mice. *Nature* **367**: 645–48.

Li Z, Bao S, Wu Q, Wang H, Eyler C, Sathornsumetee S et al. (2009). Hypoxia-inducible factors regulate tumorigenic capacity of glioma stem cells. *Cancer Cell* **15**: 501–13.

Li C, Heidt DG, Dalerba P, Burant CF, Zhang L, Adsay V et al. (2007). Identification of pancreatic cancer stem cells. *Cancer Res* **67**: 1030–37.

Li X, Lewis MT, Huang J, Gutierrez C, Osborne CK, Wu MF et al. (2008). Intrinsic resistance of tumorigenic breast cancer cells to chemotherapy. *J Natl Cancer Inst* **100**: 672–79.

Luzzi KJ, MacDonald IC, Schmidt EE, Kerkvliet N, Morris VL, Chambers AF et al. (1998). Multistep nature of metastatic inefficiency: dormancy of solitary cells after successful extravasation and limited survival of early micrometastases. *Am J Pathol* **153**: 865–73.

Ma S, Lee TK, Zheng BJ, Chan KW, Guan XY (2008). CD133+ HCC cancer stem cells confer chemoresistance by preferential expression of the Akt/PKB survival pathway. *Oncogene* **27**: 1749–58.

Miraglia S, Godfrey W, Yin AH, Atkins K, Warnke R, Holden JT et al. (1997). A novel five-transmembrane hematopoietic stem cell antigen: isolation, characterization, and molecular cloning. *Blood* **90**: 5013–21.

Mizrak D, Brittan M, Alison MR (2008). CD133: molecule of the moment. *J Pathol* **214**: 3–9.

Muller A, Homey B, Soto H, Ge N, Catron D, Buchanan ME et al. (2001). Involvement of chemokine receptors in breast cancer metastasis. *Nature* **410**: 50–56.

Nagano O, Saya H (2004). Mechanism and biological significance of CD44 cleavage. *Cancer Sci* **95**: 930–35.

O'Brien CA, Kreso A, Dick JE (2009). Cancer stem cells in solid tumors: an overview. *Semin Radiat Oncol* **19**: 71–77.

O'Brien CA, Pollett A, Gallinger S, Dick JE (2007). A human colon cancer cell capable of initiating tumour growth in immunodeficient mice. *Nature* **445**: 106–10.

Paget S (1989). The distribution of secondary growths in cancer of the breast. *Lancet* **1**: 571–73.

Pardal R, Clarke MF, Morrison SJ (2003). Applying the principles of stem-cell biology to cancer. *Nat Rev Cancer* **3**: 895–902.

Patrawala L, Calhoun T, Schneider-Broussard R, Li H, Bhatia B, Tang S et al. (2006). Highly purified CD44+ prostate cancer cells from xenograft human tumors are enriched in tumorigenic and metastatic progenitor cells. *Oncogene* **25**: 1696–708.

Prince ME, Sivanandan R, Kaczorowski A, Wolf GT, Kaplan MJ, Dalerba P et al. (2007). Identification of a subpopulation of cells with cancer stem cell properties in head and neck squamous cell carcinoma. *Proc Natl Acad Sci USA* **104**: 973–78.

Reya T, Morrison SJ, Clarke MF, Weissman IL (2001). Stem cells, cancer, and cancer stem cells. *Nature* **414**: 105–11.

Ricci-Vitiani L, Lombardi DG, Pilozzi E, Biffoni M, Todaro M, Peschle C et al. (2007). Identification and expansion of human colon-cancer-initiating cells. *Nature* **445**: 111–15.

Rosen JM, Jordan CT (2009). The increasing complexity of the cancer stem cell paradigm. *Science* **324**: 1670–73.

Sangiorgi E, Capecchi MR (2008). *Bmi1* is expressed in vivo in intestinal stem cells. *Nat Genet* **40**: 915–20.

Singh SK, Hawkins C, Clarke ID, Squire JA, Bayani J, Hide T et al. (2004). Identification of human brain tumour initiating cells. *Nature* **432**: 396–401.

Southam CM, Brunschwig A (1961). Quantitative studies of autotransplantation of human cancer: preliminary report. *Cancer* **14**: 971–78.

Staller P, Sulitkova J, Lisztwan J, Moch H, Oakeley EJ, Krek W (2003). Chemokine receptor CXCR4 downregulated by von Hippel-Lindau tumour suppressor pVHL. *Nature* **425**: 307–11.

Tan BT, Park CY, Ailles LE, Weissman IL (2006). The cancer stem cell hypothesis: a work in progress. *Lab Invest* **86**: 1203–07.

Todaro M, Alea MP, Di Stefano AB, Cammareri P, Vermeulen L, Iovino F et al. (2007). Colon cancer stem cells dictate tumor growth and resist cell death by production of interleukin-4. *Cell Stem Cell* **1**: 389–402.

Uchida N, Buck DW, He D, Reitsma MJ, Masek M, Phan TV et al. (2000). Direct isolation of human central nervous system stem cells. *Proc Natl Acad Sci USA* **97**: 14720–25.

Visvader JE, Lindeman GJ (2008). Cancer stem cells in solid tumours: accumulating evidence and unresolved questions. *Nat Rev Cancer* **8**: 755–68.

Wang JC (2007). Evaluating therapeutic efficacy against cancer stem cells: new challenges posed by a new paradigm. *Cell Stem Cell* **1**: 497–501.

Wang JC, Dick JE (2005). Cancer stem cells: lessons from leukemia. *Trends Cell Biol* **15**: 494–501.

Weichert W, Knosel T, Bellach J, Dietel M, Kristiansen G (2004). ALCAM/CD166 is overexpressed in colorectal carcinoma and correlates with shortened patient survival. *J Clin Pathol* **57**: 1160–64.

Wu C, Wei Q, Utomo V, Nadesan P, Whetstone H, Kandel R et al. (2007). Side population cells isolated from mesenchymal neoplasms have tumor initiating potential. *Cancer Res* **67**: 8216–22.

Yilmaz OH, Valdez R, Theisen BK, Guo W, Ferguson DO, Wu H et al. (2006). Pten dependence distinguishes haematopoietic stem cells from leukaemia-initiating cells. *Nature* **441**: 475–82.

Yin AH, Miraglia S, Zanjani ED, Almeida-Porada G, Ogawa M, Leary AG et al. (1997). AC133, a novel marker for human hematopoietic stem and progenitor cells. *Blood* **90**: 5002–12.

Zagzag D, Krishnamachary B, Yee H, Okuyama H, Chiriboga L, Ali MA et al. (2005). Stromal cell-derived factor-1alpha and CXCR4 expression in hemangioblastoma and clear cell-renal cell carcinoma: von Hippel-Lindau loss-of-function induces expression of a ligand and its receptor. *Cancer Res* **65**: 6178–88.

Zhu L, Gibson P, Currle DS, Tong Y, Richardson RJ, Bayazitov IT et al. (2009). Prominin 1 marks intestinal stem cells that are susceptible to neoplastic transformation. *Nature* **457**: 603–7.

Chapter 6

EPITHELIAL-MESENCHYMAL TRANSITION IN COLORECTAL CANCER

Otto Schmalhofer[1], Simone Brabletz[2] and Thomas Brabletz[3]
[1]*Department of Visceral Surgery, University of Freiburg, Freiburg, 79106, Germany, e-mail: otto.schmalhofer@uniklinik-freiburg.de*
[2]*Department of Visceral Surgery, University of Freiburg, Freiburg, 79106, Germany, e-mail: simone.spaderna@uniklinik-freiburg.de*
[3]*Department of Visceral Surgery, University of Freiburg, Freiburg, 79106, Germany, e-mail: thomas.brabletz@uniklinik-freiburg.de*

Abstract: Colorectal carcinomas are characterized by a heterogeneous differentiation pattern. Cancer cells in central regions are epithelially-differentiated, whereas disseminating tumour cells at the invasion front have undergone epithelial-mesenchymal transition and show nuclear accumulation of β-catenin. Nuclear β-catenin cooperates with transcriptional repressors of the *E-cadherin* gene to induce epithelial-mesenchymal transition and activates expression of target genes that drive malignant tumour progression.

Key words: β-catenin · E-cadherin · Colorectal cancer · Epithelial-mesenchymal transition · Tumour invasion

6.1 Introduction

Pathologists frequently observe a heterogeneous morphology in surgical specimens of well-to-moderately differentiated colorectal adenocarcinomas. The central tumour area is reminiscent of the typical glandular organization of normal colonic mucosa (Fig. 6.1, bottom). There, neoplastic cells retain an apico-basally polarized, epithelial phenotype and grow in tubular structures. The tumour margins, however, are often characterized by a transition from glandular structures to single cancer cells or small cancer cell clusters, which invade into the surrounding stroma (Fig. 6.1, top). This morphological observation is referred to as 'tumour budding'. Budding tumour cells are typically characterized by an activation of the embryonic program 'epithelial-mesenchymal transition' (EMT). During this process, epithelial

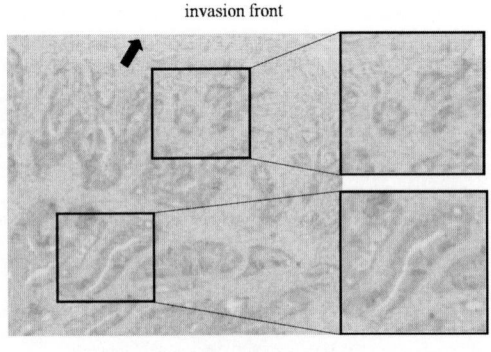

Fig. 6.1 Tumour budding at the invasion front. The tumour center (*bottom*) of well-to-moderately differentiated colorectal adenocarcinomas is typically characterized by an epithelial differentiation of tumour cells that grow in glandular structures. The tumour margins show a transition from the glandular tumour growth pattern to small clusters of cancer cells. These budding tumour cells disseminate from the main tumour mass and invade into the surrounding stroma (*top*). *Black arrow* indicates direction of invasion, insets show magnification of the tumour center and invasion front

differentiation is lost and a mesenchymal phenotype is acquired instead (Brabletz et al., 1998; Morodomi et al., 1989; Thiery, 2002; Ueno et al., 2002a). Loss of the epithelial phenotype and the local invasion of tumour cells into the host stroma are considered as the first step of the metastatic cascade (Gabbert et al., 1985). Therefore, the occurrence of budding tumour cells undergoing EMT at the invasion front is of utmost importance to physicians and colorectal cancer (CRC) patients, due to its relevance for prognosis of clinical outcome.

At the molecular level, disseminating colorectal cancer cells are characterized by an accumulation of nuclear β-catenin, the intracellular mediator of canonical Wingless/Int (WNT) signalling. The first sections of this chapter will focus on basic aspects of WNT signalling and the activated target gene program, that contributes to malignant tumour progression and EMT. Moreover, different extrinsic and intrinsic factors, that contribute to the localization of β-catenin to the nucleus and thus to the activated expression of β-catenin target genes will be discussed. A loss of E-cadherin expression is also typical for budding tumour cells in CRC. E-cadherin, the core component of adherens junctions is the most important determinant of an epithelial phenotype and its loss is a prerequisite for cancer cell invasion. Current aspects of E-cadherin loss in CRC, in particular, loss by transcriptional repression together with its involvement in nuclear β-catenin localization are discussed in the last chapter sections.

Taken together, the aim of this book chapter is to describe both the clinical aspects of EMT in colorectal cancer and the cancer cell biology that determines the mesenchymal phenotype. The chapter concentrates in particular on the contribution of nuclear β-catenin and its activated target gene program, as well as on the role of transcriptional repressors of E-cadherin in the induction of a mesenchymal phenotype.

6.2 Tumour Budding as a Prognostic Factor in CRC

To predict clinical outcome in patients diagnosed with CRC, tumour penetration depth and local lymph node involvement is routinely assessed. The staging is done predominantly according to the criteria of UICC/AJCC TNM (Union Internationale contre le Cancer/American Joint Committee on Cancer, Tumor Nodes and Metastasis). In addition to tumour staging, other CRC-associated characteristics that are relevant prognostic factors include invasion of venous as well as lymphatic vessels, perineural invasion, histological tumour grade, and lymphoid infiltration (Compton, 1999; Compton et al., 2000; Royston and Jackson, 2009; Zlobec and Lugli, 2008). Moreover, another morphological feature that appears to be important for the clinical outcome in CRC is budding tumour cells, which have undergone EMT.

First reports of budding tumour cells date back to the 1920s. However, the potential of tumour budding as an index for clinical prognosis and aggressiveness of colorectal tumours has only recently been recognized (Broders, 1921). A high degree budding was associated with adverse clinical outcome in a collective of stage I and II CRCs and was suggested as a selector for high risk patients from this group for treatment with adjuvant chemotherapy (Prall et al., 2005). In stage II CRC, a high degree of tumour budding was a predictor of adverse clinical outcome, i.e. patient survival and tumour recurrence (Tanaka et al., 2003). Also, survival of stage II patients with a high grade budding at the tumour invasion front was worse than that of stage III patients showing no or low tumour cell dissemination. Moreover, survival of stage II and stage III patients with a mild degree of budding showed no difference (Hase et al., 1993). Budding was also associated with a poor clinical outcome after curative resection of stage II and III colon carcinomas. Indeed, survival was worse in patients with tumour budding as compared to a low degree budding. Interestingly, only a marginal difference in patient survival between budding-positive stage II tumours and stage III tumours was reported (Okuyama et al., 2003a). The power of budding to select for high-risk patients within a tumour collective and for predicting poor patient survival was confirmed by other studies (Choi et al., 2007; Nakamura et al., 2008; Okuyama et al., 2002a; Okuyama et al., 2003b; Okuyama et al., 2002b; Ueno et al., 2002b; Ueno et al., 2004). Also, a high degree tumour budding at the invasive margin was correlated with increased lymphatic invasion and the presence of lymph node metastases. Moreover, tumour budding was described as a predictor of isolated tumour cells in lymph node-negative tumours (Park et al., 2005b). In addition, tumour budding was identified as a risk factor for distant metastasis to liver and lung. Furthermore, severe budding increased with tumour stage in CRC and was linked to poor tumour differentiation (Hase et al., 1993; Kazama et al., 2006; Morodomi et al., 1989; Nakamura et al., 2008; Park et al., 2005a). Also, budding was suggested as a predictor of occult metastasis in lymph node-negative CRC (Park et al., 2005b).

In summary, considerable evidence has demonstrated that tumour budding in colorectal cancer is a risk factor for tumour recurrence, lymph node and distant metastasis, as well as worse patient survival. Budding increases with tumour stage and grade and is a predictor of high-risk patients of a certain tumour stage. Budding tumour cells typically lose their epithelial differentiation, which raises the question concerning the identity of the molecular players that determine the aggressive mesenchymal phenotype in CRC. This question will be discussed/addressed in the next sections.

6.3 WNT Signalling and Nuclear β-Catenin in CRC

In recent years, core molecules and signalling pathways have been identified, which determine the dedifferentiated phenotype of budding tumour cells at the invasive front of CRCs. Typical for most sporadic colon tumours and hereditary familial adenomatous polyposis (FAP) syndrome is an aberrant activation of the canonical WNT signalling cascade. This is mostly due to mutations of the *Adenomatous polyposis coli* (APC) protein, causing nuclear localization of the transcription factor β-catenin. APC, together with the serine/threonine kinases Casein kinase 1 (CK1) and glycogen synthase kinase 3β (GSK3β), and the scaffold proteins Axin1 and Axin2, is a core component of a multiprotein complex which targets cytosolic β-catenin for proteasomal degradation in absence of a WNT signal (Fig. 6.2A) (Behrens et al.,

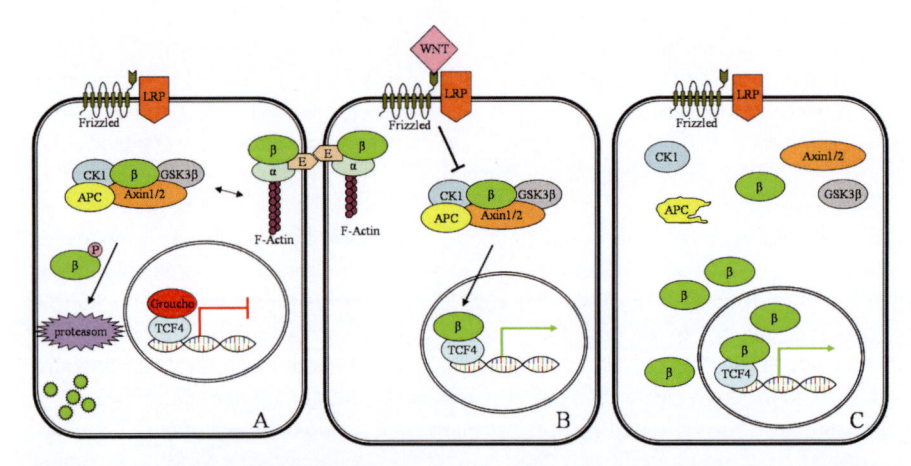

Fig. 6.2 The WNT signalling cascade in CRC. β-catenin (β) has dual functions in epithelial cells. It acts in cell-cell adhesion together with E-cadherin (E) and α-catenin (α) or as transcription factor in the nucleus (**A** and **B**). In absence of WNTs, cytosolic β-catenin is targeted for proteasomal breakdown by a multiprotein degradation complex (**A**). When WNT molecules bind to Frizzled receptors, the activity of the destruction complex is inhibited (**B**). This allows cytoplasmic β-catenin to evade degradation, to accumulate in the cytoplasm and to translocate to the nucleus. There, β-catenin interacts with TCF4, displaces factors like Groucho, and activates expression of target genes (**B**). Typical for colorectal cancers are mutations in the *APC* gene (**C**). This permanently activates the signalling cascade independently of exogenous WNTs, because the functionality of the destruction complex is inhibited. β-catenin accumulates in the cytoplasm and translocates to the nucleus. There, β-catenin aberrantly induces expression of target genes, thus driving tumour progression (**C**). Figures are adapted from Fodde et al. (2001)

1998; Fodde et al., 2001; Liu et al., 2002). When the cascade is activated by WNTs, the degradation complex is inhibited, β-catenin accumulates in the cytoplasm and finally translocates to the nucleus. There, β-catenin forms complexes with T-cell factor/lymphoid enhancer factor (TCF/LEF) proteins, in particular TCF4 or LEF1, and numerous additional factors, such as CREB-binding protein (CBP/p300) or Brahma-related gene protein 1(BRG1), to activate transcription of specific target genes (Fig. 6.2B) (Barker et al., 2001; Behrens et al., 1996; Korinek et al., 1997; Takemaru and Moon, 2000). In normal colon mucosa, this transcriptional program is restricted to the proliferation compartment at the bottom of colonic crypts. Aberrant WNT signalling however, for example due to mutations in the *APC* gene disrupts the proliferation/differentiation switch along the crypt axis and initiates colorectal carcinogenesis (Fig. 6.2C) (de Santa Barbara et al., 2003; Sancho et al., 2003). Numerous mouse models have clearly demonstrated a causal nature of activated WNT signalling in initiating and driving colorectal tumourigenesis (Taketo and Edelmann, 2009). Please refer to Chapter 3 by Drs. Kaz and Grady and to the review by J. Behrens for more detailed reading on WNT signalling in CRC (Behrens, 2005).

6.4 Intratumoural Distribution of Nuclear β-Catenin

CRCs are thought to develop from benign adenomas before becoming metastatic carcinomas. This is associated with increasing amounts of nuclear β-catenin (Brabletz et al., 2000; Inomata et al., 1996). Although all tumour cells carry mutations that activate WNT signalling, the distribution of nuclear β-catenin is very heterogeneous within CRCs (Fig. 6.3).

Nuclear β-catenin is found predominantly in the budding cells at the tumour invasion front. These cells have also lost membranous E-cadherin expression and are strong predictors of adverse clinical outcome (Fig. 6.3A) (Behrens, 2005; Bienz and Clevers, 2000; Hlubek et al., 2007b; Oving and Clevers, 2002). In contrast, central tumour areas resemble normal colonic mucosa and are characterized by an epithelial differentiation of tumour cells. There, β-catenin is localized in adherens junctions at the plasma membrane together with E-cadherin. Expression of membranous E-cadherin is the most important determinant of the epithelial phenotype. E-cadherin, the core molecule of adherens junctions, maintains epithelial cell-cell adhesion and apico-basal polarization. It also acts as a negative regulator of WNT signalling by recruiting β-catenin from the nucleus to adherens junctions. In contrast, when E-cadherin is lost, β-catenin translocates from the membrane to the nucleus, as observed in the budding tumour cells (Brabletz et al., 1998; Conacci-Sorrell et al., 2003). Thus, depending on its intracellular localization, β-catenin acts either in cell-cell adhesion together with E-cadherin or as a transcription factor (Fig. 6.2A, B). Therefore β-catenin contributes to maintain an epithelial phenotype in central tumour areas and is a transcriptional inductor of an aggressive mesenchymal phenotype in budding cancer cells at the invasion front.

Interestingly, the phenotypical appearance of metastases resembles the situation of the primary tumour. There, the central areas are again epithelially-differentiated

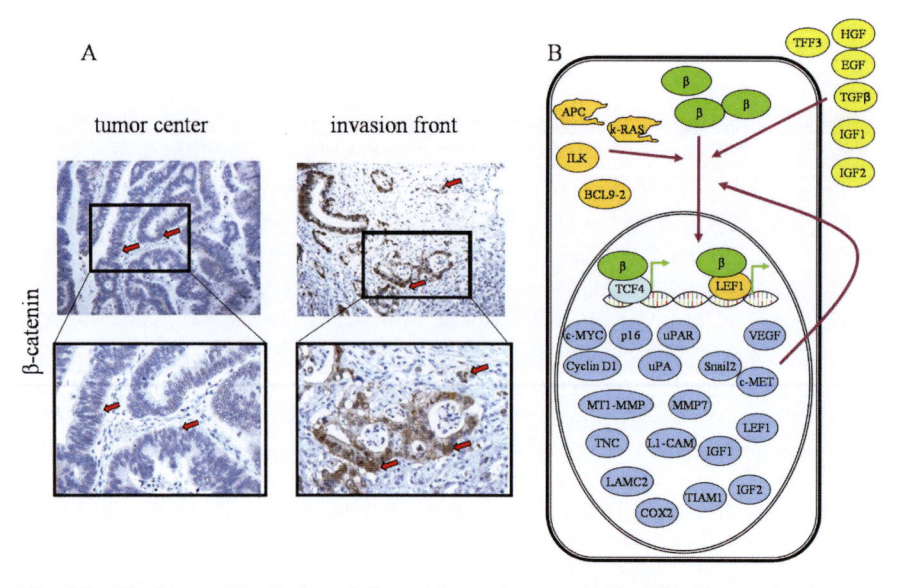

Fig. 6.3 Nuclear accumulation of β-catenin at the tumour invasion front of colorectal tumours. (**A**) A typical well-to-moderately differentiated colorectal adenocarcinoma is immunohistochemically stained for β-catenin (*red arrows*). In the tumour center, β-catenin localizes to the plasma membrane, whereas at the invasion front, it is localized in the nucleus. Insets show magnification; nuclear counterstaining in *blue*. (**B**) Experimental data suggest a model in which different molecular players cooperate to localize β-catenin (β) to the nucleus (*purple arrows*). These include endogenous (*orange*) and exogenous (*yellow*) factors. In the nucleus, β-catenin activates expression of different target genes (*blue*), including factors associated with cell proliferation, matrix components, MMPs, cytokines, and others. Moreover, many of the β-catenin-responsive target genes have been described to be activators of WNT signalling, suggesting different feed-forward loops that localize β-catenin to the nucleus

and budding cells at the invasion front display a mesenchymal phenotype. Also, similarly to its expression pattern in the primary tumour, β-catenin is heterogeneously distributed in metastases. In the central tumour areas, it is localized in adherens junctions along with re-expressed E-cadherin at the plasma membrane while in budding cells, it is present in the nucleus (Brabletz et al., 2001). This indicates that the EMT observed at the invasion front of the primary tumour is a transient and reversible event, as a mesenchymal-epithelial transition (MET) takes place during formation of metastases (Brabletz et al., 2001; Spaderna et al., 2006). The relocation of β-catenin from the nucleus of budding cells to the plasma membrane in central areas of the metastatic tumour is associated with silencing of WNT target gene expression and colonic epithelial cell differentiation. This process raises the following questions, which will be discussed in the next sections (Brabletz et al., 2005a; Hlubek et al., 2001; Mariadason et al., 2001; Naishiro et al., 2001): How does β-catenin determine a mesenchymal phenotype and contribute to malignant tumour progression? What are the regulators of the intra-tumoural β-catenin distributions? What are the regulators of E-cadherin expression in CRCs and how do they contribute to EMT and malignant tumour progression?

6.5 WNT Targets in CRC

Various reports using gene expression array analysis elucidated a considerable amount of direct and indirect WNT target genes by investigating the gene expression profiles of normal colonic mucosa, as well as colorectal tumours and cell lines (Nannini et al., 2009; Sabates-Bellver et al., 2007; van de Wetering et al., 2002; Van der Flier et al., 2007). A study by Hlubek et al. specifically addressed the question of differences in gene expression profiles between the well-differentiated central areas of CRCs and the budding cancer cells at the invasion front (Hlubek et al., 2007a). The expression profile activated by β-catenin in CRC includes genes associated with proliferation, a stem cell phenotype, as well as invasion and angiogenesis (Fig. 6.3). These genes will be discussed in this section with a special focus on their contribution to EMT in budding cancer cells. Of particular importance are WNT target genes, which contribute to localizing β-catenin to the nucleus, thus stabilizing the aggressive mesenchymal phenotype of budding tumour cells in CRC. Some of these genes are discussed in the next sections. Of note, many more target genes of β-catenin have been identified, which are not discussed here. Please visit the WNT homepage (http://www.stanford.edu/~rnusse/wntwindow.html) for a comprehensive overview on additional gene targets of β-catenin.

6.5.1 Proliferation-Associated WNT Targets

The cellular myelocytomatosis gene (*c-MYC*) was defined as a direct WNT target and plays an important role in colon cancer (He et al., 1998; Pelengaris et al., 2002). Moreover, colocalization of c-MYC and β-catenin in CRC cells has been reported (Brabletz et al., 2000). Functions of c-MYC, which were experimentally validated, include activation of proliferation and resistance to apoptosis (Hongxing et al., 2008; Zhang et al., 2009). However, the importance of c-MYC for colorectal carcinogenesis seems to go further, as indicated by the work of Sansom and collaborators who investigated the role of c-Myc activation in the intestine after loss of Apc, using Cre recombinase-mediated deletion of floxed *Apc* and *c-Myc* alleles in a compound mouse model. The observed phenotype in the mutated intestinal enterocytes consisted of impaired differentiation, migration, proliferation and apoptosis but was rescued by an additional loss of c-Myc. This indicates that c-Myc is a key player in propagating the full effects of aberrant WNT signalling thereby making it a central promoter of colorectal carcinogenesis (Sansom et al., 2007).

*Cyclin D*1 is a direct WNT target gene in vitro and is overexpressed in budding tumour cells at the invasion front of CRCs together with nuclear β-catenin. Jung et al. showed that Cyclin D1 expression is not essentially linked to proliferation, since β-catenin- and Cyclin D1-positive cell clusters at the invasion front only displayed marginal staining for KI67, a marker for cellular proliferation (Jung et al., 2001; Shtutman et al., 1999; Tetsu and McCormick, 1999). Moreover, these cells expressed the cell cycle inhibitor p16INK4A, which is a suppressor of cyclin-dependent kinase 4 and 6 activity and was recently defined as another direct target of β-catenin and predictor of adverse clinical outcome (Wassermann et al., 2009). Interestingly, low proliferation is a feature attributed to a stem cell phenotype. Another study by Mayo et al. supported the findings that Cyclin D1 expression did not necessarily correlate with proliferation after detachment of differentiated layers of the colorectal cancer cell line HT29 M6. Detachment also caused suppression of genes associated with epithelial differentiation, such as the gene coding for Mucin1 (MUC1). Moreover, ectopic expression of Cyclin D1 in differentiated HT29 M6 cells mimicked this effect. This indicates that, in addition to driving proliferation of tumour cells, overexpression of Cyclin D1 in CRCs might contribute to tumour de-differentiation by suppressing epithelial markers (Mayo and Mayol, 2009). This is in line with a previous report demonstrating that a lack of Cyclin D1 in an *Apc* mutant background is linked to increased differentiation of colonic cells and expression of epithelial marker genes, such as the gene coding for Mucin2 (MUC2) (Hulit et al., 2004). Taken together, Cyclin D1 expression in CRC seems to play a role in inhibiting epithelial differentiation in addition to its well-known function in cell cycle progression (Fig. 6.3B).

6.5.2 Stemness-Associated WNT Targets

Several WNT targets defining a stem cell-like phenotype have been reported. Indeed, tumour buds displaying a mesenchymal phenotype characterized by nuclear β-catenin were postulated to contain migrating tumour stem cells. Although this theory has not been proven yet, it is supported by the observation that metastases normally resemble the primary tumours, with respect to epithelial differentiation, presence of different cell types and tubular growth patterns. Also, there is experimental evidence that EMT promotes generation of stem-like cells (Brabletz et al., 2005b; Mani et al., 2008; Morel et al., 2008).

A recent report showed that the leucine-rich repeat-containing G protein-coupled receptor 5 (Lgr5) is a robust marker of intestinal stem cells and is regulated by WNT signalling (Barker et al., 2007). Moreover, an elegant compound mouse model revealed that selective loss of Apc in Lgr5-positive stem cells in intestinal crypts is sufficient to initiate tumourigenesis, whereas loss of Apc in other cells is not (Barker et al., 2009). This indicates that human colorectal cancers might also directly arise from stem cells of the colonic crypt. One of the WNT targets marking a subset of stem cells in gastrointestinal cell lines is the multidrug resistance protein 1 (MDR1). MDR1-positive cells showed self-renewal properties and chemoresistance to anti-cancer drugs, which are both stem cell attributes (Haraguchi et al., 2005; Longo et al., 2002; Yamada et al., 2000). Moreover, loss of *Mdr*1 in a mouse model of colorectal carcinogenesis prevented intestinal polyposis (Yamada et al., 2003). Also Survivin, which is overexpressed in CRC and predicts adverse clinical outcome, was defined as a WNT target and suggested to contribute to a stem cell phenotype of CRC cells (Kawasaki et al., 2001; Zhang et al., 2001). In addition, cluster of differentiation 133 (CD133) was suggested as a WNT target and colorectal tumours were reported to contain CD133-positive stem cells (O'Brien et al., 2007; Ricci-Vitiani et al., 2007). CD133 is also an independent marker for low survival in colorectal cancer and both CD133 and nuclear β-catenin, were defined as marker combinations to detect high risk colon cancer patients (Horst et al., 2009; Horst et al., 2008; Katoh and Katoh, 2007). Another defined WNT target and putative marker of a stem-like phenotype in CRC is CD44 (Wielenga et al., 1999). As few as 100 CD44-positive cells isolated from human CRC initiated tumour growth in nude mice. Moreover, single CD44-positive cells had the capabilitiy of sphere formation, which gave rise to tumours, when injected in nude mice. Likewise, knockdown of CD44 by means of RNA interference prevented tumour growth in a xenograft experiment (Du et al., 2008).

However, the contribution of these factors to stemness and EMT in CRC is still unclear. For example, the expression patterns of CD44 and CD133 are mutually exclusive in CRC, and knockdown of CD133 by RNA interference did not prevent growth of tumours (Du et al., 2008). This supports results from a study in which CD133-positive and CD133-negative cells were isolated from metastases of colon adenocarcinomas. Both CD133-positive and -negative cells behaved in a stem-like fashion, giving rise to tumours in grafting experiments in the mouse. Moreover, tumours arising from the CD133-negative cells grew even more aggressively than the ones arising from CD133-positive cells (Shmelkov et al., 2008). In human CRC, nuclear β-catenin-positive tumour buds at the invasion front are also negative for CD133 (Horst et al., 2008). Moreover, the expression patterns of other stemness markers like leucine-rich repeat-containing G protein-coupled receptor 5 (LGR5), MDR1, Survivin or CD44 within CRCs in general, but especially at the invasion front are not entirely clear. In summary, a considerable amount of experimental work is still required in determining whether budding cancer cells at the invasion front have a stem-like phenotype or not. Readers are encouraged to read Chapter 5 by A. Kresko et al., in this book for more information on colorectal cancer stem cells.

6.5.3 Invasion- and Neoangiogenesis-Associated WNT Targets

Degradation and remodeling of the extracellular matrix (ECM) is essential for the invasion of budding cancer cells (Liotta and Kohn, 2001; Stetler-Stevenson et al., 1993). Accordingly, disseminating colorectal cancer cells have been shown to express various proteases, including the urokinase plasminogen activator (uPA) and its receptor uPAR. Both are expressed in a β-catenin-dependent coordinated fashion in budding cancer cells. Moreover, uPAR signalling was shown to be an inducer of EMT and a promoter of migration, invasion, and intravasation (Blasi and Carmeliet, 2002; Buo et al., 1995; Hiendlmeyer et al., 2004; Lester et al., 2007). Budding cancer cells also express various metalloproteinases (MMP) in a β-catenin-dependent manner, e.g. membrane-type 1 (MT1)-MMP or MMP7, which was defined as an EMT inducer itself (Brabletz et al., 1999; Hlubek et al., 2004; Shibata et al., 2009). Also, E-cadherin may be the direct target for environmental factors like MMP7, which was shown to cleave membranous E-cadherin. Experimental evidence demonstrated that the shed ectodomain of E-cadherin inhibits E-cadherin-dependent cell-cell aggregation and promotes invasion (Fig. 6.3B) (Noe et al., 2001).

Moreover, components of the ECM which promote EMT and invasion are selectively expressed at the tumour invasion front in a β-catenin-dependent manner, such as Tenascin C (TNC) or the Laminin gamma2 chain (LAMC2) (Beiter et al., 2005; De Wever et al., 2004; Hlubek et al., 2004; Olsen et al., 2003). Factors associated with increased metastatic potential that are expressed at the invasion front, including the L1 cell adhesion molecule (L1-CAM), are markers for poor clinical outcome (Gavert et al., 2005; Gavert et al., 2007; Kaifi et al., 2007). The T-cell lymphoma invasion and metastasis 1 (TIAM1) guanine nucleotide exchange factor, which is also a WNT target and is overexpressed in colorectal cancers, was associated with increased metastatic potential. TIAM1 regulates cell migration, invasion and resistance to anoikis, a special form of apoptosis of epithelial cells. Interestingly, ectopic expression of TIAM1 caused a mesenchymal phenotype, characterized by an increase in vimentin and a decrease in E-cadherin expression (Fig. 6.3B) (Minard et al., 2006).

In addition, neo-angiogenesis is a key event during malignant tumour progression and induced under hypoxic conditions. Moreover, hypoxic conditions induced an EMT in colorectal cancer cells, which was accompanied by nuclear localization of β-catenin. Interestingly, the vascular endothelial growth factor (VEGF), a key factor mediating neoangiogenesis in CRC, not only was defined as a target of WNT signaling, but was also described as an inducer of EMT, suggesting a feed-forward-loop to stabilize the mesenchymal phenotype (see below). Of note, VEGF expression predicts a poor clinical outcome of CRC (Cannito et al., 2008; Diaz-Rubio, 2006; Easwaran et al., 2003).

6.6 Inducers of Nuclear β-Catenin Localization

Nuclear β-catenin is predominantly found in budding cancer cells. This implies that specific interactions between the tumour and the microenvironment at the site of invasion exist, as all tumour cells harbor an activated WNT signalling pathway. In addition, various tumour cell-intrinsic factors have been described, which promote translocation of β-catenin to the nucleus (Fig. 6.3B).

The tumour microenvironment comprises a variety of different cell types, such as stromal cells, e.g. fibroblasts or myofibroblasts, as well as immune cells, e.g. macrophages or lymphocytes. The role of the microenvironment in regulating tumour budding and nuclear β-catenin localization is supported by a study showing that budding takes place in orthotopically-injected tumour cell xenografts, but is not observed, when the tumour cells are injected ectopically (Sordat et al., 2000). The cells of the microenvironment were demonstrated to be a source of growth factors, cytokines and ECM components, which influence nuclear localization of β-catenin, induce EMT and promote tumour invasion (Fig. 6.3B) (De Wever et al., 2004; Le et al., 2008).

Factors secreted by the microenvironment include HGF, which was demonstrated to be an activator of WNT signalling (Muller et al., 2002; Wielenga et al., 2000). Other studies provided additional evidence that β-catenin physically interacts with the hepatocyte growth factor (HGF) receptor c-MET on colorectal cancer cells, but disassembles after binding HGF. Moreover, the HGF/c-MET complex activates β-catenin expression via the phosphatidyl inositol 3-kinase (PI3K) pathway under experimental settings, thereby simulating the conditions required for invading and metastasizing cancer cells (Rasola et al., 2007; Wielenga et al., 2000). Interestingly, the HGF receptor *c-MET* is a target gene of β-catenin, suggesting an invasion driving feed-forward loop between HGF/c-MET and β-catenin (Boon et al., 2002). This also is in line with the adverse clinical outcome of patients with c-MET-positive CRCs (Fazekas et al., 2000). Other environmental factors acting in an auto- or paracrine fashion with a putative role in the induction of nuclear β-catenin localization and EMT in CRC include epidermal growth factor, trefoil factor 3, as well as insulin-like growth factors (IGF) 1 and 2 (Freier et al., 1999; Hassan and Howell, 2000b; Liu et al., 1997; Lu et al., 2003; Morali et al., 2001; Oyama et al., 1994). Interestingly, IGF1 and IGF2 are upregulated in a WNT-dependent fashion and Igf2 was shown to enhance tumour growth in a mouse model (Fig. 6.3B) (Hassan and Howell, 2000a; Longo et al., 2002).

A recent study also implicated a role of the cyclooxygenase 2 (COX2) metabolite prostaglandin E2 (PGE2) in the nuclear localization of β-catenin (Castellone et al., 2005). This is in line with the reported role of COX2 in the malignant progression of CRCs and the reduction of tumour numbers and size in FAP patients and mouse models when non-steroidal anti-inflammatory drugs are applied, as well as the reported WNT-dependent upregulation of COX2 (Brown and DuBois, 2005; Longo et al., 2002). This point is also discussed in more detail in Chapter 10.

Hypoxic conditions cause a stabilization of the hypoxia inducible factor (HIF) 1α, which subsequently dimerizes with HIF1β, localizes to the nucleus and activates specific target genes that promote angiogenesis. One of these genes codes for VEGF and is a key factor mediating neo-angiogenesis in CRC (Cannito et al., 2008; Diaz-Rubio, 2006; Easwaran et al., 2003). Moreover, the EMT-inducer, Twist, is expressed in a HIF-dependent manner under hypoxic conditions (Yang et al., 2008). Likewise, hypoxic growth also induces expression of VEGF, and VEGF-dependent signalling was suggested to be a promoter of EMT in another study by the upregulation of Snail1, Snail2 and Twist (Cannito et al., 2008; Yang et al., 2006). This is in line with the observation that hypoxic growth conditions of colon cancer cell lines induce an EMT, characterized by nuclear localization of β-catenin and Snail1 (Cannito et al., 2008). Moreover, inhibition of VEGF signalling reduced tumour growth in a mouse model of colorectal cancer (Goodlad et al., 2006).

During malignant progression, most CRCs acquire an oncogenic mutation of K-RAS in addition to the loss of functional APC. This is associated with poor clinical outcome and was experimentally confirmed in a compound mouse model. In this model, animals carrying both mutations had a higher and more aggressive tumour burden than animals with an *Apc* mutation only. The authors provided evidence that *Apc* and *K-Ras* mutations act synergistically in the induction of WNT signalling (Fig. 6.3B) (Janssen et al., 2006; Zhang et al., 2003). There is also experimental evidence that other pathways, which are frequently altered in CRC, might contribute to nuclear localization of β-catenin, in particular, the transforming growth factor (TGF)β and phosphatase and tensin homolog on chromosome 10/v-akt murine thymoma viral oncogene homolog 1 (PTEN/Akt) pathways (Nishita et al., 2000; Persad et al., 2001).

Other factors frequently overexpressed in CRCs include the B-cell CLL/lymphoma 9-like (BCL9-2) protein, which was shown to directly interact with β-catenin. This interferes with the ability of β-catenin to act in cell-cell adhesion as part of adherens junctions. Moreover, binding of BCL9-2 to β-catenin favours β-catenin localization to the nucleus and enhances expression of WNT targets (Adachi et al., 2004; Brembeck et al., 2004; Sakamoto et al., 2007). CRCs also show overexpression of lymphoid enhancing factor 1 (LEF1), a direct partner for β-catenin in initiation of transcription. Moreover, LEF1 itself is a WNT target and traps β-catenin in the nucleus (Henderson et al., 2002; Hovanes et al., 2001). The integrin-linked kinase (ILK), an intracellular mediator of integrin signalling, additionally contributes to epithelial de-differentiation in colon cancer. ILK is activated after β-integrins 1 and 3 binding to their extracellular matrix ligands and induces EMT in two ways. First, the activation of ILK promotes expression of WNT targets by translocating β-catenin to the nucleus (Novak et al., 1998). Second, expression of the EMT-inducer Snail1 is activated by ILK in a β-catenin-independent manner (Fig. 6.3B) (Tan et al., 2001). Indeed, the role of the group of EMT-inducing transcription factors in CRC and the regulation of E-cadherin expression has received a special focus of attention and will be discussed in the next section.

Taken together, numerous tumour-stroma interactions at the invasion front of CRCs promote the translocation of β-catenin to the nucleus. Please refer to the excellent review by Le et al. for further reading (Le et al., 2008). Also a variety of intracellular factors are known to promote WNT signalling. Interestingly, some of these molecules are transcriptionally-induced by WNT signalling, indicating numerous feed-forward mechanisms that stabilize the nuclear localization of β-catenin.

6.7 Regulation of E-Cadherin Expression in CRC

Expression of membranous E-cadherin promotes an epithelial phenotype. E-cadherin suppresses invasion in various cancer cell lines and animal tumour models and its loss was demonstrated to be causal for the malignant progression from adenoma to carcinoma (Peinado et al., 2007; Tsanou et al., 2008). For numerous types of human cancers, a correlation between loss of E-cadherin expression and adverse clinical outcome has been described (Birchmeier and Behrens, 1994; Perl et al., 1998). Expression of the *E-cadherin* gene is lost by different events, including genetic alterations, epigenetic silencing, and transcriptional inhibition (Stemmler, 2008). In CRC, silencing of *E-cadherin* expression by promoter hypermethylation has been reported and reviewed in detail by F.J. Carmona and M. Esteller in Chapter 4 in this book (Garinis et al., 2002; Wheeler et al., 2001). The most frequent alteration, however, appears to be silencing of *E-cadherin* gene expression by specific transcriptional repressors. Indeed, E-cadherin is re-expressed in central areas of metastases, indicating that the loss of membranous expression of E-cadherin in budding is only a transient event. Treatment of colorectal cancer cells with tumor necrosis factor (TNF)α and TGFβ induced EMT and several transcriptional repressors of E-cadherin in colorectal cancer have been confirmed as intracellular mediators of the mesenchymal phenotype (Bates and Mercurio, 2003; Peinado et al., 2007). Amongst these are the factors Snail1 and Snail2, the zinc finger E-box-binding homeobox proteins 1 and 2 (ZEB1 and ZEB2), as well as Twist (Fig. 6.4) (Batlle et al., 2000; Bolos et al., 2003; Cano et al., 2000; Comijn et al., 2001; Eger et al., 2005; Funahashi et al., 1993; Grooteclaes and Frisch, 2000; Guaita et al., 2002; Hajra et al., 2002; Peinado et al., 2004; Takahashi et al., 2004; Yang et al., 2004).

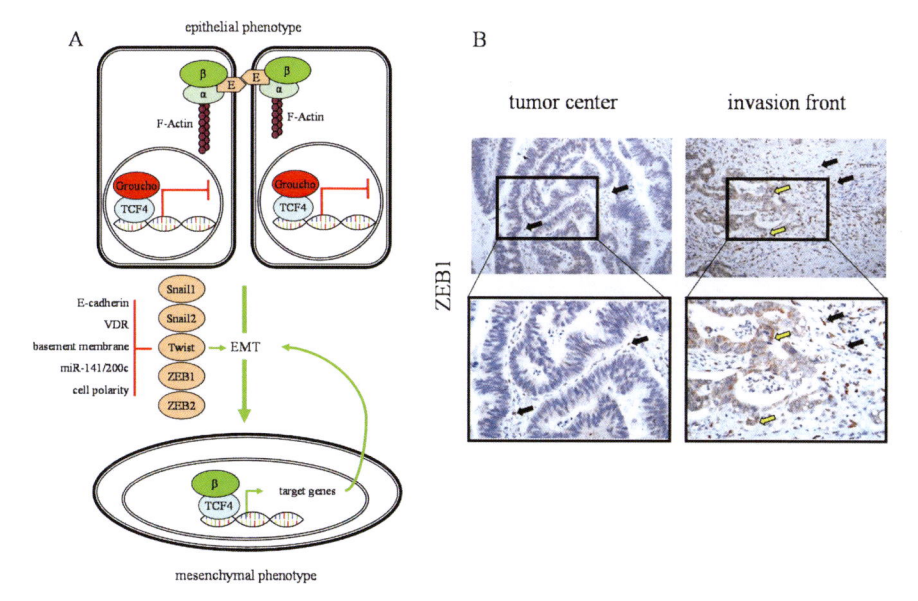

Fig. 6.4 EMT-inducing transcriptional repressors in CRC. (**A**) Many different transcriptional repressors of the *E-cadherin* gene are reported to contribute to malignant progression of colorectal cancer, including Snail1, Snail2, Twist, ZEB1 and ZEB2. Experimental data suggest a model in which these factors cooperate inter-dependently with each other and with β-catenin (β) to induce the aggressive mesenchymal phenotype of budding cancer cells. (**B**) A typical well-to-moderately differentiated colorectal adenocarcinoma is immunohistochemically stained for ZEB1. Stromal fibroblasts (*black arrows*) and budding tumour cells (*yellow arrows*) at the invasion front express ZEB1, whereas the epithelially-differentiated cancer cells in the tumour center are negative for ZEB1. Insets show magnification; nuclear counterstaining in *blue*

6.8 Snail1 and Snail2

Snail1 over-expression has been detected in CRC and is associated with distant metastasis (Olmeda et al., 2007; Roy et al., 2005). Snail1 is activated in colon cancer cell lines by an ILK-dependent mechanism, as well as by an Axin2-dependent pathway (Tan et al., 2001; Yook et al., 2006). Nuclear β-catenin activates expression of Axin2, which localizes GSK3β to the cytoplasm. This in turn leaves Snail1 in an unphosphorylated and transcriptionally-active form. Hence, Snail1 represses E-cadherin expression, induces EMT and promotes tumour invasion (Lustig et al., 2002; Yook et al., 2006). Moreover, Snail2 expression was associated with distant metastasis and poor survival (Shioiri et al., 2006). As Snail2 is a direct target of β-catenin in colon cancer, it links nuclear localization of β-catenin to the observed loss of E-cadherin at the invasion front (Conacci-Sorrell et al., 2003). One of the snail target genes in CRC is the *Vitamin D receptor* (*VDR*) gene. Snail2 cooperates with Snail1 in *VDR* repression (Larriba et al., 2009). VDR signalling was demonstrated to induce E-cadherin expression and an epithelial phenotype (Palmer et al., 2004; Pena et al., 2005; Roy et al., 2005). Moreover, VDR activation induces relocalization of β-catenin from the nucleus to the plasma membrane (Larriba et al., 2009). This highlights the direct and indirect effects of Snail1 and Snail2 on E-cadherin expression. First, it directly represses transcription of E-cadherin and second, it inhibits the transcription of factors that induce expression of E-cadherin. Strikingly, Snail1 interacts with β-catenin, and thereby promotes expression of WNT target genes in colorectal cancer cells (Roy et al., 2005; Stemmer et al., 2008). Furthermore, overexpression of Snail1 in colorectal cancer cell lines also causes up-regulation of ZEB1 (Fig. 6.4A) (Guaita et al., 2002).

6.9 ZEB1, ZEB2 and Twist

ZEB1 is expressed at the tumour invasion front of CRCs and is linked with poor patient survival (Fig. 6.4B). Furthermore, ZEB1 expression has been shown to promote migration, invasion and metastasis of tumour cells, in particular in CRC (Graham et al., 2008; Singh et al., 2008; Spaderna et al., 2006; Spaderna et al., 2008; Wang et al., 2007).

In addition, numerous signaling pathways induce ZEB1 expression. These include TGFβ and TNFα, which are important activators of EMT (Burk et al., 2008; Chua et al., 2007; Gilles et al., 1997; Gregory et al., 2008; Korpal et al., 2008; Rodrigo et al., 1999). Also, IGF1 signalling induces EMT in cancer and activates ZEB1 expression. As IGF1 is a target of β-catenin, this links ZEB1 expression indirectly to WNT signalling (Graham et al., 2008; Kawada et al., 2006; Longo et al., 2002; Miyamoto et al., 2005). In addition, EGF receptor-dependent signalling, which plays an important role in the malignant progression of CRC, induces ZEB1 and inhibits E-cadherin expression (de Castro-Carpeno et al., 2008; Verbeek et al., 1998; Yang et al., 2007). E-cadherin expression is also suppressed in a

COX2-dependent manner. Interestingly, the COX2 metabolite PGE2 induces expression of ZEB1 and Snail1 (Dohadwala et al., 2006). As COX2/PGE2 also activates nuclear localization of β-catenin in colon cancer and is itself a target of WNT signalling, this suggests another self-amplifying feed-forward loop via COX2/PGE2 in inducing and maintaining mesenchymal differentiation (Dannenberg and Zakim, 1999; Dohadwala et al., 2006; Jungck et al., 2004; Shao et al., 2005). This is in line with the observation that COX2 is over-expressed in colon cancer and is associated with poor clinical outcome (Dannenberg and Zakim, 1999; Dohadwala et al., 2002; Dohadwala et al., 2001; Jungck et al., 2004; Longo et al., 2002; Tsujii et al., 1997).

There is considerable knowledge of the molecular mechanisms by which ZEB1 induces mesenchymal differentiation. In particular, ZEB1 inhibits expression of certain components of the basement membrane, desmosomal proteins, intracellular mediators of cell polarity and E-cadherin (Aigner et al., 2007a; Aigner et al., 2007b; Spaderna et al., 2006; Spaderna et al., 2008). Breakdown of the basement membrane is a prerequisite for dissemination and metastasis of epithelial tumour cells (Barsky et al., 1983). ZEB1-mediated loss of the basement membrane contributes to tumour progression in a dual fashion: by loss of inductive signals and thus perturbation of epithelial differentiation and by overcoming a mechanical obstacle. ZEB1 also inhibits expression of cell polarity factors, such as Crumbs homolog 3 protein, subunits of the adaptor-related protein complex 1, the InaD-like protein and the lethal giant larvae homolog 2 (LGL2) protein, thus affecting basal-apical polarization of the epithelial phenotype (Aigner et al., 2007a; Marazuela and Alonso, 2004; Spaderna et al., 2008; Wodarz and Nathke, 2007). Of note, the ZEB1 target gene *LGL2* acts as a tumour suppressor, because loss of its homologue *Lgl* in Drosophila causes tumour metastasis. This is in line with the tumour-promoting functions of ZEB1 (Woodhouse et al., 1998). ZEB1 also inhibits expression of the microRNA (miR)-200 family, an important player in epithelial differentiation (Baskerville and Bartel, 2005; Lu et al., 2005). Transfection of miR-200 family members induced a MET in colorectal tumour cell lines, including up-regulation of E-cadherin expression. Furthermore, migration and invasion of undifferentiated cancer cell lines was inhibited. Strikingly, the miR-200 family targets expression of ZEB1 and other molecules that act in an invasion-promoting manner, e.g. TGFβ2, Cofilin, and the Leptin receptor. This indicates a negative feedback between miR-200 family members and ZEB1 (Burk et al., 2008; Cano and Nieto, 2008; Gregory et al., 2008; Korpal et al., 2008; Park et al., 2008). Not surprisingly, knockdown of ZEB1 in colorectal cancer cells prevented liver metastasis in nude mice xenografts (Spaderna et al., 2008). This is in line with the observation that ZEB1 expression and selective loss of basement membrane in invasive tumour regions of CRCs are strong predictors of poor patient survival and metachronous distant metastasis (Spaderna et al., 2006).

Another target of the miR-200 family is ZEB2. Strikingly, ZEB2 is also expressed at the tumour invasion front in a gene expression profiling study (Hlubek et al., 2007a). The same study identified over-expression of Twist at the tumour invasion front, which is associated with nodal invasion in CRC (Hlubek et al., 2007a; Valdes-Mora et al., 2009). Furthermore, Twist and other EMT inducers are up-regulated in a VEGF signalling-dependent manner. As VEGF is a direct WNT target, this links nuclear β-catenin to the upregulation of EMT inducers.

6.10 Conclusion

Colorectal adenocarcinomas are typically characterized by a heterogeneous differentiation pattern. Central tumour areas are epithelially-differentiated, whereas budding cancer cells at the invasion front have a mesenchymal phenotype. Tumour budding is highly predictive of adverse clinical outcome, which in part can be explained by the nuclear β-catenin accumulation in disseminating colorectal cancer cells. The non-random distribution of β-catenin within the tumour is promoted by various signals from the microenvironment, but also by intracellular factors. In the nucleus, β-catenin activates responsive target genes that contribute to induction of EMT and malignant tumour progression. Furthermore, β-catenin cooperates interdependently with a group of transcriptional repressors to suppress epithelial differentiation and to promote tumor invasion, in particular by inhibition of *E-cadherin* gene expression.

Abbreviations and Acronyms

APC	Adenomatous polyposis coli
BRG1	Brahma-related gene 1
CD133	Cluster of differentiation 133
CD44	Cluster of differentiation 44
CK1	Casein kinase 1
CREB	cAMP response element binding
c-MET	Cellular mesenchymal-epithelial transition factor
c-Myc	Cellular myelocytomatosis gene
EMT	Epithelial mesenchymal transition
GSK3β	Glycogen synthase kinase 3 β
LAMC2	Laminin gamma 2 chain
LEF1	Lymphoid enhancing factor 1
LGL2	Lethal giant larvae homolog 2
LGR5	Leucine-rich repeat-containing G protein-coupled receptor 5
MDR1	Multidrug resistance protein 1
MET	Mesenchymal epithelial transition
MMP	Metalloproteinase
MUC1	Mucin 1
PTEN	Tensin homolog deleted on chromosome 10
TCF/LEF	T-cell factor/lymphoid enhancer factor
TNC	Tenascin
UICC/AJCC, TNM	Union Internationale Contre le Cancer/American Joint Committee on Cancer, Tumour Nodes and Metastasis
uPA	Urokinase plasminogen activator

TGFβ   Transforming growth factor β
VEGF   Vascular endothelial growth factor
WNT   Wingless/int
ZEB1   Zinc finger E-box-binding protein

References

Adachi S, Jigami T, Yasui T, Nakano T, Ohwada S, Omori Y et al. (2004). Role of a BCL9-related beta-catenin-binding protein, B9L, in tumorigenesis induced by aberrant activation of Wnt signaling. *Cancer Res* **64**: 8496–501.

Aigner K, Dampier B, Descovich L, Mikula M, Sultan A, Schreiber M et al. (2007a). The transcription factor ZEB1 (deltaEF1) promotes tumour cell dedifferentiation by repressing master regulators of epithelial polarity. *Oncogene* **26**: 6979–88.

Aigner K, Descovich L, Mikula M, Sultan A, Dampier B, Bonne S et al. (2007b). The transcription factor ZEB1 (deltaEF1) represses Plakophilin 3 during human cancer progression. *FEBS Lett* **581**: 1617–24.

Barker N, Hurlstone A, Musisi H, Miles A, Bienz M, Clevers H (2001). The chromatin remodelling factor Brg-1 interacts with beta-catenin to promote target gene activation. *Embo J* **20**: 4935–43.

Barker N, Ridgway RA, van Es JH, van de Wetering M, Begthel H, van den Born M et al. (2009). Crypt stem cells as the cells-of-origin of intestinal cancer. *Nature* **457**: 608–11.

Barker N, van Es JH, Kuipers J, Kujala P, van den Born M, Cozijnsen M et al. (2007). Identification of stem cells in small intestine and colon by marker gene Lgr5. *Nature* **449**: 1003–7.

Barsky SH, Siegal GP, Jannotta F, Liotta LA (1983). Loss of basement membrane components by invasive tumors but not by their benign counterparts. *Lab Invest* **49**: 140–47.

Baskerville S, Bartel DP (2005). Microarray profiling of microRNAs reveals frequent coexpression with neighboring miRNAs and host genes. *RNA* **11**: 241–47.

Bates RC, Mercurio AM (2003). Tumor necrosis factor-alpha stimulates the epithelial-to-mesenchymal transition of human colonic organoids. *Mol Biol Cell* **14**: 1790–800.

Batlle E, Sancho E, Franci C, Dominguez D, Monfar M, Baulida J et al. (2000). The transcription factor snail is a repressor of E-cadherin gene expression in epithelial tumour cells. *Nat Cell Biol* **2**: 84–89.

Behrens J (2005). The role of the Wnt signalling pathway in colorectal tumorigenesis. *Biochem Soc Trans* **33**: 672–75.

Behrens J, Jerchow BA, Wurtele M, Grimm J, Asbrand C, Wirtz R et al. (1998). Functional interaction of an axin homolog, conductin, with beta- catenin, APC, and GSK3beta. *Science* **280**: 596–99.

Behrens J, von Kries JP, Kuhl M, Bruhn L, Wedlich D, Grosschedl R et al. (1996). Functional interaction of beta-catenin with the transcription factor LEF-1. *Nature* **382**: 638–42.

Beiter K, Hiendlmeyer E, Brabletz T, Hlubek F, Haynl A, Knoll C et al. (2005). beta-Catenin regulates the expression of tenascin-C in human colorectal tumors. *Oncogene* **24**: 8200–4.

Bienz M, Clevers H (2000). Linking colorectal cancer to Wnt signaling. *Cell* **103**: 311–20.

Birchmeier W, Behrens J (1994). Cadherin expression in carcinomas: role in the formation of cell junctions and the prevention of invasiveness. *Biochim Biophys Acta* **1198**: 11–26.

Blasi F, Carmeliet P (2002). uPAR: a versatile signalling orchestrator. *Nat Rev Mol Cell Biol* **3**: 932–43.

Bolos V, Peinado H, Perez-Moreno MA, Fraga MF, Esteller M, Cano A (2003). The transcription factor Slug represses E-cadherin expression and induces epithelial to mesenchymal transitions: a comparison with Snail and E47 repressors. *J Cell Sci* **116**: 499–511.

Boon EM, van der Neut R, van de Wetering M, Clevers H, Pals ST (2002). Wnt signaling regulates expression of the receptor tyrosine kinase met in colorectal cancer. *Cancer Res* **62**: 5126–28.

Brabletz T, Herrmann K, Jung A, Faller G, Kirchner T (2000). Expression of nuclear beta-catenin and c-myc is correlated with tumor size but not with proliferative activity of colorectal adenomas. *Am J Pathol* **156**: 865–70.

Brabletz T, Hlubek F, Spaderna S, Schmalhofer O, Hiendlmeyer E, Jung A et al. (2005a). Invasion and metastasis in colorectal cancer: epithelial-mesenchymal transition, mesenchymal-epithelial transition, stem cells and beta-catenin. *Cells Tissues Organs* **179**: 56–65.

Brabletz T, Jung A, Dag S, Hlubek F, Kirchner T (1999). beta-catenin regulates the expression of the matrix metalloproteinase-7 in human colorectal cancer. *Am J Pathol* **155**: 1033–38.

Brabletz T, Jung A, Hermann K, Gunther K, Hohenberger W, Kirchner T (1998). Nuclear overexpression of the oncoprotein beta-catenin in colorectal cancer is localized predominantly at the invasion front. *Pathol Res Pract* **194**: 701–4.

Brabletz T, Jung A, Reu S, Porzner M, Hlubek F, Kunz-Schughart L et al. (2001). Variable beta-catenin expression in colorectal cancer indicates a tumor progression driven by the tumor environment. *Proc Natl Acad Sci USA* **98**: 10356–61.

Brabletz T, Jung A, Spaderna S, Hlubek F, Kirchner T (2005b). Opinion: migrating cancer stem cells – an integrated concept of malignant tumour progression. *Nat Rev Cancer* **5**: 744–49.

Brembeck FH, Schwarz-Romond T, Bakkers J, Wilhelm S, Hammerschmidt M, Birchmeier W (2004). Essential role of BCL9-2 in the switch between {beta}-catenin's adhesive and transcriptional functions. *Genes Dev* **18**: 2225–30.

Broders AC (1921). Squamous-cell epithelioma of the skin: a study of 256 cases. *Ann Surg* **73**: 141–60.

Brown JR, DuBois RN (2005). COX-2: a molecular target for colorectal cancer prevention. *J Clin Oncol* **23**: 2840–55.

Buo L, Meling GI, Karlsrud TS, Johansen HT, Aasen AO (1995). Antigen levels of urokinase plasminogen activator and its receptor at the tumor-host interface of colorectal adenocarcinomas are related to tumor aggressiveness. *Hum Pathol* **26**: 1133–38.

Burk U, Schubert J, Wellner U, Schmalhofer O, Vincan E, Spaderna S et al. (2008). A reciprocal repression between ZEB1 and members of the miR-200 family promotes EMT and invasion in cancer cells. *EMBO Rep* **9**: 582–89.

Cannito S, Novo E, Compagnone A, Valfre di Bonzo L, Busletta C, Zamara E et al. (2008). Redox mechanisms switch on hypoxia-dependent epithelial-mesenchymal transition in cancer cells. *Carcinogenesis* **29**: 2267–78.

Cano A, Nieto MA (2008). Non-coding RNAs take centre stage in epithelial-to-mesenchymal transition. *Trends Cell Biol* **18**: 357–59.

Cano A, Perez-Moreno MA, Rodrigo I, Locascio A, Blanco MJ, del Barrio MG et al. (2000). The transcription factor snail controls epithelial-mesenchymal transitions by repressing E-cadherin expression. *Nat Cell Biol* **2**: 76–83.

Castellone MD, Teramoto H, Williams BO, Druey KM, Gutkind JS (2005). Prostaglandin E2 promotes colon cancer cell growth through a Gs-axin-beta-catenin signaling axis. *Science* **310**: 1504–10.

Choi HJ, Park KJ, Shin JS, Roh MS, Kwon HC, Lee HS (2007). Tumor budding as a prognostic marker in stage-III rectal carcinoma. *Int J Colorectal Dis* **22**: 863–68.

Chua HL, Bhat-Nakshatri P, Clare SE, Morimiya A, Badve S, Nakshatri H (2007). NF-kappaB represses E-cadherin expression and enhances epithelial to mesenchymal transition of mammary epithelial cells: potential involvement of ZEB-1 and ZEB-2. *Oncogene* **26**: 711–24.

Comijn J, Berx G, Vermassen P, Verschueren K, van Grunsven L, Bruyneel E et al. (2001). The two-handed E box binding zinc finger protein SIP1 downregulates E-cadherin and induces invasion. *Mol Cell* **7**: 1267–78.

Compton CC (1999). Pathology report in colon cancer: what is prognostically important? *Dig Dis* **17**: 67–79.

Compton CC, Fielding LP, Burgart LJ, Conley B, Cooper HS, Hamilton SR et al. (2000). Prognostic factors in colorectal cancer. College of American Pathologists Consensus Statement 1999. *Arch Pathol Lab Med* **124**: 979–94.

Conacci-Sorrell M, Simcha I, Ben-Yedidia T, Blechman J, Savagner P, Ben-Ze'ev A (2003). Autoregulation of E-cadherin expression by cadherin-cadherin interactions: the roles of beta-catenin signaling, Slug, and MAPK. *J Cell Biol* **163**: 847–57.

Dannenberg AJ, Zakim D (1999). Chemoprevention of colorectal cancer through inhibition of cyclooxygenase-2. *Semin Oncol* **26**: 499–504.

de Castro-Carpeno J, Belda-Iniesta C, Casado Saenz E, Hernandez Agudo E, Feliu Batlle J, Gonzalez Baron M (2008). EGFR and colon cancer: a clinical view. *Clin Transl Oncol* **10**: 6–13.

de Santa Barbara P, van den Brink GR, Roberts DJ (2003). Development and differentiation of the intestinal epithelium. *Cell Mol Life Sci* **60**: 1322–32.

De Wever O, Nguyen QD, Van Hoorde L, Bracke M, Bruyneel E, Gespach C et al. (2004). Tenascin-C and SF/HGF produced by myofibroblasts in vitro provide convergent pro-invasive signals to human colon cancer cells through RhoA and Rac. *FASEB J* **18**: 1016–18.

Diaz-Rubio E (2006). Vascular endothelial growth factor inhibitors in colon cancer. *Adv Exp Med Biol* **587**: 251–75.

Dohadwala M, Batra RK, Luo J, Lin Y, Krysan K, Pold M et al. (2002). Autocrine/paracrine prostaglandin E2 production by non-small cell lung cancer cells regulates matrix metalloproteinase-2 and CD44 in cyclooxygenase-2-dependent invasion. *J Biol Chem* **277**: 50828–33.

Dohadwala M, Luo J, Zhu L, Lin Y, Dougherty GJ, Sharma S et al. (2001). Non-small cell lung cancer cyclooxygenase-2-dependent invasion is mediated by CD44. *J Biol Chem* **276**: 20809–12.

Dohadwala M, Yang SC, Luo J, Sharma S, Batra RK, Huang M et al. (2006). Cyclooxygenase-2-dependent regulation of E-cadherin: prostaglandin E2 induces transcriptional repressors ZEB1 and snail in non-small cell lung cancer. *Cancer Res* **66**: 5338–45.

Du L, Wang H, He L, Zhang J, Ni B, Wang X et al. (2008). CD44 is of functional importance for colorectal cancer stem cells. *Clin Cancer Res* **14**: 6751–60.

Easwaran V, Lee SH, Inge L, Guo L, Goldbeck C, Garrett E et al. (2003). beta-Catenin regulates vascular endothelial growth factor expression in colon cancer. *Cancer Res* **63**: 3145–53.

Eger A, Aigner K, Sonderegger S, Dampier B, Oehler S, Schreiber M et al. (2005). DeltaEF1 is a transcriptional repressor of E-cadherin and regulates epithelial plasticity in breast cancer cells. *Oncogene* **24**: 2375–85.

Fazekas K, Csuka O, Koves I, Raso E, Timar J (2000). Experimental and clinicopathologic studies on the function of the HGF receptor in human colon cancer metastasis. *Clin Exp Metastasis* **18**: 639–49.

Fodde R, Smits R, Clevers H (2001). APC, signal transduction and genetic instability in colorectal cancer. *Nat Rev Cancer* **1**: 55–67.

Freier S, Weiss O, Eran M, Flyvbjerg A, Dahan R, Nephesh I et al. (1999). Expression of the insulin-like growth factors and their receptors in adenocarcinoma of the colon. *Gut* **44**: 704–08.

Funahashi J, Sekido R, Murai K, Kamachi Y, Kondoh H (1993). Delta-crystallin enhancer binding protein delta EF1 is a zinc finger-homeodomain protein implicated in postgastrulation embryogenesis. *Development* **119**: 433–46.

Gabbert H, Wagner R, Moll R, Gerharz CD (1985). Tumor dedifferentiation: an important step in tumor invasion. *Clin Exp Metastasis* **3**: 257–79.

Garinis GA, Menounos PG, Spanakis NE, Papadopoulos K, Karavitis G, Parassi I et al. (2002). Hypermethylation-associated transcriptional silencing of E-cadherin in primary sporadic colorectal carcinomas. *J Pathol* **198**: 442–49.

Gavert N, Conacci-Sorrell M, Gast D, Schneider A, Altevogt P, Brabletz T et al. (2005). L1, a novel target of {beta}-catenin signaling, transforms cells and is expressed at the invasive front of colon cancers. *J Cell Biol* **168**: 633–42.

Gavert N, Sheffer M, Raveh S, Spaderna S, Shtutman M, Brabletz T et al. (2007). Expression of L1-CAM and ADAM10 in human colon cancer cells induces metastasis. *Cancer Res* **67**: 7703–12.

Gilles C, Polette M, Birembaut P, Brunner N, Thompson EW (1997). Expression of c-ets-1 mRNA is associated with an invasive, EMT-derived phenotype in breast carcinoma cell lines. *Clin Exp Metastasis* **15**: 519–26.

Goodlad RA, Ryan AJ, Wedge SR, Pyrah IT, Alferez D, Poulsom R et al. (2006). Inhibiting vascular endothelial growth factor receptor-2 signaling reduces tumor burden in the ApcMin/+ mouse model of early intestinal cancer. *Carcinogenesis* **27**: 2133–39.

Graham TR, Zhau HE, Odero-Marah VA, Osunkoya AO, Kimbro KS, Tighiouart M et al. (2008). Insulin-like growth factor-I-dependent up-regulation of ZEB1 drives epithelial-to-mesenchymal transition in human prostate cancer cells. *Cancer Res* **68**: 2479–88.

Gregory PA, Bert AG, Paterson EL, Barry SC, Tsykin A, Farshid G et al. (2008). The miR-200 family and miR-205 regulate epithelial to mesenchymal transition by targeting ZEB1 and SIP1. *Nat Cell Biol* **10**: 593–601.

Grooteclaes ML, Frisch SM (2000). Evidence for a function of CtBP in epithelial gene regulation and anoikis. *Oncogene* **19**: 3823–8.

Guaita S, Puig I, Franci C, Garrido M, Dominguez D, Batlle E et al. (2002). Snail induction of epithelial to mesenchymal transition in tumor cells is accompanied by MUC1 repression and ZEB1 expression. *J Biol Chem* **277**: 39209–16.

Hajra KM, Chen DY, Fearon ER (2002). The SLUG zinc-finger protein represses E-cadherin in breast cancer. *Cancer Res* **62**: 1613–18.

Haraguchi N, Utsunomiya T, Inoue H, Tanaka F, Mimori K, Barnard GF et al. (2005). Characterization of a Side Population of Cancer Cells from Human Gastrointestinal System. *Stem Cells* **24**: 506–11.

Hase K, Shatney C, Johnson D, Trollope M, Vierra M (1993). Prognostic value of tumor "budding" in patients with colorectal cancer. *Dis Colon Rectum* **36**: 627–35.

Hassan AB, Howell JA (2000a). Insulin-like growth factor II supply modifies growth of intestinal adenoma in Apc(Min/+) mice. *Cancer Res* **60**: 1070–76.

Hassan AB, Howell JA (2000b). Insulin-like growth factor II supply modifies growth of intestinal adenoma in Apc(Min/+) mice. *Cancer Res* **60**: 1070–76.

He TC, Sparks AB, Rago C, Hermeking H, Zawel L, da Costa LT et al. (1998). Identification of c-MYC as a target of the APC pathway [see comments]. *Science* **281**: 1509–12.

Henderson BR, Galea M, Schuechner S, Leung L (2002). Lymphoid enhancer factor-1 blocks adenomatous polyposis coli-mediated nuclear export and degradation of beta-catenin. Regulation by histone deacetylase 1. *J Biol Chem* **277**: 24258–64.

Hiendlmeyer E, Regus S, Wassermann S, Hlubek F, Haynl A, Dimmler A et al. (2004). Beta-catenin up-regulates the expression of the urokinase plasminogen activator in human colorectal tumors. *Cancer Res* **64**: 1209–14.

Hlubek F, Brabletz T, Budczies J, Pfeiffer S, Jung A, Kirchner T (2007a). Heterogeneous expression of Wnt/beta-catenin target genes within colorectal cancer. *Int J Cancer* **121**: 1941–48.

Hlubek F, Jung A, Kotzor N, Kirchner T, Brabletz T (2001). Expression of the invasion factor laminin γ2 in colorectal carcinomas is regulated by β-catenin. *Cancer Res* **61**: 8089–93.

Hlubek F, Spaderna S, Jung A, Kirchner T, Brabletz T (2004). beta-Catenin activates a coordinated expression of the proinvasive factors laminin-5 gamma2 chain and MT1-MMP in colorectal carcinomas. *Int J Cancer* **108**: 321–6.

Hlubek F, Spaderna S, Schmalhofer O, Jung A, Kirchner T, Brabletz T (2007b). Wnt/FZD signaling and colorectal cancer morphogenesis. *Front Biosci* **12**: 458–70.

Hongxing Z, Nancai Y, Wen S, Guofu H, Yanxia W, Hanju H et al. (2008). Depletion of c-Myc inhibits human colon cancer Colo 320 cells' growth. *Cancer Biother Radiopharm* **23**: 229–37.

Horst D, Kriegl L, Engel J, Jung A, Kirchner T (2009). CD133 and nuclear beta-catenin: the marker combination to detect high risk cases of low stage colorectal cancer. *Eur J Cancer* **45**: 2034–40.

Horst D, Kriegl L, Engel J, Kirchner T, Jung A (2008). CD133 expression is an independent prognostic marker for low survival in colorectal cancer. *Br J Cancer* **99**: 1285–89.

Hovanes K, Li TW, Munguia JE, Truong T, Milovanovic T, Lawrence Marsh J et al. (2001). Beta-catenin-sensitive isoforms of lymphoid enhancer factor-1 are selectively expressed in colon cancer. *Nat Genet* **28**: 53–57.

Hulit J, Wang C, Li Z, Albanese C, Rao M, Di Vizio D et al. (2004). Cyclin D1 genetic heterozygosity regulates colonic epithelial cell differentiation and tumor number in ApcMin mice. *Mol Cell Biol* **24**: 7598–611.

Inomata M, Ochiai A, Akimoto S, Kitano S, Hirohashi S (1996). Alteration of beta-catenin expression in colonic epithelial cells of familial adenomatous polyposis patients. *Cancer Res* **56**: 2213–17.

Janssen KP, Alberici P, Fsihi H, Gaspar C, Breukel C, Franken P et al. (2006). APC and oncogenic KRAS are synergistic in enhancing Wnt signaling in intestinal tumor formation and progression. *Gastroenterology* **131**: 1096–109.

Jung A, Schrauder M, Oswald U, Knoll C, Sellberg P, Palmqvist R et al. (2001). The invasion front of human colorectal adenocarcinomas shows co-localization of nuclear beta-Catenin, cyclin D(1), and p16(INK4A) and is a region of low proliferation. *Am J Pathol* **159**: 1613–17.

Jungck M, Grunhage F, Spengler U, Dernac A, Mathiak M, Caspari R et al. (2004). E-cadherin expression is homogeneously reduced in adenoma from patients with familial adenomatous polyposis: an immunohistochemical study of E-cadherin, beta-catenin and cyclooxygenase-2 expression. *Int J Colorectal Dis* **19**: 438–45.

Kaifi JT, Reichelt U, Quaas A, Schurr PG, Wachowiak R, Yekebas EF et al. (2007). L1 is associated with micrometastatic spread and poor outcome in colorectal cancer. *Mod Pathol* **20**: 1183–90.

Katoh Y, Katoh M (2007). Comparative genomics on PROM1 gene encoding stem cell marker CD133. *Int J Mol Med* **19**: 967–70.

Kawada M, Inoue H, Masuda T, Ikeda D (2006). Insulin-like growth factor I secreted from prostate stromal cells mediates tumor-stromal cell interactions of prostate cancer. *Cancer Res* **66**: 4419–25.

Kawasaki H, Toyoda M, Shinohara H, Okuda J, Watanabe I, Yamamoto T et al. (2001). Expression of survivin correlates with apoptosis, proliferation, and angiogenesis during human colorectal tumorigenesis. *Cancer* **91**: 2026–32.

Kazama S, Watanabe T, Ajioka Y, Kanazawa T, Nagawa H (2006). Tumour budding at the deepest invasive margin correlates with lymph node metastasis in submucosal colorectal cancer detected by anticytokeratin antibody CAM5.2. *Br J Cancer* **94**: 293–98.

Korinek V, Barker N, Morin PJ, van Wichen D, de Weger R, Kinzler KW et al. (1997). Constitutive transcriptional activation by a beta-catenin-Tcf complex in APC-/- colon carcinoma [see comments]. *Science* **275**: 1784–87.

Korpal M, Lee ES, Hu G, Kang Y (2008). The miR-200 family inhibits epithelial-mesenchymal transition and cancer cell migration by direct targeting of E-cadherin transcriptional repressors ZEB1 and ZEB2. *J Biol Chem* **283**: 14910–14.

Larriba MJ, Martin-Villar E, Garcia JM, Pereira F, Pena C, de Herreros AG et al. (2009). Snail2 cooperates with Snail1 in the repression of vitamin D receptor in colon cancer. *Carcinogenesis* **30**: 1459–68.

Le NH, Franken P, Fodde R (2008). Tumour-stroma interactions in colorectal cancer: converging on beta-catenin activation and cancer stemness. *Br J Cancer* **98**: 1886–93.

Lester RD, Jo M, Montel V, Takimoto S, Gonias SL (2007). uPAR induces epithelial-mesenchymal transition in hypoxic breast cancer cells. *J Cell Biol* **178**: 425–36.

Liotta LA, Kohn EC (2001). The microenvironment of the tumour-host interface. *Nature* **411**: 375–79.

Liu C, Li Y, Semenov M, Han C, Baeg GH, Tan Y et al. (2002). Control of beta-catenin phosphorylation/degradation by a dual-kinase mechanism. *Cell* **108**: 837–47.

Liu D, el-Hariry I, Karayiannakis AJ, Wilding J, Chinery R, Kmiot W et al. (1997). Phosphorylation of beta-catenin and epidermal growth factor receptor by intestinal trefoil factor. *Lab Invest* **77**: 557–63.

Longo KA, Kennell JA, Ochocinska MJ, Ross SE, Wright WS, MacDougald OA (2002). Wnt signaling protects 3T3-L1 preadipocytes from apoptosis through induction of insulin-like growth factors. *J Biol Chem* **277**: 38239–44.

Lu J, Getz G, Miska EA, Alvarez-Saavedra E, Lamb J, Peck D et al. (2005). MicroRNA expression profiles classify human cancers. *Nature* **435**: 834–38.

Lu Z, Ghosh S, Wang Z, Hunter T (2003). Downregulation of caveolin-1 function by EGF leads to the loss of E-cadherin, increased transcriptional activity of beta-catenin, and enhanced tumor cell invasion. *Cancer Cell* **4**: 499–515.

Lustig B, Jerchow B, Sachs M, Weiler S, Pietsch T, Karsten U et al. (2002). Negative feedback loop of Wnt signaling through upregulation of conductin/axin2 in colorectal and liver tumors. *Mol Cell Biol* **22**: 1184–93.

Mani SA, Guo W, Liao MJ, Eaton EN, Ayyanan A, Zhou AY et al. (2008). The epithelial-mesenchymal transition generates cells with properties of stem cells. *Cell* **133**: 704–15.

Marazuela M, Alonso MA (2004). Expression of MAL and MAL2, two elements of the protein machinery for raft-mediated transport, in normal and neoplastic human tissue. *Histol Histopathol* **19**: 925–33.

Mariadason JM, Bordonaro M, Aslam F, Shi L, Kuraguchi M, Velcich A et al. (2001). Downregulation of beta-catenin TCF signaling is linked to colonic epithelial cell differentiation. *Cancer Res* **61**: 3465–71.

Mayo C, Mayol X (2009). Cycling D1 negatively regulates the expression of differentiation genes in HT-29 M6 mucus-secreting colon cancer cells. *Cancer Lett* **281**: 183–87.

Minard ME, Ellis LM, Gallick GE (2006). Tiam1 regulates cell adhesion, migration and apoptosis in colon tumor cells. *Clin Exp Metastasis* **23**: 301–13.

Miyamoto S, Nakamura M, Shitara K, Nakamura K, Ohki Y, Ishii G et al. (2005). Blockade of paracrine supply of insulin-like growth factors using neutralizing antibodies suppresses the liver metastasis of human colorectal cancers. *Clin Cancer Res* **11**: 3494–502.

Morali OG, Delmas V, Moore R, Jeanney C, Thiery JP, Larue L (2001). IGF-II induces rapid beta-catenin relocation to the nucleus during epithelium to mesenchyme transition. *Oncogene* **20**: 4942–50.

Morel AP, Lievre M, Thomas C, Hinkal G, Ansieau S, Puisieux A (2008). Generation of breast cancer stem cells through epithelial-mesenchymal transition. *PLoS One* **3**: e2888.

Morodomi T, Isomoto H, Shirouzu K, Kakegawa K, Irie K, Morimatsu M (1989). An index for estimating the probability of lymph node metastasis in rectal cancers. Lymph node metastasis and the histopathology of actively invasive regions of cancer. *Cancer* **63**: 539–43.

Muller T, Bain G, Wang X, Papkoff J (2002). Regulation of epithelial cell migration and tumor formation by beta-catenin signaling. *Exp Cell Res* **280**: 119–33.

Naishiro Y, Yamada T, Takaoka AS, Hayashi R, Hasegawa F, Imai K et al. (2001). Restoration of epithelial cell polarity in a colorectal cancer cell line by suppression of beta-catenin/T-cell factor 4-mediated gene transactivation. *Cancer Res* **61**: 2751–58.

Nakamura T, Mitomi H, Kanazawa H, Ohkura Y, Watanabe M (2008). Tumor budding as an index to identify high-risk patients with stage II colon cancer. *Dis Colon Rectum* **51**: 568–72.

Nannini M, Pantaleo MA, Maleddu A, Astolfi A, Formica S, Biasco G (2009). Gene expression profiling in colorectal cancer using microarray technologies: results and perspectives. *Cancer Treat Rev* **35**: 201–09.

Nishita M, Hashimoto MK, Ogata S, Laurent MN, Ueno N, Shibuya H et al. (2000). Interaction between Wnt and TGF-beta signalling pathways during formation of Spemann's organizer. *Nature* **403**: 781–85.

Noe V, Fingleton B, Jacobs K, Crawford HC, Vermeulen S, Steelant W et al. (2001). Release of an invasion promoter E-cadherin fragment by matrilysin and stromelysin-1. *J Cell Sci* **114**: 111–18.

Novak A, Hsu SC, Leung-Hagesteijn C, Radeva G, Papkoff J, Montesano R et al. (1998). Cell adhesion and the integrin-linked kinase regulate the LEF-1 and beta-catenin signaling pathways. *Proc Natl Acad Sci USA* **95**: 4374–79.

O'Brien CA, Pollett A, Gallinger S, Dick JE (2007). A human colon cancer cell capable of initiating tumour growth in immunodeficient mice. *Nature* **445**: 106–10.

Okuyama T, Nakamura T, Yamaguchi M (2003a). Budding is useful to select high-risk patients in stage II well-differentiated or moderately differentiated colon adenocarcinoma. *Dis Colon Rectum* **46**: 1400–6.

Okuyama T, Oya M, Ishikawa H (2002a). Budding as a risk factor for lymph node metastasis in pT1 or pT2 well-differentiated colorectal adenocarcinoma. *Dis Colon Rectum* **45**: 628–34.

Okuyama T, Oya M, Ishikawa H (2003b). Budding as a useful prognostic marker in pT3 well- or moderately-differentiated rectal adenocarcinoma. *J Surg Oncol* **83**: 42–47.

Okuyama T, Oya M, Yamaguchi M (2002b). Budding (sprouting) as a useful prognostic marker in colorectal mucinous carcinoma. *Jpn J Clin Oncol* **32**: 412–16.

Olmeda D, Jorda M, Peinado H, Fabra A, Cano A (2007). Snail silencing effectively suppresses tumour growth and invasiveness. *Oncogene* **26**: 1862–74.

Olsen J, Kirkeby LT, Brorsson MM, Dabelsteen S, Troelsen JT, Bordoy R et al. (2003). Converging signals synergistically activate the LAMC2 promoter and lead to accumulation of the laminin gamma 2 chain in human colon carcinoma cells. *Biochem J* **371**: 211–21.

Oving IM, Clevers HC (2002). Molecular causes of colon cancer. *Eur J Clin Invest* **32**: 448–57.

Oyama T, Kanai Y, Ochiai A, Akimoto S, Oda T, Yanagihara K et al. (1994). A truncated beta-catenin disrupts the interaction between E-cadherin and alpha-catenin: a cause of loss of intercellular adhesiveness in human cancer cell lines. *Cancer Res* **54**: 6282–87.

Palmer HG, Larriba MJ, Garcia JM, Ordonez-Moran P, Pena C, Peiro S et al. (2004). The transcription factor SNAIL represses vitamin D receptor expression and responsiveness in human colon cancer. *Nat Med* **10**: 917–19.

Park KJ, Choi HJ, Roh MS, Kwon HC, Kim C (2005a). Intensity of tumor budding and its prognostic implications in invasive colon carcinoma. *Dis Colon Rectum* **48**: 1597–602.

Park SM, Gaur AB, Lengyel E, Peter ME (2008). The miR-200 family determines the epithelial phenotype of cancer cells by targeting the E-cadherin repressors ZEB1 and ZEB2. *Genes Dev* **22**: 894–907.

Park SY, Choe G, Lee HS, Jung SY, Park JG, Kim WH (2005b). Tumor budding as an indicator of isolated tumor cells in lymph nodes from patients with node-negative colorectal cancer. *Dis Colon Rectum* **48**: 292–302.

Peinado H, Ballestar E, Esteller M, Cano A (2004). Snail mediates E-cadherin repression by the recruitment of the Sin3A/histone deacetylase 1 (HDAC1)/HDAC2 complex. *Mol Cell Biol* **24**: 306–19.

Peinado H, Olmeda D, Cano A (2007). Snail, Zeb and bHLH factors in tumour progression: an alliance against the epithelial phenotype? *Nat Rev Cancer* **7**: 415–28.

Pelengaris S, Khan M, Evan G (2002). c-MYC: more than just a matter of life and death. *Nat Rev Cancer* **2**: 764–76.

Pena C, Garcia JM, Silva J, Garcia V, Rodriguez R, Alonso I et al. (2005). E-cadherin and vitamin D receptor regulation by SNAIL and ZEB1 in colon cancer: clinicopathological correlations. *Hum Mol Genet* **14**: 3361–70.

Perl AK, Wilgenbus P, Dahl U, Semb H, Christofori G (1998). A causal role for E-cadherin in the transition from adenoma to carcinoma. *Nature* **392**: 190–93.

Persad S, Troussard AA, McPhee TR, Mulholland DJ, Dedhar S (2001). Tumor suppressor PTEN inhibits nuclear accumulation of beta-catenin and T cell/lymphoid enhancer factor 1-mediated transcriptional activation. *J Cell Biol* **153**: 1161–74.

Prall F, Nizze H, Barten M (2005). Tumour budding as prognostic factor in stage I/II colorectal carcinoma. *Histopathology* **47**: 17–24.

Rasola A, Fassetta M, De Bacco F, D'Alessandro L, Gramaglia D, Di Renzo MF et al. (2007). A positive feedback loop between hepatocyte growth factor receptor and beta-catenin sustains colorectal cancer cell invasive growth. *Oncogene* **26**: 1078–87.

Ricci-Vitiani L, Lombardi DG, Pilozzi E, Biffoni M, Todaro M, Peschle C et al. (2007). Identification and expansion of human colon-cancer-initiating cells. *Nature* **445**: 111–15.

Rodrigo I, Cato AC, Cano A (1999). Regulation of E-cadherin gene expression during tumor progression: the role of a new Ets-binding site and the E-pal element. *Exp Cell Res* **248**: 358–71.

Roy HK, Smyrk TC, Koetsier J, Victor TA, Wali RK (2005). The transcriptional repressor SNAIL is overexpressed in human colon cancer. *Dig Dis Sci* **50**: 42–46.

Royston D, Jackson DG (2009). Mechanisms of lymphatic metastasis in human colorectal adenocarcinoma. *J Pathol* **217**: 608–19.

Sabates-Bellver J, Van der Flier LG, de Palo M, Cattaneo E, Maake C, Rehrauer H et al. (2007). Transcriptome profile of human colorectal adenomas. *Mol Cancer Res* **5**: 1263–75.

Sakamoto I, Ohwada S, Toya H, Togo N, Kashiwabara K, Oyama T et al. (2007). Up-regulation of a BCL9-related beta-catenin-binding protein, B9L, in different stages of sporadic colorectal adenoma. *Cancer Sci* **98**: 83–87.

Sancho E, Batlle E, Clevers H (2003). Live and let die in the intestinal epithelium. *Curr Opin Cell Biol* **15**: 763–70.

Sansom OJ, Meniel VS, Muncan V, Phesse TJ, Wilkins JA, Reed KR et al. (2007). Myc deletion rescues Apc deficiency in the small intestine. *Nature* **446**: 676–79.

Shao J, Jung C, Liu C, Sheng H (2005). Prostaglandin E2 Stimulates the beta-catenin/T cell factor-dependent transcription in colon cancer. *J Biol Chem* **280**: 26565–72.

Shibata S, Marushima H, Asakura T, Matsuura T, Eda H, Aoki K et al. (2009). Three-dimensional culture using a radial flow bioreactor induces matrix metalloprotease 7-mediated EMT-like process in tumor cells via TGFbeta1/Smad pathway. *Int J Oncol* **34**: 1433–48.

Shioiri M, Shida T, Koda K, Oda K, Seike K, Nishimura M et al. (2006). Slug expression is an independent prognostic parameter for poor survival in colorectal carcinoma patients. *Br J Cancer* **94**: 1816–22.

Shmelkov SV, Butler JM, Hooper AT, Hormigo A, Kushner J, Milde T et al. (2008). CD133 expression is not restricted to stem cells, and both CD133+ and CD133– metastatic colon cancer cells initiate tumors. *J Clin Invest* **118**: 2111–20.

Shtutman M, Zhurinsky J, Simcha I, Albanese C, D'Amico M, Pestell R et al. (1999). The cyclin D1 gene is a target of the beta-catenin/LEF-1 pathway. *Proc Natl Acad Sci USA* **96**: 5522–27.

Singh M, Spoelstra NS, Jean A, Howe E, Torkko KC, Clark HR et al. (2008). ZEB1 expression in type I vs type II endometrial cancers: a marker of aggressive disease. *Mod Pathol* **21**: 912–23.

Sordat I, Rousselle P, Chaubert P, Petermann O, Aberdam D, Bosman FT et al. (2000). Tumor cell budding and laminin-5 expression in colorectal carcinoma can be modulated by the tissue micro-environment. *Int J Cancer* **88**: 708–17.

Spaderna S, Schmalhofer O, Hlubek F, Berx G, Eger A, Merkel S et al. (2006). A transient, EMT-linked loss of basement membranes indicates metastasis and poor survival in colorectal cancer. *Gastroenterology* **131**: 830–40.

Spaderna S, Schmalhofer O, Wahlbuhl M, Dimmler A, Bauer K, Sultan A et al. (2008). The transcriptional repressor ZEB1 promotes metastasis and loss of cell polarity in cancer. *Cancer Res* **68**: 537–44.

Stemmer V, de Craene B, Berx G, Behrens J (2008). Snail promotes Wnt target gene expression and interacts with beta-catenin. *Oncogene* **27**: 5075–80.

Stemmler MP (2008). Cadherins in development and cancer. *Mol Biosyst* **4**: 835–50.

Stetler-Stevenson WG, Aznavoorian S, Liotta LA (1993). Tumor cell interactions with the extracellular matrix during invasion and metastasis. *Annu Rev Cell Biol* **9**: 541–73.

Takahashi E, Funato N, Higashihori N, Hata Y, Gridley T, Nakamura M (2004). Snail regulates p21(WAF/CIP1) expression in cooperation with E2A and Twist. *Biochem Biophys Res Commun* **325**: 1136–44.

Takemaru KI, Moon RT (2000). The transcriptional coactivator CBP interacts with beta-catenin to activate gene expression. *J Cell Biol* **149**: 249–54.

Taketo MM, Edelmann W (2009). Mouse models of colon cancer. *Gastroenterology* **136**: 780–98.

Tan C, Costello P, Sanghera J, Dominguez D, Baulida J, de Herreros AG et al. (2001). Inhibition of integrin linked kinase (ILK) suppresses beta-catenin-Lef/Tcf-dependent transcription and expression of the E-cadherin repressor, snail, in APC-/- human colon carcinoma cells. *Oncogene* **20**: 133–40.

Tanaka M, Hashiguchi Y, Ueno H, Hase K, Mochizuki H (2003). Tumor budding at the invasive margin can predict patients at high risk of recurrence after curative surgery for stage II, T3 colon cancer. *Dis Colon Rectum* **46**: 1054–59.

Tetsu O, McCormick F (1999). Beta-catenin regulates expression of cyclin D1 in colon carcinoma cells [In Process Citation]. *Nature* **398**: 422–26.

Thiery JP (2002). Epithelial-mesenchymal transitions in tumour progression. *Nat Rev Cancer* **2**: 442–54.

Tsanou E, Peschos D, Batistatou A, Charalabopoulos A, Charalabopoulos K (2008). The E-cadherin adhesion molecule and colorectal cancer. A global literature approach. *Anticancer Res* **28**: 3815–26.

Tsujii M, Kawano S, DuBois RN (1997). Cyclooxygenase-2 expression in human colon cancer cells increases metastatic potential. *Proc Natl Acad Sci USA* **94**: 3336–40.

Ueno H, Mochizuki H, Shinto E, Hashiguchi Y, Hase K, Talbot IC (2002a). Histologic indices in biopsy specimens for estimating the probability of extended local spread in patients with rectal carcinoma. *Cancer* **94**: 2882–91.

Ueno H, Murphy J, Jass JR, Mochizuki H, Talbot IC (2002b). Tumour 'budding' as an index to estimate the potential of aggressiveness in rectal cancer. *Histopathology* **40**: 127–32.

Ueno H, Price AB, Wilkinson KH, Jass JR, Mochizuki H, Talbot IC (2004). A new prognostic staging system for rectal cancer. *Ann Surg* **240**: 832–39.

Valdes-Mora F, Gomez del Pulgar T, Bandres E, Cejas P, Ramirez de Molina A, Perez-Palacios R et al. (2009). TWIST1 overexpression is associated with nodal invasion and male sex in primary colorectal cancer. *Ann Surg Oncol* **16**: 78–87.

van de Wetering M, Sancho E, Verweij C, de Lau W, Oving I, Hurlstone A et al. (2002). The beta-catenin/TCF-4 complex imposes a crypt progenitor phenotype on colorectal cancer cells. *Cell* **111**: 241–50.

Van der Flier LG, Sabates-Bellver J, Oving I, Haegebarth A, De Palo M, Anti M et al. (2007). The Intestinal Wnt/TCF Signature. *Gastroenterology* **132**: 628–32.

Verbeek BS, Adriaansen-Slot SS, Vroom TM, Beckers T, Rijksen G (1998). Overexpression of EGFR and c-erbB2 causes enhanced cell migration in human breast cancer cells and NIH3T3 fibroblasts. *FEBS Lett* **425**: 145–50.

Wang F, Sloss C, Zhang X, Lee SW, Cusack JC (2007). Membrane-bound heparin-binding epidermal growth factor like growth factor regulates E-cadherin expression in pancreatic carcinoma cells. *Cancer Res* **67**: 8486–93.

Wassermann S, Scheel SK, Hiendlmeyer E, Palmqvist R, Horst D, Hlubek F et al. (2009). p16INK4a is a beta-catenin target gene and indicates low survival in human colorectal tumors. *Gastroenterology* **136**: 196–205.e2.

Wheeler JM, Kim HC, Efstathiou JA, Ilyas M, Mortensen NJ, Bodmer WF (2001). Hypermethylation of the promoter region of the E-cadherin gene (CDH1) in sporadic and ulcerative colitis associated colorectal cancer. *Gut* **48**: 367–71.

Wielenga VJ, Smits R, Korinek V, Smit L, Kielman M, Fodde R et al. (1999). Expression of CD44 in Apc and Tcf mutant mice implies regulation by the WNT pathway. *Am J Pathol* **154**: 515–23.

Wielenga VJ, van der Voort R, Taher TE, Smit L, Beuling EA, van Krimpen C et al. (2000). Expression of c-Met and heparan-sulfate proteoglycan forms of CD44 in colorectal cancer. *Am J Pathol* **157**: 1563–73.

Wodarz A, Nathke I (2007). Cell polarity in development and cancer. *Nat Cell Biol* **9**: 1016–24.

Woodhouse E, Hersperger E, Shearn A (1998). Growth, metastasis, and invasiveness of Drosophila tumors caused by mutations in specific tumor suppressor genes. *Dev Genes Evol* **207**: 542–50.

Yamada T, Mori Y, Hayashi R, Takada M, Ino Y, Naishiro Y et al. (2003). Suppression of intestinal polyposis in Mdr1-deficient ApcMin/+ mice. *Cancer Res* **63**: 895–901.

Yamada T, Takaoka AS, Naishiro Y, Hayashi R, Maruyama K, Maesawa C et al. (2000). Transactivation of the multidrug resistance 1 gene by T-cell factor 4/beta-catenin complex in early colorectal carcinogenesis. *Cancer Res* **60**: 4761–66.

Yang AD, Camp ER, Fan F, Shen L, Gray MJ, Liu W et al. (2006). Vascular endothelial growth factor receptor-1 activation mediates epithelial to mesenchymal transition in human pancreatic carcinoma cells. *Cancer Res* **66**: 46–51.

Yang J, Mani SA, Donaher JL, Ramaswamy S, Itzykson RA, Come C et al. (2004). Twist, a master regulator of morphogenesis, plays an essential role in tumor metastasis. *Cell* **117**: 927–39.

Yang L, Amann JM, Kikuchi T, Porta R, Guix M, Gonzalez A et al. (2007). Inhibition of epidermal growth factor receptor signaling elevates 15-hydroxyprostaglandin dehydrogenase in non-small-cell lung cancer. *Cancer Res* **67**: 5587–93.

Yang MH, Wu MZ, Chiou SH, Chen PM, Chang SY, Liu CJ et al. (2008). Direct regulation of TWIST by HIF-1alpha promotes metastasis. *Nat Cell Biol* **10**: 295–305.

Yook JI, Li XY, Ota I, Hu C, Kim HS, Kim NH et al. (2006). A Wnt-Axin2-GSK3beta cascade regulates Snail1 activity in breast cancer cells. *Nat Cell Biol* **8**: 1398–406.

Zhang B, Ougolkov A, Yamashita K, Takahashi Y, Mai M, Minamoto T (2003). beta-Catenin and ras oncogenes detect most human colorectal cancer. *Clin Cancer Res* **9**: 3073–79.

Zhang T, Otevrel T, Gao Z, Ehrlich SM, Fields JZ, Boman BM (2001). Evidence that APC regulates survivin expression: a possible mechanism contributing to the stem cell origin of colon cancer. *Cancer Res* **61**: 8664–67.

Zhang X, Ge YL, Tian RH (2009). The knockdown of c-myc expression by RNAi inhibits cell proliferation in human colon cancer HT-29 cells in vitro and in vivo. *Cell Mol Biol Lett* **14**: 305–18.

Zlobec I, Lugli A (2008). Prognostic and predictive factors in colorectal cancer. *J Clin Pathol* **61**: 561–9.

Chapter 7

CELL ADHESION MOLECULES IN COLON CANCER METASTASIS

Azadeh Arabzadeh[1] and Nicole Beauchemin[2]

[1]*Rosalind and Morris Goodman Cancer Research Centre, McGill University, Montreal, QC H3G 1Y6, Canada*
[2]*Rosalind and Morris Goodman Cancer Research Centre, McGill University, 3655 Promenade Sir-William-Osler, Lab 708, Montreal, QC, Canada, H3G 1Y6, e-mail: nicole.beauchemin@mcgill.ca*

Abstract: Cell adhesion molecules play a pivotal role in the progression and metastatic spread of epithelial malignancies including colorectal cancer. In addition to cancer cells, multiple cell populations such as endothelial, epithelial and hematopoietic cells express adhesion molecules. The expression of these molecules usually varies among primary and metastatic sites; their down-regulation contributes to tumour cell detachment from the primary site but their re-expression assists tumour cell attachment to the foreign tissue, thereby favouring colonization in the target organ. In the case of colorectal cancer cells, down-regulation of E-cadherin and the standard form of CD44 facilitates tumour cell detachment from the primary carcinoma, while the enhanced expression of various integrin subunits, selectins, CD44 variant isoforms as well as members of the immunoglobulin superfamily support tumour-host attachment, resulting in the metastatic spread of colon tumour cells to the liver. In this chapter, we present some of the best studied cell adhesion molecules in the context of colorectal cancer, and describe the dynamic nature of tumour-host interactions that heavily rely on the expression of such adhesion molecules and their ligands.

Key words: Cell adhesion molecules · Colorectal carcinoma · Metastasis · Colonization · Tumour-host interactions

7.1 Introduction

Adherent cells are characterized by a repertoire of specific cell surface receptors that enable them to interact with other cells as well as with the extracellular matrix (ECM). These adhesion receptors not only ensure the proper organization of cells in a given tissue but also actively mediate the passage of information between cells as well as between a cell and its surrounding environment.

Changes in expression and/or function of cell adhesion molecules are required for the ability of cancer cells to invade the extracellular milieu and to metastasize. In fact, a malignant cell phenotype involves several alterations in cell adhesion receptors; some that support the normal phenotype may decrease in expression while those needed for tumour invasion and metastasis can be induced (Aznavoorian et al., 1993).

Different classes of specific cell adhesion receptors responsible for cell-matrix and cell-cell interactions have been characterized (Streit et al., 1996). Some of the most studied ones include the family of integrin receptors, members of the immunoglobulin (Ig) superfamily, cadherins, cluster of differentiation 44 (CD44) receptor and its variant isoforms and selectins (lec-CAMs). The role of these molecules in growth, invasion and metastasis of gastrointestinal tumours represents an ongoing investigation. In this chapter, we have focused on the role of such adhesion proteins in malignant transformation and metastatic dissemination of colorectal carcinomas (CRC).

7.2 Integrins

Integrins are transmembrane glycoprotein receptors consisting of non-covalently associated α- and β subunits (Buck et al., 1986; Hynes, 1992). Each subunit is composed of a large extracellular domain of several hundred amino acids, a single transmembrane domain and a short cytoplasmic domain of 20–70 amino acids (Hynes, 2002). Eight β subunits can associate with 18 α subunits to form a number of distinct integrin heterodimers. Integrin heterodimers are subdivided into at least three subfamilies: $\alpha\beta1$ or VLA (very late antigen) family, $\alpha\beta2$ or LEU-CAM (leukocyte cell adhesion molecule) family, and $\alpha\beta3$ or cytoadhesion proteins (Hynes, 1987). The VLA subfamily comprises at least six related complexes, with most of them being promiscuous receptors binding to various matrix proteins including fibronectin ($\alpha3\beta1$, $\alpha4\beta1$ and $\alpha5\beta1$), laminin ($\alpha1\beta1$, $\alpha2\beta1$, $\alpha3\beta1$ and $\alpha6\beta1$) and collagen types I and IV ($\alpha1\beta1$, $\alpha2\beta1$ and $\alpha3\beta1$) (Hynes, 1987; Stallmach et al., 1992). The LEU-CAM subfamily (also termed CD18 antigens) consists of three leukocyte adhesion receptors including $\alpha L\beta2$, $\alpha M\beta2$ and $\alpha X\beta2$ (Albelda and Buck, 1990). The $\beta3$ integrin subfamily consists of two members: the vitronectin receptor ($\alpha v\beta3$) and the platelet glycoprotein IIb/IIIA complex ($\alpha IIb\beta3$) (Albelda and Buck, 1990; Stallmach et al., 1992). Other members of the integrin family include $\alpha6\beta4$ (laminin receptor), $\alpha4\beta7$ (fibronectin receptor) as well as members of the αv subfamily of integrins ($\alpha v\beta1$, $\alpha v\beta3$, $\alpha v\beta5$, $\alpha v\beta6$ and $\alpha v\beta8$). With respect to their tissue distribution, integrin heterodimers are expressed on epithelial cells, endothelial cells, leukocytes, platelets and many other normal and tumour cells. They mediate both cell-cell and cell-matrix interactions, thereby contributing to intercellular communication as well as cell response to its microenvironment. Among multiple cell functions that regulate the initiation and progression of malignancies, the interaction of tumour cells with their surrounding matrix plays a crucial role in the complex process of tumour invasion and metastasis formation. In fact, the ability of tumour cells for local and distant tissue invasion depends on the interaction of the cell surface integrins with their ligands in the surrounding ECM (Heino, 1993; Hynes, 1992; Ruoslahti, 1992; Streit et al., 1996). In the context of colorectal cancer, increasing evidence has indicated that the integrin expression is deregulated following malignant transformation of the colonic epithelium; therefore their expression tends to vary among normal colon, primary tumours and metastatic foci (Koretz et al., 1991; Pignatelli et al., 1990; Stallmach et al., 1992). In the following section, we synthesize the expression data of individual integrin chains during the transformation of normal colon mucosa through adenomas and invasive colorectal carcinomas and their liver metastases. These data also indicate the impact of alterations in integrin expression on the adoption of invasive and metastatic phenotype by colon tumour cells.

7.2.1 Integrin α-Subunits of VLA Subfamily; α2, α3, α5 and α6 Chains

Normal colonic epithelial cells uniformly and strongly express α3, α5 and α6 chains (Stallmach et al., 1992). The α2 subunit however, is only expressed on epithelial cells lining the base of the colonic crypts and is absent from the cells lining the apical part of the crypts or the surface epithelium (Koretz et al., 1991; Stallmach et al., 1992).

In colorectal adenomas, although the expression levels of the α2 and α6 chains are similar to that of normal mucosa, the α3 and α5 subunits show a somewhat reduced expression (Koretz et al., 1991; Stallmach et al., 1992). However, transformation from adenomas to colorectal carcinomas was characterized by significant loss of expression of all four α integrin chains (Stallmach et al., 1992) (Table 7.1). In particular, diminished expression of the α6-subunit (one of the known laminin receptors) exhibited a significant correlation with the transformation of adenomas into invasive carcinomas. In fact, all well-differentiated adenocarcinomas expressed the α6 integrin chain modestly, whereas in the majority of moderately- or poorly-differentiated carcinomas, there was no detectable expression of the α6 chain (Stallmach et al., 1992) (Table 7.1 and Fig. 7.1). These data indicate a sequence of changes in the expression of integrin α chains during malignant transformation of the colonic epithelium: (1) the transformation of normal mucosa into adenomas was first characterized by reduced expression of α3 and α5 chains (but not α2 and α6); (2) progression of colonic tumours from adenomas to carcinomas was accompanied by a diminished expression of α2 and α6 chains as well as nearly absent expression of α3 and α5 subunits. These results suggest that reduced expression of at least some α chain integrins may allow colon cancer cells to detach from the basement membrane thereby infiltrating the underlying mesenchyme. This may be

Table 7.1 Alterations in the expression of adhesion molecules during progression of colorectal adenocarcinoma

Adhesion receptors		Normal colon mucosa	Adenoma	Colorectal carcinoma Well-differentiated (grade 1)	Moderately-differentiated (grade 2)	Poorly-differentiated (grade 3)	Liver metastases
Integrins	α2	+ +	+ +	+	+/–	+/–	TD
	α3	+ +	+	+/–	–	–	TD
	α5	+ +	+	+/–	–	–	TD
	α6	+ +	+ +	+	+/–	+/–	TD
	αv	–	–	+	+	+ +	+ + +
	β1	+ +	+ +	+ +	+/–	+/–	TD
	β4[1]	+ +	+ +	+ +	+/–	+/–	TD
	β6	–	–	+	+ +	+ + +	+ + +
E-cadherin		+ +	+ +	+	+/–	+/–	+ + +
CD44 and variant isoforms	CD44s	+ +	+ +	+	+/–	+/–	TD
	CD44v5	–	+	+	+ +	+ + +	TD
	CD44 v6	–	+/–	+	+	+ + +	TD
	CD44v8	+/–	+	+	+ +	+ + +	TD
	CD44v9	+/–	+	+	+ +	+ + +	TD
	CD44v10	+/–	+	+	+ +	+ + +	TD
Immunoglobulin superfamily	ICAM-1	–	+/–	+ +	+	+	+/–
	CEA	–	+	+ +	+ + +	+ + + +	+ + + +

+ + Normal/relatively strong expression
+ Modest to weak expression
+/– Significant loss of expression/very low expression
– No detectable expression
+ + + Enhanced expression
+ + + + Further enhanced expression
TD To be determined
[1] Contrary results showed overexpression of this integrin subunit in well-differentiated and moderately-differentiated carcinomas while it was down-regulated only in poorly-differentiated tumors

a general phenomenon for cancer cells attaining a malignant phenotype and perhaps metastatic potential.

7.2.2 αv Integrin Subfamily

There are five members of the αv integrin subfamily (αvβ1, αvβ3, αvβ5, αvβ6 and αvβ8) that recognize RGD (arginine-glycine-aspartic acid) peptide sequences found in many ECM proteins. Amongst them, association of αv with β6 constitutes a fibronectin receptor generally not expressed on normal colonic epithelial cells, but highly expressed during tumorigenesis (Agrez et al., 1994; Agrez et al., 1996; Breuss et al., 1995) (Table 7.1 and Fig. 7.1). Immunohistochemical studies

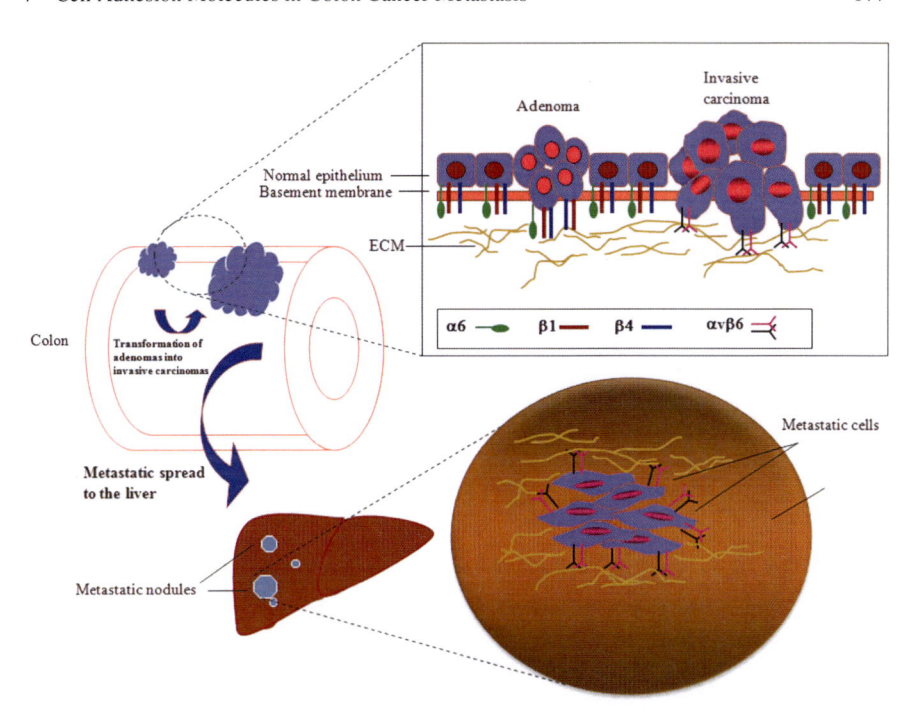

Fig. 7.1 Differential expression of integrin chains during malignant transformation of colon epithelial cells. During transition from adenomas into invasive carcinomas, some integrin subunits (e.g. α6, β1 and β4) sustain decreased expression, thereby contributing to tumor cell detachment from the primary carcinomas. Others that are not normally expressed in the colonic cells (e.g. αv and β6) gain in expression that in turn facilitates the metastatic spread of colon tumor cells to the liver

determined that αv positivity was higher in liver metastatic tissue than that in primary colon tumours (Yang et al., 2008). In addition, the results of a 3-year follow-up study of colorectal cancer patients by Yang et al. showed that patients who were αv-positive had higher liver metastasis rates than the αv-negative group. Interestingly, they further demonstrated that αv integrin expression results in secretion of matrix metalloproteinase-9 (MMP-9), the enhancement of migration on fibronectin and the survival of cancer cells in the liver, thereby contributing to the promotion of metastatic potential and survival of colon cancer cells (Yang et al., 2008). In another recent study, analysing resected liver metastases derived from primary colorectal tumours revealed that metastatic colorectal tumour subpopulations express elevated levels of αvβ3 and αvβ5 integrins (Conti et al., 2008). Indeed, both αvβ3 and αvβ5 integrins were strongly expressed within the poorly differentiated areas of metastases (areas of abundant collagen I) as compared to their low levels of expression in well-differentiated areas (areas of less dense collagen I). Further studies by Conti et al. demonstrated that protease-mediated degradation of collagen I exposes cryptic αv-binding epitopes (perhaps RGD peptide sequences) that mediate collagen I growth-promoting effects on colorectal cancer cells. Along this line, both inhibition of collagen I breakdown and antibody-directed blockade of αvβ3 and αvβ5 significantly reduced colorectal carcinoma cell proliferation and survival, particularly in cell lines with the highest metastatic potential that have also higher levels of αv integrins (Conti et al., 2008). Such in vitro findings correlated with the in vivo data showing the differential pattern of αv integrin expression within resected hepatic colorectal carcinoma metastases, thereby suggesting adhesion and signalling functions for αv integrin in regulating metastatic tumour cell growth and survival. Based on these data, it is tempting to speculate that therapeutic use of anti-integrin antibodies and/or inhibitory peptides may prove beneficial for treatment of established metastatic tumours in patients with advanced colorectal adenocarcinomas.

7.2.3 Integrin β-Subunits; β1, β4 and β6 Chains

Immunofluorescence analyses of β1 and β4 integrin chains showed strong staining in the normal colonic mucosa epithelium (Stallmach et al., 1994), whereas the β6 subunit is not expressed in normal colon (Yang et al., 2008).

In patients with colorectal adenocarcinomas, a progressive loss of the $β_1$ and β4 integrin subunits has been associated with a loss of tumour differentiation, where adenomas and well-differentiated carcinomas maintained expression of these subunits in contrast with moderately- to poorly-differentiated carcinomas that exhibited diminished or lost expression of these integrin subunits (Pignatelli et al., 1990; Stallmach et al., 1992) (Table 7.1 and Fig. 7.1). Nevertheless, the β4 (but not β1) chain expression in colon carcinomas appears to be controversial. Although being initially reported as decreased in well- to poorly-differentiated stages (Stallmach et al., 1992), the results of a more recent study demonstrated significant overexpression of this integrin chain in well-differentiated (WD) and moderately-differentiated (MD) carcinomas as compared to their corresponding normal mucosa (Ni et al., 2005). However, β4 expression was down-regulated only in poorly-differentiated primary tumours (Ni et al., 2005). Interestingly, increased levels of the β4 integrin in WD and MD tumours correlated with those of the oncogene c-MYC and such correlation was of causal nature, since c-MYC was able to stimulate integrin β4 promoter activity (Ni et al., 2005). This finding that up-regulation of c-MYC in the context of colon carcinoma cells leads to an increased transcriptional activity of the β4 integrin promoter, suggests that the β4 chain acts as another downstream target gene for c-MYC. Whether other integrin chains may also be targets of this oncogene remains to be elucidated.

Among other β integrin subunits, β6 has an important role in the progression of colon cancer cells and even serves as a novel prognostic indicator for aggressive colon carcinoma in humans (Bates et al., 2005). Expression of the β6 subunit during malignant transformation of colonic epithelium closely resembles that of its partner αv as described above, and correlates with an increase in the potential of colon cancer cells to colonize and metastasize to the liver (Yang et al., 2008) (Table 7.1

and Fig. 7.1). Along this line, Bates et al. investigated the molecular mechanism driving elevated expression of integrin β6 that in turn affects the tumorigenic properties of colon carcinoma cells (Bates et al., 2005). These investigators used an in vitro model of epithelial-mesenchymal transition (EMT) in colon carcinoma cells and demonstrated that following induction of EMT, surface expression of β6 increased dramatically with a consequent induction of the αvβ6 complex. This integrin consequently promoted the activation of autocrine TGF-β (a central mediator of the EMT process) and migration on fibronectin, thereby conferring an invasive characteristic to the cells (Bates et al., 2005). In addition, analysis of β6 expression in colorectal carcinoma samples revealed high expression of the β6 chain in poorly-differentiated infiltrating tumours as well as in liver metastases, supporting the notion that upregulation of the β6 in colorectal cancer correlates with disease progression and poorer clinical outcome (Bates et al., 2005). Given that elevated expression of this integrin is predictive of disease outcome, the β6 subunit can be an attractive therapeutic candidate for treatment of colon cancer, where its blockade may be used for early intervention and treatment. Whether the current anti-β6 antibodies (Weinreb et al., 2004) offer a promising future for the treatment of aggressive colorectal cancer still remains to be determined.

7.3 E-Cadherin

E-cadherin (epithelial-cadherin) is a transmembrane glycoprotein that functions as a calcium-dependent cell-cell adhesion receptor and plays a crucial role in maintaining the structural integrity of epithelial sheets (Kalluri and Neilson, 2003). Structurally, E-cadherin consists of an extracellular domain, a transmembrane segment and a cytoplasmic domain. The extracellular region constitutes the adhesion domain of the molecule and is composed of five repeated units of approximately 110 amino acids, with the adhesive interface located within the most amino-terminal repeat. Structural data have suggested that adhesion results from homophilic binding between extracellular domains of E-cadherin dimers on the surface of neighbouring cells that creates a zipper-like structure (Chausovsky et al., 2000; Nagar et al., 1996; Shapiro et al., 1995). The E-cadherin adhesive activity is also regulated by cytoplasmic signalling events, via its highly conserved cytoplasmic domain interacting with the catenins that connect it to the actin cytoskeleton. In fact, the carboxy-terminal part of the cytoplasmic domain directly associates with β-catenin or plakoglobin (also called γ-catenin) whereas the juxtamembrane part binds to p120 catenin (Ozawa et al., 1990; Yap et al., 1998). Both β-catenin and γ-catenin bind to the vinculin-related protein α-catenin via their amino-terminal domains. α-catenin in turn connects with actin filaments (Herrenknecht et al., 1991; Watabe-Uchida et al., 1998; Weiss et al., 1998) (Fig. 7.2).

Changes in intercellular adhesion are among the most prominent features of malignant cells, and therefore E-cadherin has long been known as the major target of such alterations in tumour cells of epithelial origin (Behrens et al., 1989; Behrens et al., 1993; Chen and Obrink, 1991; Frixen et al., 1991). Indeed, decreased

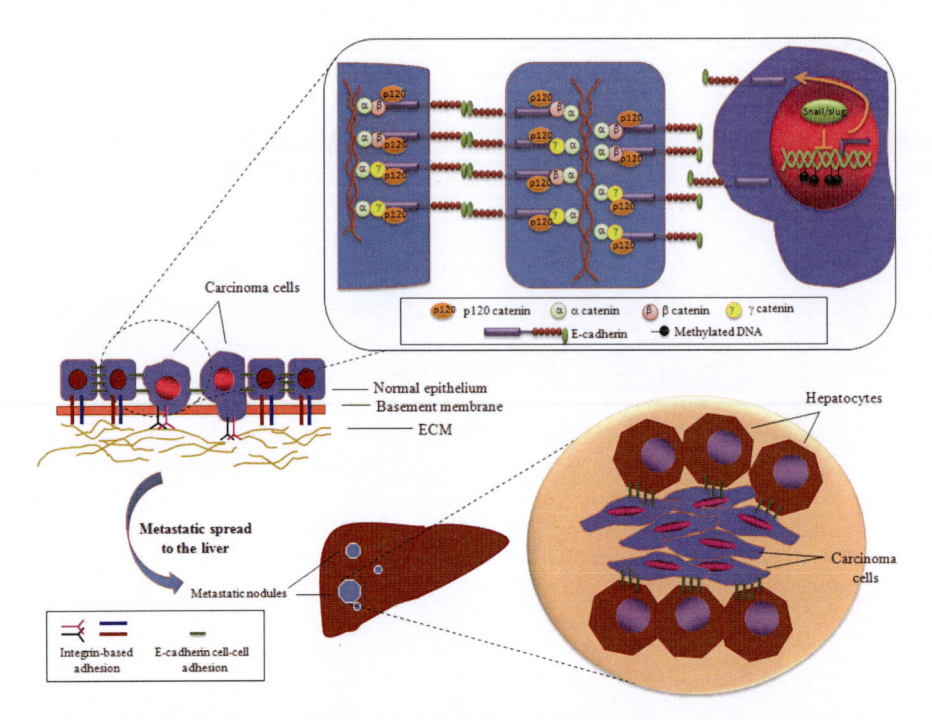

Fig. 7.2 Down-regulation E-cadherin is one of the most prominent features of colon carcinoma cells. This occurs as the result of several mechanisms such as transcriptional repression by Snail/Slug transcription factors and/or E-cadherin promoter hypermethylation. Loss of E-cadherin-based cell adhesion along with enhanced integrin-based adhesion is associated with tumor cell invasion and metastasis to the liver. However, following the initial seeding in the liver, E-cadherin gain of expression in colon tumor cells is required for their hepatic colonization and establishment of secondary tumours

expression or loss of membrane localization of E-cadherin has been recognized in breast, esophageal, gastric, colon, pancreatic and other carcinomas (Hajra et al., 2002; Ikeguchi et al., 2001; Krishnadath et al., 1997; Oda et al., 1994; Pignatelli et al., 1994; Tamura et al., 1996). Such loss of E-cadherin in epithelial malignancies is associated with invasion, tumour metastasis and an unfavourable prognosis (Behrens et al., 1989; Behrens et al., 1993; Brabletz et al., 2001; Ikeguchi et al., 2000; Kanazawa et al., 2002a, b; Kimura et al., 2000a, b; Vleminckx et al., 1991).

In colorectal carcinoma, significant down-regulation of E-cadherin has been observed in moderately- to poorly-differentiated primary tumours (Frixen et al., 1991; Kinsella et al., 1993) (Table 7.1). Recently, immunohistochemistry analysis of E-cadherin expression in a tissue microarray of 577 colon tumours with 10 years of clinical follow-up revealed that around 34% of samples exhibited cytoplasmic immunolocalization of E-cadherin and 23% showed complete absence of E-cadherin immunostaining, whereas normal membranous localization of E-cadherin was present in only 38% of samples (Bellovin et al., 2005). Notably, the 10-year survival rates were significantly less for those patients with aberrant or absent expression of E-cadherin in tumours (Bellovin et al., 2005). In another study, immunohistochemical localization of E-cadherin at the site of deepest tumour invasion in specimens of advanced colorectal carcinomas revealed that patients with reduced E-cadherin expression showed a significantly poorer prognosis (Kimura et al., 2000b). E-cadherin reduced expression was also frequently associated with a high Ki-67 labelling index, mucin-positivity, higher microvessel density in tumour lesions as well as lymph node metastases (Kimura et al., 2000b).

Although loss of E-cadherin is associated with loss of differentiation, and with invasion and metastasis of colon primary tumours, and is therefore a prognostic factor in patients with colorectal carcinoma (Ghadimi et al., 1999; Gofuku et al., 1999), the pattern of E-cadherin expression in metastatic foci seems to deviate from that observed in primary tumours. Comparison of expression levels of E-cadherin in primary colon tumours with those in metastatic tumours revealed increased levels of expression in both metastatic lymph nodes and metastatic liver tumours, whereas primary ones exhibited reduced expression of the E-cadherin-β-catenin complex (Ikeguchi et al., 2001) (Table 7.1 and Fig. 7.2). Interestingly, although reduced expression of the E-cadherin-β-catenin complex in primary carcinomas correlated with higher incidence of lymph node metastasis, patients who had metastatic tumours that expressed E-cadherin more strongly than primary tumours showed unfavourable prognosis and shorter survival (Ikeguchi et al., 2001). Increased expression levels of adhesion molecules including E-cadherin in metastatic foci have also been noticed in other tumour types such as gastric and breast cancer (Bukholm et al., 2000; Mayer et al., 1993). Based on these data, it has been suggested that cancer cells transiently lose E-cadherin expression in metastasis, and then re-express this molecule at a distant metastatic site in order to adhere in that remote organ.

Several mechanisms are operative for down-regulation of E-cadherin in colorectal primary tumours (Fig. 7.2), including gene mutations (Efstathiou et al., 1999), promoter hypermethylation (Wheeler et al., 2001) as well as transcriptional repression by Snail and Slug transcription factors (Roy et al., 2005; Shioiri et al., 2006) (for more details, refer to Chapter 6 by O. Schmalhofer et al., in this book). The last one is the predominant mechanism responsible for E-cadherin silencing and in a recent publication, wild-type p53 (a known tumour suppressor) was shown to suppress E-cadherin down-regulation and cancer invasion by inducing Slug degradation (Wang et al., 2009). Moreover, Src-induced de-regulation of E-cadherin in colorectal cancer cells was shown to require signalling through integrins αv and β1 (Avizienyte et al., 2002), demonstrating interdependence between integrin-induced signals and E-cadherin-associated adhesion changes at cell-cell contacts, thereby facilitating cancer cell migration and metastatic dissemination.

Taken together, alterations of E-cadherin expression demonstrate profound effects on the invasive and metastatic potential of colorectal cancer cells. Such effects are believed to occur through disruption of cell-cell junctions thereby facilitating the epithelial-mesenchymal transition, a process required for adoption of invasive characteristics (Thiery, 2003) (for more details, refer to Chapter 6 in this book). The hope of identifying new treatments that will improve the survival of colon cancer patients lies in a better understanding of the effector signalling pathways downstream of E-cadherin that contribute to metastasis.

7.4 CD44 and Its Variant Isoforms

CD44 was originally discovered as a leukocyte antigen in 1982 (Trowbridge et al., 1982) and later on, it was assigned several functions including lymphocyte activation and homing, hematopoiesis, cell migration and tumour metastasis (Lesley et al., 1993). CD44 is a cell surface glycoprotein with an N-terminal region that is structurally related to several hyaluronate binding proteins (Underhill, 1992). This protein is widely expressed and serves as an adhesion molecule in cell-cell and cell-extracellular matrix interactions (Lesley et al., 1993). Some of the known ligands for CD44 include hyaluronate, collagen (type I, IV and VI) and fibronectin which constitute major ECM components (Jalkanen and Jalkanen, 1992; Underhill, 1992). Notably, a recent study identified the sialofucosylated CD44 variant isoforms as the major functional P-selectin ligands on colon carcinoma cells (Napier et al., 2007; Thomas et al., 2008), suggesting its role in the selectin-mediated adhesion, a process that will be discussed later. CD44 has a standard form (CD44s) and several variant isoforms (CD44v) generated by alternative splicing of ten exons (Gunthert, 1993; Mackay et al., 1994). Several splice variants of CD44 are expressed on the surface of rat mammary and pancreatic carcinoma cell lines, where their expression correlates with the metastatic potential of these cells (Gunthert et al., 1991; Rudy et al., 1993). In fact, CD44 encoded by variant exon 6 (CD44v6) confers metastatic potential to non-metastasizing pancreatic carcinoma cells in rats (Gunthert et al., 1991; Rudy et al., 1993). In addition, a monoclonal antibody against rat CD44v6 inhibited invasion of these carcinoma cells into the lung and regional lymph nodes (Matzku et al., 1989).

Expression of CD44v isoforms in human tissues is also associated with tumour progression and more particularly with the metastatic potential of some carcinomas (Zoller, 1995). For example, analysis of human breast and colon carcinomas showed a significant up-regulation of CD44v6 or CD44v8–v10 while normal tissues only express the standard form of CD44 (Heider et al., 1993; Matsumura and Tarin, 1992; Sneath and Mangham, 1998; Tanabe et al., 1993).

In the context of colon mucosa, CD44s is broadly expressed in epithelial cells and its expression is associated with proliferation of both normal and neoplastic human colorectal epithelial cells (Abbasi et al., 1993; Mackay et al., 1994). Other than weak expression of CD44v8–v10 in only a few cells at the base of the colonic crypts, none of the other CD44 splice variants are expressed in the normal colorectal mucosa (Terpe et al., 1994; Wielenga et al., 1993) (Table 7.1). However, samples from various stages of colorectal carcinogenesis exhibited changes in the expression of CD44 variant proteins (Heider et al., 1993; Wielenga et al., 1993). Elevated levels of CD44v5 were observed at the very early stage of colorectal tumour progression (i.e. early adenomas) with further increase towards more advanced stages (Wielenga et al., 1993) (Table 7.1). Similarly, expression of epitopes encoded by exons v8–v10 was increased at the adenoma stage and underwent further enhancement upon tumour progression (Wielenga et al., 1993) (Table 7.1). Interestingly, the expression of variants carrying exon v6 sequences (CD44v6) was largely restricted to the advanced stages of colon tumour development (Table 7.1). Indeed, early (9%) and advanced (45%) polyps as well as invasive carcinomas (68%) were variably positive for the CD44v6 isoform (Wielenga et al., 1993). In addition, patients with CD44v6-positive carcinomas showed poorer prognosis than those with negative tumours (Herrlich et al., 1995), suggesting that tumours carrying this CD44 isoform may acquire a selective advantage during tumour progression and metastasis formation. As another studied variant of CD44 in colorectal cancer progression, CD44v8–10 (an isoform containing exons 8–10) was also introduced as an independent prognostic factor for colorectal carcinoma patients. In fact, Yamaguchi et al. found a significant correlation between the incidence of both lymph node and hematogenous metastasis with CD44v8–10 immunoreactivity (Yamaguchi et al., 1996). Moreover, patients with CD44v8–10-positive tumours exhibited shorter survival than those with CD44v8–10-negative tumours, and CD44v8–10 expression also correlated with a high recurrence rate in those patients who underwent curative resection (Yamaguchi et al., 1996). These results suggest that CD44v8–10 also plays an important role in metastasis of colorectal cancer and may be of prognostic value in this disease.

Overall, it appears from these observations that expression of the CD44v isoforms can be exploited for diagnosis purposes. For example, since exon v5-encoded epitopes appear early in colorectal carcinogenesis (i.e. most polyps carry the epitope), these could represent early indicators of colorectal epithelium transformation. On the other hand, the occurrence of epitopes encoded by exon v6 would indicate the presence of more aggressive tumours as well as a possibility of metastasis development in patients. In addition to the overexpression of several CD44 splice variants in colonic tumours, CD44s expression may also be associated with transformation of the colon mucosa to carcinoma. Along this line, Takahashi et al. (1995) found that CD44s expression is down-regulated in colon carcinomas compared to that in normal mucosa. Intriguingly, re-expression of CD44s in the carcinoma cells reduced both in vitro and in vivo growth rate and tumorigenicity of the cancer cells. Such growth reduction was directly correlated with enhanced hyaluronate binding of colon carcinoma cells (Takahashi et al., 1995). Moreover, the authors reported that the hyaluronate binding ability was less pronounced in highly metastatic cell lines compared to poorly metastatic ones. These observations imply that CD44s down-regulation is associated with colonic mucosa transformation and might be just as important as up-regulation of CD44v isoforms in the diagnosis of colonic tumours.

7.5 Selectins

In the last decades, dissecting the metastatic cascade (Ahmad and Hart, 1997; Fidler, 2003; Pantel and Brakenhoff, 2004) has revealed a step-wise process that is initiated by detachment of cells from the primary tumour and their penetration into the extracellular matrix. A fraction of the invading cells are shed into lymphatics or into the systemic circulation (intravasation). The tumour cells in the blood often aggregate with platelets and leukocytes in order to form emboli that are arrested in the capillary bed of new organs. Trapped cancer cells interact with endothelial cells and migrate into the surrounding tissue (extravasation) where they will proliferate and form secondary neoplasm. While most cancer cells do not survive this series of events, a small number of them (~0.01%) succeed in passing through all these steps to form metastases (for more details, refer to Chapter 1 by N. Porquet et al., in this book). According to the scenario described above, interactions of cancer cells with components of their microenvironment determine whether cancer cells will progress towards metastasis or whether they will stay dormant. In this context, the selectin-selectin ligand-mediated interactions are particularly pivotal to intravasation, extravasation and emboli formation of tumour cells thereby playing a crucial role in tumour progression and metastasis.

Selectins form a family of adhesion proteins composed of three members: L-, P- and E-selectin (Sperandio, 2006; Varki, 1992; Vestweber, 1993b). L-selectin is constitutively expressed by leukocytes, whereas E-selectin is exclusively expressed by activated endothelial cells and P-selectin by activated platelets and endothelial cells (Zarbock et al., 2007). Structurally, selectins are membrane proteins whose extracellular portion contains an N-terminal C-type lectin domain, followed by an EGF-type domain and a series of short consensus repeats. Selectins are anchored into the membrane through a single transmembrane domain that is followed by a short cytoplasmic tail. Selectin ligands are cell surface glycoconjugates such as P-selectin glycoprotein ligand-1 (PSGL-1), E-selectin ligand-1 (ESL-1), CD24, sialyl-Lewis^a, sialyl-Lewis^x, CD34, mucosal addressin cell adhesion molecule-1 (MAdCAM-1), lysosome-associated membrane proteins (LAMP-1 and LAMP-2), sulfatides, hematopoietic cell E-/L-selectin ligand (HCELL) and CD44 variant isoforms (Brandley et al., 1990; Burdick et al., 2006; Hanley et al., 2005; Kansas, 1996; Lasky, 1994; Lowe, 2002; Napier et al., 2007; Swiedler, 1991; Tomlinson et al., 2000; Varki, 1992; Varki, 1994; Vestweber, 1993a, b, 1996; Witz, 2006a). These ligands are composed of a protein or a lipid core modified by glycosylation (Vestweber and Blanks, 1999). Selectin-selectin ligand interactions mediate tethering, rolling and adhesion of several types of cells. Accumulating evidence indicates that cancer cells, particularly those of epithelial origin, express high levels of selectin ligands whose interaction with the corresponding selectins is involved in their metastatic dissemination (Brodt et al., 1997; Witz, 2006b). Among these ligands, sialylated fucosylated glycans such as sialyl-Lewis^a and sialyl-Lewis^x are highly expressed by carcinoma cells and their expression correlates with poor prognosis due to tumour progression and metastatic dissemination (Dennis and Laferte, 1987; Hakomori, 1996). In the following section, we discuss the involvement of individual selectins in colorectal carcinoma progression and metastasis. Such involvement is reflected in at least two major events: (1) formation of circulating emboli that results from the interaction of tumour cells with platelets (via P-selectin) and/or leukocytes (via L-selectin); (2) extravasation that is caused by the interaction of tumour cells with endothelial cells (via E-selectin).

7.5.1 P-Selectin

A large body of evidence indicates that tumour metastasis is facilitated by blood platelets that form emboli resulting from the interactions of platelets with tumour cells and leukocytes (Gasic, 1984; Honn et al., 1992; Karpatkin and Pearlstein, 1981). Such emboli structures can more easily get arrested in the vasculature of distant organs in order to establish secondary tumours (i.e. metastasis). In addition, aggregation of platelets around tumour cells has been suggested to physically interfere with the access of leukocytes to tumour cells, thereby playing an immune protective effect (Borsig et al., 2001; Nieswandt et al., 1999). Absence of such surface shielding by platelet aggregates can no longer impede tumour cell lysis by Natural Killer cells, resulting in less colonization of target organs by metastasizing cells that eventually leads to a dramatic reduction in the number of metastatic foci (Nieswandt et al., 1999). Moreover, experimental reduction of blood platelets (thrombocytopenia) before tumour cell injection decreases tumour metastasis (Gasic, 1984). In essence, it is believed that expression of P-selectin on activated platelets serves as a mediator of pathological interactions between platelets and carcinoma cells, explaining to some degree the protective effect of platelets on circulating cancer cells thereby contributing to the promotion of metastasis (Fig. 7.3).

In the context of colon cancer metastasis, the importance of P-selectin-mediated interactions is deduced from the study of P-selectin-deficient mice by Kim et al. (1998). In this study, P-selectin-deficient mice generated fewer lung metastases upon intravenous injection of human colon carcinoma cells. Indeed, it was shown that P-selectin can recognize sialyl-Lewis$^{x/a}$-containing mucins on the surface of LS180 colon carcinoma cells and facilitate their initial seeding into the lungs, therefore promoting progression to the metastatic phenotype (Kim et al., 1998). More recently, P-selectin ligands of non-mucin origin were found on the surface of MC38 mouse colon carcinoma cells (Borsig et al., 2002; Garcia et al., 2007) and also facilitated experimental metastasis in a syngeneic mouse model (Garcia et al., 2007). Corresponding ligands were sulfoglycolipids and enzymatic removal of sulfation resulted in decreased P-selectin binding of MC38 cells and led to attenuation of their metastatic spread (Garcia et al., 2007). Whether non-mucin P-selectin ligands also contribute to the metastatic potential of human colon cancer cells has yet to be determined in future studies.

Without ruling out additional roles for other selectins in the metastatic cascade, P-selectin-mediated interactions potentially provide a mechanistic explanation for several other observations, including: the presence of platelet-rich thromboemboli in patients with mucin producing carcinomas (Gasic, 1984; Honn et al., 1992; Karpatkin and Pearlstein, 1981), correlation of mucin production with poor clinical prognosis (You et al., 2006) as well as the strong correlation of sialyl-Lewis$^{x/a}$ expression with tumour progression and metastatic spread in colorectal cancer patients (Hoff et al., 1989; Izumi et al., 1995; Matsushita et al., 1990; Nakamori et al., 1993; Nakayama et al., 1995).

Such cancer mucin-endogenous lectin interaction can bear clinical implications including intervention using anti-P-selectin therapeutics. In this regard, the

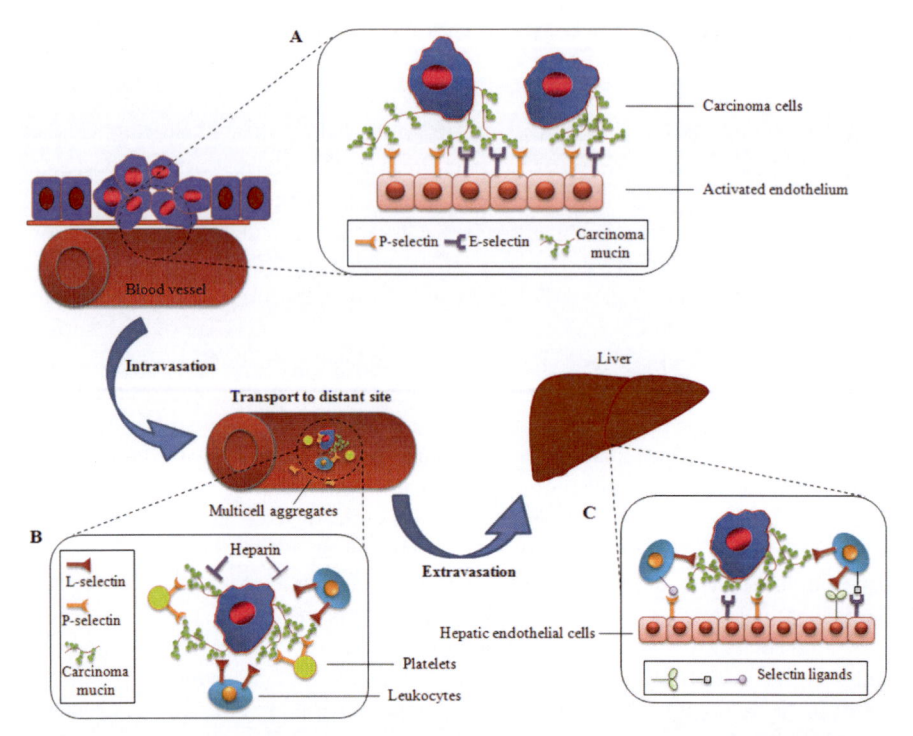

Fig. 7.3 Selectin-selectin ligand interactions are pivotal to the metastatic dissemination of colorectal carcinomas, by affecting three major events of the metastatic cascade. (**a**) during the first phase, recognition of sialylated mucins on the surface of carcinoma cells by P-selectin and E-selectin, that are expressed by activated endothelial cells, facilitates tumor cell intravasation into the blood vessels; (**b**) once in the circulation, aggregates of tumor cells with leukocytes and platelets form as the result of interactions between leukocyte L-selectin and platelet P-selectin with carcinoma mucins. Such emboli structures protect tumor cells from the shear stress as well as impede tumor cell lysis by natural killer cells. Interestingly, the anticoagulant agent heparin inhibits principally P-selectin-dependent interactions and to a lesser extent L-selectin-based contacts, thereby attenuating metastasis of colon cancer cells; (**c**) arriving at the distant site, carcinoma cell surface mucins are recognized by E-selectin expressed on hepatic endothelial cells. This, in concert with leukocyte-endothelial cell interactions, leads to the extravasation of tumor cells out of the blood vessels and into the liver parenchyma

antithrombotic agent heparin has been widely used for its anticoagulant effects. However, heparin also functions as a potent inhibitor of P-selectin binding to its natural ligands (Koenig et al., 1998) (Fig. 7.3). Notably, this interaction was inhibited by heparin at concentrations ~50 fold lower than those recommended for effective anticoagulation in vivo (Koenig et al. 1998). In addition, in the presence of heparin, P-selectin-positive platelets showed significantly reduced binding to mucin-containing human colon adenocarcinoma cells both in vitro and in vivo (Borsig et al., 2001). More interestingly, injection of a single heparin dose attenuated lung metastasis of colon carcinoma cells in P-selectin-positive mice but had no further effect on P-selectin-deficient mice, suggesting that P-selectin deficiency and heparin likely act via a common mechanism (Borsig et al., 2001). In summary, these data indicate that the early platelet-tumour cell interactions are P-selectin-dependent and correlate with later metastatic progression that can be significantly inhibited by heparin. Therefore, heparin therapy for prevention of metastasis in humans remains to be explored. Whether low-dose heparin may be utilized to abolish primary adhesive interaction involved in formation of later metastases in colon cancer patients awaits further investigations and should be addressed in a clinical setting.

7.5.2 L-Selectin

The well-known physiological function of L-selectin is to facilitate leukocyte rolling along the vessel wall, one of the earliest responses to inflammatory stimuli or tissue damage (Butcher, 1991; Girard and Springer, 1995; Kansas, 1996; Ley and Tedder, 1995; Lowe, 1997). In addition, L-selectin mediates homing of normal lymphocytes to lymph nodes and in a transgenic model of carcinogenesis, ectopic expression of L-selectin in non-lymphoma tumour cells facilitated their lymph node metastasis (Qian et al., 2001).

Evidence to the role of L-selectin in promoting metastasis of colon cancer cells comes from a study by Borsig et al. using experimental metastasis of colorectal carcinoma cells in L-selectin knockout mice (Borsig et al., 2002). Both human and mouse colon carcinoma cells were used in these experiments and indicated a very significant reduction in terms of metastatic burden in the lungs of L-selectin-deficient ($L^{-/-}$) mice. Notably, combined deficiency of P- and L-selectins ($PL^{-/-}$ mice) further reduced lung metastasis of colon cancer cells, suggesting synergistic function of L- and P-selectin in facilitating colon cancer metastasis (Borsig et al., 2002). Moreover, injection of a single dose of heparin prior to injection of cancer cells resulted in a further reduction in the incidence of metastasis in $L^{-/-}$ mice but had no additional effect in $P^{-/-}$ or $PL^{-/-}$ mice. This suggests that although heparin is also an inhibitor of L-selectin, its function is primarily exerted via P-selectin inhibition (Borsig et al., 2002; Koenig et al., 1998; Xie et al., 2000) (Fig. 7.3). Although certain possibilities for the involvement of L-selectin in the metastatic cascade have been proposed based on the current knowledge (e.g. interaction of L-selectin-positive leukocytes with platelet-tumour cell emboli to promote tumour cell extravasation (Fig. 7.3), release of cytokines in the microenvironment of tumour emboli to support tumour cell survival and/or extravasation), the exact mechanism by which this endogenous lectin contributes to the metastatic spread of colon cancer cells is not yet known and needs further investigations.

7.5.3 E-Selectin

Carcinoma cell surface mucins carrying sialyl-Lewis$^{x/a}$ can be recognized by all three selectins (Fig. 7.3) including endothelial-specific selectin (E-selectin)

(Fukuda, 1996; Hakomori, 1996; Kannagi, 1997; Kim et al., 1999; Kim and Varki, 1997; Kim et al., 1996; Mannori et al., 1995; Takada et al., 1993). The notion that E-selectin expressed on activated endothelial cells may facilitate metastatic dissemination is supported by overexpression of E-selectin in the mouse liver, which was able to redirect metastasis of melanoma cells bearing E-selectin ligands to this organ (Biancone et al., 1996).

E-selectin mediates adhesion of tumour cells to liver endothelial cells in colon cancer metastasis and promotes metastatic spread (Brodt et al., 1997) (Fig. 7.3). Moreover, blockade of hepatic endothelial E-selectin expression, using antisense oligonucleotides, abrogated E-selectin-dependent adhesion of human colorectal cancer cells in vitro as well as reduced their liver metastasis by 86% in vivo (Khatib et al., 2002). Similarly, interfering with the binding of colon carcinoma cells to activated vascular endothelium, by using a soluble form of E-selectin, blocked the retention of these cells in the lungs, thereby impairing lung metastasis (Mannori et al., 1997). These results suggest that disruption of E-selectin-dependent adhesion of tumour cells to endothelium might represent a therapeutic approach to the metastatic diffusion of colon tumours. Along this line, a study by Kobayashi et al. demonstrated for the first time that cimetidine, a drug with beneficial effects on the survival of colorectal carcinoma patients, can block the adhesion of colorectal carcinoma cells to endothelial cells in vitro and it can also suppress their metastasis in a nude mouse model (Kobayashi et al., 2000). In fact, the anti-metastatic effect of cimetidine occurs through down-regulation of the cell surface expression of E-selectin on endothelial cells (Kobayashi et al., 2000). In a separate clinical study, the effects of cimetidine treatment on survival and recurrence of CRC patients were investigated (Matsumoto et al., 2002). The results clearly indicated that cimetidine treatment dramatically improved CRC survival and was particularly effective in patients whose tumour cells expressed higher levels of sialyl-Lewis^x and sialyl-Lewis^a (both are ligands for E-selectin) (Matsumoto et al., 2002). Moreover, Kakiuchi et al. showed that treatment of colon tumour cells with Celecoxib (an anti-inflammatory agent acting by cyclooxygenase 2 (COX-2) inhibition) decreased sialyl-Lewis^a expression as well as adherence to liver endothelial cells, and therefore reduced the metastatic potential of colon tumour cells in vivo, further verifying the importance of E-selectin-mediated interactions as a therapeutic target in colon cancer metastasis (Kakiuchi et al., 2002). However, therapeutic usefulness of such drug for prevention of metastasis in CRC patients remains to be elucidated by further studies particularly in a clinical setting.

In summary, cancer cells including colorectal carcinoma cells usurp at least some of the functional properties of the selectin-selectin ligand axis in order to progress towards metastasis. For this to happen, selectins and their ligands are involved in at least two major events during metastatic dissemination: (1) in the formation of circulating emboli where tumour cells form aggregates with platelets (P-selectin-mediated interactions) and leukocytes (likely via L-selectin). In such aggregates tumour cells are protected from shear stress and their binding to the vascular endothelium is facilitated by the leukocyte component of the emboli; (2) in extravasation of tumour cells, where selectin-selectin ligand interactions (involvement of E-selectin-mediated interactions) initiate the contact between extravasating metastatic cells and endothelial cells. Interfering with selectin-mediated interactions (e.g. heparin treatment, use of cimetidine, Celecoxib or other anti-inflammatory agents) introduces new paradigms in the prevention of human colon carcinoma metastasis and deserves further evaluation in clinical trials.

7.6 Immunoglobulin (IG) Superfamily

Proteins that belong to the Ig superfamily share a common structural feature of Ig molecules, i.e. a 70–110 amino acid domain organized into several beta-pleated sheets, each stabilized by a single disulfide bond (Springer, 1990). In this section, we focus on two members of the Ig superfamily whose expression is not only important for the metastatic potential of colorectal carcinomas but also predictive of the recurrence and prognosis of gastrointestinal malignancies including colon cancer.

7.6.1 Intercellular Adhesion Molecule-1 (ICAM-1)

ICAM-1 (or CD54) was identified more than 20 years ago as a cytokine-inducible cell adhesion molecule (Rothlein et al., 1986). It is a 90 kDa transmembrane glycoprotein with an extracellular region containing five Ig-like domains, a predicted transmembrane segment and a cytoplasmic tail of 28 amino acids (Makgoba et al., 1988). This molecule is constitutively expressed on the surface of a wide variety of cell types including vascular endothelial cells and some leukocytes (Long, 1992; Springer, 1990). Interaction of endothelial ICAM-1 with leukocyte integrins supports adhesion and transmigration of leukocytes and is integral to many adhesion-dependent leukocyte functions (Makgoba et al., 1989). ICAM-1 expression is markedly elevated in the presence of active inflammation in vivo as well as through the action of inflammatory cytokines in vitro (Roebuck and Finnegan, 1999; Springer, 1994). As for the role of this adhesion molecule in cancer metastasis, expression of ICAM-1 on many human tumour cells is required for their interaction with leukocytes. Therefore, low expression of ICAM-1 on tumour cells may impair their lysis by immunocompetent effector cells (Anichini et al., 1990; Vanky et al., 1990).

In the context of colon cancer, although normal colonic epithelial cells lack ICAM-1, tumour cells demonstrate focal expression of ICAM-1 with the highest levels detected in well-differentiated tumours (Table 7.1). The expression of ICAM-1 in colonic cancer cells can be induced by inflammatory cytokines and supports the adhesion of cancer cells to the tumour infiltrating lymphocytes and lymphokine-activated killer (LAK) cells (Kelly et al., 1992). In a study by Rivoltini et al., the high lysability by LAK cells of human colon carcinoma cells was attributed to high surface expression of ICAM-1 receptor (Rivoltini et al., 1991). In this study, doxorubicin-resistant human colon carcinoma subline (LoVo/Dx) bore a higher amount of adhesion molecules including ICAM-1 and displayed a less differentiated phenotype. Intriguingly, treatment of LoVo/Dx cells with differentiating agents resulted in reduced expression of ICAM-1 and led to an increased resistance to LAK-mediated lysis. Similarly, use of anti-ICAM-1 monoclonal antibodies caused a reduction in lysis by LAK cells (Rivoltini et al., 1991). These data indicate that susceptibility of colon carcinoma cells to activated immune cells' lytic activity depends on the level of expression of adhesion molecules, including ICAM-1, and is related to the differentiation stage. Association of elevated ICAM-1 expression and increased lysability by immune cells has important implications in formation of colorectal metastases. Along this line, pre-treatment of CT-26 colon cancer cells with anti-ICAM-1 monoclonal antibody suppressed natural killer activity (NK activity) of leukocytes and significantly increased the number of metastatic nodules in the murine liver (Kaihara et al., 1998). Given that ICAM-1 is a ligand for leukocyte function antigen-1 (LFA-1) receptor, present on the surface of leukocytes (Staunton et al., 1988), binding of ICAM-1 to LFA-1 may explain leukocytes NK activity and their cytotoxicity towards colon tumour cells that express ICAM-1 ligand (Kaihara et al., 1998). The impact of ICAM-1 expression on the metastatic potential of colon tumour cells is further verified by this observation that lower numbers of ICAM-1-positive cells were found in metastasizing tumours of colon (Wimmenauer et al., 1997) (Table 7.1). This may also be the reason why pronounced lymphocytic infiltration in colorectal tumours is associated with improved prognosis (Baeten et al., 2006; Koch et al., 2006). However, the role of other ICAM-1-expressing liver resident cells is reflected in other studies. Indeed, murine experiments have revealed that CRC cells induce production of inflammatory cytokines by Kupffer cells which in turn stimulate sinusoidal endothelial cells to express high levels of ICAM-1 and VCAM-1; these adhesion molecules mediate cancer cell adhesion and support subsequent extravasation of CRC cells during the metastatic cascade (Khatib et al., 2005).

7.6.2 Carcinoembryonic Antigen (CEA)

CEA was first identified by Gold and Freedman in 1965 (Gold and Freedman, 1965). CEA is a 180–200 kDa glycoprotein expressing approximately 60% carbohydrate. The peptide chain consists of a 108 amino acid Ig-V-like N-terminus domain followed by six Ig-C2-like repeating loop domains. Covalent attachment of a glycosylphosphatidylinositol (GPI) moiety to the CEA C-terminus anchors the molecule to the cell membrane prior to its secretion (Hefta et al., 1988). The protein is present in extracts of human adult colon adenocarcinoma as well as in fetal colon, but not in extracts of normal adult colon (Table 7.1). However, it is now known that CEA is expressed in many different normal tissues, albeit at a lower level than in carcinomas. In adenocarcinoma of colon, CEA is highly expressed throughout the cellular surface of tumour cells which is in contrast to its strict localization on the apical luminal surface of normal colonocytes (Hammarstrom, 1999). Such deregulated cell surface expression of CEA inversely correlates with the degree of tumour differentiation (Table 7.1), suggesting that CEA directly contributes to colon tumour progression by inhibiting colonocyte differentiation (Ilantzis et al., 2002; Ilantzis et al., 1997). Moreover upon transition of colonic adenomas into invasive carcinomas, CEA serum concentration substantially increases, making a useful marker in assessing prognosis of colorectal carcinoma (Hammarstrom, 1999). In fact, an elevated serum CEA level in the blood of CRC patients predicts an increased risk of disease recurrence (Jessup and Thomas, 1989). Serum CEA level also increases prior to the appearance of clinical metastasis (Kimura et al., 1986), indicative of the potential role of CEA in the development of CRC metastasis (Table 7.1). In support of such role, Jessup and Thomas showed that intravenous injection of CEA prior to the intrasplenic injection of human colon cancer cells enhanced the metastatic potential of two weakly metastatic CRC cell lines. However, it did not render a non-metastatic line metastatic or a highly metastatic one further aggressive (Jessup and Thomas, 1989). Up to now, several groups have investigated the mechanism through which CEA can enhance metastasis by certain CRC cells. On one hand, CEA may promote hepatic metastasis of CRC cells throughout the circulatory phase, a phase during which tumour cells survive in the blood circulation while traveling to a distant site. Two mechanisms have been suggested by which CEA exerts this function. First, as shown by Benchimol et al. (1989), transfection of CEA was sufficient to cause aggregation of fibroblasts expressing normally glycosylated CEA and anti-CEA antibodies inhibited CEA-induced fibroblast aggregation. Given that homotypic and heterotypic aggregation of CEA has been demonstrated in vitro (Jessup and Thomas, 1989; Lisowska et al., 1983; Toth et al., 1988), it seems that CEA may function as an aggregant where it can cause formation of large emboli by tumour cells, thereby facilitating their entrapment in the microvasculature. The second aspect of the circulatory phase that might be affected by CEA is the host immune response. CEA may be an immunosuppressant, directly or indirectly inhibiting humoral and cell-mediated immunity. It has been shown that CEA inhibits both proliferation and antibody production of lymphocytes in vitro (Hakim, 1984). In addition, CEA induces suppressor T cells from CRC patients to release a factor that inhibits DNA synthesis of normal T cells (Medoff et al., 1984). Therefore, such CEA-mediated immunosuppression may be involved in inhibition of host defence responses during the circulatory phase that might otherwise prevent metastasis.

On the other hand, facilitation of intercellular adhesion by CEA during the tumour implantation phase is another suggested mechanism accounting for the effect of this molecule on metastatic dissemination. Metastasizing CRC cells enter the liver through the portal vein and traverse hepatic sinusoids. Tumour cells within the hepatic sinusoids may interact with endothelial cells, Kupffer cells or hepatocytes. This binding phase would be followed by extravasation of tumour cells out of the sinusoids and their implantation and proliferation among the hepatocytes. Jessup et al. (1993) used an experimental hepatic metastasis model to determine whether CEA promoted the implantation of CRC cells. In fact, athymic nude mice pre-treated with CEA showed enhanced retention of two metastatic colon cancer cell lines in the liver. The authors further demonstrated that their tested CRC cells specifically bound to CEA (Jessup et al., 1993). Given that CEA is also bound to

Kupffer cells and hepatocytes and displayed on cell membranes (Byrn et al., 1985; Thomas et al., 1992; Thomas and Toth, 1989, 1990), the enhanced retention of metastasizing CRC cells in the liver could be at least partly explained by increased attachment of the metastatic tumour cells in terms of Kupffer cell/hepatocyte-tumour cell interactions (Jessup et al., 1993; Jessup and Thomas, 1989). Binding of CEA to Kupffer cells has other consequences as well. Amongst them, production of cytokines by CEA-stimulated Kupffer cells has been known for a while and is believed to mediate tumour cell adhesion induced by CEA (Gangopadhyay et al., 1998; Minami et al., 2001). Indeed, activation of Kupffer cells by CEA resulted in release of IL-1β, TNF-α and IL-6 (Gangopadhyay et al., 1998). Such Kupffer cell-derived cytokines induced endothelial cells to overexpress several adhesion molecules including ICAM-1 that in turn led to a significant enhancement in the adhesion of colorectal carcinoma cells to the endothelial cells (Gangopadhyay et al., 1998; Minami et al., 2001). These phenomena were blocked by the addition of cytokine inhibitors as well as an antibody to ICAM-1 (Gangopadhyay et al., 1998; Minami et al., 2001). These results suggest a mechanism by which CEA indirectly modulates CRC cell adhesion to the hepatic endothelium, thereby contributing to the metastasis of malignant cells to the liver. Recently, additional mechanisms have been suggested for metastasis-promoting function of CEA in colorectal carcinomas. For example, Jessup's group demonstrated that CEA promoted survival of colon tumour cells in the liver and therefore enhanced CRC metastasis to this organ (Jessup et al., 2004). CEA exerted this function by inducing IL-10 which in turn inhibited iNOS (inducible nitric oxide synthase) up-regulation and nitric oxide production in host liver, that would otherwise kill the metastatic CRC cells (Jessup et al., 2004). In addition, CEA was reported to directly interact with TRAIL-R2 (DR5) death receptor on the surface of colorectal carcinoma cells, thereby inhibiting anoikis through the extrinsic pathway and increasing metastatic potential of CRC cells (Samara et al., 2007).

Collectively, the positive influence of CEA on the metastatic cascade in colorectal carcinomas can be explained by different mechanisms. During the circulatory phase, its aggregating function may contribute to formation of large emboli promoting entrapment of tumour cells in microvasculature. In addition, CEA's immunosuppressive function may affect several host defence mechanisms that would otherwise inhibit metastasis. During the implantation phase, CEA adhesive properties as well as its stimulatory effect on Kupffer cells may also facilitate extravasation of tumour cells out of the circulation and into the metastatic site. Interaction of CEA with a variety of cell surface receptors at the metastatic site may also provide survival signals promoting metastatic potential of tumour cells.

Given that CEA is overexpressed in the majority of human colon carcinomas and that it already constitutes one of the most extensively used clinical tumour markers, its value as a therapeutic target is being increasingly recognized as well. Indeed, several vaccination approaches against CEA have been proven safe and capable of inducing humoral, CD4$^+$ helper T-cell as well as CD8$^+$ cytotoxic T-cell responses (Fong et al., 2001; Horig et al., 2000; Marshall et al., 2000; Mosolits et al., 2005; Samanci et al., 1998; Ullenhag et al., 2004). For example, in a phase I clinical trial, colorectal carcinoma patients were immunized using recombinant human CEA protein in combination with recombinant granulocyte-macrophage colony-stimulating factor (GM-CSF) as an adjuvant (Samanci et al., 1998). All these patients developed a strong CEA-specific immune response where both humoral and cellular elements of the response were induced (Samanci et al., 1998). In addition, a 6-year follow-up study demonstrated that vaccination with recombinant CEA and GM-CSF was also non-toxic and elicited a durable antibody and T-cell response that correlated with increased patient survival (Ullenhag et al., 2004). Recently in a study by Hallermalm et al. (2007), a DNA prime/protein boost vaccination strategy was tested on animals with the aim of further improving the results of the protein vaccination trials (Samanci et al., 1998; Ullenhag et al., 2004). In this study, repeated intradermal administration of a plasmid DNA vaccine, namely CEA66, was used for the priming and the boosting was performed using recombinant CEA protein. Interestingly, the CEA DNA prime/CEA protein boost vaccination elicited a more potent immune response (evidenced by further augmented anti-CEA antibody titres and more pronounced $CD4^+$ and $CD8^+$ T-cell responses) than repeated administration of CEA protein as a single modality vaccine (Hallermalm et al., 2007). These results along with the finding that CEA66 DNA vaccine showed no toxicity in mice, warrant further clinical evaluation of this vaccination strategy in humans. In spite of all the promising results coming from testing of CEA vaccines in different settings, one recent clinical study on the treatment of CRC liver metastases showed similar recurrence-free survival in post-hepatic resection patients treated with a CEA vaccine (39%), as compared to those who underwent hepatic resection alone (40%) (Posner et al., 2008). Therefore, it seems that separate clinical trials should be set to prove the immunotherapeutic value of CEA vaccines in comparison to other therapeutic modalities such as curative surgery, radiotherapy and chemotherapy.

7.7 Conclusion

The importance of cell adhesion molecules in the progression of colorectal cancer and its metastatic dissemination to the liver has been increasingly recognized over the last three decades. Multiple cell types in the body as well as colon tumour cells per se express and/or secrete adhesion molecules. In the course of colon cancer progression and following ill-defined molecular pathways, expression of such adhesion proteins undergoes alterations in the primary and/or metastatic sites. These alterations are indeed suited towards adhesive and migratory abilities of cancer cells in such a way that they promote detachment of tumour cells from the primary carcinomas while assisting their attachment to the metastatic organ. Although only a handful of cell adhesion molecules were discussed in this chapter, the clinical outcome of modulating the expression of the abovementioned proteins remains as an important question in the field which has yet to be answered. In fact, future research needs to be more targeted towards therapeutic intervention of tumour cell-host interactions. In this context, use of anti-integrin antibodies (Weinreb et al., 2004) or integrin inhibitors such as Cilengitide (Reardon et al., 2008; Stupp et al., 2007;

Stupp and Ruegg, 2007), interfering with selectin-mediated interactions (through for example, heparin, cimetidine, Celecoxib, etc.), application of ICAM-1 antibodies as well as CEA vaccines may be considered as part of the anti-adhesion treatment against colorectal cancer and their therapeutic value will hopefully be addressed in clinical trials.

Acknowledgments The work described in this chapter was supported by the Canadian Institutes of Health Research and the Canadian Cancer Society Research Institute.

Abbreviations and Acronyms

CD44	Cluster of differentiation 44
CEA	Carcinoembryonic antigen
COX2	Cyclooxygenase 2
EMT	Epithelial mesenchymal transition
ESL-1	E-selectin ligand-1
GPI	Glycosylphosphatidylinositol
HCELL	Hematopoietic cell E-/L-selectin ligand
ICAM-1	Intercellular adhesion molecule-1
LAK cells	Lymphokine-activated killer cells
LAMP-1	Lysosome-associated membrane protein 1
LEU-CAM	Leukocyte cell adhesion molecule
MAdCAM-1	Mucosal addressin cell adhesion molecule-1
MMP9	Matrix metalloproteinase-9
PSGL1	P-selectin glycoprotein ligand-1
RGD	Arginine-glycine-aspartic acid
VCAM	Vascular cell adhesion molecule
VLA	Very late antigen

References

Abbasi AM, Chester KA, Talbot IC, Macpherson AS, Boxer G, Forbes A et al. (1993). CD44 is associated with proliferation in normal and neoplastic human colorectal epithelial cells. *Eur J Cancer* **29A**: 1995–2002.

Agrez M, Chen A, Cone RI, Pytela R, Sheppard D (1994). The alpha v beta 6 integrin promotes proliferation of colon carcinoma cells through a unique region of the beta 6 cytoplasmic domain. *J Cell Biol* **127**: 547–56.

Agrez MV, Bates RC, Mitchell D, Wilson N, Ferguson N, Anseline P et al. (1996). Multiplicity of fibronectin-binding alpha V integrin receptors in colorectal cancer. *Br J Cancer* **73**: 887–92.

Ahmad A, Hart IR (1997). Mechanisms of metastasis. *Crit Rev Oncol Hematol* **26**: 163–73.

Albelda SM, Buck CA (1990). Integrins and other cell adhesion molecules. *FASEB J* **4**: 2868–80.

Anichini A, Mortarini R, Supino R, Parmiani G (1990). Human melanoma cells with high susceptibility to cell-mediated lysis can be identified on the basis of ICAM-1 phenotype, VLA profile and invasive ability. *Int J Cancer* **46**: 508–15.

Avizienyte E, Wyke AW, Jones RJ, McLean GW, Westhoff MA, Brunton VG et al. (2002). Src-induced de-regulation of E-cadherin in colon cancer cells requires integrin signalling. *Nat Cell Biol* **4**: 632–38.

Aznavoorian S, Murphy AN, Stetler-Stevenson WG, Liotta LA (1993). Molecular aspects of tumor cell invasion and metastasis. *Cancer* **71**: 1368–83.

Baeten CI, Castermans K, Hillen HF, Griffioen AW (2006). Proliferating endothelial cells and leukocyte infiltration as prognostic markers in colorectal cancer. *Clin Gastroenterol Hepatol* **4**: 1351–57.

Bates RC, Bellovin DI, Brown C, Maynard E, Wu B, Kawakatsu H et al. (2005). Transcriptional activation of integrin beta6 during the epithelial-mesenchymal transition defines a novel prognostic indicator of aggressive colon carcinoma. *J Clin Invest* **115**: 339–47.

Behrens J, Mareel MM, Van Roy FM, Birchmeier W (1989). Dissecting tumor cell invasion: epithelial cells acquire invasive properties after the loss of uvomorulin-mediated cell-cell adhesion. *J Cell Biol* **108**: 2435–47.

Behrens J, Vakaet L, Friis R, Winterhager E, Van Roy F, Mareel MM et al. (1993). Loss of epithelial differentiation and gain of invasiveness correlates with tyrosine phosphorylation of the E-cadherin/beta-catenin complex in cells transformed with a temperature-sensitive v-SRC gene. *J Cell Biol* **120**: 757–66.

Bellovin DI, Bates RC, Muzikansky A, Rimm DL, Mercurio AM (2005). Altered localization of p120 catenin during epithelial to mesenchymal transition of colon carcinoma is prognostic for aggressive disease. *Cancer Res* **65**: 10938–45.

Benchimol S, Fuks A, Jothy S, Beauchemin N, Shirota K, Stanners CP (1989). Carcinoembryonic antigen, a human tumor marker, functions as an intercellular adhesion molecule. *Cell* **57**: 327–34.

Biancone L, Araki M, Araki K, Vassalli P, Stamenkovic I (1996). Redirection of tumor metastasis by expression of E-selectin in vivo. *J Exp Med* **183**: 581–87.

Borsig L, Wong R, Feramisco J, Nadeau DR, Varki NM, Varki A (2001). Heparin and cancer revisited: mechanistic connections involving platelets, P-selectin, carcinoma mucins, and tumor metastasis. *Proc Natl Acad Sci USA* **98**: 3352–57.

Borsig L, Wong R, Hynes RO, Varki NM, Varki A (2002). Synergistic effects of L- and P-selectin in facilitating tumor metastasis can involve non-mucin ligands and implicate leukocytes as enhancers of metastasis. *Proc Natl Acad Sci USA* **99**: 2193–98.

Brabletz T, Jung A, Reu S, Porzner M, Hlubek F, Kunz-Schughart LA et al. (2001). Variable beta-catenin expression in colorectal cancers indicates tumor progression driven by the tumor environment. *Proc Natl Acad Sci USA* **98**: 10356–61.

Brandley BK, Swiedler SJ, Robbins PW (1990). Carbohydrate ligands of the LEC cell adhesion molecules. *Cell* **63**: 861–63.

Breuss JM, Gallo J, DeLisser HM, Klimanskaya IV, Folkesson HG, Pittet JF et al. (1995). Expression of the beta 6 integrin subunit in development, neoplasia and tissue repair suggests a role in epithelial remodeling. *J Cell Sci* **108(Pt 6)**: 2241–51.

Brodt P, Fallavollita L, Bresalier RS, Meterissian S, Norton CR, Wolitzky BA (1997). Liver endothelial E-selectin mediates carcinoma cell adhesion and promotes liver metastasis. *Int J Cancer* **71**: 612–19.

Buck CA, Shea E, Duggan K, Horwitz AF (1986). Integrin (the CSAT antigen): functionality requires oligomeric integrity. *J Cell Biol* **103**: 2421–28.

Bukholm IK, Nesland JM, Borresen-Dale AL (2000). Re-expression of E-cadherin, alpha-catenin and beta-catenin, but not of gamma-catenin, in metastatic tissue from breast cancer patients [seecomments]. *J Pathol* **190**: 15–19.

Burdick MM, Chu JT, Godar S, Sackstein R (2006). HCELL is the major E- and L-selectin ligand expressed on LS174T colon carcinoma cells. *J Biol Chem* **281**: 13899–905.

Butcher EC (1991). Leukocyte-endothelial cell recognition: three (or more) steps to specificity and diversity. *Cell* **67**: 1033–36.

Byrn RA, Medrek P, Thomas P, Jeanloz RW, Zamcheck N (1985). Effect of heterogeneity of carcinoembryonic antigen on liver cell membrane binding and its kinetics of removal from circulation. *Cancer Res* **45**: 3137–42.

Chausovsky A, Bershadsky AD, Borisy GG (2000). Cadherin-mediated regulation of microtubule dynamics. *Nat Cell Biol* **2**: 797–804.

Chen WC, Obrink B (1991). Cell-cell contacts mediated by E-cadherin (uvomorulin) restrict invasive behavior of L-cells. *J Cell Biol* **114**: 319–27.

Conti JA, Kendall TJ, Bateman A, Armstrong TA, Papa-Adams A, Xu Qet al. (2008). The desmoplastic reaction surrounding hepatic colorectal adenocarcinoma metastases aids tumor growth and survival via alphav integrin ligation. *Clin Cancer Res* **14**: 6405–13.

Dennis JW, Laferte S (1987). Tumor cell surface carbohydrate and the metastatic phenotype. *Cancer Metastasis Rev* **5**: 185–204.

Efstathiou JA, Liu D, Wheeler JM, Kim HC, Beck NE, Ilyas Met al. (1999). Mutated epithelial cadherin is associated with increased tumorigenicity and loss of adhesion and of responsiveness to the motogenic trefoil factor 2 in colon carcinoma cells. *Proc Natl Acad Sci USA* **96**: 2316–21.

Fidler IJ (2003). The pathogenesis of cancer metastasis: the 'seed and soil' hypothesis revisited. *Nat Rev Cancer* **3**: 453–8.

Fong L, Hou Y, Rivas A, Benike C, Yuen A, Fisher GAet al. (2001). Altered peptide ligand vaccination with Flt3 ligand expanded dendritic cells for tumor immunotherapy. *Proc Natl Acad Sci USA* **98**: 8809–14.

Frixen UH, Behrens J, Sachs M, Eberle G, Voss B, Warda Aet al. (1991). E-cadherin-mediated cell-cell adhesion prevents invasiveness of human carcinoma cells. *J Cell Biol* **113**: 173–85.

Fukuda M (1996). Possible roles of tumor-associated carbohydrate antigens. *Cancer Res* **56**: 2237–44.

Gangopadhyay A, Lazure DA, Thomas P (1998). Adhesion of colorectal carcinoma cells to the endothelium is mediated by cytokines from CEA stimulated Kupffer cells. *Clin Exp Metastasis* **16**: 703–12.

Garcia J, Callewaert N, Borsig L (2007). P-selectin mediates metastatic progression through binding to sulfatides on tumor cells. *Glycobiology* **17**: 185–96.

Gasic GJ (1984). Role of plasma, platelets, and endothelial cells in tumor metastasis. *Cancer Metastasis Rev* **3**: 99–114.

Ghadimi BM, Behrens J, Hoffmann I, Haensch W, Birchmeier W, Schlag PM (1999). Immunohistological analysis of E-cadherin, alpha-, beta- and gamma-catenin expression in colorectal cancer: implications for cell adhesion and signaling. *Eur J Cancer* **35**: 60–65.

Girard JP, Springer TA (1995). High endothelial venules (HEVs): specialized endothelium for lymphocyte migration. *Immunol Today* **16**: 449–57.

Gofuku J, Shiozaki H, Tsujinaka T, Inoue M, Tamura S, Doki Yet al. (1999). Expression of E-cadherin and alpha-catenin in patients with colorectal carcinoma. Correlation with cancer invasion and metastasis. *Am J Clin Pathol* **111**: 29–37.

Gold P, Freedman SO (1965). Demonstration of Tumor-Specific Antigens in Human Colonic Carcinomata by Immunological Tolerance and Absorption Techniques. *J Exp Med* **121**: 439–62.

Gunthert U (1993). CD44: a multitude of isoforms with diverse functions. *Curr Top Microbiol Immunol* **184**: 47–63.

Gunthert U, Hofmann M, Rudy W, Reber S, Zoller M, Haussmann Iet al. (1991). A new variant of glycoprotein CD44 confers metastatic potential to rat carcinoma cells. *Cell* **65**: 13–24.

Hajra KM, Chen DY, Fearon ER (2002). The SLUG zinc-finger protein represses E-cadherin in breast cancer. *Cancer Res* **62**: 1613–18.

Hakim AA (1984). Carcinoembryonic antigen, a tumor-associated glycoprotein induces defective lymphocyte function. *Neoplasma* **31**: 385–97.

Hakomori S (1996). Tumor malignancy defined by aberrant glycosylation and sphingo(glyco)lipid metabolism. *Cancer Res* **56**: 5309–18.

Hallermalm K, Johansson S, Brave A, Ek M, Engstrom G, Boberg Aet al. (2007). Pre-clinical evaluation of a CEA DNA prime/protein boost vaccination strategy against colorectal cancer. *Scand J Immunol* **66**: 43–51.

Hammarstrom S (1999). The carcinoembryonic antigen (CEA) family: structures, suggested functions and expression in normal and malignant tissues. *Semin Cancer Biol* **9**: 67–81.

Hanley WD, Burdick MM, Konstantopoulos K, Sackstein R (2005). CD44 on LS174T colon carcinoma cells possesses E-selectin ligand activity. *Cancer Res* **65**: 5812–17.

Hefta SA, Hefta LJ, Lee TD, Paxton RJ, Shively JE (1988). Carcinoembryonic antigen is anchored to membranes by covalent attachment to a glycosylphosphatidylinositol moiety: identification of the ethanolamine linkage site. *Proc Natl Acad Sci USA* **85**: 4648–52.

Heider KH, Hofmann M, Hors E, van den Berg F, Ponta H, Herrlich Pet al. (1993). A human homologue of the rat metastasis-associated variant of CD44 is expressed in colorectal carcinomas and adenomatous polyps. *J Cell Biol* **120**: 227–33.

Heino J (1993). Integrin-type extracellular matrix receptors in cancer and inflammation. *Ann Med* **25**: 335–42.

Herrenknecht K, Ozawa M, Eckerskorn C, Lottspeich F, Lenter M, Kemler R (1991). The uvomorulin-anchorage protein alpha catenin is a vinculin homologue. *Proc Natl Acad Sci USA* **88**: 9156–60.

Herrlich P, Pals S, Ponta H (1995). CD44 in colon cancer. *Eur J Cancer* **31A**: 1110–12.

Hoff SD, Matsushita Y, Ota DM, Cleary KR, Yamori T, Hakomori Set al. (1989). Increased expression of sialyl-dimeric LeX antigen in liver metastases of human colorectal carcinoma. *Cancer Res* **49**: 6883–88.

Honn KV, Tang DG, Crissman JD (1992). Platelets and cancer metastasis: a causal relationship? *Cancer Metastasis Rev* **11**: 325–51.

Horig H, Lee DS, Conkright W, Divito J, Hasson H, LaMare Met al. (2000). Phase I clinical trial of a recombinant canarypoxvirus (ALVAC) vaccine expressing human carcinoembryonic antigen and the B7.1 co-stimulatory molecule. *Cancer Immunol Immunother* **49**: 504–14.

Hynes RO (1987). Integrins: a family of cell surface receptors. *Cell* **48**: 549–54.

Hynes RO (1992). Integrins: versatility, modulation, and signaling in cell adhesion. *Cell* **69**: 11–25.

Hynes RO (2002). Integrins: bidirectional, allosteric signaling machines. *Cell* **110**: 673–87.

Ikeguchi M, Makino M, Kaibara N (2001). Clinical significance of E-cadherin-catenin complex expression in metastatic foci of colorectal carcinoma. *J Surg Oncol* **77**: 201–7.

Ikeguchi M, Taniguchi T, Makino M, Kaibara N (2000). Reduced E-cadherin expression and enlargement of cancer nuclei strongly correlate with hematogenic metastasis in colorectal adenocarcinoma. *Scand J Gastroenterol* **35**: 839–46.

Ilantzis C, DeMarte L, Screaton RA, Stanners CP (2002). Deregulated expression of the human tumor marker CEA and CEA family member CEACAM6 disrupts tissue architecture and blocks colonocyte differentiation. *Neoplasia* **4**: 151–63.

Ilantzis C, Jothy S, Alpert LC, Draber P, Stanners CP (1997). Cell-surface levels of human carcinoembryonic antigen are inversely correlated with colonocyte differentiation in colon carcinogenesis. *Lab Invest* **76**: 703–16.

Izumi Y, Taniuchi Y, Tsuji T, Smith CW, Nakamori S, Fidler IJet al. (1995). Characterization of human colon carcinoma variant cells selected for sialyl Lex carbohydrate antigen: liver colonization and adhesion to vascular endothelial cells. *Exp Cell Res* **216**: 215–21.

Jalkanen S, Jalkanen M (1992). Lymphocyte CD44 binds the COOH-terminal heparin-binding domain of fibronectin. *J Cell Biol* **116**: 817–25.

Jessup JM, Petrick AT, Toth CA, Ford R, Meterissian S, O'Hara CJet al. (1993). Carcinoembryonic antigen: enhancement of liver colonisation through retention of human colorectal carcinoma cells. *Br J Cancer* **67**: 464–70.

Jessup JM, Samara R, Battle P, Laguinge LM (2004). Carcinoembryonic antigen promotes tumor cell survival in liver through an IL-10-dependent pathway. *Clin Exp Metastasis* **21**: 709–17.

Jessup JM, Thomas P (1989). Carcinoembryonic antigen: function in metastasis by human colorectal carcinoma. *Cancer Metastasis Rev* **8**: 263–80.

Kaihara A, Iwagaki H, Gouchi A, Hizuta A, Isozaki H, Takakura Net al. (1998). Soluble intercellular adhesion molecule-1 and natural killer cell activity in gastric cancer patients. *Res Commun Mol Pathol Pharmacol* **100**: 283–300.

Kakiuchi Y, Tsuji S, Tsujii M, Murata H, Kawai N, Yasumaru Met al. (2002). Cyclooxygenase-2 activity altered the cell-surface carbohydrate antigens on colon cancer cells and enhanced liver metastasis. *Cancer Res* **62**: 1567–72.

Kalluri R, Neilson EG (2003). Epithelial-mesenchymal transition and its implications for fibrosis. *J Clin Invest* **112**: 1776–84.

Kanazawa N, Oda T, Gunji N, Nozue M, Kawamoto T, Todoroki Tet al. (2002a). E-cadherin expression in the primary tumors and metastatic lymph nodes of poorly differentiated types of rectal cancer. *Surg Today* **32**: 123–28.

Kanazawa T, Watanabe T, Kazama S, Tada T, Koketsu S, Nagawa H (2002b). Poorly differentiated adenocarcinoma and mucinous carcinoma of the colon and rectum show higher rates of loss of heterozygosity and loss of E-cadherin expression due to methylation of promoter region. *Int J Cancer* **102**: 225–29.

Kannagi R (1997). Carbohydrate-mediated cell adhesion involved in hematogenous metastasis of cancer. *Glycoconj J* **14**: 577–84.

Kansas GS (1996). Selectins and their ligands: current concepts and controversies. *Blood* **88**: 3259–87.

Karpatkin S, Pearlstein E (1981). Role of platelets in tumor cell metastases. *Ann Intern Med* **95**: 636–41.

Kelly CP, O'Keane JC, Orellana J, Schroy PC 3rd, Yang S, LaMont JTet al. (1992). Human colon cancer cells express ICAM-1 in vivo and support LFA-1-dependent lymphocyte adhesion in vitro. *Am J Physiol* **263**: G864–70.

Khatib AM, Auguste P, Fallavollita L, Wang N, Samani A, Kontogiannea Met al. (2005). Characterization of the host proinflammatory response to tumor cells during the initial stages of liver metastasis. *Am J Pathol* **167**: 749–59.

Khatib AM, Fallavollita L, Wancewicz EV, Monia BP, Brodt P (2002). Inhibition of hepatic endothelial E-selectin expression by C-raf antisense oligonucleotides blocks colorectal carcinoma liver metastasis. *Cancer Res* **62**: 5393–98.

Kim YJ, Borsig L, Han HL, Varki NM, Varki A (1999). Distinct selectin ligands on colon carcinoma mucins can mediate pathological interactions among platelets, leukocytes, and endothelium. *Am J Pathol* **155**: 461–72.

Kim YJ, Borsig L, Varki NM, Varki A (1998). P-selectin deficiency attenuates tumor growth and metastasis. *Proc Natl Acad Sci USA* **95**: 9325–30.

Kim YJ, Varki A (1997). Perspectives on the significance of altered glycosylation of glycoproteins in cancer. *Glycoconj J* **14**: 569–76.

Kim YS, Gum J Jr, Brockhausen I (1996). Mucin glycoproteins in neoplasia. *Glycoconj J* **13**: 693–707.

Kimura K, Endo Y, Yonemura Y, Heizmann CW, Schafer BW, Watanabe Yet al. (2000a). Clinical significance of S100A4 and E-cadherin-related adhesion molecules in non-small cell lung cancer. *Int J Oncol* **16**: 1125–31.

Kimura O, Kaibara N, Nishidoi H, Okamoto T, Takebayashi M, Kawasumi Het al. (1986). Carcinoembryonic antigen slope analysis as an early indicator for recurrence of colorectal carcinoma. *Jpn J Surg* **16**: 106–11.

Kimura T, Tanaka S, Haruma K, Sumii K, Kajiyama G, Shimamoto Fet al. (2000b). Clinical significance of MUC1 and E-cadherin expression, cellular proliferation, and angiogenesis at the deepest invasive portion of colorectal cancer. *Int J Oncol* **16**: 55–64.

Kinsella AR, Green B, Lepts GC, Hill CL, Bowie G, Taylor BA (1993). The role of the cell-cell adhesion molecule E-cadherin in large bowel tumour cell invasion and metastasis. *Br J Cancer* **67**: 904–9.

Kobayashi K, Matsumoto S, Morishima T, Kawabe T, Okamoto T (2000). Cimetidine inhibits cancer cell adhesion to endothelial cells and prevents metastasis by blocking E-selectin expression. *Cancer Res* **60**: 3978–84.

Koch M, Beckhove P, Op den Winkel J, Autenrieth D, Wagner P, Nummer D et al. (2006). Tumor infiltrating T lymphocytes in colorectal cancer: tumor-selective activation and cytotoxic activity in situ. *Ann Surg* **244**: 986–92; discussion 992–3.

Koenig A, Norgard-Sumnicht K, Linhardt R, Varki A (1998). Differential interactions of heparin and heparan sulfate glycosaminoglycans with the selectins. Implications for the use of unfractionated and low molecular weight heparins as therapeutic agents. *J Clin Invest* **101**: 877–89.

Koretz K, Schlag P, Boumsell L, Moller P (1991). Expression of VLA-alpha 2, VLA-alpha 6, and VLA-beta 1 chains in normal mucosa and adenomas of the colon, and in colon carcinomas and their liver metastases. *Am J Pathol* **138**: 741–50.

Krishnadath KK, Tilanus HW, van Blankenstein M, Hop WC, Kremers ED, Dinjens WNet al. (1997). Reduced expression of the cadherin-catenin complex in oesophageal adenocarcinoma correlates with poor prognosis. *J Pathol* **182**: 331–8.

Lasky LA (1994). Sialomucin ligands for selectins: a new family of cell adhesion molecules. *Princess Takamatsu Symp* **24**: 81–90.

Lesley J, Hyman R, Kincade PW (1993). CD44 and its interaction with extracellular matrix. *Adv Immunol* **54**: 271–335.

Ley K, Tedder TF (1995). Leukocyte interactions with vascular endothelium. New insights into selectin-mediated attachment and rolling. *J Immunol* **155**: 525–28.

Lisowska E, Krop-Watorek A, Sedlaczek P (1983). The dimeric structure of carcinoembryonic antigen (CEA). *Biochem Biophys Res Commun* **115**: 206–11.

Long MW (1992). Blood cell cytoadhesion molecules. *Exp Hematol* **20**: 288–301.

Lowe JB (1997). Selectin ligands, leukocyte trafficking, and fucosyltransferase genes. *Kidney Int* **51**: 1418–26.

Lowe JB (2002). Glycosyltransferases and glycan structures contributing to the adhesive activities of L-, E- and P-selectin counter-receptors. *Biochem Soc Symp* **69**: 33–45.

Mackay CR, Terpe HJ, Stauder R, Marston WL, Stark H, Gunthert U (1994). Expression and modulation of CD44 variant isoforms in humans. *J Cell Biol* **124**: 71–82.

Makgoba MW, Sanders ME, Ginther Luce GE, Dustin ML, Springer TA, Clark EAet al. (1988). ICAM-1 a ligand for LFA-1-dependent adhesion of B, T and myeloid cells. *Nature* **331**: 86–88.

Makgoba MW, Sanders ME, Shaw S (1989). The CD2-LFA-3 and LFA-1-ICAM pathways: relevance to T-cell recognition. *Immunol Today* **10**: 417–22.

Mannori G, Crottet P, Cecconi O, Hanasaki K, Aruffo A, Nelson RMet al. (1995). Differential colon cancer cell adhesion to E-, P-, and L-selectin: role of mucin-type glycoproteins. *Cancer Res* **55**: 4425–31.

Mannori G, Santoro D, Carter L, Corless C, Nelson RM, Bevilacqua MP (1997). Inhibition of colon carcinoma cell lung colony formation by a soluble form of E-selectin. *Am J Pathol* **151**: 233–43.

Marshall JL, Hoyer RJ, Toomey MA, Faraguna K, Chang P, Richmond Eet al. (2000). Phase I study in advanced cancer patients of a diversified prime-and-boost vaccination protocol using recombinant vaccinia virus and recombinant nonreplicating avipox virus to elicit anti-carcinoembryonic antigen immune responses. *J Clin Oncol* **18**: 3964–73.

Matsumoto S, Imaeda Y, Umemoto S, Kobayashi K, Suzuki H, Okamoto T (2002). Cimetidine increases survival of colorectal cancer patients with high levels of sialyl Lewis-X and sialyl Lewis-A epitope expression on tumour cells. *Br J Cancer* **86**: 161–67.

Matsumura Y, Tarin D (1992). Significance of CD44 gene products for cancer diagnosis and disease evaluation. *Lancet* **340**: 1053–58.

Matsushita Y, Cleary KR, Ota DM, Hoff SD, Irimura T (1990). Sialyl-dimeric Lewis-X antigen expressed on mucin-like glycoproteins in colorectal cancer metastases. *Lab Invest* **63**: 780–91.

Matzku S, Wenzel A, Liu S, Zoller M (1989). Antigenic differences between metastatic and non-metastatic BSp73 rat tumor variants characterized by monoclonal antibodies. *Cancer Res* **49**: 1294–99.

Mayer B, Johnson JP, Leitl F, Jauch KW, Heiss MM, Schildberg FWet al. (1993). E-cadherin expression in primary and metastatic gastric cancer: down-regulation correlates with cellular dedifferentiation and glandular disintegration. *Cancer Res* **53**: 1690–95.

Medoff JR, Jegasothy BV, Roche JK (1984). Carcinoembryonic antigen-induced release of a suppressor factor from normal human lymphocytes in vitro. *Cancer Res* **44**: 5822–27.

Minami S, Furui J, Kanematsu T (2001). Role of carcinoembryonic antigen in the progression of colon cancer cells that express carbohydrate antigen. *Cancer Res* **61**: 2732–35.

Mosolits S, Ullenhag G, Mellstedt H (2005). Therapeutic vaccination in patients with gastrointestinal malignancies. A review of immunological and clinical results. *Ann Oncol* **16**: 847–62.

Nagar B, Overduin M, Ikura M, Rini JM (1996). Structural basis of calcium-induced E-cadherin rigidification and dimerization. *Nature* **380**: 360–64.

Nakamori S, Kameyama M, Imaoka S, Furukawa H, Ishikawa O, Sasaki Yet al. (1993). Increased expression of sialyl Lewisx antigen correlates with poor survival in patients with colorectal carcinoma: clinicopathological and immunohistochemical study. *Cancer Res* **53**: 3632–37.

Nakayama T, Watanabe M, Katsumata T, Teramoto T, Kitajima M (1995). Expression of sialyl Lewis(a) as a new prognostic factor for patients with advanced colorectal carcinoma. *Cancer* **75**: 2051–56.

Napier SL, Healy ZR, Schnaar RL, Konstantopoulos K (2007). Selectin ligand expression regulates the initial vascular interactions of colon carcinoma cells: the roles of CD44v and alternative sialofucosylated selectin ligands. *J Biol Chem* **282**: 3433–41.

Ni H, Dydensborg AB, Herring FE, Basora N, Gagne D, Vachon PHet al. (2005). Upregulation of a functional form of the beta4 integrin subunit in colorectal cancers correlates with c-Myc expression. *Oncogene* **24**: 6820–29.

Nieswandt B, Hafner M, Echtenacher B, Mannel DN (1999). Lysis of tumor cells by natural killer cells in mice is impeded by platelets. *Cancer Res* **59**: 1295–300.

Oda T, Kanai Y, Oyama T, Yoshiura K, Shimoyama Y, Birchmeier Wet al. (1994). E-cadherin gene mutations in human gastric carcinoma cell lines. *Proc Natl Acad Sci USA* **91**: 1858–62.

Ozawa M, Ringwald M, Kemler R (1990). Uvomorulin-catenin complex formation is regulated by a specific domain in the cytoplasmic region of the cell adhesion molecule. *Proc Natl Acad Sci USA* **87**: 4246–50.

Pantel K, Brakenhoff RH (2004). Dissecting the metastatic cascade. *Nat Rev Cancer* **4**: 448–56.

Pignatelli M, Ansari TW, Gunter P, Liu D, Hirano S, Takeichi Met al. (1994). Loss of membranous E-cadherin expression in pancreatic cancer: correlation with lymph node metastasis, high grade, and advanced stage. *J Pathol* **174**: 243–48.

Pignatelli M, Smith ME, Bodmer WF (1990). Low expression of collagen receptors in moderate and poorly differentiated colorectal adenocarcinomas. *Br J Cancer* **61**: 636–38.

Posner MC, Niedzwiecki D, Venook AP, Hollis DR, Kindler HL, Martin EWet al. (2008). A phase II prospective multi-institutional trial of adjuvant active specific immunotherapy following curative resection of colorectal cancer hepatic metastases: cancer and leukemia group B study 89903. *Ann Surg Oncol* **15**: 158–64.

Qian F, Hanahan D, Weissman IL (2001). L-selectin can facilitate metastasis to lymph nodes in a transgenic mouse model of carcinogenesis. *Proc Natl Acad Sci USA* **98**: 3976–81.

Reardon DA, Nabors LB, Stupp R, Mikkelsen T (2008). Cilengitide: an integrin-targeting arginine-glycine-aspartic acid peptide with promising activity for glioblastoma multiforme. *Expert Opin Investig Drugs* **17**: 1225–35.

Rivoltini L, Cattoretti G, Arienti F, Mastroianni A, Melani C, Colombo MPet al. (1991). The high lysability by LAK cells of colon-carcinoma cells resistant to doxorubicin is associated with a high expression of ICAM-1, LFA-3, NCA and a less-differentiated phenotype. *Int J Cancer* **47**: 746–54.

Roebuck KA, Finnegan A (1999). Regulation of intercellular adhesion molecule-1 (CD54) gene expression. *J Leukoc Biol* **66**: 876–88.

Rothlein R, Dustin ML, Marlin SD, Springer TA (1986). A human intercellular adhesion molecule (ICAM-1) distinct from LFA-1. *J Immunol* **137**: 1270–74.

Roy HK, Smyrk TC, Koetsier J, Victor TA, Wali RK (2005). The transcriptional repressor SNAIL is overexpressed in human colon cancer. *Dig Dis Sci* **50**: 42–46.

Rudy W, Hofmann M, Schwartz-Albiez R, Zoller M, Heider KH, Ponta Het al. (1993). The two major CD44 proteins expressed on a metastatic rat tumor cell line are derived from different splice variants: each one individually suffices to confer metastatic behavior. *Cancer Res* **53**: 1262–68.

Ruoslahti E (1992). The Walter Herbert Lecture. Control of cell motility and tumour invasion by extracellular matrix interactions. *Br J Cancer* **66**: 239–42.
Samanci A, Yi Q, Fagerberg J, Strigard K, Smith G, Ruden U et al. (1998). Pharmacological administration of granulocyte/macrophage-colony-stimulating factor is of significant importance for the induction of a strong humoral and cellular response in patients immunized with recombinant carcinoembryonic antigen. *Cancer Immunol Immunother* **47**: 131–42.
Samara RN, Laguinge LM, Jessup JM (2007). Carcinoembryonic antigen inhibits anoikis in colorectal carcinoma cells by interfering with TRAIL-R2 (DR5) signaling. *Cancer Res* **67**: 4774–82.
Shapiro L, Fannon AM, Kwong PD, Thompson A, Lehmann MS, Grubel G et al. (1995). Structural basis of cell–cell adhesion by cadherins. *Nature* **374**: 327–37.
Shioiri M, Shida T, Koda K, Oda K, Seike K, Nishimura M et al. (2006). Slug expression is an independent prognostic parameter for poor survival in colorectal carcinoma patients. *Br J Cancer* **94**: 1816–22.
Sneath RJ, Mangham DC (1998). The normal structure and function of CD44 and its role in neoplasia. *Mol Pathol* **51**: 191–200.
Sperandio M (2006). Selectins and glycosyltransferases in leukocyte rolling in vivo. *FEBS J* **273**: 4377–89.
Springer TA (1990). Adhesion receptors of the immune system. *Nature* **346**: 425–34.
Springer TA (1994). Traffic signals for lymphocyte recirculation and leukocyte emigration: the multistep paradigm. *Cell* **76**: 301–14.
Stallmach A, von Lampe B, Matthes H, Bornhoft G, Riecken EO (1992). Diminished expression of integrin adhesion molecules on human colonic epithelial cells during the benign to malign tumour transformation. *Gut* **33**: 342–46.
Stallmach A, von Lampe B, Orzechowski HD, Matthes H, Riecken EO (1994). Increased fibronectin-receptor expression in colon carcinoma-derived HT 29 cells decreases tumorigenicity in nude mice. *Gastroenterology* **106**: 19–27.
Staunton DE, Marlin SD, Stratowa C, Dustin ML, Springer TA (1988). Primary structure of ICAM-1 demonstrates interaction between members of the immunoglobulin and integrin supergene families. *Cell* **52**: 925–33.
Streit M, Schmidt R, Hilgenfeld RU, Thiel E, Kreuser ED (1996). Adhesion receptors in malignant transformation and dissemination of gastrointestinal tumors. *J Mol Med* **74**: 253–68.
Stupp R, Hegi ME, Gilbert MR, Chakravarti A (2007). Chemoradiotherapy in malignant glioma: standard of care and future directions. *J Clin Oncol* **25**: 4127–36.
Stupp R, Ruegg C (2007). Integrin inhibitors reaching the clinic. *J Clin Oncol* **25**: 1637–38.
Swiedler SJ (1991). Reverse glycobiology: the LEC-CAMs and their carbohydrate ligands. *Glycobiology* **1**: 237–38.
Takada A, Ohmori K, Yoneda T, Tsuyuoka K, Hasegawa A, Kiso M et al. (1993). Contribution of carbohydrate antigens sialyl Lewis A and sialyl Lewis X to adhesion of human cancer cells to vascular endothelium. *Cancer Res* **53**: 354–61.
Takahashi K, Stamenkovic I, Cutler M, Saya H, Tanabe KK (1995). CD44 hyaluronate binding influences growth kinetics and tumorigenicity of human colon carcinomas. *Oncogene* **11**: 2223–32.
Tamura S, Shiozaki H, Miyata M, Kadowaki T, Inoue M, Matsui S et al. (1996). Decreased E-cadherin expression is associated with haematogenous recurrence and poor prognosis in patients with squamous cell carcinoma of the oesophagus. *Br J Surg* **83**: 1608–14.
Tanabe KK, Ellis LM, Saya H (1993). Expression of CD44R1 adhesion molecule in colon carcinomas and metastases. *Lancet* **341**: 725–26.
Terpe HJ, Stark H, Prehm P, Gunthert U (1994). CD44 variant isoforms are preferentially expressed in basal epithelial of non-malignant human fetal and adult tissues. *Histochemistry* **101**: 79–89.
Thiery JP (2003). Epithelial-mesenchymal transitions in development and pathologies. *Curr Opin Cell Biol* **15**: 740–46.

Thomas P, Petrick AT, Toth CA, Fox ES, Elting JJ, Steele G, Jr. (1992). A peptide sequence on carcinoembryonic antigen binds to a 80kD protein on Kupffer cells. *Biochem Biophys Res Commun* **188**: 671–77.
Thomas P, Toth CA (1989). Site of carcinoembryonic antigen binding to Kupffer cells. *Biochem Soc Trans* **17**: 1121–22.
Thomas P, Toth CA (1990). Carcinoembryonic antigen binding to Kupffer cells is via a peptide located at the junction of the N-terminal and first loop domains. *Biochem Biophys Res Commun* **170**: 391–96.
Thomas SN, Zhu F, Schnaar RL, Alves CS, Konstantopoulos K (2008). Carcinoembryonic antigen and CD44 variant isoforms cooperate to mediate colon carcinoma cell adhesion to E- and L-selectin in shear flow. *J Biol Chem* **283**: 15647–55.
Tomlinson J, Wang JL, Barsky SH, Lee MC, Bischoff J, Nguyen M (2000). Human colon cancer cells express multiple glycoprotein ligands for E-selectin. *Int J Oncol* **16**: 347–53.
Toth CA, Haagensen DE Jr, Davis S, Zamcheck N, Thomas P (1988). Hepatic clearance and metabolism in the rat of a human breast cancer associated glycoprotein (GCDFP-15). *Breast Cancer Res Treat* **12**: 235–43.
Trowbridge IS, Lesley J, Schulte R, Hyman R, Trotter J (1982). Biochemical characterization and cellular distribution of a polymorphic, murine cell-surface glycoprotein expressed on lymphoid tissues. *Immunogenetics* **15**: 299–312.
Ullenhag GJ, Frodin JE, Jeddi-Tehrani M, Strigard K, Eriksson E, Samanci A et al. (2004). Durable carcinoembryonic antigen (CEA)-specific humoral and cellular immune responses in colorectal carcinoma patients vaccinated with recombinant CEA and granulocyte/macrophage colony-stimulating factor. *Clin Cancer Res* **10**: 3273–81.
Underhill C (1992). CD44: the hyaluronan receptor. *J Cell Sci* **103(Pt 2)**: 293–98.
Vanky F, Wang P, Patarroyo M, Klein E (1990). Expression of the adhesion molecule ICAM-1 and major histocompatibility complex class I antigens on human tumor cells is required for their interaction with autologous lymphocytes in vitro. *Cancer Immunol Immunother* **31**: 19–27.
Varki A (1992). Selectins and other mammalian sialic acid-binding lectins. *Curr Opin Cell Biol* **4**: 257–66.
Varki A (1994). Selectin ligands. *Proc Natl Acad Sci USA* **91**: 7390–97.
Vestweber D (1993a). Glycoprotein ligands of the two endothelial selectins. *Res Immunol* **144**: 704–8; discussion 754–62.
Vestweber D (1993b). The selectins and their ligands. *Curr Top Microbiol Immunol* **184**: 65–75.
Vestweber D (1996). Ligand-specificity of the selectins. *J Cell Biochem* **61**: 585–91.
Vestweber D, Blanks JE (1999). Mechanisms that regulate the function of the selectins and their ligands. *Physiol Rev* **79**: 181–213.
Vleminckx K, Vakaet L, Jr., Mareel M, Fiers W, van Roy F (1991). Genetic manipulation of E-cadherin expression by epithelial tumor cells reveals an invasion suppressor role. *Cell* **66**: 107–19.
Wang SP, Wang WL, Chang YL, Wu CT, Chao YC, Kao SH et al. (2009). p53 controls cancer cell invasion by inducing the MDM2-mediated degradation of Slug. *Nat Cell Biol* **11**: 694–704.
Watabe-Uchida M, Uchida N, Imamura Y, Nagafuchi A, Fujimoto K, Uemura T et al. (1998). alpha-Catenin-vinculin interaction functions to organize the apical junctional complex in epithelial cells. *J Cell Biol* **142**: 847–57.
Weinreb PH, Simon KJ, Rayhorn P, Yang WJ, Leone DR, Dolinski BM et al. (2004). Function-blocking integrin alphavbeta6 monoclonal antibodies: distinct ligand-mimetic and nonligand-mimetic classes. *J Biol Chem* **279**: 17875–87.
Weiss EE, Kroemker M, Rudiger AH, Jockusch BM, Rudiger M (1998). Vinculin is part of the cadherin-catenin junctional complex: complex formation between alpha-catenin and vinculin. *J Cell Biol* **141**: 755–64.
Wheeler JM, Kim HC, Efstathiou JA, Ilyas M, Mortensen NJ, Bodmer WF (2001). Hypermethylation of the promoter region of the E-cadherin gene (CDH1) in sporadic and ulcerative colitis associated colorectal cancer. *Gut* **48**: 367–71.

Wielenga VJ, Heider KH, Offerhaus GJ, Adolf GR, van den Berg FM, Ponta Het al. (1993). Expression of CD44 variant proteins in human colorectal cancer is related to tumor progression. *Cancer Res* **53**: 4754–56.

Wimmenauer S, Keller H, Ruckauer KD, Rahner S, Wolff-Vorbeck G, Kirste Get al. (1997). Expression of CD44, ICAM-1 and N-CAM in colorectal cancer. Correlation with the tumor stage and the phenotypical characteristics of tumor-infiltrating lymphocytes. *Anticancer Res* **17**: 2395–400.

Witz IP (2006a). The involvement of selectins and their ligands in tumor-progression. *Immunol Lett* **104**: 89–93.

Witz IP (2006b). Tumor-microenvironment interactions: the selectin-selectin ligand axis in tumor-endothelium cross talk. *Cancer Treat Res* **130**: 125–40.

Xie X, Rivier AS, Zakrzewicz A, Bernimoulin M, Zeng XL, Wessel HPet al. (2000). Inhibition of selectin-mediated cell adhesion and prevention of acute inflammation by nonanticoagulant sulfated saccharides. Studies with carboxyl-reduced and sulfated heparin and with trestatin a sulfate. *J Biol Chem* **275**: 34818–25.

Yamaguchi A, Urano T, Goi T, Saito M, Takeuchi K, Hirose Ket al. (1996). Expression of a CD44 variant containing exons 8–10 is a useful independent factor for the prediction of prognosis in colorectal cancer patients. *J Clin Oncol* **14**: 1122–27.

Yang GY, Xu KS, Pan ZQ, Zhang ZY, Mi YT, Wang JSet al. (2008). Integrin alpha v beta 6 mediates the potential for colon cancer cells to colonize in and metastasize to the liver. *Cancer Sci* **99**: 879–87.

Yap AS, Niessen CM, Gumbiner BM (1998). The juxtamembrane region of the cadherin cytoplasmic tail supports lateral clustering, adhesive strengthening, and interaction with p120ctn. *J Cell Biol* **141**: 779–89.

You JF, Hsieh LL, Changchien CR, Chen JS, Chen JR, Chiang JMet al. (2006). Inverse effects of mucin on survival of matched hereditary nonpolyposis colorectal cancer and sporadic colorectal cancer patients. *Clin Cancer Res* **12**: 4244–50.

Zarbock A, Polanowska-Grabowska RK, Ley K (2007). Platelet-neutrophil-interactions: linking hemostasis and inflammation. *Blood Rev* **21**: 99–111.

Zoller M (1995). CD44: physiological expression of distinct isoforms as evidence for organ-specific metastasis formation. *J Mol Med* **73**: 425–38.

Chapter 8

EPITHELIAL CELL SIGNALLING IN COLORECTAL CANCER METASTASIS

Caroline Saucier[1] and Nathalie Rivard[2]
[1]Département d'Anatomie et de Biologie Cellulaire, Faculté de Médecine et des Sciences de la Santé, Université de Sherbrooke, Sherbrooke, QC, Canada
e-mail: Caroline.Saucier@USherbrooke.ca
[2]Département d'Anatomie et de Biologie Cellulaire, Faculté de Médecine et des Sciences de la Santé, Université de Sherbrooke, Sherbrooke, QC, Canada
e-mail: Nathalie.Rivard@USherbrooke.ca

Abstract: The development of metastatic tumours is a complex process that consists of a series of cellular events that shift neoplastic cells from the primary tumour to a distant location (Chambers et al., 2002). Cancer cells must first detach from the primary tumour and invade the surrounding stroma, degrade the basement membrane, disseminate and survive into the circulatory systems, and ultimately extravasate and colonize a new microenvironment. Research of the past decades has revealed that complex and redundant signalling pathways in both tumour and the microenvironment govern tumour cell invasion at the primary site, survival in the bloodstream, and progressive outgrowth at distant sites. In this chapter, we highlight the role of growth factor receptor tyrosine kinase (RTK) signalling pathways in progression of colorectal cancer (CRC) to advanced metastatic disease, with a particular focus on those leading to activation of the proliferative RAS/Mitogen-activated protein kinase (MAPK) and survival Phosphatidylinositol 3-kinase (PI3K)/AKT pathways in epithelial colorectal cancer cells.

Keywords: Receptor tyrosine kinase · RAS · RAF · ERK · PI3K · PTEN · AKT · MAPK

8.1 Receptor Tyrosine Kinase Signalling in Colorectal Cancer Metastases

As normal intestinal epithelial cells evolve to become highly malignant colorectal cancer (CRC) cells, they acquire peculiar hallmarks, which enable them to aberrantly grow, to disregard normal growth inhibitory and death signals, to sustain angiogenesis as well as to invade tissue (Hanahan and Weinberg, 2000). Remarkably, these are all biological attributes featured during normal embryonic development and wound healing, which are to a large extent orchestrated by growth factor receptor tyrosine kinase (RTKs) signalling networks in a tightly regulated manner. Not surprisingly, experimental and clinical evidences entailing a role for deregulation of RTKs in the etiology and progression of human cancers are abundant and compelling, including colorectal malignancies. In this respect, RTKs have been evidenced to control key cellular processes involved in cancer metastases. For instance, metastatic relevant biological characteristics foreseen to be ascribed in part to the deregulation of RTKs in cancer include proliferation, survival, epithelial-mesenchymal transition (EMT), anchorage-independent growth, migration and invasion as well as angiogenesis, the formation of new blood vessels from the preexisting vasculature (Blume-Jensen and Hunter, 2001). It is now well-recognized that RTK signalling pathways represent promising therapeutic targets in metastatic CRC. In this section, we highlight evidence that links deregulation of RTKs to colorectal metastases and the mechanisms by which RTKs engage the mitogenic RAS/Mitogen-activated protein kinase (MAPK) and survival Phosphatidylinositol 3-kinase (PI3K)/AKT signalling cascades.

8.1.1 Receptor Tyrosine Kinase Structure and Mechanisms of Activation

Growth factor receptor tyrosine kinases are cell surface receptors relaying extracellular cues to achieve alterations in cell fate. These receptors typically present an extracellular segment that binds a ligand (growth factors), a single hydrophobic transmembrane spanning domain, and a cytoplasmic domain containing an intrinsic tyrosine-specific kinase activity (Fig. 8.1). The initial event in activation of RTKs consists in the association of the ligand to the extracellular domain of the receptor that promotes receptor dimerization and/or oligomerization. This, in turn, releases auto-inhibitory constraints allowing the binding of ATP within the intracellular catalytic domain, leading consequently to the activation of the tyrosine kinase and autophosphorylation of the receptor on specific tyrosine residues. Whereas the phosphorylated tyrosine residues located within the activation loop of the catalytic domain stabilize the receptor in an active state, those located outside the catalytic domain create specific binding sites for a variety of signalling proteins, which contain Src homology 2 (SH2) or phosphotyrosine-binding (PTB) domains that recognize phosphorylated tyrosine residues in the context of their surrounding amino acids. Among the variety of signalling proteins directly recruited

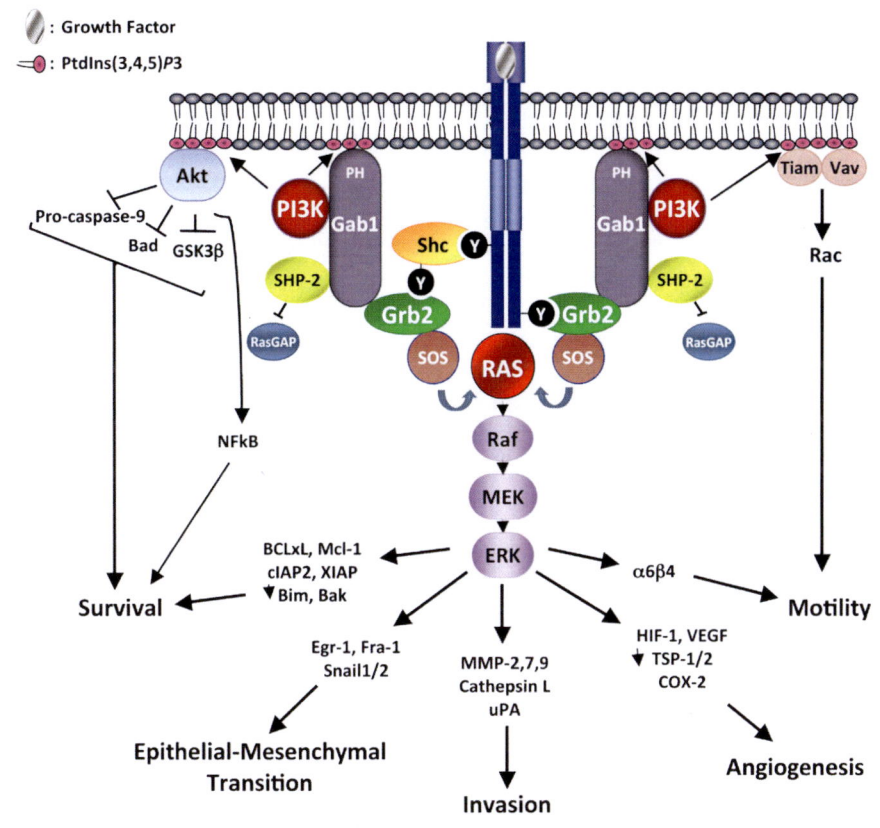

8 Epithelial Cell Signalling in Colorectal Cancer Metastasis

Fig. 8.1 Schematic representation of distinct signalling pathways activated downstream of RTKs involved in colorectal metastasis. Activation of RTKs following ligand stimulation or ligand-independent dimerization promotes their phosphorylation on multiple tyrosine residues (Y; only two are depicted here for simplicity). Those located in the C-terminal portion and primarily outside of the kinase domain of RTKs represent binding motifs for the recruitment of signalling protein effectors, such as Grb2 and/or Shc adaptor proteins. These, in turn, lead to the activation of the Ras/Raf/MEK/ERK pathway through the formation of Grb2/SOS and/or Grb2/Gab1/SHP-2 protein complexes. RTK-mediated signalling also activates the PI3K/AKT pathway, which mediates anti-apoptotic effects of RTK activation and alters Rho GTPases activity that remodels actin cytoskeleton. The coordinated activation of Ras/MAPK and PI3K/AKT signalling cascades by RTKs regulates the expression of key proteins involved in metastasis-relevant cellular responses including tumour-cell proliferation, EMT, protection from apoptosis, migration, invasion and angiogenesis. Abbreviations used are: Receptor tyrosine kinase, RTK; growth factor receptor-bound protein 2, Grb2; Shc Src-homology collagen protein, Shc; Grb2-associated binding protein-1; tyrosine phosphatase SHP-2; phosphatidylinositol 3-kinase, PI3K and epithelial-mesenchymal transition, EMT

to RTKs in a phosphotyrosine-dependent manner, these include molecules with intrinsic enzymatic activity as well as adaptor or scaffold proteins such as Shc (Src-homology collagen protein), Grb2 (growth factor receptor-bound protein 2), or Gab1 (Grb2-associated binding protein-1), that even though they lack enzymatic activity themselves, they encompass protein–protein interaction motifs and domains driving the formation of multiprotein complexes to the activated receptor. RTKs therefore act as docking proteins to assemble specific networks of signalling proteins that relay and amplify a series of downstream signals within the interior of the cell that culminate in specific biological responses (reviewed in Pawson and Nash, 2000). As anticipated, activation of RTKs is subsequently overridden by negative regulation under normal physiological settings. This involves in most cases ligand-mediated ubiquitination of the RTK through the Grb2-dependent recruitment of Cbl (Casitas B-cell lymphoma) protein. This is a substrate of RTKs that possesses E3-ubiquitin-protein ligase activity that mediates rapid internalization and trafficking of active ligand-receptor complexes inside the cell into endocytic cellular compartments, where they can either be sorted for lysosomal degradation or recycled back to the cell surface. It is worth mentioning that once internalized, RTK complexes do continue to signal along the endocytic pathway, thereby contributing to spatio-temporal regulation of RTK signal transduction in cells (reviewed in Abella and Park, 2009).

8.1.2 Deregulation of Receptor Tyrosine Kinase, a Common Feature in Colon Metastases

Oncogenic activation of RTKs in human malignancies can be evoked as a result of gain-of-function type of gene alterations conferring ligand-independent receptor activation, such as point mutations, deletions or chromosomal rearrangements fusing the cytoplasmic domain of RTKs to dimerization motifs, or by mutations that reduce degradation of the receptor. However, such RTK alterations appear to be relatively rare in human colorectal malignancies (Barber et al., 2004; Lenz et al., 2006; Nagahara et al., 2005; Tsuchihashi et al., 2005; Zeng et al., 2008). Dysregulation of RTKs in human CRC rather implicates the creation of autocrine/paracrine ligand-receptor activation loops. It also involves RTK over-expression through gene amplification or increased transcription/translation, thereby lowering the threshold response of cells to growth factor stimulation and even leading to receptor activation in the absence of ligand. Among RTKs family members, those that are aberrantly activated in this manner in CRC include members of the epidermal growth factor receptor family (EGFR/HER/ErbB 1-4), the hepatocyte growth factor receptor (Met/HGF RTK), the receptor for the type I insulin-like growth factor (IGF-1R), the platelet-derived growth factor (PDGFR) and the vascular endothelial growth factor (VEGFR) (Cohen et al., 2005). Herein, we briefly highlight evidence underscoring the importance of EGFR and Met/HGF receptor deregulation in colorectal metastases.

8.1.2.1 EGFR

EGFR is a member of the HER family that, upon interaction with EGF-related ligands, such as the epidermal growth factor (EGF) and transforming growth factor-α (TGF-α), transmits intracellular signals playing pivotal roles in the development and tissue homeostasis of various organs, including the intestine (Miettinen et al., 1995). In CRC, EGFR overexpression in colonic tumours and its association with an advanced disease stage is well-documented, with colorectal-derived liver metastases expressing EGFR levels by far superior than the corresponding primary tumour (Goldstein and Armin, 2001; Kluftinger et al., 1992; Spano et al., 2005b). Although the clinical prognostic value of EGFR expression in terms of survival in CRC remains a controversial issue (Spano et al., 2005a), the EGFR expression level has been reported to predict poor survival outcome and lower response rates in locally-advanced rectal cancer patients undergoing radiotherapy (Giralt et al., 2005; Zlobec et al., 2007). Incidentally, it has been shown that human colorectal tumour specimens display greater expression levels of EGFR ligands, such as TGF-α and EGF, and of EGFR relative to adjacent normal mucosa (Liu et al., 1990). Co-expression of both EGFR and TGF-α represents a common feature of more advanced human colorectal tumours (Barozzi et al., 2002; De Jong et al., 1998). Experimentally, the extent of EGFR expression in human colon carcinoma cells isolated from surgical specimens or in CRC-derived cell lines was shown to predict their proficiency to produce experimental liver metastasis following their intrasplenic injection into mice (Radinsky et al., 1995). Furthermore, EGFR phosphorylation levels, reflecting its state of activation, are increased in human colorectal carcinoma cells of liver metastases relative to primary tumours growing orthotopically in the caecum or ectopically in the spleen of nude mice (Parker et al., 1998). Thus, this suggests that communication between the tumour cells and their microenvironment impacts on the EGFR activation status in CRC cells and on the formation of metastases. Consistent with this notion, both tumour cells and tumour-associated endothelial cells in surgical specimens of human colon adenocarcinoma growing orthotopically in nude mice were shown to display TGF-α/EGFR and VEGF/VEGFR autocrine/paracrine activating loops, hence phosphorylated EGFR and VEGFR (Kuwai et al., 2008a; Yokoi et al., 2005). Importantly, EGFR activation in tumour-associated endothelial cells is greatly dependent on the production of TGF-α by the tumour cells, and represents a major determinant in colorectal tumour responses to EGFR-specific targeted therapy (Kuwai et al., 2008a). Moreover, in a model of HT29 human CRC cells implanted in the caecum of nude mice, treatment with a small molecule inhibiting both EGFR and VEGFR tyrosine kinases (AEE788) inhibits EGFR and VEGFR phosphorylation in tumour cells and in tumour-associated endothelial cells, and reduces primary tumour growth and the incidence of lymph node metastases (Yokoi et al., 2005). A recent study provided part of the mechanistic basis underlying the importance of autocrine/paracrine EGFR signalling in colon cancer cells in promoting metastases. Namely, EGFR activation in tumour cells by TGF-α was shown to engage tumour-stromal signalling networks, thereby creating a primary tumour microenvironment favourable to the metastatic dissemination of cancer cells, i.e. by increasing the production of pro-angiogenic regulators, such as VEGF, IL-8, and matrix degrading enzymes (MMP-2 & 9), and by promoting the recruitment of macrophages, hence the formation of blood and lymphatic vessels (Sasaki et al., 2008).

8.1.2.2 Met/HGF Receptor

HGF is a pleiotropic cytokine of mesenchymal origin that, depending on the cell context, can promote proliferation, differentiation, survival, migration, invasion and tissue-specific morphogenic programs via activation of the Met/HGF RTK in a wide spectrum of epithelial cells (Birchmeier et al., 2003; Peschard and Park, 2007). Compelling evidence infers an important role of the Met/HGF receptor-signalling axis in CRC metastasis. In occurrence, the expression of the Met/HGF receptor and of its ligand, HGF, is enhanced in the majority of CRCs at the earliest stages of the disease. Moreover the Met/HGF receptor is over-expressed in virtually all invasive colorectal carcinomas and amplified in 10% of colorectal liver metastases (Di Renzo et al., 1995; Fazekas et al., 2000; Hiscox et al., 1997; Liu et al., 1992; Otte et al., 2000). Incidentally, increased expression of Met/HGF receptor is recognized as a powerful indicator for early stages of invasion and metastasis of colorectal human tumours, and the co-expression of Met and HGF in primary colon cancers represents a predictor of tumour staging and clinical outcome (Di Renzo et al., 1995; Fazekas et al., 2000; Kammula et al., 2007; Takeuchi et al., 2003). Interestingly, the c-*Met* gene was identified as a transcriptional target of β-catenin, HIF-1 (Hypoxia-inducible factor-1) and MACC1 (metastasis associated in colon cancer 1), which provides potential basis for the up-regulation of Met/HGF receptor expression in CRC (Pennacchietti et al., 2003; Rasola et al., 2007; Stein et al., 2009). In this respect, expression of MACC1 was recently identified as an independent prognostic indicator of metastasis in primary CRC specimens (Stein et al., 2009).

Several studies have documented that HGF stimulation or over-expression of the Met/HGF receptor can confer metastatic properties to human and mouse colorectal tumour-derived cell lines, including cell scattering migration and invasion in culture (Fassetta et al., 2006; Kataoka et al., 2000; Kermorgant et al., 2001; Long et al., 2003; Stein et al., 2009). Conversely, inhibition of Met/HGF receptor signalling through various approaches in highly metastatic CRC-derived cell lines was shown to reduce their metastatic activities in vitro, i.e.: blocking cell motility and invasiveness, and to impair their capacity to form metastases in animal models (Arena et al., 2007; Herynk et al., 2003; Parr et al., 2000; Stein et al., 2009; van der Horst et al., 2009; Wen et al., 2004, 2007). More recently, constitutive activation of the Met/HGF receptor in normal-derived intestinal or colonic epithelial cells was shown to be sufficient to evoke EMT-like morphological transformation and a loss of E-cadherin expression, and to enhance proliferation and anchorage-independent cell growth (Bernier et al., 2010; Boon et al., 2005). Notably, oncogenic activation of the Met/HGF receptor endows non-cancerous intestinal epithelial cells with the capacity to produce VEGF and elicit angiogenic responses, and to form sub-cutaneous tumours and experimental lung metastases in mice (Bernier et al., 2010). These results further substantiate the importance of Met/HGF receptor signalling in CRC metastasis, but further advocate that deregulation of the Met/HGF receptor, may itself be an initiating event in malignant progression of CRC.

8.1.2.3 Receptor Tyrosine Kinase-Targeted Therapy

Because of their relevance in the progression of CRC, RTK-targeting agents are viewed as a promising therapeutic approach in human CRC. Whereas several therapeutic agents targeting RTKs are at various clinical trial phases (clinicaltrials.gov), monoclonal antibodies targeting EGFR (Cetuximab/Erbitux and Panitumumab/Vectibix) and VEGFR (Bevacizumab/Avastin), have received Food and Drug Administration (FDA) approval in 2004 as treatment for metastatic CRCs. However, marginal clinical benefits have been observed so far with agents targeting a single RTK in CRC. One possible reason, among others, for this mitigated success is the manifest heterogeneity of RTKs in CRC. Hence, targeting multiple RTKs simultaneously may achieve better therapeutic effects than targeting a specific RTK (Cohen and Hochster, 2007; Kaulfuss et al., 2009; Kuwai et al., 2008b). Another alternative may reside on targeting downstream signalling effectors of RTKs representing converging critical nodes, i.e.: cellular effectors that are engaged by all, or at least several growth factor RTKs and which are regulating biological processes essential for the initiation and/or malignant progression of CRC. This concept has been already supported experimentally with Grb2-SH2 domain-binding antagonists that were shown to block Met/HGF receptor-induced motility and invasion, to reduce angiogenesis in endothelial cell culture models and to diminish the ability of a human prostate cancer cell line to form experimental metastases in mice (Giubellino et al., 2008). Hence, one of the challenges in the development of new CRC therapies may rely on the identification of these potential targets, and therefore on a better understanding of the role of RTK downstream signalling effectors in CRC progression.

8.1.3 The Role of RTK-Proximal Signalling Effectors: Road Maps to the Activation of RAS/MAPK and PI3K/AKT

The Grb2 molecule is a small adaptor protein widely expressed and essential for a wide spectrum of cellular activities (Cheng et al., 1998; Saxton et al., 2001). It is structurally composed of a single SH2 domain flanked on each side by an SH3 domain. While the Grb2-SH2 domain binds directly to tyrosine-phosphorylated sequences found in many activated receptors, each of the Grb2-SH3 domains interacts with distinct sets of proline-rich containing proteins, thereby directing the translocation of specific multiprotein complexes to RTK at the plasma membrane (Fig. 8.1) (Pawson and Nash, 2003). In addition to physically interacting directly with activated RTKs, Grb2 is also recruited to some RTKs through an indirect mechanism implicating the Shc adaptor protein (referring herein to the ShcA protein isoforms). The Shc protein interacts with activated RTKs mainly via the ability of its N-terminal PTB domain to recognize NPXpY sequence motifs found within many RTKs. The recruitment of Shc to RTKs results in phosphorylation of tyrosine residues (Y239/240/317) within the collagen-homology domain 1 (CH1) of Shc, which represent consensus-binding sites for the Grb2 adaptor protein SH2 domain, thereby engaging Grb2-dependent signalling pathways (Fig. 8.1) (reviewed in Ravichandran, 2001).

The best-characterized mechanism by which Grb2 couples RTKs to the activation of the RAS/MAPK signalling pathway involves the translocation of the cytosolic RAS-specific guanine nucleotide exchange factor SOS (Son of sevenless) in close proximity of RAS localized at the plasma membrane. This is mediated by the virtue of SOS to be constitutively associated with the Grb2 N-SH3 domain (Fig. 8.1). On the other hand, the C-terminal SH3 domain of Grb2 associates with members of the Grb2-associated binder scaffold protein family, such as Gab1, thereby providing an alternative mechanism by which Grb2 couples RTKs to the RAS/MAPK pathway. In addition, this association represents a means to activate the anti-apoptotic PI3K/AKT signalling pathway (Gu and Neel, 2003). The importance of these two oncogenic signalling pathways in CRC is described in details in Sections 8.2.1 and 8.2.2 of this chapter.

Gab1 belongs to a family of large docking/scaffolding proteins that function as amplifiers and integrators for signals of growth factor RTKs. They do so by mobilizing multimeric signalling complexes which, depending on the receptor and cellular contexts, regulate proliferation, survival, migration and morphogenesis (Gu and Neel, 2003). The Gab1 protein encompasses an N-terminal pleckstrin homology (PH) domain, two proline-rich Grb2 binding sites, in addition to multiple tyrosine residues, which, when phosphorylated, represent binding sites for multiple SH2 domain containing signalling effectors, including the tyrosine phosphatase SHP-2, the regulatory subunit of the PI3K and the RAS-GTPase activating protein (RAS-GAP), a negative regulator of RAS (Gu and Neel, 2003; Montagner et al., 2005). The interaction of the Gab protein with virtually all RTKs involves Grb2-dependent mediated events. Whereas the Grb2-SH2 domain binds to tyrosine-phosphorylated motifs found within activated receptors, the C-terminal SH3 domain of Grb2 constitutively associates with proline-rich domains in Gab proteins (Fig. 8.1) (Gu and Neel, 2003). However, the association of Gab1 with the Met/HGF receptor is unique, since it also takes place via a direct interaction involving a central 19-amino acid sequence (referred as the Met-binding site) found exclusively within Gab1. This dual mode of recruitment of Gab1 to the Met/HGF receptor is critical for Met-induced sustained activation of MAPK and branching morphogenesis of epithelial MDCK cells, as well as placenta development and liver growth in mice. Yet, the direct or the Grb2-dependent recruitment of Gab1 to the Met/HGF receptor are sufficient for induction of cell-cycle progression and muscle precursor cell migration in mice (Birchmeier et al., 2003; Gu and Neel, 2003; Mood et al., 2006a; Peschard and Park, 2007; Schaeper et al., 2007).

The current model for activation of the RAS/MAPK downstream of Gab1 involves the targeting of phospho-Gab1/SHP-2 multiprotein complex at the plasma membrane. SHP-2 promotes dephosphorylation of specific tyrosine residues in Gab1, representing RASGAP binding sites, a negative regulator of RAS, thereby enabling sustained activation of the RAS/MAPK pathway (Fig. 8.1) (Montagner et al., 2005). The importance of SHP-2 in RTK-mediated activation and biological functions of RAS/MAPK is underscored by studies showing that the expression of a Gab1 mutant defective in SHP-2-binding or of a SHP-2 dominant negative mutant greatly hinders activation of RAS/MAPK pathway and Gab1-mediated responses downstream of a variety of RTKs. This includes oncogenic transformation induced by RTK-derived oncoproteins (Gu and Neel, 2003; Holgado-Madruga and Wong, 2004; Mood et al., 2006a; Peschard and Park, 2007).

A critical role for Gab1 in activation of PI3K/AKT survival signalling pathway triggered by RTKs, such as for the Met/HGF receptor, EGFR and VEGFR, is also well established (Dance et al., 2006; Gu and Neel, 2003; Mattoon et al., 2004; Peschard and Park, 2007). In addition to its interaction with cell surface receptors, the preferential binding of the Gab1 PH domain to phosphatidylinositol 3-4-5 triphosphate (PIP3), the lipid product of PI3K, is proposed to participate in the targeting of Gab1-associated protein complexes to the plasma membrane and PIP3-rich micro-domains in cells (Fig. 8.1) (Maroun et al., 1999; Rodrigues et al., 2000). Hence, the ability of Gab1 to recruit the PI3K enzyme provides a positive-feedback mechanism for increasing the PIP3 amount at the cell membrane, thereby further facilitating Gab1 mobilization into receptor complex as well as its subsequent tyrosine phosphorylation and activation of downstream signalling pathways. Therefore, activation of PI3K downstream of RTKs is not only a major regulatory step leading to the activation of AKT-dependent survival pathways in cells, but also acts in conjunction with Gab1 and SHP-2 to enable sustained activation of the RAS/MAPK pathway. Consistent with this notion, inhibition of PI3K activity has often been reported to reduce RAS/MAPK activation and proliferation induced by a variety of RTKs, including the Met/HGF receptor. However, the engagement of PI3K-dependent signals is apparently not sufficient to trigger cell proliferation downstream of RTKs and Gab1 (Mood et al., 2006a, b; Schaeper et al., 2007).

The shared capacity of Grb2, Shc and Gab1 to engage RAS/MAPK and PI3K/AKT signalling pathways downstream of RTKs, among others, implies that targeting these RTK effectors may represent a promising strategy in the treatment of CRC. However, this warrants further investigation to determine the specific roles of these effectors as integrators of PI3K/AKT and RAS/MAPK in CRC metastasis.

8.1.3.1 The Role of Grb2, Shc, and Gab1 Adaptor Proteins in Colorectal Cancer: An Open Question

Structure/function studies performed predominantly in breast cancer and fibroblast cell models have unveiled key roles for Grb2, Shc and Gab1 adaptor proteins downstream of RTKs in biological events contributing to the development and progression of cancers. For instance, the exclusive oncogenic engagement of either the Grb2 or Shc-dependent signals by RTKs is sufficient to promote cell-cycle progression, morphological oncogenic transformation and anchorage-independent growth in fibroblast culture models as well as tumourigenesis and experimental lung metastasis in nude mice (Dankort et al., 1997; Mood et al., 2006b; Saucier et al., 2002). However, signalling pathways engaged by the Shc adaptor protein play a unique and critical role in promoting VEGF production and early onset of tumour angiogenesis downstream of the Met/HGF and ErbB2 (EGFR2/HER2) receptors

(Saucier et al., 2004; Ursini-Siegel et al., 2008). On the other hand, the docking protein Gab1 is essential for Met/HGF receptor-mediated invasive branching morphogenesis of MDCK epithelial cells, EGFR-dependent proliferation and migration as well as for cellular transformation induced by a variety of RTK-derived oncogenes, including oncogenic forms of the EGFR and of the Met/HGF receptor (Gu and Neel, 2003; Holgado-Madruga and Wong, 2004; Peschard and Park, 2007; Seiden-Long et al., 2008).

Although, the deregulation of RTK signalling pathways is regarded as a major determinant in malignant CRC progression, very few studies have directly addressed the roles of the RTK-proximal signalling effectors in CRC. Nonetheless, Yu et al. have recently demonstrated greater levels of *Grb2* gene expression in CRC metastatic cells relative to primary tumour cells (Yu et al., 2008). As well, Yu et al. showed an association between immunohistochemical detection of Grb2 in human colorectal carcinoma specimens and distant metastases, and demonstrated that treatment with a Grb2-SH2 antagonist reduced the migration of the SW620 human CRC cells in vitro (Yu et al., 2008). Moreover, results of a study by Seiden-Long et al. suggest that over-expression of the Met/HGF receptor in human DLD-1 CRC cells that harbour a *K-RAS* activating mutation, accelerates tumour growth by mechanisms dependent on Gab1 signals, but not on those of Grb2 or Shc (Seiden-Long et al., 2008). On the other hand, elevated expression of the p66Shc protein isoform in tumour was found to predict disease relapse and survival in stage IIA colon cancer (Grossman et al., 2007). In mammals, the *ShcA* gene encodes three distinct isoforms (p66, p52 & p46Shc). The p66Shc isoform was characterized, among the other Shc isoforms, to uniquely promote apoptosis in response to cellular oxygen stress (Giorgio et al., 2005; Nemoto and Finkel, 2002) and to negatively regulate MAPK activation triggered by growth factor RTKs, partly by counteracting p52Shc-mediated activation of this pathway (Migliaccio et al., 1997; Okada et al., 1997).

Overall, these results point to a potential central role for the Grb2, Shc and Gab1 adaptor/scaffolding proteins in CRC metastasis. Incidentally, these effectors have in common the property to integrate RTK signalling pathways leading to the activation of RAS/MAPK and PI3K/AKT that represent two critical signalling cascades in progression of CRC.

8.2 The K-RAS Oncogene and Its Downstream Signalling

As discussed in Chapter 5 in this book, activating mutations of the RAS family members are among the most common genetic events in human tumourigenesis (Bos, 1989). Specifically, *K-RAS* is mutated in nearly 50% of colorectal tumours at a relatively early stage of the carcinogenic process (Malumbres and Barbacid, 2003), and despite extensive research, the primary reason for this high frequency remains unclear. Genetic and biochemical studies have firmly established the central role of RAS GTPases in regulating cell proliferation, growth and survival (Pretlow and Pretlow, 2005). Recent studies suggest that RAS signalling may contribute to metastasis formation in CRC (Smakman et al., 2005). A large population-based study involving 1,413 CRC patients showed that *K-RAS* codon 12 mutations were more frequently detected in advanced stage CRC with regional lymph node involvement and distant metastases than in non-metastatic tumours (Samowitz et al., 2000). However, the downstream effector pathways directly involved remain unclear. More than ten distinct classes of RAS effectors have been identified to date, several of which are associated with oncogenic signalling pathways (Malumbres and Barbacid, 2003). Two classes of RAS effectors are now well-established (Fig. 8.1): the Raf family of protein kinases leading to sequential phosphorylation and activation of the MAPKs MEK1/MEK2 and ERK1/ERK2, and the type 1 PI3K, leading to phosphorylation and activation of the AKT kinases (Malumbres and Barbacid, 2003).

8.2.1 The ERK MAPK Signalling Pathway

Upon activation by growth factor-stimulated receptors, activated RAS complexes promote and activate Raf kinases, which in turn activate MEK1 and MEK2, resulting in activation of ERK1 and ERK2. Activated ERKs then translocate into the nucleus where they phosphorylate and activate nuclear transcription factors such as Elk-1, ATF-2 and ETS1/2 resulting in immediate-early gene induction. Studies on cultured intestinal epithelial cells have revealed a close correlation between ERK activation and DNA synthesis, while pharmacological or molecular inhibition of cellular ERK activity has been shown to block cell cycle progression (Meloche and Pouyssegur, 2007; Ramos, 2008; Rivard et al., 1999). Notably, the phosphorylated and activated forms of ERK1/2 have mostly been detected in the nucleus of undifferentiated proliferative crypt cells in human fetal small intestine (Aliaga et al., 1999), hence supporting the role of these kinases in the control of cell proliferation in intestinal crypts. The critical involvement of this MAPK cascade in intestinal tumourigenesis is supported by a number of experimental observations. Firstly, mutations of B-RAF, a member of the Raf family, are associated with increased kinase activity and have been found in 10–15% of CRCs; many of those with such mutations are at early Dukes' stage (A and B) (Davies et al., 2002; Rajagopalan et al., 2002). Furthermore, B-RAF mutations are frequently identified in sporadic CRC with microsatellite instability (Deng et al., 2004). Secondly, it has been demonstrated that MEK is phosphorylated and activated in 30–40% of adenomas and in 76% of colorectal tumours (Eggstein et al., 1999; Lee et al., 2004). Thirdly, CRCs exhibit particularly high frequencies of ERK activation (Hoshino et al., 1999) and some studies have reported that ERK1/2 activities are elevated in intestinal tumours (Kuno et al., 1998; Licato and Brenner, 1998). Fourthly, treatment with synthetic MEK1/2 inhibitors markedly attenuates the proliferation of colon carcinoma cells in vitro and in mouse xenografts (Sebolt-Leopold et al., 1999). Fifthly, we and others have recently shown that expression of constitutively active MEK1 in non-transformed rat intestinal epithelial crypt cell lines is sufficient to induce growth factor relaxation for DNA synthesis and to promote morphological transformation and growth in soft agar (Boucher et al., 2004; Komatsu et al., 2005). Therefore, much emphasis has been placed on treatment strategies that target this protein kinase cascade (Roberts and Der, 2007). In particular, potent and selective inhibitors of MEK1 and MEK2 have been developed and are currently in phase I/II clinical trials (AZD6244, XL51, and ARRY-162) (Haigis et al., 2008). Interestingly, an early study reported that the enzymatic activity of ERK1/ERK2 is markedly up-regulated during late progression of carcinogen-induced colon carcinomas (Licato et al., 1997). More importantly, we and others have also reported that activation of MEK1 and MEK2 is sufficient to fully transform intestinal epithelial cells and to induce invasive and metastatic tumours in nude mice (Lemieux et al., 2009; Voisin et al., 2008). Together, these observations strengthen the idea that ERK1/2 MAP kinase signalling may play a critical role in CRC progression (Fang and Richardson, 2005).

8.2.2 The PI3K Signalling Pathway

The PI3K, a ubiquitous lipid kinase involved in RTKs signal transduction as mentioned above, comprises a large and complex family that includes 3 classes with multiple subunits and isoforms (Anderson and Jackson, 2003). The class I PI3Ks are composed of a SH2 domain-containing the 85 kDa regulatory subunit (p85) and a 110-kDa catalytic subunit (p110), which catalyze the phosphorylation of phosphoinositol 4-phosphate and phosphoinositol 4,5-phosphate at their D3 position (PIP3). The PI3K regulatory subunits include p85α and its truncated splice variants p50α and p55α, as well as p85β and p55γ; the catalytic subunits include p110α, p110β, and p110Δ for class IA and p110γ for class IB. The regulatory subunits p85α, p50α, and p55α are encoded by the *Pik3r1* gene; p85α is the most abundantly expressed regulatory isoform of PI3K, and p55α and p50α are two additional minor alternative splicing isoforms. The type I enzymes have been extensively studied and were originally identified in association with tyrosine kinases such as growth factor receptors and products of oncogenes such as K-RAS (Zhao and Vogt, 2008). Most studies evaluating the type I PI3Ks have focused on the α form. In particular, class IA PI3Ks are strongly expressed in colonic epithelial carcinoma cell lines (Shao et al., 2004). The gene coding for p110α (*Pik3cα*) is amplified in ovarian and breast tumours (Campbell et al., 2004) implicating *Pik3cα* as a potential oncogene in these cancers. The *Pik3ca* gene is also mutated in 20–25% of CRCs. *Pik3ca* mutations occurring in hotspots located in exon 9 and exon 20 are oncogenic in CRC cell models (Ikenoue et al., 2005). *Pik3ca* gene abnormalities seem to occur at relatively late stages of neoplasia, when tumours begin to invade and metastasize (Samuels et al., 2005). The implication of PI3K in different steps of carcinogenesis is also strongly suggested by the expression of PTEN, a lipid phosphatase that keeps phosphatidylinositol 3-4 biphosphate (PIP2) and PIP3 in their dephosphorylated forms (Wu et al., 1998). This phosphatase is encoded by the *PTEN* gene (phosphatase and tensin homolog deleted on chromosome 10), which is a tumour-suppressor gene located on chromosomal band 10q23. The *PTEN* mutations have an important role in sporadic colorectal tumourigenesis, where *PTEN* expression is moderate or lost in more that 70% of CRC patients (Colakoglu et al.,

2008; Zhou et al., 2002). Although inherited hamartoma polyposis syndromes like Cowden disease generally show germ-line mutations of *PTEN* (Chi et al., 1998; Eng, 2003), there are very few data supporting a role for PTEN in adenomatous polyps. Interestingly, Colakoglu et al. (2008) noted no PTEN expression in 40% of patients with polyps, a higher percentage than in tumour patients (5.3%). Although this relationship remains to be elucidated in prospective studies, PTEN loss may be important for the adenoma-colon cancer sequence. More recently, loss of PTEN expression has been associated with CRC liver metastasis and poor patient survival (Eng, 2003).

In addition to the regulation of normal intestinal epithelial cell proliferation and differentiation (Laprise et al., 2002; Sheng et al., 2003; Wang et al., 2001), the promotion of cell survival by the activation of PI3K occurs by the inhibition of pro-apoptotic signals and the induction of survival signals, which contribute to malignant transformation and tumour progression (Blume-Jensen and Hunter, 2001). In this regard, there is a growing body of evidence to support the notion that the activation of PI3K/AKT is associated with colorectal carcinoma and can convert differentiated human gastric or colonic carcinoma cells to a less differentiated and more malignant phenotype (Semba et al., 2002). *Pik3ca* mutations in CRC cell lines result in the capacity of cells to migrate and invade in vitro and are also essential for the formation of metastases in an orthotopic cancer mouse model (Guo et al., 2007; Samuels et al., 2005). The effects of PI3K on tumour growth and progression are thought to be mediated by AKT, a downstream effector of PI3K (Fresno Vara et al., 2004). The AKT family defines a family of closely related highly conserved cellular homologs of the viral oncoprotein v-akt. In humans, there are three members of the *Akt* gene family, designated *Akt1*, *Akt2* and *Akt3*, which are located on different chromosomes. The *Akt* gene products, cytoplasmic serine/threonine (Ser/Thr)-specific protein kinases, are major downstream targets of numerous RTK signalling via PI3K (reviewed in Engelman et al., 2006). In CRC, AKT is over-expressed (Roy et al., 2002), and it has been reported that AKT phosphorylation in human colon carcinomas correlates with cell proliferation and apoptosis inhibition as well as with different clinico-pathological parameters, such as invasion grade, vessel infiltration, metastasis to lymph nodes and tumour stage (Itoh et al., 2002; Khaleghpour et al., 2004). More importantly, the following evidence recently highlighted the critical role of AKT2 in the establishment of CRC metastasis: First, AKT2 is over-expressed in late-stage CRC and metastatic tumours (Rychahou et al., 2006, 2008). Second, suppression of AKT2 expression in highly metastatic colorectal carcinoma cells inhibits their ability to metastasize in an experimental liver metastasis model (Rychahou et al., 2008). More importantly, AKT2 over-expression in the tumourigenic, but non-metastatic and wild-type PTEN-carrying SW480 CRC line, led to the formation of micrometastases (Rychahou et al., 2008). Taken together, these data support a role for AKT2 over-expression in metastatic colorectal cancer.

In the next section, we will discuss the specific influence of K-RAS and of its effectors MAPK and PI3K signalling on overcoming each of the distinct barriers that protect an organism against metastatic tumour growth.

8.2.3 Oncogenic K-RAS Signalling Inhibits Epithelial Cell Polarity

During the development of CRC, epithelial cells may loose their polarity and acquire a fibroblastic morphology (Smakman et al., 2005). This process is generally referred to as epithelial-mesenchymal transition (EMT) (see Chapter 6 by O. Schmalhofer et al., in this book). However, the degree of CRC de-differentiation varies greatly between tumours. Furthermore, the differentiation state of tumour cells within a single tumour may not be homogeneous: de-differentiated cells that have lost their polarization and their contact with other tumour cells are usually only observed at the invasive front of carcinomas, where single tumour cells detach from the primary tumour (Prall, 2007). Such 'budding' tumour cell clusters identify tumours with a high propensity to form haematogenous and regional metastases in CRC patients (Hase et al., 1993; Ono et al., 1996; Shinto et al., 2006).

Epithelial cell polarity largely depends on the Ca^{2+}-dependent cadherin-based adherens junctions (Nejsum and Nelson, 2009). Over-expression of H-RASG12V in rat intestinal epithelial cells or in MDCK cells leads to reduced cell–cell adhesion and adherens junction formation, which is accompanied by mis-localization and/or reduced expression of E-cadherin (Fujimoto et al., 2001; Potempa and Ridley, 1998; Schmidt et al., 2004, 2003). Conversely, it was found that deletion of the endogenous K-RASG13D oncogene from HCT-116 CRC cells did not affect E-cadherin expression or adherens junction formation, but restored their ability to assemble stress fibers and focal adhesions/complexes, accompanied by increased cell-matrix adhesion to collagens I and IV, to laminin and to fibronectin, and reduced motility (Pollock et al., 2005). Over-expression of the RAS target, c-Raf1, also causes MDCK cell depolarization and loss of intercellular contacts (Lehmann et al., 2000), whereas inhibition of MEK prevents it (Chen et al., 2000; Lehmann et al., 2000; Potempa and Ridley, 1998). Moreover, we and others have recently demonstrated that the expression of an activated MEK1 mutant is sufficient for the induction of EMT in intestinal epithelial crypt cells (Lemieux et al., 2009; Voisin et al., 2008). Indeed, expression of an activated MEK1 is sufficient to markedly down-regulate E-cadherin, occludin and ZO-1 expression, whereas an induction in N-cadherin and vimentin, two mesenchymal markers, was noted. In recent years, several direct transcriptional repressors of E-cadherin (Snail1, Snail2, deltaEF1, SIP1 and E47) have been identified (Batlle et al., 2000; Bolos et al., 2003; Cano et al., 2000; Comijn et al., 2001; Eger et al., 2005; Perez-Moreno et al., 2001). These proteins act downstream in EMT-inducing signal transduction pathways activated by transforming growth factor-β (TGF-β), fibroblast growth factor (FGF), EGF, integrin engagement and hypoxia (De Craene et al., 2005; Imamichi et al., 2007; Krishnamachary et al., 2006; Peinado et al., 2004a, b). Snail family members directly interact with the E-box response elements in the proximal *E-cadherin* gene promoter and could actively repress transcription by recruiting transcriptional co-repressors such as mSin3A (Peinado et al., 2004a). In addition, Snail1/Snail2 and deltaEF1/SIP1 proteins mediate up-regulation of genes implicated in cell invasion and motility (e.g., vimentin, members of the MMP family of proteases, fibronectin). We have shown that the transcription factors Egr-1 and Fra-1, an AP-1-like protein, are respectively responsible for MEK1-induced *Snail1* and *Snail2* gene expression (Lemieux et al., 2009), hence providing a mechanistic insight into how K-RAS signalling and MEK1 triggers EMT (Fig. 8.1). In this respect, transformation of intestinal epithelial cells by oncogenic RAS is blocked by MEK/ERK inhibition, but not by PI3K inhibition (Schmidt et al., 2003). Hence, this indicates that abnormal activation of K-RAS-Raf/MEK/ERK may disrupt epithelial cell polarity by destabilizing adherens junctions. Furthermore, abnormal activation of this pathway also reduces cell–matrix interactions probably through modulation of integrin expression, maturation and activity (Hughes et al., 1997; Schramm et al., 2000; Yan et al., 1997a), hence providing another mechanism by which this pathway may disrupt epithelial polarity. On the other hand, previous studies have also reported that the PI3K/AKT pathway may also promote EMT in intestinal epithelial cells. For example, PRL-3, a metastasis-associated phosphatase, down-regulates PTEN expression and signals through PI3K to promote EMT in the DLD-1 CRC cell line (Wang et al., 2007). Aside from these observations, it has been also demonstrated that expression of K-RASG12V up-regulates carcino-embryonic antigen (CEA) expression in CRC cells, with improper membrane localization and loss of basolateral polarity (Yan et al., 1997b). CEA is a cell surface glycoprotein that mediates homotypic Ca^{2+}-independent cell–cell interactions (Paschos et al., 2009) (please see Chapter 7 by Arabzadeh and Beauchemin, in this book). Its localization at the apical luminal membrane in polarized colonocytes is essential for maintaining basolateral polarity.

To what extent are all these phenomena associated with the occurrence of K-RAS mutations in human CRC remains to be established (Smakman et al., 2005). It is important to note that the epithelial cells in aberrant crypt foci (ACF), the earliest recognizable precursor lesions in CRC, usually retain their polarization and intercellular adhesion, yet frequently contain mutant K-RAS (Pretlow and Pretlow, 2005). This suggests that an acquired mutation in K-RAS during CRC development is not sufficient for a complete loss of epithelial cell polarity and for cell detachment. Another point is that local de-differentiation of tumour cells in the primary carcinoma is often reversed in distant metastases. This suggests that microenvironmental cues are important determinants of carcinoma cell differentiation, and that mutational activation or over-expression of RAS oncogenes may not be sufficient to induce de-differentiation of epithelial cells (Smakman et al., 2005). Signalling by TGF-β can cooperate with activated RAS to induce epithelial de-differentiation (Davies et al., 2005; Janda et al., 2002; Oft et al., 2002, 1998, 1996). In colonic epithelial cells, K-RASG12V, but not H-RASG12V, induces TGF-β-independent epithelial de-differentiation (Yan et al., 1997a). Interestingly, it has been recently demonstrated in mice that the combination of TGF-β signalling pathway inactivation and expression of oncogenic K-RAS leads to formation of invasive intestinal neoplasms and metastases (Trobridge et al., 2009). Therefore, this result supports the assumption that the de-differentiation of colonic epithelial cells during CRC development requires the cooperative action of TGF-β and oncogenic K-RAS (smakman et al., 2005).

8.2.4 Oncogenic K-RAS Signalling Promotes Cell Invasion, Migration and Intravasation

An essential process in forming distant metastases is the degradation of the extracellular matrix allowing tumour cells to invade local tissue, intravasate and extravasate blood vessels and build new metastatic sites (please see Chapter 1, in this book, for more details). This process is primarily influenced by the activity of proteinases secreted by the tumour. Currently, at least four classes of proteinases are known: serine proteinases (e.g.: urokinase plasminogen activator; uPA), aspartatic proteinases, cysteine proteinases (e.g.: cathepsins B, H and L) and matrix metalloproteinases (MMPs) (Berger, 2002; Jedeszko and Sloane, 2004; Wagenaar-Miller et al., 2004). Collectively, these proteinases are capable of breaking down all components of the extracellular matrix. Under physiological conditions, such as tissue remodelling, angiogenesis, ovulation or wound healing, there is a precise regulation between proteolytic degradation and regulatory inhibition of proteolysis. This physiological balance seems to be disrupted in cancer.

Laminin and collagen IV are the major constituents of epithelial basement membranes and are readily degraded by a variety of proteolytic enzymes. Degradation of the basal membrane (BM) not only removes a physical barrier for tumour cell dissemination, but also leads to the generation of laminin and collagen IV fragments that actively stimulate tumour cell migration and angiogenesis (Giannelli et al., 1997; Xu et al., 2001). MMPs are a family of zinc-dependent endopeptidases that are collectively capable of cleaving virtually all extracellular matrix substrates and play an important role in diverse physiological and pathological processes. In addition, MMPs cleave a plethora of non-ECM substrates, including cell surface- and matrix-bound growth factors and cytokines, growth factor receptors, proteases and their inhibitors and cell adhesion molecules (reviewed in Cauwe et al., 2007), thus creating a microenvironment that is conducive to local tumour outgrowth and angiogenesis. Several MMPs are up-regulated in almost every type of cancers and their expression is often associated with a poor prognosis for patients suffering of cancers including CRC (Cauwe et al., 2007; Curran et al., 2004). As mentioned above, K-RAS mutations are found already in pre-malignant lesions (ACF and adenomas) that usually contain intact BMs (Cheng and Lai, 2003). Thus, an acquired mutation in K-RAS alone is apparently not sufficient for the loss of BM integrity (Smakman et al., 2005). Nevertheless, mutant K-RAS may contribute to BM breakdown by stimulating the expression and/or activity of MMPs, cathepsins and uPA (see below). For example, MMP-7 (Matrilysin-1) is expressed early during CRC development (Newell et al., 1994) and its expression is correlated with metastatic potential (Adachi et al., 1999; Masaki et al., 2001). MMP-7 expression correlates with the presence of K-RAS mutations in pancreatic carcinomas (Fukushima et al., 2001), but not in colorectal carcinomas, where it correlates with nuclear β-catenin (Ougolkov et al., 2002). However, mutant K-RAS and EGF can stimulate MMP-7 expression in colorectal carcinoma cells through the ERK/MAPK pathway (Lynch et al., 2004; Yamamoto et al., 1995). MMP-7 is also highly expressed in APC-deficient polyps (with active β-catenin) in the mouse intestine and promotes intestinal polyp formation (Wilson et al., 1997). Thus, MMP-7 expression is a determinant of metastatic potential that is controlled by both K-RAS and β-catenin signalling. The early detection of MMP-7 in pre-malignant lesions during CRC development may therefore be the direct result of APC loss and/or mutational activation of K-RAS (Smakman et al., 2005). Recent studies revealed that the constitutive activation of MEK1 in normal intestinal crypt cells is sufficient to induce migration through Matrigel and expression of several other MMPs including MT1-MMP, MMP-2, MMP-3, MMP-9, MMP-10 and MMP-13 (Lemieux et al., 2009; Voisin et al., 2008). Other studies have also suggested a link between the ERK pathway and CRC cell invasion (Brand et al., 2005; Huang et al., 2009; Zhang et al., 2004). Hence, these provide a first molecular explanation for the regulation of invasion by activation of K-RAS (Fig. 8.1).

Urokinase plasminogen activator (uPA) is a serine protease whose major substrate is the zymogen plasminogen, which is cleaved and activated to form plasmin. By activating plasminogen, uPA is at the top of a proteolytic cascade that ends up in the cleavage, degradation, and sometimes activation of a myriad of proteins, including other proteases. Plasmin has broad substrate specificity and degrades fibrin and extracellular matrix components, but it can also activate MMPs resulting in further ECM breakdown. Tumour-associated uPA is produced both by stromal cells (Grondahl-Hansen et al., 1991; Pyke et al., 1991) and by tumour cells (Harvey et al., 1999). On tumour cells, the uPA receptor (uPAR) localizes uPA to the cell surface, thereby promoting pericellular proteolysis and tumour cell migration through BMs and extracellular matrices (Andreasen et al., 1997). Expression of K-RASG13D is required for high level expression of the uPA receptor in a human CRC cell line (Allgayer et al., 1999). In the same cells, K-RASG13D is also required to maintain co-localization of uPA with cathepsin B in caveolae at the cell surface (Cavallo-Medved et al., 2003, 2005). Expression of uPA has been found in tumours resulting from the subcutaneous injection of caMEK-expressing intestinal cells (Lemieux et al., 2009). Conversely, interactions between the cell-surface uPAR and integrins are crucial for tumour invasion and metastasis, and uPA increases basal ERK activation in colon cancer cells (Ahmed et al., 2003). Thus, oncogenic RAS signalling regulates a proteolytic cascade by promoting uPA and uPAR expression. Levels of components of the uPA/uPAR system correlate with metastatic potential of cell lines in vitro and with tumour progression and patient survival in vivo (Andreasen et al., 1997; Yang et al., 2000).

The cysteine cathepsins are a class of lysosomal proteases involved in intracellular protein degradation. However, cathepsins are also found outside the lysosomes, notably in the cytoplasm, in the nucleus and at the cell surface. Furthermore, cathepsins may be secreted into the extracellular space. Secreted and cell surface-localized cathepsins B, L and H control CRC progression (Jedeszko and Sloane, 2004), presumably by degrading BM components like laminin and collagen IV. Early studies have shown that in fibroblasts expressing either H-RASG12V or K-RASG12V, cathepsin L mRNA and protein is most abundantly induced (Joseph et al., 1987; Mason et al., 1987). Furthermore, K-RAS mutations in CRC are associated with increased cathepsin L expression (Kim et al., 1998). As mentioned above, K-RASG13D promotes the association of cathepsin B with caveolae in human CRC cells, where it may control uPA activity and pericellular proteolysis. In line with this, cathepsin B is found at the BM of colorectal adenomas and carcinomas (Campo et al., 1994) where it is ideally positioned to degrade BM components. In addition, cathepsin B expression has been closely associated with local colorectal tumour invasion ('budding') and areas of BM disruption, and may therefore be a critical factor in controlling metastasis formation (Guzinska-Ustymowicz et al., 2004; Hirai et al., 1999). Interestingly, genetic ablation of cathepsin B results in suppression of tumour-infiltrating pro-inflammatory cells and in notable attenuation of polyposis in Apc^{Min} mice (Gounaris et al., 2008). The modulation of cathepsin B/L expression and localization by mutant K-RAS signalling is likely contributing to the metastatic phenotype of CRC cells (Fig. 8.1) (Smakman et al., 2005).

Previous studies have indicated the involvement of the RAS effector, PI3K, in invasion of CRC. For example, in SW480 and RKO CRC cell lines, activation of AKT/NF-κB pathway promotes expression of angiogenic and metastatic genes including uPA, COX2 (see below), MMP-9, cathepsin B and galectin-3 (Agarwal et al., 2005; Kang et al., 2008). Finally, the protein signature derived from PI3K/AKT pathway suggests a promising multiplex biomarker for hepatic metastasis in CRC (Kang et al., 2008).

Another major feature of RAS-transformed cells is that they have a remodelled actin cytoskeleton which contributes to poor adhesion, increased motility, invasiveness and contact-independent growth (Charest and Firtel, 2007). For example, deletion of the endogenous K-RASG13D oncogene from HCT-116 CRC cells markedly reduced cell motility by restoring stress fibers and focal adhesions/complexes and by increasing cell matrix adhesion (Pollock et al., 2005). The Rho GTPases, Rho, Rac and Cdc42, are key regulators of actin cytoskeleton and are required for RAS-mediated transformation (Malliri and Collard, 2003; Sahai and Marshall, 2002). At the leading edge of migrating cells, Rac regulates the formation of lamellipodial protrusions, whereas Cdc42 induces filopodial extensions by activating the actin polymerization apparatus at these sites. In contrast, Rho regulates the formation of stress fibers and focal adhesions. In CRC cells, oncogenic K-RAS uses the MEK-ERK-Fra-1 pathway to deregulate Rho signalling and thus maintain a disrupted actin cytoskeleton (Vial et al., 2003). This contributes to the poor cell-matrix adhesion and enhanced motility of these cells. Furthermore, elevated RhoC expression has been found to correlate with poor outcome in colorectal carcinoma and may be used as a prognostic marker of colorectal carcinoma, where increased levels of RhoA expression was observed in Asian patients with colorectal carcinoma (Bellovin et al., 2006; Wang et al., 2009). Reduction in RhoA and RhoC expression markedly inhibits the invasion and migration potentials of CRC cells (Liu et al., 2009). Conversely, expression of activated RhoA in intestinal epithelial cell line cooperates with Raf to transform cells and to induce growth resistance to TGF-β (Du et al., 2004).

Oncogenic RAS signalling may also be involved in CRC progression by altering adhesion of colorectal cells to extracellular matrix. Indeed, inappropriate synthesis or degradation of any ECM molecules due to degradation by proteolytic enzymes and/or a lack of biosynthesis is often correlated with tumour progression. Expression of oncogenic MEK1 in intestinal crypt cells induces expression of integrin α6 (Lemieux et al., 2009) (Fig. 8.1). Enns et al. (2004) showed that α6β1 and α6β4 integrins are crucial for cancer cell adhesion in liver sinusoids (see Chapter 7 in this book for more information). Furthermore, α6β4 integrin has been identified as a tumour antigen, also designated as TSP-180 or A9 (Kennel et al., 1989; Van Waes et al., 1991) and increased expression of α6β4 and changes in its distribution correlate with increased aggressiveness of tumours and poor prognosis (Falcioni et al., 1986; Wolff et al., 1990). In colon carcinoma, the α6β4 integrin promotes cell migration on laminin-1, since it induces and stabilizes actin-containing motility structures, instead of being associated with hemi-desmosomes to support stable adhesive structures (Rabinovitz and Mercurio, 1997).

Once tumour cells have invaded through the epithelial BM and surrounding ECM and migrated through the stromal compartment, they will eventually come into contact with tumour-associated microvasculature. Tumour cells must then traverse any BM surrounding the vessel. This is achieved through adhesive interactions between the tumour cells and the endothelial cell BM through integrin-mediated interactions and dissolution of the BM by proteolytic enzymes (see before). The process is aided by the defective architecture, fenestrations and 'leakiness' of the newly formed tumour-associated vasculature. Once the tumour cells have passed the BM barrier and reached the vasculature, they are able to adhere to the vascular endothelial cells. Evidence for an intravasation-promoting effect of oncogenic K-RAS signalling during CRC development is currently lacking. However, it seems likely that the K-RAS-induced changes in peri-cellular proteolysis promote the degradation of both tumour- and endothelium-associated BM (Smakman et al., 2005).

8.2.5 Oncogenic K-RAS Signalling Prevents Anoikis

Resistance of solid tumour cells to anoikis, apoptosis induced by cell detachment from the ECM, is thought to be critical for the ability of these cells to grow in an anchorage-independent fashion within three-dimensional tumour masses and to form metastases. Intravasated tumour cells are carried via the mesenteric veins into the portal system of the liver. During this phase, tumour cells are devoid of contact with extracellular matrices, are exposed to shear stress and encounter cytotoxic immune cells. Therefore, metastasis formation requires the development of anoikis-resistance in circulating tumour cells. RAS oncogenes can induce both pro- and anti-apoptotic signalling (Smakman et al., 2005). In carcinoma cells, anti-apoptotic signalling prevails. Deletion of K-RASG13D in CRC cells sensitizes these cells to anoikis (Rosen et al., 2000; Zhang et al., 2000). In addition, the death of intestinal epithelial cells in suspension culture can be attenuated or aborted by the expression of oncogenic RAS (Rosen et al., 1998, 2000). Several RAS-activated signalling pathways may mediate protection against apoptosis (Cox and Der, 2003). Thus far, oncogenic RAS blocks anoikis (Rak et al., 1995b) of intestinal epithelial cells by three mechanisms. One mechanism involves reversal of detachment-induced inhibition of Bcl-xL expression (Rosen et al., 2000). The second one is driven by RAS-induced down-regulation of Bak (Rosen et al., 1998). The third one is through the up-regulation of cIAP2 and XIAP, two inhibitors of caspases (Liu et al., 2005). Moreover, the Raf/MEK/ERK signalling cascade may contribute to the protective action of oncogenic RAS against anoikis (Coll et al., 2002; Loza-Coll et al., 2005). Indeed, it has been recently demonstrated that constitutive activation of MEK1 or MEK2 in intestinal epithelial cells resulted in the up-regulation of the pro-survival proteins Mcl-1, Bcl-2 and, to a lesser extent, Bcl-xL (Boucher et al., 2004; Voisin et al., 2008). Reciprocally, induction of the pro-apoptotic proteins Bim (Voisin et al., 2008) and Bak (Boucher et al., 2004) was suppressed in cells expressing the oncogenic MEKs. This finding is consistent with previous reports documenting the role of the ERK1/2 MAP kinase pathway in promoting anoikis resistance in other cell types (Galante et al., 2008; Le Gall et al., 2000). Together, these data support the notion that the RAS/Raf/MEK/ERK pathway is a key regulator of intestinal epithelial and colorectal carcinoma cell anoikis (Fig. 8.1). Nevertheless, several studies have reported that the PI3K/AKT pathway may also be involved in the induction of anoikis resistance in CRC cells (Golubovskaya et al., 2003; Loza-Coll et al., 2005; Rychahou et al., 2006; Sekharam et al., 2003; Wee et al., 2008; Windham et al., 2002). PI3K/AKT may regulate cell survival by blocking the pro-apoptotic protein Bad to increase anti-apoptotic Bcl-x_L for the increase of cell survival. AKT can phosphorylate Bad for degradation and thus increase Bcl-x_L and Bcl2 activity. PI3K/AKT also phosphorylates several downstream targets (Blume-Jensen and Hunter, 2001), including IκB, the inhibitor of NF-κB, to up-regulate cellular survival signal pathway (Fig. 8.1). NF-κB not only increases tumour cell resistance to apoptosis but also regulates its angiogenesis and invasiveness (Boye et al., 2008).

8.2.6 Oncogenic K-RAS Signalling in Extravasation, Proliferation and Angiogenesis

The adhesion of cancer cells to endothelial cells is a prerequisite for extravasation of circulating cancer cells during metastatic dissemination. It requires specific interactions between adhesion receptors present on vascular endothelial cells and their counter-receptors on cancer cells (please see Chapter 11 by T. Winder and H.-J. Lenz, in this book for more information). E-selectin is a specific endothelial adhesion receptor that is induced by pro-inflammatory stimuli such as tumour necrosis factor-α and interleukin-1β (Gout and Huot, 2008). Typically, the colon cancer cell/endothelial cell interactions in the liver imply first a selectin-mediated initial attachment and rolling of the circulating cancer cells on the endothelium (please see Chapter 1 by Porquet et al. and Chapter 10 by P. Brodt, in this book for more details). The rolling cancer cells then become activated by locally released chemokines present at the surface of endothelial cells. This triggers the activation of integrins from the cancer cells allowing their firmer adhesion to members of the Ig-CAM family such as ICAM and VCAM, initiating the transendothelial migration and extravasation processes (Gout and Huot, 2008) (please see Chapter 7 by A. Arabzadeh and N. Beauchemin, in this book for more details on adhesion). A new E-selectin counter-receptor has been recently identified in colon carcinoma cells, the death receptor-3 (DR-3). Activation of this receptor by E-selectin triggers the activation of p38 and ERK MAP Kinases, conferring migration and survival advantages to colon carcinoma cells (Gout et al., 2006; Tremblay et al., 2006). Moreover, signalling from DR3 in the colon cancer cells is a pre-requisite for their transendothelial migration (Gout et al., 2006).

Once extravasated, tumour cells need to adapt to their new microenvironment. Under continuous attack of liver-associated immune cells, they have to survive and start proliferating to form new tumours (Smakman et al., 2005). The effect of mutant K-RAS on normal intestinal epithelial cell proliferation is well documented (Cheng and Lai, 2003). In addition, hyperplasic ACF are induced in transgenic mice expressing K-RAS in intestinal epithelial cells (Janssen et al., 2002; Tuveson et al., 2004). Whether mutant K-RAS is still required for CRC proliferation in liver metastases has not been formally shown and is difficult to assess. However, the persistence of mutant K-RAS in liver metastases suggests that it is required for this process (Smakman et al., 2005).

Developing tumours stimulate the formation of and are dependent on a new vascular network (angiogenesis) to supply it with nutrients and oxygen. Tumour-derived cell lines expressing activated K-RAS, as well as cell lines transfected with an activated H-RAS gene show increased synthesis and production of VEGF-A (Arbiser et al., 1997; Matsuo et al., 2009; Okada et al., 1998; Rak et al., 1995a), but not VEGF-B or VEGF-C (Enholm et al., 1997; Milanini et al., 1998). Conversely, inhibition of mutant *K-RAS* gene expression in human colon cancer cells reversed the up-regulation of VEGF expression (Rak et al., 1995a; Ross et al., 2001; Tokunaga et al., 2000). Thus, activated K-RAS is instrumental in elevating VEGF expression in colon cancer cells. The classical RAS>Raf>MEK>ERK1/2 kinase cascade and the RAS>PI3K>AKT pathway may be both involved independently in the control of VEGF transcription in cells expressing oncogenic RAS, probably through the regulation of HIF-1 expression (Blancher et al., 2001; Sodhi et al., 2001) and trans-activation potential for the VEGF promoter (Milanini et al., 1998; Richard et al., 1999) (Fig. 8.1). Is the stimulation of VEGF synthesis essential for RAS-stimulated angiogenesis and tumour growth? Okada et al. (1998) showed that down-regulation of VEGF transcription by anti-sense technology in human colon cancer cells harbouring an activated *K-RAS* gene greatly reduces their tumourigenic potential in vivo. Conversely, over-expression of VEGF in cells with a deleted K-RAS oncogene is not sufficient to fully restore tumourigenic potential (Okada et al., 1998). This indicates that additional RAS-regulated factors are likely to cooperate with VEGF during these processes (Kranenburg et al., 2004). Interestingly, specific inhibitors of MEK and PI3K inhibited HGF-induced expression of VEGF in CRC cells, indicating that these pathways are indeed involved in VEGF production by CRC cells (Zhang et al., 2007). In addition, it has been found that PI3K/AKT regulated VEGF and HIF-1 expression through HDM2 and p70S6K1 activation. Whereas tumour cells expressing activated RAS show elevated levels of VEGF, the levels of thrombospondin-1 (TSP-1) (Lawler, 2002; Volpert et al., 1995) and thrombospondin-2 (TSP-2) are dramatically reduced. TSP-1 and TSP-2 are extracellular matrix glycoproteins that are negative regulators of angiogenesis (Adams, 2001). Interestingly, in a mouse model for the development of intestinal adenomas, endogenous TSP-1 expression is down-regulated in regions of dysplasia that undergo extensive neo-vascularisation. Importantly, TSP-1 deficiency promotes the initiation and progression of tumour growth, thus establishing a critical inhibitory role for TSP-1 in the early stages of intestinal tumour development (Gutierrez et al., 2003).

In another line of ideas, chronic inflammation has been associated with the development of various common types of cancer and creates a pro-angiogenic environment (Dalgleish and O'Byrne, 2002). In line with this notion and as described in Chapter 10, in this book, the regular intake of non-steroidal anti-inflammatory drugs (NSAIDs) like aspirin reduces the risk for developing colon cancer by 40–50% (Smalley and Dubois, 1997) and may even cause regression of pre-existing adenomas (Giardiello et al., 1995). NSAIDs inhibit cyclooxygenases (COX-1 and COX-2), enzymes that convert arachidonic acid into prostaglandin H2 (PG-H2) which is further converted into inflammatory mediators like PG-F2a, PG-D2, PG-E2, PG-I2 and thromboxane A2 (TX-A2) (Subbaramaiah and Dannenberg, 2003). COX-1 is ubiquitously expressed and controls prostaglandin synthesis under physiological conditions. In contrast, COX-2 expression is inducible by growth factors and oncogenes and is highly expressed in many solid and haematologic tumours as well as in inflamed tissue (Kranenburg et al., 2004). As a result, high PG levels are found under these pathological conditions (Dubois et al., 1998). The importance of elevated COX-2 expression for tumour-associated angiogenesis and tumour progression has been reported in several studies demonstrating inhibitory effects of COX inhibitors on angiogenesis and tumour development (Dubois et al., 1998; Kranenburg et al., 2004; Masferrer et al., 2000; Subbaramaiah and Dannenberg, 2003). In addition, COX-deficient mice are refractory to tumour development in the intestines (Chulada et al., 2000; Oshima et al., 1996). *COX-2* gene expression in CRC cells is regulated by a variety of signals that are involved in either initiation or promotion of colorectal tumour growth, including deregulation of the Wnt pathway (Araki et al., 2003; Howe et al., 2001) and signalling by oncogenic RAS (Araki et al., 2003; Komatsu et al., 2005; Repasky et al., 2007; Sheng et al., 2001). Different RAS-activated signalling pathways have been implicated in the control of COX-2 expression including the ERK/MAPK (Komatsu et al., 2005; Lemieux et al., 2009) and the PI3K/AKT pathways (Sheng et al., 2001) (Fig. 8.1). Finally, COX-2 expression is required for the transforming effect of oncogenic K-RAS and MEK1 in intestinal epithelial cells (Komatsu et al., 2005; Repasky et al., 2007). Therefore, as suggested by Kranenburg et al., (2004), oncogenic RAS signalling may promote tumour angiogenesis by at least three independent mechanisms: (i) by stimulating the production of pro-angiogenic growth factors; (ii) by reducing the production of anti-angiogenic factors; and (iii) by ensuring the availability of pro-angiogenic growth factors through local degradation of the ECM (see above).

8.3 Conclusions

Experimental and clinical research from the past decades has greatly advanced our understanding of the biological processes implicated in cancer metastasis and shed light on some of the key regulatory signals governing the metastatic cascade. In this chapter, we have placed particular emphasis on the role of deregulated growth factor RTK signalling pathways in CRC metastatic progression. Although, it is clear that deregulation of RTKs is implicated in virtually all facets of malignant progression of CRCs, and that targeting RTKs represents one of the most promising therapeutic approaches for the treatment of CRC metastasis, several issues remain to be tackled. For instance, the realization of the extent of RTK heterogeneity in colorectal tumours represents an important issue. As well, the status of PI3K/PTEN, K-RAS and B-RAF mutations are important determinants of therapeutic responses to CRC EGFR therapies (Walther et al., 2009); this supports not only a causal role for deregulation of RTK signaling pathways in CRC, but also highlights its complexity and redundancy of signals engaged by these receptors. In this respect, RTK signalling pathways are subjected to complex regulation that we are only just beginning to fully understand. Hence, in order to identify RTK signalling components that hold promises to achieving meaningful inhibition of CRC metastasis, one of the challenges may rely on a better understanding of the specific biological relevance of RTK proximal events that trigger and integrate signals leading to the activation of RAS/MAPK and PI3K/AKT signalling cascades in colorectal tumour cells. It has also become apparent that in order to metastasize, cancer cells must not only adapt in the new microenvironment of distant organs, but also subvert their primary tumour microenvironment, in such a way that it becomes permissive for their dissemination. Thus, a better understanding of the regulatory signalling networks engaged by RTKs in both tumour cells and tumour-associated stromal cells that govern colorectal tumour metastasis, and how each of these influence each other, warrants further investigation. This is a pre-requisite to gain full insight into the role of RTK signalling cascades in CRC progression, and to provide new knowledge of the mechanisms behind the biology of CRC metastasis. It will also likely help in the identification of promising molecular targets for anti-metastatic CRC therapy and in the design of strategies to circumvent key obstacles to their clinical development for the benefit of patients afflicted by metastatic colorectal malignancies.

Acknowledgments We are thankful to members of our laboratories for their research work and helpful discussions. We are particularly grateful to Véronique Pomerleau and Sébastien Cagnol for their critical reading of the chapter. We apologize to the authors whose work was not cited because of space limitation. Our cancer research program is supported by grants from the Canadian

Institutes of Health (C.S., MOP-84382; N.R., MOP-14405) and the Cancer Research Society (to N.R.). The authors are members of the FRSQ-funded Centre de Recherche Clinique Étienne LeBel and of the CIHR team on the Digestive Epithelium. C.S. is a scholar from the Fonds de la Recherche en Santé du Québec and N.R. is a recipient of a Canadian Research Chair in Signalling and Digestive Physiopathology.

Abbreviations and Acronyms

ACF	Aberrant crypt foci
Bcl-2	B-cell lymphoma protein 2
Bcl-x_L	B-cell lymphoma extra-large protein
BM	Basal membrane
Cbl	Casitas B-cell lymphoma protein
CEA	Carcinoembryonic antigen
CRC	Colorectal cancer
COX	Cyclooxygenase
EGFR	Epidermal growth factor receptor
EMT	Epithelial-mesenchymal transition
Gab1	Grb2-associated binding protein-1
Grb2	Growth factor receptor-bound protein 2
HGF	Hepatocyte growth factor
HIF-1	Hypoxia-inducible factor-1
IGFR	Insulin-like growth factor
MACC1	Metastasis-associated in colon cancer 1
MAPK	Mitogen-activated protein kinase
Mcl-1	Myeloid leukemia cell differentiation protein
MMP2	Metalloproteinase 2
NF-κB	Nuclear factor kappa light chain in activated B cells
NSAIDs	Non-steroidal anti-inflammatory drugs
PDGFR	Platelet-derived growth factor
PIP3	Phosphatidylinositol 3,4,5-triphosphate
PI3K	Phosphatidyl inositol 3-kinase
PTEN	Phosphatase and tensin homolog deleted on chromosome 10
PRL-3	Phosphatase of regenerating liver 3
RTK	Receptor tyrosine kinase
PTB	Phosphotyrosine binding domain
RAS-GAP	RAS-GTPase activating protein
Shc	Src-homology collagen protein
SH2	Src homology domain 2
SOS	Son of Sevenless
TGF	Transforming growth factor
TSP	Thrombospondin
uPA	Urokinase plasminogen activator
uPAR	uPA receptor
VEGFR	Vascular endothelial growth factor receptor

References

Abella JV, Park M (2009). Breakdown of endocytosis in the oncogenic activation of receptor tyrosine kinases. *Am J Physiol Endocrinol Metab* **296**: E973–84.

Adachi Y, Yamamoto H, Itoh F, Hinoda Y, Okada Y, Imai K (1999). Contribution of matrilysin (MMP-7) to the metastatic pathway of human colorectal cancers. *Gut* **45**: 252–58.

Adams JC (2001). Thrombospondins: multifunctional regulators of cell interactions. *Annu Rev Cell Dev Biol* **17**: 25–51.

Agarwal A, Das K, Lerner N, Sathe S, Cicek M, Casey G et al. (2005). The AKT/I kappa B kinase pathway promotes angiogenic/metastatic gene expression in colorectal cancer by activating nuclear factor-kappa B and beta-catenin. *Oncogene* **24**: 1021–31.

Ahmed N, Oliva K, Wang Y, Quinn M, Rice G (2003). Downregulation of urokinase plasminogen activator receptor expression inhibits Erk signalling with concomitant suppression of invasiveness due to loss of uPAR-beta1 integrin complex in colon cancer cells. *Br J Cancer* **89**: 374–84.

Aliaga JC, Deschenes C, Beaulieu JF, Calvo EL, Rivard Nd (1999). Requirement of the MAP kinase cascade for cell cycle progression and differentiation of human intestinal cells. *Am J Physiol* **277**: G631–41.

Allgayer H, Wang H, Shirasawa S, Sasazuki T, Boyd D (1999). Targeted disruption of the K-RAS oncogene in an invasive colon cancer cell line down-regulates urokinase receptor expression and plasminogen-dependent proteolysis. *Br J Cancer* **80**: 1884–91.

Anderson KE, Jackson SP (2003). Class I phosphoinositide 3-kinases. *Int J Biochem Cell Biol* **35**: 1028–33.

Andreasen PA, Kjoller L, Christensen L, Duffy MJ (1997). The urokinase-type plasminogen activator system in cancer metastasis: a review. *Int J Cancer* **72**: 1–22.

Araki Y, Okamura S, Hussain SP, Nagashima M, He P, Shiseki M et al. (2003). Regulation of cyclooxygenase-2 expression by the Wnt and ras pathways. *Cancer Res* **63**: 728–34.

Arbiser JL, Moses MA, Fernandez CA, Ghiso N, Cao Y, Klauber N et al. (1997). Oncogenic H-ras stimulates tumor angiogenesis by two distinct pathways. *Proc Natl Acad Sci USA* **94**: 861–66.

Arena S, Pisacane A, Mazzone M, Comoglio PM, Bardelli A (2007). Genetic targeting of the kinase activity of the Met receptor in cancer cells. *Proc Natl Acad Sci USA* **104**: 11412–17.

Barber TD, Vogelstein B, Kinzler KW, Velculescu VE (2004). Somatic mutations of EGFR in colorectal cancers and glioblastomas. *N Engl J Med* **351**: 2883.

Barozzi C, Ravaioli M, D'Errico A, Grazi GL, Poggioli G, Cavrini G et al. (2002). Relevance of biologic markers in colorectal carcinoma: a comparative study of a broad panel. *Cancer* **94**: 647–57.

Batlle E, Sancho E, Franci C, Dominguez D, Monfar M, Baulida J et al. (2000). The transcription factor snail is a repressor of E-cadherin gene expression in epithelial tumour cells. *Nat Cell Biol* **2**: 84–89.

Bellovin DI, Simpson KJ, Danilov T, Maynard E, Rimm DL, Oettgen P et al. (2006). Reciprocal regulation of RhoA and RhoC characterizes the EMT and identifies RhoC as a prognostic marker of colon carcinoma. *Oncogene* **25**: 6959–67.

Berger DH (2002). Plasmin/plasminogen system in colorectal cancer. *World J Surg* **26**: 767–71.

Bernier J, Chababi W, Pomerleau V, Saucier C (2010). Oncogenic engagement of the Met receptor tyrosine kinase is sufficient to evoke angiogenic, tumorigenic and metastatic activities in intestinal epithelial cells. *Am J Physiol Gastrointest Liver Physiol*, 2010 Jun 10. [Epub ahead of print]

Birchmeier C, Birchmeier W, Gherardi E, Vande Woude GF (2003). Met, metastasis, motility and more. *Nat Rev Mol Cell Biol* **4**: 915–25.

Blancher C, Moore JW, Robertson N, Harris AL (2001). Effects of ras and von Hippel-Lindau (VHL) gene mutations on hypoxia-inducible factor (HIF)-1alpha, HIF-2alpha, and vascular endothelial growth factor expression and their regulation by the phosphatidylinositol 3'-kinase/Akt signaling pathway. *Cancer Res* **61**: 7349–55.

Blume-Jensen P, Hunter T (2001). Oncogenic kinase signalling. *Nature* **411**: 355–65.
Bolos V, Peinado H, Perez-Moreno MA, Fraga MF, Esteller M, Cano A (2003). The transcription factor Slug represses E-cadherin expression and induces epithelial to mesenchymal transitions: a comparison with Snail and E47 repressors. *J Cell Sci* **116**: 499–511.
Boon EM, Kovarikova M, Derksen PW, van der Neut R (2005). MET signalling in primary colon epithelial cells leads to increased transformation irrespective of aberrant Wnt signalling. *Br J Cancer* **92**: 1078–83.
Bos JL (1989). Ras oncogenes in human cancer: a review. *Cancer Res* **49**: 4682–89.
Boucher MJ, Jean D, Vezina A, Rivard N (2004). Dual role of MEK/ERK signaling in senescence and transformation of intestinal epithelial cells. *Am J Physiol Gastrointest Liver Physiol* **286**: G736–46.
Boye K, Grotterod I, Aasheim HC, Hovig E, Maelandsmo GM (2008). Activation of NF-kappaB by extracellular S100A4: analysis of signal transduction mechanisms and identification of target genes. *Int J Cancer* **123**: 1301–10.
Brand S, Dambacher J, Beigel F, Olszak T, Diebold J, Otte JM et al. (2005). CXCR4 and CXCL12 are inversely expressed in colorectal cancer cells and modulate cancer cell migration, invasion and MMP-9 activation. *Exp Cell Res* **310**: 117–30.
Campbell IG, Russell SE, Choong DY, Montgomery KG, Ciavarella ML, Hooi CS et al. (2004). Mutation of the PIK3CA gene in ovarian and breast cancer. *Cancer Res* **64**: 7678–81.
Campo E, Munoz J, Miquel R, Palacin A, Cardesa A, Sloane BF et al. (1994). Cathepsin B expression in colorectal carcinomas correlates with tumor progression and shortened patient survival. *Am J Pathol* **145**: 301–9.
Cano A, Perez-Moreno MA, Rodrigo I, Locascio A, Blanco MJ, del Barrio MG et al. (2000). The transcription factor snail controls epithelial-mesenchymal transitions by repressing E-cadherin expression. *Nat Cell Biol* **2**: 76–83.
Cauwe B, Van den Steen PE, Opdenakker G (2007). The biochemical, biological, and pathological kaleidoscope of cell surface substrates processed by matrix metalloproteinases. *Crit Rev Biochem Mol Biol* **42**: 113–85.
Cavallo-Medved D, Dosescu J, Linebaugh BE, Sameni M, Rudy D, Sloane BF (2003). Mutant K-RAS regulates cathepsin B localization on the surface of human colorectal carcinoma cells. *Neoplasia* **5**: 507–19.
Cavallo-Medved D, Mai J, Dosescu J, Sameni M, Sloane BF (2005). Caveolin-1 mediates the expression and localization of cathepsin B, pro-urokinase plasminogen activator and their cell-surface receptors in human colorectal carcinoma cells. *J Cell Sci* **118**: 1493–503.
Chambers AF, Groom AC, MacDonald IC (2002). Dissemination and growth of cancer cells in metastatic sites. *Nat Rev Cancer* **2**: 563–72.
Charest PG, Firtel RA (2007). Big roles for small GTPases in the control of directed cell movement. *Biochem J* **401**: 377–90.
Chen Y, Lu Q, Schneeberger EE, Goodenough DA (2000). Restoration of tight junction structure and barrier function by down-regulation of the mitogen-activated protein kinase pathway in ras-transformed Madin-Darby canine kidney cells. *Mol Biol Cell* **11**: 849–62.
Cheng AM, Saxton TM, Sakai R, Kulkarni S, Mbamalu G, Vogel W et al. (1998). Mammalian Grb2 regulates multiple steps in embryonic development and malignant transformation. *Cell* **95**: 793–803.
Cheng L, Lai MD (2003). Aberrant crypt foci as microscopic precursors of colorectal cancer. *World J Gastroenterol* **9**: 2642–49.
Chi SG, Kim HJ, Park BJ, Min HJ, Park JH, Kim YW et al. (1998). Mutational abrogation of the PTEN/MMAC1 gene in gastrointestinal polyps in patients with Cowden disease. *Gastroenterology* **115**: 1084–89.
Chulada PC, Thompson MB, Mahler JF, Doyle CM, Gaul BW, Lee C et al. (2000). Genetic disruption of Ptgs-1, as well as Ptgs-2, reduces intestinal tumorigenesis in Min mice. *Cancer Res* **60**: 4705–8.
Cohen DJ, Hochster HS (2007). Update on clinical data with regimens inhibiting angiogenesis and epidermal growth factor receptor for patients with newly diagnosed metastatic colorectal cancer. *Clin Colorectal Cancer* **7**(**Suppl 1**): S21–7.

Cohen SJ, Cohen RB, Meropol NJ (2005). Targeting signal transduction pathways in colorectal cancer – more than skin deep. *J Clin Oncol* **23**: 5374–85.

Colakoglu T, Yildirim S, Kayaselcuk F, Nursal TZ, Ezer A, Noyan T et al. (2008). Clinicopathological significance of PTEN loss and the phosphoinositide 3-kinase/Akt pathway in sporadic colorectal neoplasms: is PTEN loss predictor of local recurrence? *Am J Surg* **195**: 719–25.

Coll ML, Rosen K, Ladeda V, Filmus J (2002). Increased Bcl-xL expression mediates v-Src-induced resistance to anoikis in intestinal epithelial cells. *Oncogene* **21**: 2908–13.

Comijn J, Berx G, Vermassen P, Verschueren K, van Grunsven L, Bruyneel E et al. (2001). The two-handed E box binding zinc finger protein SIP1 downregulates E-cadherin and induces invasion. *Mol Cell* **7**: 1267–78.

Cox AD, Der CJ (2003). The dark side of Ras: regulation of apoptosis. *Oncogene* **22**: 8999–9006.

Curran S, Dundas SR, Buxton J, Leeman MF, Ramsay R, Murray GI (2004). Matrix metalloproteinase/tissue inhibitors of matrix metalloproteinase phenotype identifies poor prognosis colorectal cancers. *Clin Cancer Res* **10**: 8229–34.

Dalgleish AG, O'Byrne K Jr (2002). Chronic immune activation and inflammation in the pathogenesis of AIDS and cancer. *Adv Cancer Res* **84**: 231–76.

Dance M, Montagner A, Yart A, Masri B, Audigier Y, Perret B et al. (2006). The adaptor protein Gab1 couples the stimulation of vascular endothelial growth factor receptor-2 to the activation of phosphoinositide 3-kinase. *J Biol Chem* **281**: 23285–95.

Dankort DL, Wang Z, Blackmore V, Moran MF, Muller WJ (1997). Distinct tyrosine autophosphorylation sites negatively and positively modulate neu-mediated transformation. *Mol Cell Biol* **17**: 5410–25.

Davies H, Bignell GR, Cox C, Stephens P, Edkins S, Clegg S et al. (2002). Mutations of the B-RAF gene in human cancer. *Nature* **417**: 949–54.

Davies M, Robinson M, Smith E, Huntley S, Prime S, Paterson I (2005). Induction of an epithelial to mesenchymal transition in human immortal and malignant keratinocytes by TGF-beta1 involves MAPK, Smad and AP-1 signalling pathways. *J Cell Biochem* **95**: 918–31.

De Craene B, van Roy F, Berx G (2005). Unraveling signalling cascades for the Snail family of transcription factors. *Cell Signal* **17**: 535–47.

De Jong KP, Stellema R, Karrenbeld A, Koudstaal J, Gouw AS, Sluiter WJ et al. (1998). Clinical relevance of transforming growth factor alpha, epidermal growth factor receptor, p53, and Ki67 in colorectal liver metastases and corresponding primary tumors. *Hepatology* **28**: 971–79.

Deng G, Bell I, Crawley S, Gum J, Terdiman JP, Allen BA et al. (2004). B-RAF mutation is frequently present in sporadic colorectal cancer with methylated hMLH1, but not in hereditary nonpolyposis colorectal cancer. *Clin Cancer Res* **10**: 191–95.

Di Renzo MF, Olivero M, Giacomini A, Porte H, Chastre E, Mirossay L et al. (1995). Overexpression and amplification of the met/HGF receptor gene during the progression of colorectal cancer. *Clin Cancer Res* **1**: 147–54.

Du J, Jiang B, Coffey RJ, Barnard J (2004). Raf and RhoA cooperate to transform intestinal epithelial cells and induce growth resistance to transforming growth factor beta. *Mol Cancer Res* **2**: 233–41.

Dubois RN, Abramson SB, Crofford L, Gupta RA, Simon LS, Van De Putte LB et al. (1998). Cyclooxygenase in biology and disease. *Faseb J* **12**: 1063–73.

Eger A, Aigner K, Sonderegger S, Dampier B, Oehler S, Schreiber M et al. (2005). DeltaEF1 is a transcriptional repressor of E-cadherin and regulates epithelial plasticity in breast cancer cells. *Oncogene* **24**: 2375–85.

Eggstein S, Franke M, Kutschka I, Manthey G, von Specht BU, Ruf G et al. (1999). Expression and activity of mitogen activated protein kinases in human colorectal carcinoma. *Gut* **44**: 834–38.

Eng C (2003). Constipation, polyps, or cancer? Let PTEN predict your future. *Am J Med Genet A* **122A**: 315–22.

Engelman JA, Luo J, Cantley LC (2006). The evolution of phosphatidylinositol 3-kinases as regulators of growth and metabolism. *Nat Rev Genet* **7**: 606–19.

Enholm B, Paavonen K, Ristimaki A, Kumar V, Gunji Y, Klefstrom J et al. (1997). Comparison of VEGF, VEGF-B, VEGF-C and Ang-1 mRNA regulation by serum, growth factors, oncoproteins and hypoxia. *Oncogene* **14**: 2475–83.

Enns A, Gassmann P, Schluter K, Korb T, Spiegel HU, Senninger N et al. (2004). Integrins can directly mediate metastatic tumor cell adhesion within the liver sinusoids. *J Gastrointest Surg* **8**: 1049–59; discussion 1060.

Falcioni R, Kennel SJ, Giacomini P, Zupi G, Sacchi A (1986). Expression of tumor antigen correlated with metastatic potential of Lewis lung carcinoma and B16 melanoma clones in mice. *Cancer Res* **46**: 5772–78.

Fang JY, Richardson BC (2005). The MAPK signalling pathways and colorectal cancer. *Lancet Oncol* **6**: 322–27.

Fassetta M, D'Alessandro L, Coltella N, Di Renzo MF, Rasola A (2006). Hepatocyte growth factor installs a survival platform for colorectal cancer cell invasive growth and overcomes p38 MAPK-mediated apoptosis. *Cell Signal* **18**: 1967–76.

Fazekas K, Csuka O, Koves I, Raso E, Timar J (2000). Experimental and clinicopathologic studies on the function of the HGF receptor in human colon cancer metastasis. *Clin Exp Metastasis* **18**: 639–49.

Fresno Vara JA, Casado E, de Castro J, Cejas P, Belda-Iniesta C, Gonzalez-Baron M (2004). PI3K/Akt signalling pathway and cancer. *Cancer Treat Rev* **30**: 193–204.

Fujimoto K, Sheng H, Shao J, Beauchamp RD (2001). Transforming growth factor-beta1 promotes invasiveness after cellular transformation with activated Ras in intestinal epithelial cells. *Exp Cell Res* **266**: 239–49.

Fukushima H, Yamamoto H, Itoh F, Nakamura H, Min Y, Horiuchi S et al. (2001). Association of matrilysin mRNA expression with K-RAS mutations and progression in pancreatic ductal adenocarcinomas. *Carcinogenesis* **22**: 1049–52.

Galante JM, Mortenson MM, Bowles TL, Virudachalam S, Bold RJ (2008). ERK/BCL-2 pathway in the resistance of pancreatic cancer to anoikis. *J Surg Res* **152**: 18–25.

Giannelli G, Falk-Marzillier J, Schiraldi O, Stetler-Stevenson WG, Quaranta V (1997). Induction of cell migration by matrix metalloprotease-2 cleavage of laminin-5. *Science* **277**: 225–28.

Giardiello FM, Offerhaus GJ, DuBois RN (1995). The role of nonsteroidal anti-inflammatory drugs in colorectal cancer prevention. *Eur J Cancer* **31A**: 1071–76.

Giorgio M, Migliaccio E, Orsini F, Paolucci D, Moroni M, Contursi C et al. (2005). Electron transfer between cytochrome c and p66Shc generates reactive oxygen species that trigger mitochondrial apoptosis. *Cell* **122**: 221–33.

Giralt J, de las Heras M, Cerezo L, Eraso A, Hermosilla E, Velez D et al. (2005). The expression of epidermal growth factor receptor results in a worse prognosis for patients with rectal cancer treated with preoperative radiotherapy: a multicenter, retrospective analysis. *Radiother Oncol* **74**: 101–8.

Giubellino A, Burke TR Jr., Bottaro DP (2008). Grb2 signaling in cell motility and cancer. *Expert Opin Ther Targets* **12**: 1021–33.

Goldstein NS, Armin M (2001). Epidermal growth factor receptor immunohistochemical reactivity in patients with American Joint Committee on Cancer Stage IV colon adenocarcinoma: implications for a standardized scoring system. *Cancer* **92**: 1331–46.

Golubovskaya VM, Gross S, Kaur AS, Wilson RI, Xu LH, Yang XH et al. (2003). Simultaneous inhibition of focal adhesion kinase and SRC enhances detachment and apoptosis in colon cancer cell lines. *Mol Cancer Res* **1**: 755–64.

Gounaris E, Tung CH, Restaino C, Maehr R, Kohler R, Joyce JA et al. (2008). Live imaging of cysteine-cathepsin activity reveals dynamics of focal inflammation, angiogenesis, and polyp growth. *PLoS One* **3**: e2916.

Gout S, Huot J (2008). Role of cancer microenvironment in metastasis: focus on colon cancer. *Cancer Microenviron* **1**: 69–83.

Gout S, Morin C, Houle F, Huot J (2006). Death receptor-3, a new E-Selectin counter-receptor that confers migration and survival advantages to colon carcinoma cells by triggering p38 and ERK MAPK activation. *Cancer Res* **66**: 9117–24.

Grondahl-Hansen J, Ralfkiaer E, Kirkeby LT, Kristensen P, Lund LR, Dano K (1991). Localization of urokinase-type plasminogen activator in stromal cells in adenocarcinomas of the colon in humans. *Am J Pathol* **138**: 111–17.

Grossman SR, Lyle S, Resnick MB, Sabo E, Lis RT, Rosinha E et al. (2007). p66 Shc tumor levels show a strong prognostic correlation with disease outcome in stage IIA colon cancer. *Clin Cancer Res* **13**: 5798–804.

Gu H, Neel BG (2003). The "Gab" in signal transduction. *Trends Cell Biol* **13**: 122–30.

Guo XN, Rajput A, Rose R, Hauser J, Beko A, Kuropatwinski K et al. (2007). Mutant PIK3CA-bearing colon cancer cells display increased metastasis in an orthotopic model. *Cancer Res* **67**: 5851–58.

Gutierrez LS, Suckow M, Lawler J, Ploplis VA, Castellino FJ (2003). Thrombospondin 1 – a regulator of adenoma growth and carcinoma progression in the APC(Min/+) mouse model. *Carcinogenesis* **24**: 199–207.

Guzinska-Ustymowicz K, Zalewski B, Kasacka I, Piotrowski Z, Skrzydlewska E (2004). Activity of cathepsin B and D in colorectal cancer: relationships with tumour budding. *Anticancer Res* **24**: 2847–51.

Haigis KM, Kendall KR, Wang Y, Cheung A, Haigis MC, Glickman JN et al. (2008). Differential effects of oncogenic K-RAS and N-Ras on proliferation, differentiation and tumor progression in the colon. *Nat Genet* **40**: 600–8.

Hanahan D, Weinberg RA (2000). The hallmarks of cancer. *Cell* **100**: 57–70.

Harvey SR, Sait SN, Xu Y, Bailey JL, Penetrante RM, Markus G (1999). Demonstration of urokinase expression in cancer cells of colon adenocarcinomas by immunohistochemistry and in situ hybridization. *Am J Pathol* **155**: 1115–20.

Hase K, Shatney C, Johnson D, Trollope M, Vierra Ma (1993). Prognostic value of tumor "budding" in patients with colorectal cancer. *Dis Colon Rectum* **36**: 627–35.

Herynk MH, Stoeltzing O, Reinmuth N, Parikh NU, Abounader R, Laterra J et al. (2003). Down-regulation of c-Met inhibits growth in the liver of human colorectal carcinoma cells. *Cancer Res* **63**: 2990–96.

Hirai K, Yokoyama M, Asano G, Tanaka S (1999). Expression of cathepsin B and cystatin C in human colorectal cancer. *Hum Pathol* **30**: 680–86.

Hiscox SE, Hallett MB, Puntis MC, Nakamura T, Jiang WG (1997). Expression of the HGF/SF receptor, c-met, and its ligand in human colorectal cancers. *Cancer Invest* **15**: 513–21.

Holgado-Madruga M, Wong AJ (2004). Role of the Grb2-associated binder 1/SHP-2 interaction in cell growth and transformation. *Cancer Res* **64**: 2007–15.

Hoshino R, Chatani Y, Yamori T, Tsuruo T, Oka H, Yoshida O et al. (1999). Constitutive activation of the 41-/43-kDa mitogen-activated protein kinase signaling pathway in human tumors. *Oncogene* **18**: 813–22.

Howe LR, Crawford HC, Subbaramaiah K, Hassell JA, Dannenberg AJ, Brown AM (2001). PEA3 is up-regulated in response to Wnt1 and activates the expression of cyclooxygenase-2. *J Biol Chem* **276**: 20108–15.

Huang J, Che MI, Huang YT, Shyu MK, Huang YM, Wu YM et al. (2009). Overexpression of MUC15 activates extracellular signal-regulated kinase 1/2 and promotes the oncogenic potential of human colon cancer cells. *Carcinogenesis* **30**: 1452–58.

Hughes PE, Renshaw MW, Pfaff M, Forsyth J, Keivens VM, Schwartz MA et al. (1997). Suppression of integrin activation: a novel function of a Ras/Raf-initiated MAP kinase pathway. *Cell* **88**: 521–30.

Ikenoue T, Kanai F, Hikiba Y, Obata T, Tanaka Y, Imamura J et al. (2005). Functional analysis of PIK3CA gene mutations in human colorectal cancer. *Cancer Res* **65**: 4562–67.

Imamichi Y, Konig A, Gress T, Menke A (2007). Collagen type I-induced Smad-interacting protein 1 expression downregulates E-cadherin in pancreatic cancer. *Oncogene* **26**: 2381–85.

Itoh N, Semba S, Ito M, Takeda H, Kawata S, Yamakawa M (2002). Phosphorylation of Akt/PKB is required for suppression of cancer cell apoptosis and tumor progression in human colorectal carcinoma. *Cancer* **94**: 3127–34.

Janda E, Lehmann K, Killisch I, Jechlinger M, Herzig M, Downward J et al. (2002). Ras and TGF[beta] cooperatively regulate epithelial cell plasticity and metastasis: dissection of Ras signaling pathways. *J Cell Biol* **156**: 299–313.

Janssen KP, el-Marjou F, Pinto D, Sastre X, Rouillard D, Fouquet C et al. (2002). Targeted expression of oncogenic K-RAS in intestinal epithelium causes spontaneous tumorigenesis in mice. *Gastroenterology* **123**: 492–504.

Jedeszko C, Sloane BF (2004). Cysteine cathepsins in human cancer. *Biol Chem* **385**: 1017–27.

Joseph L, Lapid S, Sukhatme V (1987). The major ras induced protein in NIH3T3 cells is cathepsin L. *Nucleic Acids Res* **15**: 3186.

Kammula US, Kuntz EJ, Francone TD, Zeng Z, Shia J, Landmann RG et al. (2007). Molecular co-expression of the c-Met oncogene and hepatocyte growth factor in primary colon cancer predicts tumor stage and clinical outcome. *Cancer Lett* **248**: 219–28.

Kang B, Hao C, Wang H, Zhang J, Xing R, Shao J et al. (2008). Evaluation of hepatic-metastasis risk of colorectal cancer upon the protein signature of PI3K/AKT pathway. *J Proteome Res* **7**: 3507–15.

Kataoka H, Hamasuna R, Itoh H, Kitamura N, Koono M (2000). Activation of hepatocyte growth factor/scatter factor in colorectal carcinoma. *Cancer Res* **60**: 6148–59.

Kaulfuss S, Burfeind P, Gaedcke J, Scharf JG (2009). Dual silencing of insulin-like growth factor-I receptor and epidermal growth factor receptor in colorectal cancer cells is associated with decreased proliferation and enhanced apoptosis. *Mol Cancer Ther* **8**: 821–33.

Kennel SJ, Foote LJ, Falcioni R, Sonnenberg A, Stringer CD, Crouse C et al. (1989). Analysis of the tumor-associated antigen TSP-180. Identity with alpha 6-beta 4 in the integrin superfamily. *J Biol Chem* **264**: 15515–21.

Kermorgant S, Aparicio T, Dessirier V, Lewin MJ, Lehy T (2001). Hepatocyte growth factor induces colonic cancer cell invasiveness via enhanced motility and protease overproduction. Evidence for PI3 kinase and PKC involvement. *Carcinogenesis* **22**: 1035–42.

Khaleghpour K, Li Y, Banville D, Yu Z, Shen SH (2004). Involvement of the PI 3-kinase signaling pathway in progression of colon adenocarcinoma. *Carcinogenesis* **25**: 241–48.

Kim K, Cai J, Shuja S, Kuo T, Murnane MJ (1998). Presence of activated ras correlates with increased cysteine proteinase activities in human colorectal carcinomas. *Int J Cancer* **79**: 324–33.

Kluftinger AM, Robinson BW, Quenville NF, Finley RJ, Davis NL (1992). Correlation of epidermal growth factor receptor and c-erbB2 oncogene product to known prognostic indicators of colorectal cancer. *Surg Oncol* **1**: 97–105.

Komatsu K, Buchanan FG, Katkuri S, Morrow JD, Inoue H, Otaka M et al. (2005). Oncogenic potential of MEK1 in rat intestinal epithelial cells is mediated via cyclooxygenase-2. *Gastroenterology* **129**: 577–90.

Kranenburg O, Gebbink MF, Voest EE (2004). Stimulation of angiogenesis by Ras proteins. *Biochim Biophys Acta* **1654**: 23–37.

Krishnamachary B, Zagzag D, Nagasawa H, Rainey K, Okuyama H, Baek JH et al. (2006). Hypoxia-inducible factor-1-dependent repression of E-cadherin in von Hippel-Lindau tumor suppressor-null renal cell carcinoma mediated by TCF3, ZFHX1A, and ZFHX1B. *Cancer Res* **66**: 2725–31.

Kuno Y, Kondo K, Iwata H, Senga T, Akiyama S, Ito K et al. (1998). Tumor-specific activation of mitogen-activated protein kinase in human colorectal and gastric carcinoma tissues. *Jpn J Cancer Res* **89**: 903–9.

Kuwai T, Nakamura T, Sasaki T, Kim SJ, Fan D, Villares GJ et al. (2008a). Phosphorylated epidermal growth factor receptor on tumor-associated endothelial cells is a primary target for therapy with tyrosine kinase inhibitors. *Neoplasia* **10**: 489–500.

Kuwai T, Nakamura T, Sasaki T, Kitadai Y, Kim JS, Langley RR et al. (2008b). Targeting the EGFR, VEGFR, and PDGFR on colon cancer cells and stromal cells is required for therapy. *Clin Exp Metastasis* **25**: 477–89.

Laprise P, Chailler P, Houde M, Beaulieu JF, Boucher MJ, Rivard N (2002). Phosphatidylinositol 3-kinase controls human intestinal epithelial cell differentiation by promoting adherens junction assembly and p38 MAPK activation. *J Biol Chem* **277**: 8226–34.

Lawler J (2002). Thrombospondin-1 as an endogenous inhibitor of angiogenesis and tumor growth. *J Cell Mol Med* **6**: 1–12.

Le Gall M, Chambard JC, Breittmayer JP, Grall D, Pouyssegur J, Van Obberghen-Schilling E (2000). The p42/p44 MAP kinase pathway prevents apoptosis induced by anchorage and serum removal. *Mol Biol Cell* **11**: 1103–12.

Lee SH, Lee JW, Soung YH, Kim SY, Nam SW, Park WS et al. (2004). Colorectal tumors frequently express phosphorylated mitogen-activated protein kinase. *Apmis* **112**: 233–38.

Lehmann K, Janda E, Pierreux CE, Rytomaa M, Schulze A, McMahon M et al. (2000). Raf induces TGFbeta production while blocking its apoptotic but not invasive responses: a mechanism leading to increased malignancy in epithelial cells. *Genes Dev* **14**: 2610–22.

Lemieux E, Bergeron S, Durand V, Asselin C, Saucier C, Rivard N (2009). Constitutively active MEK1 is sufficient to induce epithelial-to-mesenchymal transition in intestinal epithelial cells and to promote tumor invasion and metastasis. *Int J Cancer* **125**: 1575–86.

Lenz HJ, Van Cutsem E, Khambata-Ford S, Mayer RJ, Gold P, Stella P et al. (2006). Multicenter phase II and translational study of cetuximab in metastatic colorectal carcinoma refractory to irinotecan, oxaliplatin, and fluoropyrimidines. *J Clin Oncol* **24**: 4914–21.

Licato LL, Brenner DA (1998). Analysis of signaling protein kinases in human colon or colorectal carcinomas. *Dig Dis Sci* **43**: 1454–64.

Licato LL, Keku TO, Wurzelmann JI, Murray SC, Woosley JT, Sandler RS et al. (1997). In vivo activation of mitogen-activated protein kinases in rat intestinal neoplasia. *Gastroenterology* **113**: 1589–98.

Liu C, Park M, Tsao MS (1992). Overexpression of c-met proto-oncogene but not epidermal growth factor receptor or c-erbB-2 in primary human colorectal carcinomas. *Oncogene* **7**: 181–85.

Liu C, Woo A, Tsao MS (1990). Expression of transforming growth factor-alpha in primary human colon and lung carcinomas. *Br J Cancer* **62**: 425–29.

Liu XP, Wang HB, Yang K, Sui AH, Shi Q, Qu S (2009). Inhibitory effects of adenovirus mediated tandem expression of RhoA and RhoC shRNAs in HCT116 cells. *J Exp Clin Cancer Res* **28**: 52.

Liu Z, Li H, Derouet M, Filmus J, LaCasse EC, Korneluk RG et al. (2005). ras Oncogene triggers up-regulation of cIAP2 and XIAP in intestinal epithelial cells: epidermal growth factor receptor-dependent and -independent mechanisms of ras-induced transformation. *J Biol Chem* **280**: 37383–92.

Long IS, Han K, Li M, Shirasawa S, Sasazuki T, Johnston M et al. (2003). Met receptor overexpression and oncogenic Ki-ras mutation cooperate to enhance tumorigenicity of colon cancer cells in vivo. *Mol Cancer Res* **1**: 393–401.

Loza-Coll MA, Perera S, Shi W, Filmus J (2005). A transient increase in the activity of Src-family kinases induced by cell detachment delays anoikis of intestinal epithelial cells. *Oncogene* **24**: 1727–37.

Lynch CC, Crawford HC, Matrisian LM, McDonnell S (2004). Epidermal growth factor upregulates matrix metalloproteinase-7 expression through activation of PEA3 transcription factors. *Int J Oncol* **24**: 1565–72.

Malliri A, Collard JG (2003). Role of Rho-family proteins in cell adhesion and cancer. *Curr Opin Cell Biol* **15**: 583–89.

Malumbres M, Barbacid M (2003). RAS oncogenes: the first 30 years. *Nat Rev Cancer* **3**: 459–65.

Maroun CR, Holgado-Madruga M, Royal I, Naujokas MA, Fournier TM, Wong AJ et al. (1999). The Gab1 PH domain is required for localization of Gab1 at sites of cell-cell contact and epithelial morphogenesis downstream from the met receptor tyrosine kinase. *Mol. Cell. Biol.* **19**: 1784–99.

Masaki T, Matsuoka H, Sugiyama M, Abe N, Goto A, Sakamoto A et al. (2001). Matrilysin (MMP-7) as a significant determinant of malignant potential of early invasive colorectal carcinomas. *Br J Cancer* **84**: 1317–21.

Masferrer JL, Leahy KM, Koki AT, Zweifel BS, Settle SL, Woerner BM et al. (2000). Antiangiogenic and antitumor activities of cyclooxygenase-2 inhibitors. *Cancer Res* **60**: 1306–11.

Mason RW, Gal S, Gottesman MM (1987). The identification of the major excreted protein (MEP) from a transformed mouse fibroblast cell line as a catalytically active precursor form of cathepsin L. *Biochem J* **248**: 449–54.

Matsuo Y, Campbell PM, Brekken RA, Sung B, Ouellette MM, Fleming JB et al. (2009). K-RAS promotes angiogenesis mediated by immortalized human pancreatic epithelial cells through mitogen-activated protein kinase signaling pathways. *Mol Cancer Res* **7**: 799–808.

Mattoon DR, Lamothe B, Lax I, Schlessinger J (2004). The docking protein Gab1 is the primary mediator of EGF-stimulated activation of the PI-3 K/Akt cell survival pathway. *BMC Biol* **2**: 24.

Meloche S, Pouyssegur J (2007). The ERK1/2 mitogen-activated protein kinase pathway as a master regulator of the G1- to S-phase transition. *Oncogene* **26**: 3227–39.

Miettinen PJ, Berger JE, Meneses J, Phung Y, Pedersen RA, Werb Z et al. (1995). Epithelial immaturity and multiorgan failure in mice lacking epidermal growth factor receptor. *Nature* **376**: 337–41.

Migliaccio E, Mele S, Salcini AE, Pelicci G, Lai K-A V, Superti-Furga G et al. (1997). Opposite effects of the p52shc/p46shc and p66shc splicing isoforms on the EGF receptor-Map kinase-fos signalling pathway. *EMBO J.* **16**: 706–16.

Milanini J, Vinals F, Pouyssegur J, Pages G (1998). p42/p44 MAP kinase module plays a key role in the transcriptional regulation of the vascular endothelial growth factor gene in fibroblasts. *J Biol Chem* **273**: 18165–72.

Montagner A, Yart A, Dance M, Perret B, Salles JP, Raynal P (2005). A novel role for Gab1 and SHP2 in epidermal growth factor-induced Ras activation. *J Biol Chem* **280**: 5350–60.

Mood K, Saucier C, Bong YS, Lee HS, Park M, Daar IO (2006a). Gab1 is required for cell cycle transition, cell proliferation, and transformation induced by an oncogenic met receptor. *Mol Biol Cell* **17**: 3717–28.

Mood K, Saucier C, Ishimura A, Bong YS, Lee HS, Park M et al. (2006b). Oncogenic met receptor induces cell-cycle progression in Xenopus oocytes independent of direct Grb2 and Shc binding or mos synthesis, but requires phosphatidylinositol 3-kinase and raf signaling. *J Cell Physiol* **207**: 271–85.

Nagahara H, Mimori K, Ohta M, Utsunomiya T, Inoue H, Barnard GF et al. (2005). Somatic mutations of epidermal growth factor receptor in colorectal carcinoma. *Clin Cancer Res* **11**: 1368–71.

Nejsum LN, Nelson WJ (2009). Epithelial cell surface polarity: the early steps. *Front Biosci* **14**: 1088–98.

Nemoto S, Finkel T (2002). Redox regulation of forkhead proteins through a p66shc-dependent signaling pathway. *Science* **295**: 2450–52.

Newell KJ, Witty JP, Rodgers WH, Matrisian LM (1994). Expression and localization of matrix-degrading metalloproteinases during colorectal tumorigenesis. *Mol Carcinog* **10**: 199–206.

Oft M, Akhurst RJ, Balmain A (2002). Metastasis is driven by sequential elevation of H-ras and Smad2 levels. *Nat Cell Biol* **4**: 487–94.

Oft M, Heider KH, Beug H (1998). TGFbeta signaling is necessary for carcinoma cell invasiveness and metastasis. *Curr Biol* **8**: 1243–52.

Oft M, Peli J, Rudaz C, Schwarz H, Beug H, Reichmann E (1996). TGF-beta1 and Ha-Ras collaborate in modulating the phenotypic plasticity and invasiveness of epithelial tumor cells. *Genes Dev* **10**: 2462–77.

Okada F, Rak JW, Croix BS, Lieubeau B, Kaya M, Roncari L et al. (1998). Impact of oncogenes in tumor angiogenesis: mutant K-RAS up-regulation of vascular endothelial growth factor/vascular permeability factor is necessary, but not sufficient for tumorigenicity of human colorectal carcinoma cells. *Proc Natl Acad Sci USA* **95**: 3609–14.

Okada S, Kao AW, Ceresa BP, Blaikie P, Margolis B, Pessin JE (1997). The 66-kDa Shc isoform is a negative regulator of the epidermal growth factor-stimulated mitogen-activated protein kinase pathway. *J Biol Chem* **272**: 28042–49.

Ono M, Sakamoto M, Ino Y, Moriya Y, Sugihara K, Muto T et al. (1996). Cancer cell morphology at the invasive front and expression of cell adhesion-related carbohydrate in the primary lesion of patients with colorectal carcinoma with liver metastasis. *Cancer* **78**: 1179–86.

Oshima M, Dinchuk JE, Kargman SL, Oshima H, Hancock B, Kwong E et al. (1996). Suppression of intestinal polyposis in Apc delta716 knockout mice by inhibition of cyclooxygenase 2 (COX-2). *Cell* **87**: 803–9.

Otte JM, Schmitz F, Kiehne K, Stechele HU, Banasiewicz T, Krokowicz P et al. (2000). Functional expression of HGF and its receptor in human colorectal cancer. *Digestion* **61**: 237–46.

Ougolkov AV, Yamashita K, Mai M, Minamoto Ts (2002). Oncogenic beta-catenin and MMP-7 (matrilysin) cosegregate in late-stage clinical colon cancer. *Gastroenterology* **122**: 60–71.

Parker C, Roseman BJ, Bucana CD, Tsan R, Radinsky R (1998). Preferential activation of the epidermal growth factor receptor in human colon carcinoma liver metastases in nude mice. *J Histochem Cytochem* **46**: 595–602.

Parr C, Hiscox S, Nakamura T, Matsumoto K, Jiang WG (2000). Nk4, a new HGF/SF variant, is an antagonist to the influence of HGF/SF on the motility and invasion of colon cancer cells. *Int J Cancer* **85**: 563–70.

Paschos KA, Canovas D, Bird NC (2009). The role of cell adhesion molecules in the progression of colorectal cancer and the development of liver metastasis. *Cell Signal* **21**: 665–74.

Pawson T, Nash P (2000). Protein-protein interactions define specificity in signal transduction. *Genes Dev* **14**: 1027–47.

Pawson T, Nash P (2003). Assembly of cell regulatory systems through protein interaction domains. *Science* **300**: 445–52.

Peinado H, Ballestar E, Esteller M, Cano AI (2004a). Snail mediates E-cadherin repression by the recruitment of the Sin3A/histone deacetylase 1 (HDAC1)/HDAC2 complex. *Mol Cell Biol* **24**: 306–19.

Peinado H, Marin F, Cubillo E, Stark HJ, Fusenig N, Nieto MA et al. (2004b). Snail and E47 repressors of E-cadherin induce distinct invasive and angiogenic properties in vivo. *J Cell Sci* **117**: 2827–39.

Pennacchietti S, Michieli P, Galluzzo M, Mazzone M, Giordano S, Comoglio PM (2003). Hypoxia promotes invasive growth by transcriptional activation of the met protooncogene. *Cancer Cell* **3**: 347–61.

Perez-Moreno MA, Locascio A, Rodrigo I, Dhondt G, Portillo F, Nieto MA et al. (2001). A new role for E12/E47 in the repression of E-cadherin expression and epithelial-mesenchymal transitions. *J Biol Chem* **276**: 27424–31.

Peschard P, Park M (2007). From Tpr-Met to Met, tumorigenesis and tubes. *Oncogene* **26**: 1276–85.

Pollock CB, Shirasawa S, Sasazuki T, Kolch W, Dhillon AS (2005). Oncogenic K-RAS is required to maintain changes in cytoskeletal organization, adhesion, and motility in colon cancer cells. *Cancer Res* **65**: 1244–50.

Potempa S, Ridley AJ (1998). Activation of both MAP kinase and phosphatidylinositide 3-kinase by Ras is required for hepatocyte growth factor/scatter factor-induced adherens junction disassembly. *Mol Biol Cell* **9**: 2185–200.

Prall F (2007). Tumour budding in colorectal carcinoma. *Histopathology* **50**: 151–62.

Pretlow TP, Pretlow TG (2005). Mutant KRAS in aberrant crypt foci (ACF): initiation of colorectal cancer? *Biochim Biophys Acta* **1756**: 83–96.

Pyke C, Kristensen P, Ralfkiaer E, Grondahl-Hansen J, Eriksen J, Blasi F et al. (1991). Urokinase-type plasminogen activator is expressed in stromal cells and its receptor in cancer cells at invasive foci in human colon adenocarcinomas. *Am J Pathol* **138**: 1059–67.

Rabinovitz I, Mercurio AM (1997). The integrin alpha6beta4 functions in carcinoma cell migration on laminin-1 by mediating the formation and stabilization of actin-containing motility structures. *J Cell Biol* **139**: 1873–84.

Radinsky R, Risin S, Fan D, Dong Z, Bielenberg D, Bucana CD et al. (1995). Level and function of epidermal growth factor receptor predict the metastatic potential of human colon carcinoma cells. *Clin Cancer Res* **1**: 19–31.

Rajagopalan H, Bardelli A, Lengauer C, Kinzler KW, Vogelstein B, Velculescu VE (2002). Tumorigenesis: RAF/RAS oncogenes and mismatch-repair status. *Nature* **418**: 934.

Rak J, Mitsuhashi Y, Bayko L, Filmus J, Shirasawa S, Sasazuki T et al. (1995a). Mutant ras oncogenes upregulate VEGF/VPF expression: implications for induction and inhibition of tumor angiogenesis. *Cancer Res* **55**: 4575–80.

Rak J, Mitsuhashi Y, Erdos V, Huang SN, Filmus J, Kerbel RS (1995b). Massive programmed cell death in intestinal epithelial cells induced by three-dimensional growth conditions: suppression by mutant c-H-ras oncogene expression. *J Cell Biol* **131**: 1587–98.

Ramos JW (2008). The regulation of extracellular signal-regulated kinase (ERK) in mammalian cells. *Int J Biochem Cell Biol* **40**: 2707–19.

Rasola A, Fassetta M, De Bacco F, D'Alessandro L, Gramaglia D, Di Renzo MF et al. (2007). A positive feedback loop between hepatocyte growth factor receptor and beta-catenin sustains colorectal cancer cell invasive growth. *Oncogene* **26**: 1078–87.

Ravichandran KS (2001). Signaling via Shc family adapter proteins. *Oncogene* **20**: 6322–30.

Repasky GA, Zhou Y, Morita S, Der CJ (2007). Ras-mediated intestinal epithelial cell transformation requires cyclooxygenase-2-induced prostaglandin E2 signaling. *Mol Carcinog* **46**: 958–70.

Richard DE, Berra E, Gothie E, Roux D, Pouyssegur J (1999). p42/p44 mitogen-activated protein kinases phosphorylate hypoxia-inducible factor 1alpha (HIF-1alpha) and enhance the transcriptional activity of HIF-1. *J Biol Chem* **274**: 32631–37.

Rivard N, Boucher MJ, Asselin C, L'Allemain G (1999). MAP kinase cascade is required for p27 downregulation and S phase entry in fibroblasts and epithelial cells. *Am J Physiol* **277**: C652–64.

Roberts PJ, Der CJ (2007). Targeting the Raf-MEK-ERK mitogen-activated protein kinase cascade for the treatment of cancer. *Oncogene* **26**: 3291–310.

Rodrigues GA, Falasca M, Zhang Z, Ong SH, Schlessinger J (2000). A novel positive feedback loop mediated by the docking protein Gab1 and phosphatidylinositol 3-kinase in epidermal growth factor receptor signaling. *Mol Cell Biol* **20**: 1448–59.

Rosen K, Rak J, Jin J, Kerbel RS, Newman MJ, Filmus J (1998). Downregulation of the pro-apoptotic protein Bak is required for the ras-induced transformation of intestinal epithelial cells. *Curr Biol* **8**: 1331–34.

Rosen K, Rak J, Leung T, Dean NM, Kerbel RS, Filmus J (2000). Activated Ras prevents downregulation of Bcl-X(L) triggered by detachment from the extracellular matrix. A mechanism of Ras-induced resistance to anoikis in intestinal epithelial cells. *J Cell Biol* **149**: 447–56.

Ross PJ, George M, Cunningham D, DiStefano F, Andreyev HJ, Workman P et al. (2001). Inhibition of Kirsten-ras expression in human colorectal cancer using rationally selected Kirsten-ras antisense oligonucleotides. *Mol Cancer Ther* **1**: 29–41.

Roy HK, Olusola BF, Clemens DL, Karolski WJ, Ratashak A, Lynch HT et al. (2002). AKT proto-oncogene overexpression is an early event during sporadic colon carcinogenesis. *Carcinogenesis* **23**: 201–5.

Rychahou PG, Jackson LN, Silva SR, Rajaraman S, Evers BM (2006). Targeted molecular therapy of the PI3K pathway: therapeutic significance of PI3K subunit targeting in colorectal carcinoma. *Ann Surg* **243**: 833–42; discussion 843–4.

Rychahou PG, Kang J, Gulhati P, Doan HQ, Chen LA, Xiao SY et al. (2008). Akt2 overexpression plays a critical role in the establishment of colorectal cancer metastasis. *Proc Natl Acad Sci USA* **105**: 20315–20.

Sahai E, Marshall CJ (2002). RHO-GTPases and cancer. *Nat Rev Cancer* **2**: 133–42.

Samowitz WS, Curtin K, Schaffer D, Robertson M, Leppert M, Slattery ML (2000). Relationship of Ki-ras mutations in colon cancers to tumor location, stage, and survival: a population-based study. *Cancer Epidemiol Biomarkers Prev* **9**: 1193–97.

Samuels Y, Diaz LA Jr, Schmidt-Kittler O, Cummins JM, Delong L, Cheong I et al. (2005). Mutant PIK3CA promotes cell growth and invasion of human cancer cells. *Cancer Cell* **7**: 561–73.

Sasaki T, Nakamura T, Rebhun RB, Cheng H, Hale KS, Tsan RZ et al. (2008). Modification of the primary tumor microenvironment by transforming growth factor alpha-epidermal growth factor receptor signaling promotes metastasis in an orthotopic colon cancer model. *Am J Pathol* **173**: 205–16.

Saucier C, Khoury H, Lai K-MV, Peschard P, Dankort D, Naujokas MA et al. (2004). The Shc adaptor protein is critical for VEGF induction by Met and ErbB2 receptors and for early onset of tumor angiogenesis. *Proc Natl Acad Sci USA* **101**: 2345–50.

Saucier C, Papavasiliou V, Palazzo A, Naujokas MA, Kremer R, Park M (2002). Use of signal specific receptor tyrosine kinase oncoproteins reveals that pathways downstream from Grb2 or Shc are sufficient for cell transformation and metastasis. *Oncogene* **21**: 1800–11.

Saxton TM, Cheng AM, Ong SH, Lu Y, Sakai R, Cross JC et al. (2001). Gene dosage-dependent functions for phosphotyrosine-Grb2 signaling during mammalian tissue morphogenesis. *Curr Biol* **11**: 662–70.

Schaeper U, Vogel R, Chmielowiec J, Huelsken J, Rosario M, Birchmeier W (2007). Distinct requirements for Gab1 in Met and EGF receptor signaling in vivo. *Proc Natl Acad Sci USA* **104**: 15376–81.

Schmidt CR, Gi YJ, Coffey RJ, Beauchamp RD, Pearson AS (2004). Oncogenic Ras dominates overexpression of E-cadherin in malignant transformation of intestinal epithelial cells. *Surgery* **136**: 303–9.

Schmidt CR, Washington MK, Gi YJ, Coffey RJ, Beauchamp RD, Pearson AS (2003). Dysregulation of E-cadherin by oncogenic Ras in intestinal epithelial cells is blocked by inhibiting MAP kinase. *Am J Surg* **186**: 426–30.

Schramm K, Krause K, Bittroff-Leben A, Goldin-Lang P, Thiel E, Kreuser ED (2000). Activated K-RAS is involved in regulation of integrin expression in human colon carcinoma cells. *Int J Cancer* **87**: 155–64.

Sebolt-Leopold JS, Dudley DT, Herrera R, Van Becelaere K, Wiland A, Gowan RC et al. (1999). Blockade of the MAP kinase pathway suppresses growth of colon tumors in vivo. *Nat Med* **5**: 810–16.

Seiden-Long I, Navab R, Shih W, Li M, Chow J, Zhu CQ et al. (2008). Gab1 but not Grb2 mediates tumor progression in Met overexpressing colorectal cancer cells. *Carcinogenesis* **29**: 647–55.

Sekharam M, Zhao H, Sun M, Fang Q, Zhang Q, Yuan Z et al. (2003). Insulin-like growth factor 1 receptor enhances invasion and induces resistance to apoptosis of colon cancer cells through the Akt/Bcl-x(L) pathway. *Cancer Res* **63**: 7708–16.

Semba S, Itoh N, Ito M, Youssef EM, Harada M, Moriya T et al. (2002). Down-regulation of PIK3CG, a catalytic subunit of phosphatidylinositol 3-OH kinase, by CpG hypermethylation in human colorectal carcinoma. *Clin Cancer Res* **8**: 3824–31.

Shao J, Evers BM, Sheng H (2004). Roles of phosphatidylinositol 3'-kinase and mammalian target of rapamycin/p70 ribosomal protein S6 kinase in K-RAS-mediated transformation of intestinal epithelial cells. *Cancer Res* **64**: 229–35.

Sheng H, Shao J, Dubois RN (2001). K-RAS-mediated increase in cyclooxygenase 2 mRNA stability involves activation of the protein kinase B1. *Cancer Res* **61**: 2670–75.

Sheng H, Shao J, Townsend CM Jr., Evers BM (2003). Phosphatidylinositol 3-kinase mediates proliferative signals in intestinal epithelial cells. *Gut* **52**: 1472–78.

Shinto E, Jass JR, Tsuda H, Sato T, Ueno H, Hase K et al. (2006). Differential prognostic significance of morphologic invasive markers in colorectal cancer: tumor budding and cytoplasmic podia. *Dis Colon Rectum* **49**: 1422–30.

Smakman N, Borel Rinkes IH, Voest EE, Kranenburg O (2005). Control of colorectal metastasis formation by K-RAS. *Biochim Biophys Acta* **1756**: 103–14.

Smalley WE, DuBois RN (1997). Colorectal cancer and nonsteroidal anti-inflammatory drugs. *Adv Pharmacol* **39**: 1–20.

Sodhi A, Montaner S, Miyazaki H, Gutkind JS (2001). MAPK and Akt act cooperatively but independently on hypoxia inducible factor-1alpha in rasV12 upregulation of VEGF. *Biochem Biophys Res Commun* **287**: 292–300.

Spano JP, Fagard R, Soria JC, Rixe O, Khayat D, Milano G (2005a). Epidermal growth factor receptor signaling in colorectal cancer: preclinical data and therapeutic perspectives. *Ann Oncol* **16**: 189–94.

Spano JP, Lagorce C, Atlan D, Milano G, Domont J, Benamouzig R et al. (2005b). Impact of EGFR expression on colorectal cancer patient prognosis and survival. *Ann Oncol* **16**: 102–8.

Stein U, Walther W, Arlt F, Schwabe H, Smith J, Fichtner I et al. (2009). MACC1, a newly identified key regulator of HGF-MET signaling, predicts colon cancer metastasis. *Nat Med* **15**: 59–67.
Subbaramaiah K, Dannenberg AJ (2003). Cyclooxygenase 2: a molecular target for cancer prevention and treatment. *Trends Pharmacol Sci* **24**: 96–102.
Takeuchi H, Bilchik A, Saha S, Turner R, Wiese D, Tanaka M et al. (2003). c-MET expression level in primary colon cancer: a predictor of tumor invasion and lymph node metastases. *Clin Cancer Res* **9**: 1480–88.
Tokunaga T, Tsuchida T, Kijima H, Okamoto K, Oshika Y, Sawa N et al. (2000). Ribozyme-mediated inactivation of mutant K-RAS oncogene in a colon cancer cell line. *Br J Cancer* **83**: 833–39.
Tremblay PL, Auger FA, Huot J (2006). Regulation of transendothelial migration of colon cancer cells by E-selectin-mediated activation of p38 and ERK MAP kinases. *Oncogene* **25**: 6563–73.
Trobridge P, Knoblaugh S, Washington MK, Munoz NM, Tsuchiya KD, Rojas A et al. (2009). TGF-beta receptor inactivation and mutant Kras induce intestinal neoplasms in mice via a beta-catenin-independent pathway. *Gastroenterology* **136**: 1680–88.
Tsuchihashi Z, Khambata-Ford S, Hanna N, Janne PA (2005). Responsiveness to cetuximab without mutations in EGFR. *N Engl J Med* **353**: 208–9.
Tuveson DA, Shaw AT, Willis NA, Silver DP, Jackson EL, Chang S et al. (2004). Endogenous oncogenic K-RAS(G12D) stimulates proliferation and widespread neoplastic and developmental defects. *Cancer Cell* **5**: 375–87.
Ursini-Siegel J, Hardy WR, Zuo D, Lam SH, Sanguin-Gendreau V, Cardiff RD et al. (2008). ShcA signalling is essential for tumour progression in mouse models of human breast cancer. *Embo J* **27**: 910–20.
van der Horst EH, Chinn L, Wang M, Velilla T, Tran H, Madrona Y et al. (2009). Discovery of fully human anti-MET monoclonal antibodies with antitumor activity against colon cancer tumor models in vivo. *Neoplasia* **11**: 355–64.
Van Waes C, Kozarsky KF, Warren AB, Kidd L, Paugh D, Liebert M et al. (1991). The A9 antigen associated with aggressive human squamous carcinoma is structurally and functionally similar to the newly defined integrin alpha 6 beta 4. *Cancer Res* **51**: 2395–402.
Vial E, Sahai E, Marshall CJ (2003). ERK-MAPK signaling coordinately regulates activity of Rac1 and RhoA for tumor cell motility. *Cancer Cell* **4**: 67–79.
Voisin L, Julien C, Duhamel S, Gopalbhai K, Claveau I, Saba-El-Leil MK et al. (2008). Activation of MEK1 or MEK2 isoform is sufficient to fully transform intestinal epithelial cells and induce the formation of metastatic tumors. *BMC Cancer* **8**: 337.
Volpert OV, Tolsma SS, Pellerin S, Feige JJ, Chen H, Mosher DF et al. (1995). Inhibition of angiogenesis by thrombospondin-2. *Biochem Biophys Res Commun* **217**: 326–32.
Wagenaar-Miller RA, Gorden L, Matrisian LM (2004). Matrix metalloproteinases in colorectal cancer: is it worth talking about? *Cancer Metastasis Rev* **23**: 119–35.
Walther A, Johnstone E, Swanton C, Midgley R, Tomlinson I, Kerr D (2009). Genetic prognostic and predictive markers in colorectal cancer. *Nat Rev Cancer* **9**: 489–99.
Wang H, Quah SY, Dong JM, Manser E, Tang JP, Zeng Q (2007). PRL-3 down-regulates PTEN expression and signals through PI3K to promote epithelial-mesenchymal transition. *Cancer Res* **67**: 2922–26.
Wang HB, Liu XP, Liang J, Yang K, Sui AH, Liu YJ (2009). Expression of RhoA and RhoC in colorectal carcinoma and its relations with clinicopathological parameters. *Clin Chem Lab Med* **47**: 811–17.
Wang Q, Wang X, Hernandez A, Kim S, Evers BM (2001). Inhibition of the phosphatidylinositol 3-kinase pathway contributes to HT29 and Caco-2 intestinal cell differentiation. *Gastroenterology* **120**: 1381–92.
Wee S, Wiederschain D, Maira SM, Loo A, Miller C, deBeaumont R et al. (2008). PTEN-deficient cancers depend on PIK3CB. *Proc Natl Acad Sci USA* **105**: 13057–62.
Wen J, Matsumoto K, Taniura N, Tomioka D, Nakamura T (2004). Hepatic gene expression of NK4, an HGF-antagonist/angiogenesis inhibitor, suppresses liver metastasis and invasive growth of colon cancer in mice. *Cancer Gene Ther* **11**: 419–30.

Wen J, Matsumoto K, Taniura N, Tomioka D, Nakamura T (2007). Inhibition of colon cancer growth and metastasis by NK4 gene repetitive delivery in mice. *Biochem Biophys Res Commun* **358**: 117–23.

Wilson CL, Heppner KJ, Labosky PA, Hogan BL, Matrisian LM (1997). Intestinal tumorigenesis is suppressed in mice lacking the metalloproteinase matrilysin. *Proc Natl Acad Sci USA* **94**: 1402–7.

Windham TC, Parikh NU, Siwak DR, Summy JM, McConkey DJ, Kraker AJ et al. (2002). Src activation regulates anoikis in human colon tumor cell lines. *Oncogene* **21**: 7797–807.

Wolff WL, Shinya H, Cwern M, Hsu M (1990). Cancerous colonic polyps. "Hands on" or "hands off?" *Am Surg* **56**: 148–52.

Wu X, Senechal K, Neshat MS, Whang YE, Sawyers CL (1998). The PTEN/MMAC1 tumor suppressor phosphatase functions as a negative regulator of the phosphoinositide 3-kinase/Akt pathway. *Proc Natl Acad Sci USA* **95**: 15587–91.

Xu J, Rodriguez D, Petitclerc E, Kim JJ, Hangai M, Moon YS et al. (2001). Proteolytic exposure of a cryptic site within collagen type IV is required for angiogenesis and tumor growth in vivo. *J Cell Biol* **154**: 1069–79.

Yamamoto H, Itoh F, Senota A, Adachi Y, Yoshimoto M, Endoh T et al. (1995). Expression of matrix metalloproteinase matrilysin (MMP-7) was induced by activated Ki-ras via AP-1 activation in SW1417 colon cancer cells. *J Clin Lab Anal* **9**: 297–301.

Yan Z, Chen M, Perucho M, Friedman E (1997a). Oncogenic Ki-ras but not oncogenic Ha-ras blocks integrin beta1-chain maturation in colon epithelial cells. *J Biol Chem* **272**: 30928–36.

Yan Z, Deng X, Chen M, Xu Y, Ahram M, Sloane BF et al. (1997b). Oncogenic c-Ki-ras but not oncogenic c-Ha-ras up-regulates CEA expression and disrupts basolateral polarity in colon epithelial cells. *J Biol Chem* **272**: 27902–7.

Yang JL, Seetoo D, Wang Y, Ranson M, Berney CR, Ham JM et al. (2000). Urokinase-type plasminogen activator and its receptor in colorectal cancer: independent prognostic factors of metastasis and cancer-specific survival and potential therapeutic targets. *Int J Cancer* **89**: 431–39.

Yokoi K, Thaker PH, Yazici S, Rebhun RR, Nam DH, He J et al. (2005). Dual inhibition of epidermal growth factor receptor and vascular endothelial growth factor receptor phosphorylation by AEE788 reduces growth and metastasis of human colon carcinoma in an orthotopic nude mouse model. *Cancer Res* **65**: 3716–25.

Yu GZ, Chen Y, Long YQ, Dong D, Mu XL, Wang JJ (2008). New insight into the key proteins and pathways involved in the metastasis of colorectal carcinoma. *Oncol Rep* **19**: 1191–204.

Zeng ZS, Weiser MR, Kuntz E, Chen CT, Khan SA, Forslund A et al. (2008). c-Met gene amplification is associated with advanced stage colorectal cancer and liver metastases. *Cancer Lett* **265**: 258–69.

Zhang J, Anastasiadis PZ, Liu Y, Thompson EA, Fields AP (2004). Protein kinase C (PKC) betaII induces cell invasion through a Ras/Mek-, PKC iota/Rac 1-dependent signaling pathway. *J Biol Chem* **279**: 22118–23.

Zhang YA, Nemunaitis J, Scanlon KJ, Tong AW (2000). Anti-tumorigenic effect of a K-RAS ribozyme against human lung cancer cell line heterotransplants in nude mice. *Gene Ther* **7**: 2041–50.

Zhang YH, Wei W, Xu H, Wang YY, Wu WX (2007). Inducing effects of hepatocyte growth factor on the expression of vascular endothelial growth factor in human colorectal carcinoma cells through MEK and PI3K signaling pathways. *Chin Med J (England)* **120**: 743–48.

Zhao L, Vogt PK (2008). Class I PI3K in oncogenic cellular transformation. *Oncogene* **27**: 5486–96.

Zhou XP, Loukola A, Salovaara R, Nystrom-Lahti M, Peltomaki P, de la Chapelle A et al. (2002). PTEN mutational spectra, expression levels, and subcellular localization in microsatellite stable and unstable colorectal cancers. *Am J Pathol* **161**: 439–47.

Zlobec I, Vuong T, Hayashi S, Haegert D, Tornillo L, Terracciano L et al. (2007). A simple and reproducible scoring system for EGFR in colorectal cancer: application to prognosis and prediction of response to preoperative brachytherapy. *Br J Cancer* **96**: 793–800.

Chapter 9

ANGIOGENESIS AND LYMPHANGIOGENESIS IN COLON CANCER METASTASIS

Delphine Garnier[1] and Janusz Rak[2]
[1] *Montreal Children's Hospital Research Institute, McGill University, Montreal, QC, Canada*
[2] *Montreal Children's Hospital Research Institute, McGill University, Montreal, QC, Canada, e-mail: janusz.rak@mcgill.ca*

Abstract: The vascular system markedly contributes to the pathogenesis of colorectal cancer (CRC). Indeed, agents targeting angiogenesis (bevacizumab) exhibit considerable efficacy in treatment of metastatic CRC, but less so in other (adjuvant) settings. These unexpected outcomes indicate that, to make further progress, a more complete understanding is required of the relationship between the tumour cell compartment and various facets of the vasculature. Here, we review the general mechanisms involved in angiogenesis and lymphangiogenesis during formation, growth and metastatic dissemination of CRC. We discuss several levels at which blood vessel growth is regulated, namely through local growth factor networks, circulating effectors, coagulation system, microvesicles and bone marrow-derived cells, the latter acting at the systemic level. We survey the mechanisms triggering the proangiogenic state in cancer, including microenvironment and oncogenic pathways, and discuss the developments in anti-angiogenic therapy.

Key words: Angiogenesis · Bone marrow · Colorectal cancer · Lymphangiogenesis · Metastasis

9.1 Introduction: Tumour-Vascular Interface in Progression and Metastasis of Colorectal Cancer

The wall of the normal colon is richly supplied with blood and lymphatic vessels, the architecture of which differs from that of the small intestine and between more proximal and distal colonic segments (Tomita, 2008; Konerding et al., 2001). While colonic lymphatics form slender endothelial insertions positive for lymphatic vessel endothelial hyaluronan receptor 1 (LYVE-1) into the *muscularis mucosa* and around the bases of the crypts (Tomita, 2008), blood vessel capillaries are organized into orderly honeycomb-like patterns around the crypts (Konerding et al., 2001), and lie in one or more layers immediately underneath the basement membrane of the colonic epithelium (Tomita, 2008). In spite of this proximity, there is, however, a strict micro-anatomical separation between these compartments, mainly afforded by basement membranes and layers of extracellular matrix (ECM) that prevent a direct physical contact between endothelium and blood on the one hand, and colonocytes and intestinal content on the other. This serves to preserve the barrier, absorptive and other functions of the large intestine, intricate spatial relationships that undergo dramatic changes during the course of colonic pathology, and especially in colorectal cancer (CRC).

Indeed, one of the most striking features in progression of CRC, and human malignancies in general, is the emergence of multiple new and abnormal points of direct contact between the cellular compartments, from which the tumour originates (e.g. epithelia, cancer stem cells), and the various facets of the host vascular system. As a result, the initial barriers separating these respective compartments become compromised due to the onset of several processes, including: blood vessel cooption by cancer cells and vascular invasion, onset of capillary hyperpermeability and leakage of plasma macromolecules into the interstitium, formation of new vascular and lymphatic structures through processes of vasculogenesis, angiogenesis and lymphangiogenesis. This is accompanied by onset of local and systemic coagulation, intravasation of cancer cells, as well as embolisation and modification of vascular wall during the process of regional and distant metastasis (Folkman and Kalluri, 2003; Holash et al., 1999; Dvorak and Rickles, 2006; Carmeliet, 2005).

These processes progressively change the vascular micro-anatomy (Konerding et al., 2001), and the positioning of cancer cells vis-à-vis their adjacent vascular structures, as well as the scope and nature of their related functional interactions (Rak, 2009). A more heterogeneous and dynamic state that emerges in the process could be collectively described as *tumour-vascular interface* (TVI) (Rak, 2009), and in many ways it represents both the outcome and the causal element in the pathogenesis of CRC (Ellis, 2004).

Indeed, tumour vascular interface is critical not only in control of growth, survival, metabolic activity, invasion, endocrine and paracrine stimulation and dissemination of cancer cells (Folkman and Kalluri, 2003), but also exerts a potent influence on cancer stem cell compartment (Bao et al., 2006; Calabrese et al., 2007; Rak et al., 2008), on drug delivery, responsiveness to therapy, on composition and distribution of disease biomarkers, and is also a source of para-neoplastic syndromes (e.g. cachexia, thrombosis). These processes also modulate bone marrow responses, immunity and a plethora of other critical events, both local and systemic in nature. Several aspects of this relationship are illustrated by the continuum of vascular processes leading through tumour angiogenesis, lymphangiogenesis and invasion to metastasis and disseminated disease, all of which accompany the development of full blown CRC and tumour progression in general (Folkman, 1985; Fidler, 2003;

Ellis, 2004). These constituents will be described in the remainder of this chapter along with some of their therapeutic implications.

9.2 Mechanisms of Vascular and Lymphatic Growth

Blood vessels and lymphatics play distinct, but complementary roles in regulating tissue and systemic homeostasis, namely as conduits and regulators of sustained and directional circulation of fluids, blood cells, nutrients and regulatory molecules within and between organs (Alitalo et al., 2005; Carmeliet, 2005; Jimeno et al., 2007). While the central cellular constituent of both of these systems are endothelial cells, the properties of these cells differ between the vascular and lymphatic microcirculation, as do structural and functional features of the corresponding capillaries, and processes of their generation (Carmeliet, 2005). The latter occurs most robustly during development, but also accompanies tissue repair, tissue mass and organ enlargement, both in health and disease, including cancer. It is increasingly clear that, in all these contexts, blood and lymphatic vessels are programmed to evolve to meet the local tissue requirements, and this is associated, at least to some extent, with the expression of organ/site-specific features (Seaman et al., 2007). Such features are also found during blood vessel formation accompanying CRC (St. Croix et al., 2000; van Beijnum and Griffioen, 2005). This site-specificity is, however, superimposed with a more generic program of blood vessel growth and remodelling, the molecular understanding of which is increasingly well understood (Carmeliet, 2005).

9.2.1 Formation of Microvascular Networks

Blood vessel networks associated with cancer progression are highly abnormal from the structural (Folkman and Kalluri, 2003; Jain et al., 2006; Konerding et al., 2001; McDonald and Choyke, 2003), cellular (McDonald and Choyke, 2003) and molecular (Seaman et al., 2007; van Beijnum and Griffioen, 2005; St. Croix et al., 2000) points of view. This is likely a consequence of a deregulation of vascular homeostasis by tumour-related, oncogenic and micro-environmental factors (Rak et al., 2000b; Bouck et al., 1996; Rak and Kerbel, 2003). These are linked to the emergence of new cellular masses and/or replacement of the pre-existing normal vascularised tissue structures. Both of these processes necessitate a corresponding expansion and remodelling of the microvasculature (Folkman and Kalluri, 2003).

Indeed, the access to the vasculature is essential for tumour cell growth, survival, formation of cancer stem cell niches and metastasis (Folkman and Kalluri, 2003; Gilbertson and Rich, 2007; Fidler, 2003; Ellis, 2004). This access may also influence a number of fundamentally important tumour properties, such as extent of metabolic and hypoxic stress (Harris, 2002), paracrine effects of vascular cells on the tumour cell population (Rak et al., 1996), access of inflammatory cells to the tumour interior (Karin, 2005), selection of cancer cell subpopulations according to their vascular proximity (Yu et al., 2001), regional heterogeneity of cancer cells and the resulting changes in tumour aggressiveness (Rak et al., 2002; Yu et al., 2002b), or invasiveness (Ebos et al., 2009; Paez-Ribes et al., 2009; Skobe et al., 1997) as well as the regulation of drug delivery, responses to radiation (Jain, 1990), genetic instability of cancer cells and various manifestations of therapeutic resistance (Shahrzad et al., 2005, 2008; Rak, 2009), to mention only the more studied properties.

Cancer cells may secure the access to the local microcirculation either by actively moving towards, and invading, the existing vasculature (vascular cooption or invasion, respectively (Folkman and Kalluri, 2003; Holash et al., 1999)), and sometimes by forming the lining of the perfused spaces within the tumour mass (vasculogenic mimicry (Hendrix et al., 2003)). However, the most predominant biological process whereby tumours develop and modulate their 'private' vascular supply is by the recruitment of host vascular cells and formation of endothelial channels through several processes, which depending on their nature are referred to as: angiogenesis, vasculogenesis, vascular remodelling, vascular regression (pruning), vessel maturation/stabilization (Carmeliet, 2000; Kerbel, 2008), and neo-arteriogenesis (an aberrant formation of larger feeding vessels) (Yu and Rak, 2003).

Endothelial cells are central to all these processes, along with their supporting mural cells (pericytes), inflammatory cells and other bone marrow-derived progenitor and regulatory cellular populations (Folkman and Kalluri, 2003; Carmeliet, 2005; Kerbel, 2008). Thus, endothelial cell tubes may, in principle, emerge through a self assembly and differentiation of endothelial progenitor cells (EPCs), during the sequence of events known as vasculogenesis (Risau, 1997). There are likely several subsets of EPCs that may contribute to this process and they mostly express distinct, or overlapping molecular markers (Asahara et al., 1997; Lyden et al., 2001; Bertolini et al., 2006), including: CD34+, VEGFR2+, CD45–, CD133+, CD117+, and possibly other characteristics. Prenatally, such cells and their precursors emanate from the embryonal mesenchyme and certain preformed vascular structures, while the main sources of their postnatal counterparts are in the bone marrow (Risau, 1997; Carmeliet, 2005; Ema and Rossant, 2003; Coultas et al., 2005), and possibly in some subsets of peripheral endothelial cells (Pacilli and Pasquinelli, 2009). A major structural involvement of EPCs in blood vessel assembly is observed during vascular development (Carmeliet, 2000), while this contribution appears to be much less consistent and less pronounced in adulthood, and during tumour neo-vascularization (Peters et al., 2005; Lyden et al., 2001). However, this does not preclude an increasingly well-understood and prominent role of circulating endothelial progenitors (CEPs) under more specific circumstances, namely during vascular repair and re-endothelialization of vascular structures or grafts (Shantsila et al., 2007), and also during vascular re-growth in tumours, for instance after successful antivascular therapy (Shaked et al., 2006).

Mobilization, recruitment and retention of such progenitor cells in the tumour microcirculation is regulated by a number of factors, such as the expression of DNA-binding protein inhibitor 1 (Id1) Id3 family of transcriptional repressors and a network of paracrine, endocrine and adhesive influences, involving: vascular endothelial growth factor (VEGF), stromal-derived factor 1 (SDF1), colony stimulating factors (CSFs), α4β1 integrins, amongst many other less-studied mechanisms (Rafii et al., 2002; Asahara et al., 1999; Shaked et al., 2006; Kerbel, 2008; Avraamides et al., 2008; Carmeliet, 2005). The levels of CEPs are negatively affected by aging and atherosclerosis (Shantsila et al., 2007), a circumstance that may have an impact on age-related aspects of tumour angiogenesis and anti-angiogenesis (Klement et al., 2007).

In contrast to vasculogenesis, the process of angiogenesis begins from the preformed capillary network, and leads to its enlargement and formation of new vascular loops (Folkman and Kalluri, 2003; Carmeliet, 2000). This can be achieved through a number of mechanisms, such as for example, a longitudinal division of larger capillaries into several lower calibre vessels. These become separated by septa formed through the action of extra-vascular (intussusceptive) (Burri, 1991), or intra-vascular (splitting) cellular pillars, which ultimately divide the vascular lumen (Carmeliet, 2000). Such events have, indeed, been observed in some experimental colorectal tumours (Patan et al., 1996), but the main pathway of new blood vessel formation in this and other cancer-related circumstances is believed to entail another form of angiogenesis. The latter relies upon mobilization and directional deployment of endothelial cell cohorts, and is commonly known as vascular sprouting (Carmeliet, 2000).

The morphological and molecular events associated with vascular sprouting are relatively well described (Paku and Paweletz, 1991; Paweletz and Knierim, 1989; Dvorak et al., 1991; Carmeliet and Jain, 2000; Gerhardt et al., 2003). They are believed to represent a microvascular response to formation of regulatory gradients of pro- and anti-angiogenic growth factors that are thought to trigger the 'angiogenic switch' upon reaching certain biological thresholds around the pre-existing vessels (Folkman and Kalluri, 2003). Due to the destructive nature of vascular growth per se, most adult tissues are programmed to resist the angiogenic stimulation, notably by low constitutive levels of angiogenic growth factors, expression of anti-angiogenic molecules and by structural constrains (pericyte coverage, basement membrane development or extracellular matrix), all of which maintain endothelial cells in a quiescent state (Folkman and Kalluri, 2003).

The relief from this endothelial growth arrest and the onset of the perpetual angiogenesis cycles are amongst the most consistent hallmarks of cancer (Hanahan and Weinberg, 2000). Although the nature of the underlying process is highly complex, multifactorial, as well as site- and tumour-specific, the related key events may, for simplicity, be illustrated here by the description of the well-studied responses of blood vessels to vascular endothelial growth factor A (VEGF-A/VEGF), which is the central regulator of angiogenesis, vasculogenesis and vascular development, and a well established therapeutic target in metastatic CRC (Ferrara, 2005; Dvorak, 2002). Please see Table 9.1, Figs. 9.1 and 9.2 for a summary of angiogenic and lymphangiogenic regulators.

These events have been recently described by Dvorak (Dvorak, 2002; Pettersson et al., 2000) and others (Gerhardt et al., 2003; Thurston et al., 2007; Uyttendaele et al., 1996; Carmeliet, 2005; Kerbel, 2008) and begin with the VEGF-dependent

Table 9.1 Examples of angiogenesis and lymphangiogenesis regulators (see text Carmeliet, 2005; Lohela et al., 2009; Alitalo et al., 2005)

	Angiogenesis	Lymphangiogenesis
Growth factors and receptors	VEGF-A binds VEGFR1, VEGFR2	VEGF-C and VEGF-D bind VEGFR3
	Tie-2 receptor binds Ang-1 (promotes sprouting and maturation) and Ang-2 (destabilizes vessels and conditions them for angiogenesis)	
	Neuropilin NRP1 (arteries), NRP2 (veins)	NRP2, a receptor for VEGF-C, can interact with VEGFR3
	EphrinB2, FGF-2, PDGF-B	
	PlGF, HGF, TGF-beta	HGF, IGF1 and IGF2
Other membrane proteins	Notch receptors and Delta-like-4 (DLL4) ligand	Podoplanin
	CD44 hyaluronan receptor	LYVE-1 hyaluronan receptor
Transcription factors	Foxc2, forkhead transcription factor	Prox-1 homeobox transcription factor
Adhesion molecules	$\alpha_v\beta_3$, $\alpha_v\beta_5$, $\alpha_5\beta_1$, $\alpha_6\beta_4$ integrins	Desmoplakin, α_9, β_1 integrins

initial circumferential enlargement of the capillary (or venule) (Pettersson et al., 2000), resulting in formation of a thin-walled structure called a 'mother vessel' (Pettersson et al., 2000). This is followed by a focal dissolution of the basement membrane, detachment of the pericytes from the endothelial tube, increase in vascular permeability and activation of migratory, proliferative and morphogenetic programs of those endothelial cells that are most directly exposed to the highest VEGF concentrations (Pettersson et al., 2000). These cells form an organized multicellular projection/column (sprout), which moves in a direction defined by the VEGF gradient (Dvorak, 2002).

Sprouts are heterogenous, as each contains a leading endothelial cell (tip cell) containing numerous filopodia, rich in receptors for VEGF, platelet-derived growth factor B (PDGF-B) and other factors, all of which are required for detection of the angiogenic gradients (Gerhardt et al., 2003). Tip cells also express high levels of the endothelial-specific Notch ligand, delta-like 4 (Dll-4), which ensures their 'leadership' position in the endothelial hierarchy (Uyttendaele et al., 1996). The following endothelial cells (stalk cells) participate in the extension of the vascular sprout by directional and highly coordinated migration and proliferative responses, the latter most intense at the base of the sprout (Carmeliet, 2005), as well as by formation of the capillary lumen through connections between intracellular vacuoles (Kamei et al., 2006).

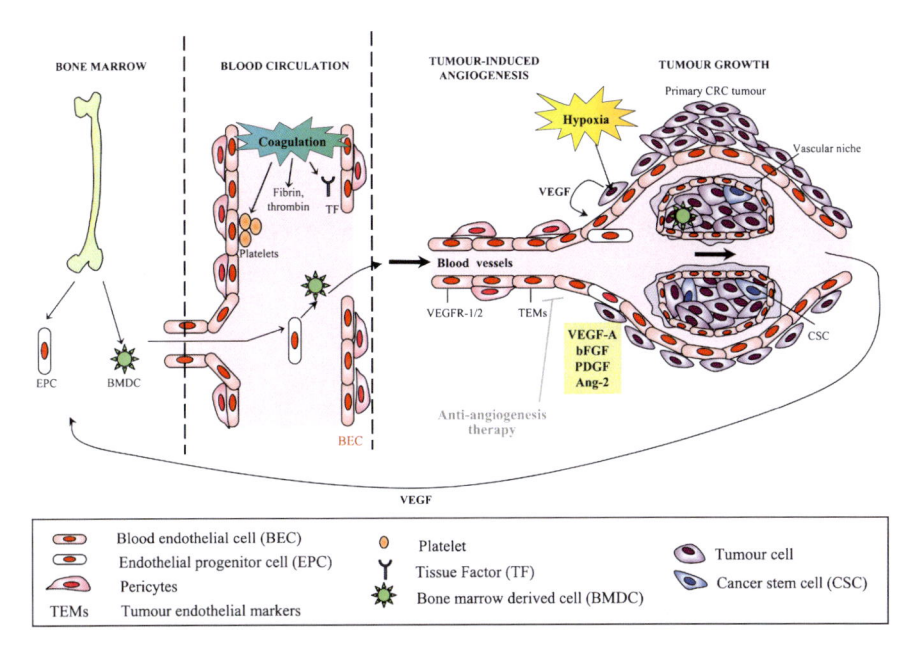

9 Angiogenesis and Lymphangiogenesis in Colon Cancer Metastasis 249

Fig. 9.1 Cell types and molecular mediators involved in angiogenesis. Tumour angiogenesis is triggered by gradients of angiogenic factors (e.g. members of the VEGF family) the levels of which are deregulated by hypoxia, inflammation, oncogenic events and other influences. These processes act locally, to mobilize blood vessel resident endothelial (BEC) and mural cells (pericytes), but also cells in the bone marrow. The latter include hematopoietic (HSC) and endothelial progenitor cells (EPC), and bone marrow derived cells (BMDC) with regulatory properties, which contribute to a further secretion of angiogenic factors, tumour angiogenesis and tumour growth

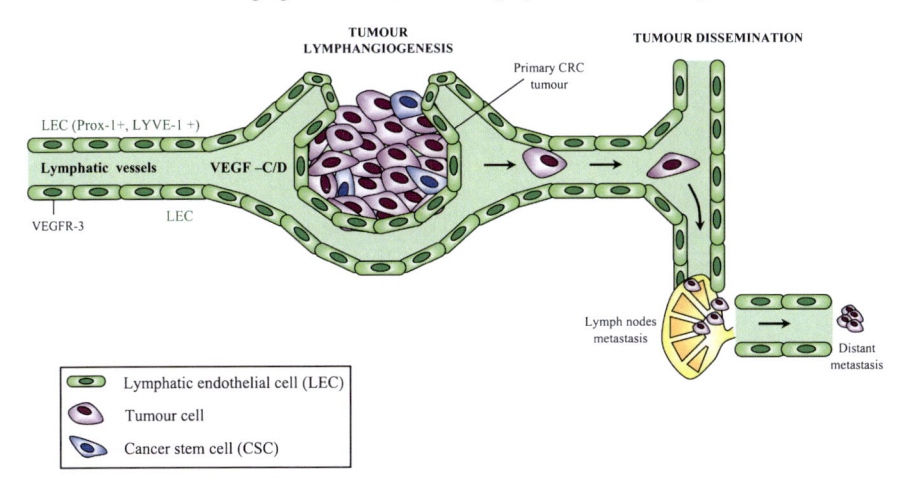

Fig. 9.2 Lymphangiogenesis in tumour. Formation of tumour-related lymphatics involves a distinct set of cell types and molecular mediators. The production of lymphangiogenic factors such as VEGF-C or D by tumour cells and other elements stimulates growth of lymphatic endothelial cells (LECs) and formation of thin walled lymphatic channels that drain fluids from perfused tissues. In cancer, robust formation of peritumoural lymphatics contributes to the dissemination of tumour cells to lymph nodes and distant organs

It should be mentioned in this context that, while VEGF acts directly on endothelial cells, mainly through the signalling receptor known as vascular endothelial growth factor receptor 2 (VEGFR2)/kinase insert domain-containing receptor (KDR)/fetal liver kinase 1 (Flk-1), other growth factor cascades also help orchestrate the angiogenic process (Shibuya, 2006). Some of these factors emanate from endothelial cells, while others could be supplied by their non-endothelial counterparts surrounding vascular sprouts and loops (Carmeliet, 2000). Of those, some cells express another functional VEGF receptor, VEGFR1/fms-related tyrosine kinase 1 (Flt-1), which is involved in cellular migration and recruitment, including in the case of certain types of cancer cells of colorectal and pancreatic origin (Fan et al., 2005). VEGFR-1 is also expressed by macrophages, myeloid cells and hematopoietic stem cells (HSCs) involved in angiogenesis (see below) (Rafii et al., 2002; Bertolini et al., 2006; Ellis, 2004; Shibuya, 2006). Interestingly, the arrival of VEGFR1$^+$ bone marrow-derived cells may precede angiogenic switch activating endothelial cells, at least in certain experimental settings (Lyden et al., 2001). Cells with similar characteristics are also involved in formation of pre-metastatic niches, micro-environmental sites to which metastatic cancer cells subsequently lodge (Kaplan et al., 2005), all of which is suggestive of the involvement of bone marrow in these otherwise local processes.

At least two out of several VEGF-triggered endothelial growth factors appear to be obligatory during the course of the sprouting angiogenesis, namely: angiopoietin-2 (Ang-2) and Dll-4 (Yancopoulos et al., 2000; Thurston et al., 2007; Uyttendaele et al., 1996). Ang-2 is a natural antagonist of the blood vessel stabilizing ligand, angiopoietin 1 (Ang-1), which interacts with the endothelial receptor tyrosine kinase, known as tyrosine kinase with Ig-like loops and epidermal growth factor homology domains-2 (Tie-2)/Tek (Dumont et al., 1992; Yancopoulos et al., 2000; Augustin et al., 2009). While Ang-1 triggers a robust phosphorylation of Tie-2 and exhibits pro-survival and pro-angiogenic functions itself, in so doing this mediator appears to also be involved in orchestrating the coverage of endothelial tubes with pericytes and in counteracting vascular permeability effects induced by VEGF. These effects of Ang-1 are of considerable importance for vascular maturation, mechanical resistance and functionality of the newly formed capillaries (Thurston et al., 2007; Hanahan, 1997; Carmeliet, 2005). In contrast to Ang-1, VEGF-driven upregulation of Ang-2 in endothelial cells reverses some of these stabilizing effects rendering endothelial tubes more fragile, but also more susceptible to sprout forming influences of VEGF and other ligands (Yancopoulos et al., 2000; Hanahan, 1997).

As mentioned earlier, in the presence of VEGF some endothelial cells assume the role of tip cells and begin to express high levels of Dll-4 (Uyttendaele et al., 1996; Noguera-Troise et al., 2006). This selective expression of Dll-4 by the leading cells at the tip of each sprout, regulates the number of tip cells via signals mediated through the Notch receptor pathway (Uyttendaele et al., 1996). Indeed, blockade of Dll-4 leads to exuberant formation of new tip cells, excessive sprouting and branching, and to formation of hyper-dense microvascular networks that are functionally deficient, poorly perfused, and unable to support proper tissue oxygenation and tumour growth, an effect known as *non-productive angiogenesis* (Thurston et al., 2007; Noguera-Troise et al., 2006).

Aberrant formation and movement of tip cells and their associated sprouts could also be influenced by the characteristics of the VEGF gradient itself (Gerhardt et al., 2003). In this regard, it was long known that several molecular VEGF isoforms are produced in various tissues, resulting from the alternative splicing of the transcript produced from a single *VEGF-A* gene (Ferrara, 2005). Several such splice variants have been described and accordingly designated on the basis of the number of their constituent amino acids, for instance as: VEGF121, VEGF165 and VEGF189 (VEGF120, VEGF164 and VEGF188 in mice) (Ferrara, 2005).

This diversity of protein products is highly consequential. For instance, formation of the shortest VEGF species (VEGF121) leads to exclusion of neuropilin 1 (NRP1) binding sites from the molecule, which does not contain sequences encoded by the exon 7 of VEGF (Soker et al., 1998). VEGF121 also does not bind to heparin due to the absence of sites encoded by exons 6–7 (Ferrara, 2005). This property renders VEGF121 highly soluble and unable to be retained on the scaffold of the ECM, or on cellular surfaces, both of which are required for the formation of a stable VEGF gradient in the angiogenic tissue (Gerhardt et al., 2003). In contrast, VEGF189 contains an abundance of heparin binding sites and is almost entirely retained on the cell surface, which makes it virtually indiffusible and poorly angiogenic (Yu et al., 2002a). VEGF165 exhibits intermediate properties, in that it binds efficiently to ECM, but is also readily diffusible, whereby it forms robust pericellular gradients and stimulates florid angiogenic responses (Ferrara, 2002).

It is unclear why various cancer cells express one, or more VEGF isoforms, but the resulting vascular patterns are markedly different (Yu et al., 2002a; Grunstein et al., 2000). Similarly, a selective removal of VEGF isoforms in mice suggests the differential roles of these ligands in angiogenesis and vascular homeostasis in different organs (Stalmans et al., 2002). A recent ground-breaking study demonstrated that proper formation and guidance of tip cells depends on the gradient of VEGF165, while the exposure to highly soluble VEGF121 may perturb this process (Gerhardt et al., 2003).

VEGF/VEGF-A and its isoforms are not the only members of this family of angiogenic proteins (Ferrara, 2002; Ladomery et al., 2007). Indeed, at least five additional factors share a partial sequence homology, including: VEGF-B, VEGF-C, VEGF-D, VEGF-E and PlGF (placenta growth factor) (Ferrara, 2002). In spite of this, the role of VEGF-A in the vascular system is rather unique, even though other members of this family may also activate VEGF receptors, including: VEGFR1 (PlGF, VEGF-B), VEGFR2 (VEGF-E), VEGFR3/Flt-4 (VEGF-C, VEGF-D), NRP1 (VEGF-A165), or are known to participate in pathological angiogenesis, lymphangiogenesis (VEGF-C/D) and other aspects of vascular regulation (Fischer et al., 2008; Alitalo et al., 2005; Ferrara, 2005). While the receptors involved in these events are usually activated by the respective biologically active homodimers (e.g. of VEGF-A), heteromerization of some of these ligands has also been described (Carmeliet, 2000).

Under physiological conditions newly formed vascular sprouts eventually anastomose with each other, or connect with target capillary vessels, events which permit blood flow to commence. They also mature by attracting pericytes and smooth muscle cells, and by developing their basement membranes (Carmeliet and Jain, 2000; Carmeliet, 2000). Functionality of such an emerging microvascular network depends on its ability to maintain a directional and unperturbed blood flow, properties that are as a function of the structural stability, vascular patency and architectural hierarchy (arborisation). The latter involves the removal of excessive capillary vessels (pruning) and definition of the arterial and venous sides of the microcirculation. The expression of ephrin B2 and its EphB4 receptor (Wang et al., 1998), respectively, and the mechanosensory stimulation by the moving blood (Swift and Weinstein, 2009) ensure the integrity and completion of these processes. In CRC, these processes are largely deregulated leading to abnormal and dysfunctional vascular patterns and often poor arterio-venous definition (Carmeliet, 2005; Jain, 2001).

In addition to soluble growth factors (e.g. VEGF/VEGFR) and juxtacrine interactions (e.g. Dll-4/Notch), blood vessel forming processes are dependent on a timely resolution and restoration of intercellular junctions, as well as on the proper attachment to, and stimulation of endothelial cells by the ECM (Avraamides et al., 2008). In this regard, homotypic interactions via the endothelial specific member of the cadherin family, VE-cadherin (CD144), are central to these processes, including the very functionality of various growth factor receptors (Dejana, 2004). VEGF signal transduction depends also on the ligation of integrins, many of which play significant, but often complex (Reynolds et al., 2002) roles in tumour angiogenesis, including such receptors as: $\alpha_v\beta_3$, $\alpha_v\beta_5$, $\alpha_5\beta_1$, $\alpha_6\beta_4$ (Dejana, 2004; Silva et al., 2008; Rivoltini et al., 1989; Eliceiri and Cheresh, 2001) (see Chapter 7 by A. Arabzadeh and N. Beauchemin, in this book). This plethora of molecular interactions presents itself as an opportunity for the corresponding therapeutic efforts aimed at the various constituents of pathological angiogenesis (Folkman and Kalluri, 2003; Kerbel, 2008).

9.2.2 Lymphangiogenesis and Molecular Mediators of Lymphatic Development

In the same way as angiogenesis is responsible for blood vessel formation, another process (lymphangiogenesis) allows formation of lymphatic vessels from the pre-existing lymphatics (Alitalo et al., 2005; Das and Skobe, 2008; Cueni and Detmar, 2008; Makinen and Alitalo, 2007; Skobe et al., 2001; Alitalo and Carmeliet, 2002; Jain and Padera, 2002). Although only 2% of genes are differentially expressed between lymphatic (LECs) and blood vascular endothelial cells (BECs) (Hirakawa et al., 2003) the properties of these cells, their function and the underlying regulatory events are vastly different (Alitalo et al., 2005).

The lymphatic network is present in almost all organs, except for the central nervous system (CNS), bone marrow (BM) and avascular tissues, such as cartilage, cornea and epidermis. Lymphatics drain extravasated fluid, macromolecules and cells coming from tissues, and direct them to lymph nodes, after which they may enter the general blood circulation. Lymphatic networks are also involved in the immune response by virtue of their role in the transport of lymphocytes and antigen-presenting cells to and from lymphoid organs. Moreover, these vessels participate in the absorption of dietary fat, secreted by enterocytes as chylomicrons. Besides their physiological roles, lymphatics also contribute to several human diseases, such as lymphedema, inflammation and tumour metastasis (Karpanen and Alitalo, 2008; Lazarus et al., 2004; Alitalo et al., 2005).

Despite some common properties, lymphatic capillaries differ structurally from their corresponding blood capillaries. Generally, the capillary lymphatics are open-ended thin-walled endothelial tubes with a discontinuous or absent basement membrane, and mostly (though with some exceptions) with no pericytes or smooth muscle cell coverage. Lymphatic endothelial cells are connected to the surrounding ECM by specialized fibrillin-containing anchoring filaments and thereby are equipped to collect interstitial fluid (Alitalo et al., 2005).

Even though the first description of lymphatics dates back to 400 years ago, their better understanding is very recent owing to discovery of specific markers of LECs and their stimulating lymphangiogenic factors. The former include the prospero homeobox transcription factor (Prox-1), podoplanin and LYVE-1 (Alitalo et al., 2005). Prox-1 is essential during embryonic development, as illustrated by the absence of the lymphatic vasculature observed upon its genetic deletion (Wigle et al., 2002; Petrova et al., 2002). Podoplanin, a transmembrane mucin-like protein, is also highly expressed in LECs, and the respective knock-out mice lacking this gene product exhibit defects in lymphatic pattern formation (Schacht et al., 2003). LYVE-1 is a homolog of the hyaluronan receptor CD44, and an early marker of LEC differentiation (Jackson, 2004).

The unique regulatory pathway involved in lymphangiogenesis consists of the aforementioned VEGF-related ligands, VEGF-C and VEGF-D, and their receptor expressed preferentially (though not exclusively) on LECs, known as VEGFR3/Flt-4 (Alitalo et al., 2005). Deletion of VEGF-C results in the absence of lymphatic vasculature, as does disruption of forkhead box C2 (Foxc2) during later stages of lymphangiogenesis (Lohela et al., 2009). Moreover, co-expression of ephrin-B2 and its receptor EphB in LECs was found to control their sprouting, as well as their interaction with smooth muscle cells, and is essential for the remodelling of lymphatic vasculature (Lohela et al., 2009). Finally, unlike during angiogenesis, Ang-2 can act as an agonist of Tie2 receptor on LECs and functions as a crucial regulator of lymphangiogenesis. Lymphatic defects resulting from Ang-2 deletion can be rescued by Ang-1 (Gale et al., 2002; Morisada et al., 2005).

Proliferation, migration and survival of LECs are mainly controlled by VEGF-C, and to a lesser extent by VEGF-D, following their interactions with VEGFR3 (Lohela et al., 2009). It is noteworthy that, whereas immature VEGF-C and VEGF-D bind VEGFR3, the mature (proteolytically processed) forms of these factors can also bind VEGFR2, introducing angiogenesis into this circuitry (Lohela et al., 2009). Moreover, VEGF-A also contributes to lymphangiogenesis through its interaction with VEGFR2 on LECs (Lohela et al., 2009). VEGF-C binds not only to VEGFR3 but also to Neuropilin-2 (NRP-2), a semaphorin receptor, which interacts with VEGFR3, and this process is also essential for lymphangiogenesis (Lohela et al., 2009). Moreover, $\beta 1$ and $\alpha 9$ integrins participate in VEGFR3 activation and VEGF-C/D binding, respectively (Vlahakis et al., 2005). Other growth factors were also found to induce lymphangiogenesis, including: hepatocyte growth factor (HGF), insulin-like growth factors 1 and 2 (IGF-1 and IGF-2), PDGF-B, and fibroblast growth factor (FGF) (Lohela et al., 2009; Alitalo et al., 2005).

In order to maintain its function, the lymphatic capillary network must be strictly separated from its vascular counterpart, to prevent the mixing of lymph and blood. In this regard, the tyrosine kinase Syk and its substrate adaptor molecule Slp76, are essential regulators of this functional divide. Indeed, the deficiency in one or the other of these molecules leads to the formation of mixed blood and lymphatic endothelial networks and to aberrant vascular-lymphatic anasthomosis (Abtahian et al., 2003).

9.3 Oncogenic and Microenvironmental Inducers of Tumour Angiogenesis in Colon Cancer

9.3.1 Aberrations of Vascular Growth in Cancer

In cancer, the formation of endothelial sprouts is profoundly altered, leading to unscheduled and perpetual cycles of growth, branching, dilatation, regional enlargement, directionless extension, paradoxical anasthomosis, remodelling and other changes within the tumour microvascular network (Jain, 2001). These anomalies result in structural and molecular alterations (Jain, 2001; McDonald and Choyke, 2003; Seaman et al., 2007; St. Croix et al., 2000; Folkman and Kalluri, 2003) that distinguish tumour blood vessels from their normal counterparts and reveal potential targets for a direct anti-angiogenic therapy, as originally postulated by Folkman (Folkman, 1971; Folkman and Kalluri, 2003). As such, these changes are also a stark manifestation of the abnormal signalling circuitry that operates in the tumour microenvironment. The related regulatory processes themselves could also serve as (indirect) therapeutic targets, e.g. by agents designed to block the onset, modify the course, and otherwise alter the nature of tumour-associated vascular growth inducing stimuli (Kerbel and Folkman, 2002; Kerbel, 2008; Rak and Kerbel, 2003). The validity of this latter approach is documented by the recent approval of bevacizumab (Avastin), a humanized neutralizing monoclonal antibody against VEGF-A, which is used as a frontline therapy in the treatment of metastatic CRC (Hurwitz et al., 2004), and in other human malignancies (Grothey and Ellis, 2008).

9.3.2 Genesis of the Pro-angiogenic Phenotype in Colorectal Cancer

While targeting vascular events in cancer has been already validated as a viable therapeutic avenue (Folkman and Kalluri, 2003; Ferrara, 2005; Kerbel, 2008), impacting the causation of these processes requires a better understanding of how do tumours induce angiogenesis and lymphangiogenesis (Bouck et al., 1996). The angiogenic phenotype may emerge in both cancer cells and their surrounding stroma (Folkman and Kalluri, 2003). The major causative influences in this regard include: (i) hypoxia and metabolic deprivation (Shweiki et al., 1992; Harris, 2002; Fraisl et al., 2009); (ii) oncogenic transformation of cancer cells and its impact on tumour stroma (Bouck et al., 1996; Rak et al., 2000b; Kalas et al., 2005) and (iii) inflammatory processes associated with cancer progression (Mantovani et al., 2008; Yu and Rak, 2003; Ancrile et al., 2007).

Hypoxia is the major trigger of physiological angiogenesis (Harris, 2002; Semenza, 2003; Fraisl et al., 2009), and is well documented in CRC (Rasheed et al., 2008). This response may be precipitated by perturbations in vascular patency (e.g. embolization), changes in ambient oxygen levels, increases in tissue mass without an adequate increase in vascularity, non-productive angiogenesis (Thurston et al., 2007) and by other factors. This state becomes resolved upon adequate vascular growth and blood flow restoration, followed by increase in oxygen supply and normoxia. Alternatively, if flow is not restored, hypoxia may result in cell death and tissue necrosis (Harris, 2002). These cycles of events commonly occur during tissue repair. Similar events also occur in malignancy, but are of more chronic and recurrent nature, owing to the functional inefficiency, architectural anomalies, thrombosis and flow perturbations in the tumour microcirculation (Harris, 2002). Hence, hypoxia and necrosis may paradoxically accompany exuberant angiogenesis in various cancers, including CRC (Harris, 2002; Rasheed et al., 2009).

Several signalling pathways serve as sensors of oxygen supply in stromal, parenchymal and endothelial cells (Boutin et al., 2008; Tang et al., 2004), and their molecular details have been exhaustively reviewed elsewhere (Harris, 2002; Semenza, 2003; Rasheed et al., 2008; Mizukami et al., 2007). In this regard, the regulation of VEGF by the hypoxia inducible factor (HIF)-dependent transcription illustrates the salient mechanisms of this circuitry (Ferrara, 2002; Tang et al., 2004). While hypoxia exerts several effects on VEGF expression (Harris, 2002), the transcriptional control of the VEGF gene is amongst the most recognized, and is known to be executed by the hypoxia-responsive element (HRE) in the 3' untranslated region (UTR) of the VEGF gene. This motif serves as a binding site of HIFs (Tischer et al., 1991), a family of transcription factors, which are dimeric and consist of a common beta subunit, also known as aryl hydrocarbon nuclear translocator (ARNT), and a regulated alpha subunit (HIF-1 alpha or HIF-2 alpha). ARNT is constitutively expressed in most cell types, often in a DNA-bound state, where it interacts with the respective HIF alpha subunits (Harris, 2002; Semenza, 2003).

HIF alpha proteins are synthesized constitutively and then rapidly degraded by the ubiquitin pathway. This mechanism is driven by the recognition of this factor by the von Hippel Lindau (VHL) protein, which acts as the ubiquitin ligase (Semenza, 2003; Kaelin, 2008). Interactions between HIF alpha and VHL are dependent upon the modification of the former partner by the specific prolyl- and aspargyl hydroxylases, the activity of which is oxygen-dependent (Kaelin, 2008; Semenza,

2003; Harris, 2002). Consequently, under hypoxic conditions this hydroxylation is impaired, ubiquitination and degradation of HIF alpha is abolished, the increased levels of HIF alpha protein accumulate in the cell. This leads to nuclear translocation and binding of HIF alpha and ARNT, followed by the onset of transcription of hypoxia inducible genes (Harris, 2002). Among those, VEGF and several other factors involved in angiogenesis and metabolic responses to hypoxia are prominent targets of HIF (Harris, 2002), and thereby important regulators of tumour angiogenesis and growth (Shweiki et al., 1992).

In 1995, we have demonstrated that VEGF expression is elevated in cancer cells also under normoxic conditions (in culture), and as a function of their oncogenic transformation with mutant H-RAS, K-RAS and Src (Rak et al., 1995), and other oncogenes, e.g. epidermal growth factor receptor (EGFR) and human epidermal growth factor receptor-2 (HER-2) (Viloria-Petit et al., 1997; Rak et al., 2000b). These findings came on the heels of the groundbreaking work of Noel Bouck and her colleagues who demonstrated that the status of *p53* tumour suppressor influences the constitutive angiogenic phenotype of cancer cells through an 'intrinsic' and cancer-specific, rather than microenvironmental control of thrombospondin 1 (TSP-1), a potent endogenous angiogenesis inhibitor (Rastinejad et al., 1989; Dameron et al., 1994; Bouck et al., 1996).

Recent studies have extended these findings and directly implicated over 20 different oncogenic lesions in the regulation of the angiogenic phenotype of cancer cells (Rak and Kerbel, 2003). In addition, these studies revealed that multiple direct-acting angiogenesis regulators may remain under control of each of these oncogenic pathways (Rak and Kerbel, 2003). This includes not only VEGF, TSP-1, Ang-2, or pigment epithelium-derived factor (PEDF) (Rak and Kerbel, 2003), but also systemically acting angiogenesis inhibitors (arresten, endostatin, tumstatin) (Teodoro et al., 2006), molecular regulators of bone marrow-derived pro-angiogenic cells (VEGF), and various effectors of the haemostatic system, which are also involved in tumour angiogenesis, metastasis and cancer coagulopathy (Rak et al., 2000b, 2008) (see below). The regulatory events involved include oncogene-dependent changes in gene transcription (Semenza, 2003), translation (Kevil et al., 1996), deregulation of micro RNA species (Dews et al., 2006), mRNA stability and other effects (Rak, 2009).

It was recently realized that oncogenic pathways may also influence some of the less studied mechanisms of angiogenesis regulation, notably molecular exchanges between the cells via tumour-derived vesicles, microvesicles and exosomes (Al-Nedawi et al., 2009a; Dolo et al., 2005; Ratajczak et al., 2006; Gesierich et al., 2006). Indeed, recent studies suggest that oncogenic mutation of K-RAS, EGFR or *p53* lead to an increase in the release of microvesicles harbouring the pro-coagulant receptor known as tissue factor (TF) (Yu and Rak, 2004; Yu et al., 2005; Milsom et al., 2008). Microvesicles generated in this manner can transfer their cargo (e.g. TF or other receptors) from cell to cell, resulting in the intercellular propagation of various biological activities (del Conde et al., 2005; Yu et al., 2008). Several membrane receptors and cellular proteins may undergo such microvesicular propagation with various consequences (Mack et al., 2000; Al-Nedawi et al., 2009a), including several angiogenic proteins (e.g. VEGF, proteases, active phospholipids and adhesion molecules) (Taraboletti et al., 2006; Ratajczak et al., 2006; Gesierich et al., 2006).

Interestingly, this oncogene-driven, microvesicular, intercellular transfer process often affects oncoproteins themselves (Al-Nedawi et al., 2009b). We have recently uncovered evidence that members of the EGFR family (e.g. EGFR and mutant EGFRvIII) can move between tumour and endothelial cells via specific microvesicles (oncosomes), resulting in pro-angiogenic changes in the phenotype of their cellular recipients (Al-Nedawi et al., 2008, 2009a). More recently, these kinds of events have been found to occur also in various tumours including: brain (Skog et al., 2008) and prostate cancer (Di Vizio et al., 2009), and may prove to have a significant biological role in tumour progression and angiogenesis. Circulating oncosomes could also serve as prognostic and predictive biomarker (Al-Nedawi et al., 2008), possibly also in CRC (Choi et al., 2007; Valenti et al., 2007) and in other tumours (Al-Nedawi et al., 2009b).

The involvement of constitutively activated oncogenic pathways in various effector mechanisms of angiogenesis does not preclude the impact of the microenvironment, inflammation or other 'extracellular' processes (Giaccia, 2003). Indeed, several downstream events triggered by activated oncogenes converge upon hypoxia-regulated pathways, including HIF (Berra et al., 2000), whereby they can mimic, or exacerbate the respective cellular responses. For instance, the loss of the VHL tumour suppressor gene in renal cancer precipitates conditions of protracted HIF-mediated transcription, and VEGF upregulation, which is similar in nature to that induced by hypoxia (Escudier et al., 2007; Kaelin, 2008). Hypoxia can also synergize with oncogenic events through various signalling cross-talks, e.g. via co-activation of the phosphatidyl inositol kinase 3 (PI3K) pathway (Mazure et al., 1997).

Oncogenic regulation of the angiogenic phenotype converges also upon the inflammatory pathway. In particular, mutant RAS, and possibly other oncogenes as well, trigger the expression of inflammatory chemokines (interleukin-8 – IL-8) (Sparmann and Bar-Sagi, 2004) and cytokines (IL-6) (Ancrile et al., 2007), which are able to impact both endothelial cells and also the pro-angiogenic subsets of inflammatory cells (Ancrile et al., 2007).

CRC is driven by the sequence of genetic lesions (Fearon and Vogelstein, 1990) and their variation associated with different forms of the disease, e.g. those occurring with or without preceding polyposis, in sporadic colorectal cancer, or in malignancy coupled with the inflammatory bowel disease (IBD) (Itzkowitz and Yio, 2004). These events may create a complex combinatorial network, where the impact of individual mutations would be modified by various confounders. Nonetheless, certain molecular switches are beginning to emerge in this context, as a function of their respective genetic triggering mechanisms, such as mutant Adenomatous polyposis coli (APC), K-RAS, *p53* and epigenetic changes in various genes (Fig. 9.3) (Fearon and Vogelstein, 1990; Itzkowitz and Yio, 2004). In this context, it is noteworthy that in sporadic colorectal cancer the threshold event (angiogenic switch) appears to occur relatively early during adenoma stage of disease progression

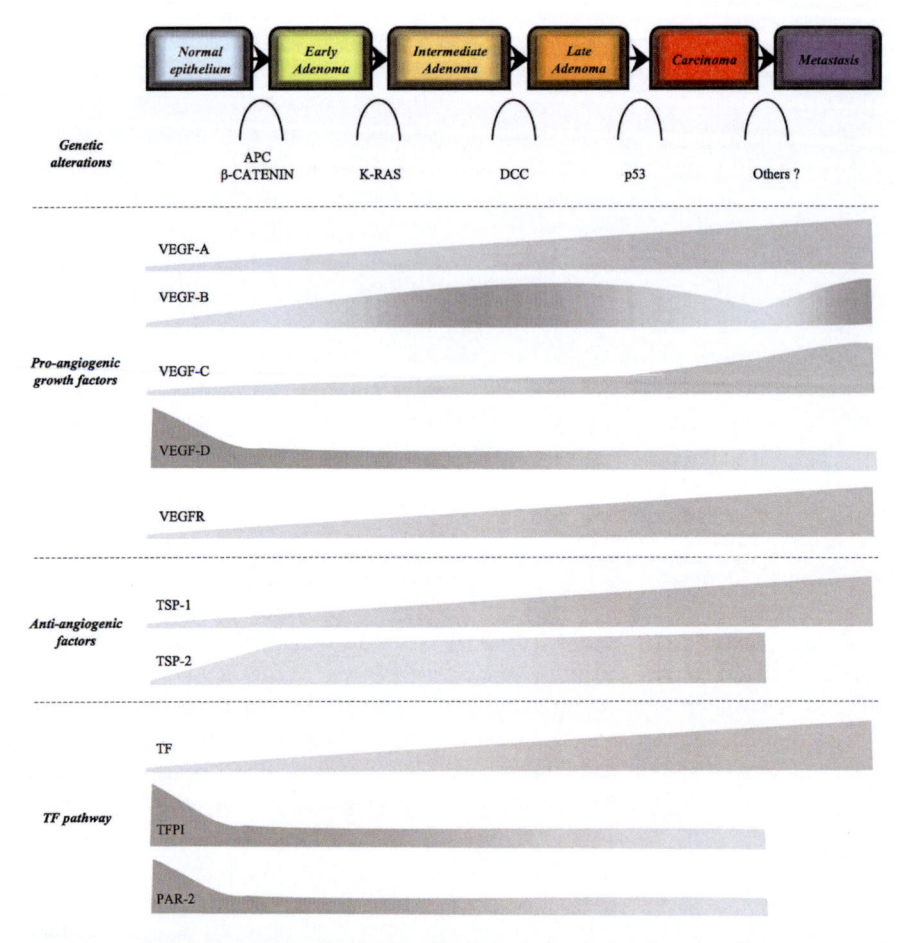

Fig. 9.3 Angiogenesis progression during the course of colorectal cancer. The sequence of genetic hits and the associated microenvironmental changes in CRC are paralleled by sequential changes in expression of angiogenic factors and the evolution of the angiogenic phenotype (see text)

(Staton et al., 2007), which suggests that some genetic events may be more directly involved in this event than others. It is tempting to speculate that the angiogenic switch in CRC may be coincidental with K-RAS mutations (Rak et al., 1995), which are known to drive the expression of several angiogenesis-related genes (Rak and Kerbel, 2003), and are often detectable at the stage of intermediate adenoma (Fearon and Vogelstein, 1990). On the other hand, in colitis-related cancer the early involvement of *p53* may contribute to the onset of angiogenesis, as predicted from preclinical studies on the effects of this tumour suppressor (Bouck et al., 1996). This could be combined with pro-angiogenic effects of inflammatory events themselves (Zumsteg and Christofori, 2009), though more studies are needed to establish these relationships more firmly.

9.3.3 Cellular, Molecular and Systemic Triggers of Tumour Angiogenesis

The onset and progression of tumour angiogenesis are regulated at both the local and the systemic levels, and by the intricate network of molecular queues (Folkman and Kalluri, 2003; Carmeliet, 2005; Kerbel, 2008). While the concept of the 'angiogenic switch' (Folkman and Kalluri, 2003) captures the cumulative and discrete nature of the observable onset of blood vessel formation process in cancer, the preceding and following events may also influence the important characteristics of this continuum (Hanahan and Folkman, 1996; Relf et al., 1997; Bergers et al., 1999). This can be referred to collectively as 'angiogenesis progression' (Rak et al., 1996) and entails not only quantitative, but also qualitative changes in the mechanisms governing blood vessel formation, and the steps in molecular progression of the underlying disease (Rak et al., 1996). Such a linkage is often reflected by the changing repertoire of angiogenic influences detectable in a given tumour over time (Relf et al., 1997) (vascular supply), but also by the level of dependence of the angiogenic process on a specific factor (Viloria-Petit et al., 2003; Casanovas et al., 2005; Shojaei and Ferrara, 2008), or for that matter, dependence of cancer cells on the vascular supply in general (vascular demand) (Rak and Kerbel, 1996; Yu et al., 2002b; Rak and Yu, 2004). Collectively, these changing properties may also define the changing level of responsiveness/resistance of tumours to specific anti-angiogenic therapies, as initially postulated by us (Rak and Kerbel, 1996) and others (Kerbel et al., 2001; Broxterman et al., 2003; Bergers and Hanahan, 2008), and later documented experimentally (Bergers et al., 1999; Bergers and Hanahan, 2008).

The number of pro-angiogenic molecules that may participate in the angiogenic continuum includes several polypeptide growth factors (VEGF, basic fibroblast growth factor bFGF, HGF), cytokines (IL-6), chemokines (IL-8), phospholipids (sphingosine-1-phosphate), ribonucleases (angiogenin) and other entities that can stimulate endothelial cell growth directly, or through upregulation of VEGF in the surrounding cells (e.g. pericytes, fibroblasts or inflammatory cells) (Folkman and Kalluri, 2003). Some of these factors act through the recruitment of stromal and circulating cells that are capable of releasing VEGF and other mediators into the tumour microenvironment (Folkman and Kalluri, 2003; Rak and Kerbel, 2003; Kerbel, 2008), or may act via secretion of proteolytic activities, such as matrix metalloproteinases (MMP-2, MMP-9) (Bergers et al., 2000).

These positive effector mechanisms can overcome endogenous angiogenesis inhibitors, the levels of which may also be synchronously down-regulated e.g. by hypoxia or oncogenic influences (Folkman and Kalluri, 2003). Many of such inhibitory molecules have recently been identified, and include entities of such diverse nature as: soluble splice isoforms of angiogenic growth factor receptors (sVEGFR1/Flt-1), certain VEGF isoforms (VEGF165b) (Woolard et al., 2004), proteolytic fragments of plasma proteins (angiostatin, antithrombin), fragments of extracellular matrix molecules (endostatin, tumstatin, arresten), secretable matricellular proteins (TSP-1, -2), anti-angiogenic chemokines (platelet factor 4 – PF4), fragments of regulatory proteins such as prolactin (16 Kd), or factors present in the neuroectodermal tissues (brain-specific angiogenesis inhibitor 1 – BAI1, or PEDF) (Folkman and Kalluri, 2003; Kalluri, 2003; Kerbel, 2008; Fischer et al., 2008).

Although traditionally angiogenesis was thought to be regulated mainly at the local level, many of the aforementioned angiogenesis regulators are present systemically, in the circulating blood. Such circulating angiogenesis regulators can be found in complexes with their soluble receptors (e.g. VEGF/VEGFR), as cargo of microvesicles (Taraboletti et al., 2006), or within the content of platelet granules, the latter recently proposed to selectively accumulate angiogenesis stimulators and inhibitors in separate vesicular compartments (Klement et al., 2009). The consequences of such a systemic control of angiogenesis could be demonstrated through perturbations in the metastatic growth and cessation of tumour dormancy following surgery or other manipulations. As these interventions affect the primary lesion, they may lead to changes in the level of circulating angiogenic effectors and changes in tumour growth (Gimbrone et al., 1972; Folkman and Kalluri, 2003; Holmgren et al., 1995; Naumov et al., 2001).

The systemic angiogenesis regulation also has an important cellular component. This came to light with the increasing understanding of the involvement the various populations of bone marrow-derived cells have in the regulation of vascular integrity, repair and in pathology (Carmeliet et al., 2001; Rafii et al., 2002; Kerbel, 2008; Shojaei et al., 2008; Coussens and Werb, 2002). Such cells include the aforementioned endothelial progenitor-like cells (EPCs/CEPs; VEGFR2+), which may play a dual role, namely as structural and regulatory elements in angiogenesis/vasculogenesis (Bertolini et al., 2006; Shaked et al., 2006; Rafii et al., 2002; Asahara et al., 1997; Gao et al., 2008).

Other bone marrow-derived cells (BMDCs) are also involved (De Palma and Naldini, 2006; Staton et al., 2007). Thus, transient accumulation of hematopoietic progenitor cells (HPCs, VEGFR1+) often precedes angiogenic reaction (Rafii et al., 2002), and appears to play a role in metastasis (Kaplan et al., 2005). Inflammatory cells, such as M2 macrophages and granulocytic cells (Shojaei et al., 2008) may be recruited to the tumour site by cancer cell-, or stromal-derived cytokines and chemokines (Sparmann and Bar-Sagi, 2004; Ancrile et al., 2007). The influx of these cells is often indispensable for efficient angiogenesis, and results in production of new angiogenic factors (e.g. Bv8), which in some cases can account for resistance to anti-angiogenic therapies targeting VEGF (Shojaei and Ferrara, 2008). There is also mounting evidence that several types of bone marrow-derived cells may play important regulatory roles in this context including: VEGFR1+/CXCR4+/CD11b+ cells (RBCCs), Tie-2-expressing CD11b+ monocytes (TEMs), VEGFR1+/CXCR4+ hemangiocytes, CD11b+/VE-cadherin+ vascular leukocytes, Gr1+/CD11b+ neutrophils and myeloid suppressor cells (De Palma and Naldini, 2006; Kerbel, 2008). The extent to which these cells are involved in angiogenesis in CRC is presently poorly understood.

9.3.4 Tumour Angiogenesis Metastasis and the Haemostatic System

In addition of the aforementioned cellular circuitry, tumour angiogenesis, progression and metastasis are also under the influence of blood itself, especially the coagulation and fibrinolytic systems (Dvorak and Rickles, 2006). These mechanisms engage haemostatic elements of the vascular wall (e.g. TF, thrombomodulin – TM, endothelial protein C receptor – EPCR, and protease activated receptors – PARs), but also blood platelets and plasma protease cascades, which are involved in formation of thrombin, fibrin, and recruitment of fibrin degrading enzymes (plasmin) (Dvorak and Rickles, 2006).

Over 90% of disseminated malignancies in humans are reportedly associated with various levels of symptomatic, or asymptomatic dysfunction of the clotting system (coagulopathy), a notion indicative of a profound (albeit often subclinical) deregulation of haemostasis in cancer (Dvorak and Rickles, 2006; Rickles, 2009; Falanga, 2005). These events are relatively common in CRC (Iversen and Thorlacius-Ussing, 2003; Lykke and Nielsen, 2004; Seto et al., 2000; Nakasaki et al., 2002), and in other tumours of the gastrointestinal (GI) tract, especially in pancreatic cancer (Kakkar et al., 1995; Khorana et al., 2007). Some manifestations of this condition have been known for over 140 years, and were often described as Trousseau's syndrome (Varki, 2007). Thrombotic abnormalities are also amongst the most important contributing factors to morbidity and mortality associated with human malignancies (Rickles, 2009; Buller et al., 2007; Fotopoulou et al., 2008).

It is noteworthy that several effectors of the coagulation system are also involved in angiogenesis (Dvorak and Rickles, 2006). The most studied of those include: platelets (Pinedo et al., 1998), fibrin (Dvorak and Rickles, 2006), thrombin (Nierodzik and Karpatkin, 2006; Tsopanoglou and Maragoudakis, 2004), but also other coagulation factors, such as factor VIIa (FVIIa) and tissue factor (TF) (Nierodzik and Karpatkin, 2006; Rak et al., 2006; Belting et al., 2005; Versteeg et al., 2008). TF is a unique, high affinity cell membrane-associated receptor for FVIIa, and the central initiator of the coagulation cascade. The genetic and pharmacological manipulations of TF expression and function were found to exert potent anti-angiogenic, anti-tumour and anti-metastatic effects in experimental settings (Zhang et al., 1994; Abe et al., 1999; Hembrough et al., 2003; Yu et al., 2005; Palumbo et al., 2007; Versteeg et al., 2008; Milsom et al., 2008), while downstream-acting anti-coagulants exhibited anticancer effect in recent clinical trials (Falanga, 2005; Kakkar et al., 2004; Lee et al., 2005; Altinbas et al., 2004; Klerk et al., 2005).

At the mechanistic level, these effects could be attributed to at least two main TF properties. First, the canonical proteolytic activity of the TF/VIIa complex is known to trigger formation of coagulation factors Xa and thrombin (IIa), resulting in the activation of the entire coagulation cascade, deposition of the pro-angiogenic fibrin matrix, as well as release of angiogenic factors from activated platelets (Dvorak and Rickles, 2006). Second, TF may act as a 'sensor' of plasma, and transducer of responses to cellular exposure to plasma-associated FVIIa, a property mediated by a series of intracellular signalling events that may mimic a 'healing reaction' of injured tissues (Dvorak and Rickles, 2006). These intracellular signals are evoked in endothelial, stromal, inflammatory and cancer cells via interactions of TF with integrins and growth factor receptors, but mainly by PARs, especially PAR-1 (thrombin receptor) and PAR-2 (Coughlin, 2000).

PARs (PAR-1, -2, -3 and -4) transmit signals elicited by specific proteolytic cleavage events within their respective N-termini, an effect that is catalyzed by the TF/VIIa complex (PAR-2), factor Xa (PAR-1) and thrombin (PAR-1, -3 and -4) (Coughlin, 2000). The significance of the resulting signalling is illustrated by the altered profiles of gene expression (Camerer et al., 2000; Albrektsen et al., 2007), changes in tumour growth in mice hypomorphic for TF (Yu et al., 2008), or deficient for PAR-2 (Versteeg et al., 2008). These responses involve changes in the expression of angiogenesis-related genes, and alterations in the function of vascular cells, as illustrated by developmental defects induced by manipulation of *PAR-1* in the endothelium (Griffin et al., 2001).

It is of note that TF upregulation (and the potential to activate both coagulation and the PAR pathway) is frequently observed in cancer, including CRC (Lykke and Nielsen, 2004; Iversen and Thorlacius-Ussing, 2003). This expression is also linked to poor prognosis (Seto et al., 2000), expression of VEGF (Shigemori et al., 1998) and evidence of robust angiogenesis in colorectal lesions (Nakasaki et al., 2002). Inhibition of the TF pathway reduces angiogenic activity of human CRC cells in mice (Yu et al., 2005), inhibits growth of spontaneous intestinal tumours in Min mice (Zhao et al., 2009), and impairs metastatic dissemination of CRC cells in experimental settings (Zerbib et al., 2009; Zhao et al., 2009; Hembrough et al., 2003; Ngo et al., 2007; Palumbo et al., 2007; Versteeg et al., 2008). Other elements of the coagulation and fibrinolytic systems have also been implicated in these processes, and their role has been reviewed elsewhere, at length (Rickles, 2006; Ruf, 2007; Nierodzik and Karpatkin, 2006; Carmeliet, 2001). Nonetheless, these studies suggest that angiogenesis-regulating signals can emanate from both the 'outside' and the 'inside' of the blood vessel system, and that the respective therapeutic targets do exist in both compartments, including agents that may be effective in CRC (Yu et al., 2005; Zhao et al., 2009; Zerbib et al., 2009).

Coagulation system also emerges as one of the key regulators of metastasis (Rickles, 2006). This is due to the causative continuum between the angiogenesis and lymphangiogenesis in and around the primary tumour and the access of cancer cells to the systemic circulation, the main conduit of dissemination (Fidler, 2003). In this regard, deregulation of angiogenesis- (*VEGF, IL-8*) and lymphangiogenesis-related (*VEGF-C*) genes by TF/PAR signalling pathway (Albrektsen et al., 2007), involvement of fibrin and platelets in supporting and shielding metastatic cancer cells and other effects play significant roles in metastasis, and have been described previously (Rickles, 2006; Dvorak and Rickles, 2006; Palumbo et al., 2007; Francis and Amirkhosravi, 2002). In addition, thrombosis is often associated with a more aggressive disease in a general sense, and the expression of some of the key effectors of this condition, e.g. TF, are found to correlate with metastasis and poor survival in CRC patients (Shigemori et al., 1998; Nakasaki et al., 2002; Seto et al., 2000).

One element that is infrequently discussed in this context is the vascular aspect of cancer cell heterogeneity, including the metastatic and tumour initiating cell subsets. It is of note, for example, that in several experimental systems metastatic growth appears to be particularly susceptible to manipulations that affect TF and the coagulation system, and similar treatments directed against established tumour masses produce less dramatic consequences (Versteeg et al., 2008; Rak et al., 2008). One distinguishing feature in this regard is the fact that formation of metastases, incipient tumours and repopulation of cancer cell masses post cytoreductive therapies occurs from the threshold numbers, or single cancer cells, especially those described as tumour initiating cells (TICs) or cancer stem cells (CSCs) (Reya et al., 2001; Dick, 2009; Gilbertson and Rich, 2007). Such cells have also been described in settings of GI malignancies (Zhu et al., 2009). Notably, CSCs are thought to utilize the vascular system as their protective 'niche' (Gilbertson and Rich, 2007), express high levels of VEGF (Bao et al., 2006), and sometimes markedly up-regulate TF (Milsom et al., 2007). Moreover, targeting TF genetically (Palumbo et al., 2007), or by administration of neutralizing antibodies appears to dampen tumour initiating potential of various tumours (Milsom et al., 2008; Rak et al., 2008). Whether these effects play a role in CRC remains to be elucidated, but anti-TF agents appear to be more effective against clonal growth of liver metastases than against massive experimental primary lesions formed by colorectal cancer cells injected in large numbers into animals (Zerbib et al., 2009).

9.4 Effectors of Angiogenesis and Lymphangiogenesis in Primary and Metastatic Colorectal Tumours

Development of colorectal cancer profoundly alters the expression, function and biological role of several effectors of angiogenesis and lymphangiogenesis, as described in the previous sections. The resulting molecular abnormalities and florid tumour angiogenesis have already been validated, as viable therapeutic targets, a notion borne out in the advent of anti-VEGF/VEGR agents that are now commonly used in the treatment of metastatic CRC (Hurwitz et al., 2004; Ferrara, 2005). As the advantages achieved with these relatively simple approaches become exhausted, further progress in this area will likely depend on a better understanding of the complexity, 'druggability' and context-dependent properties of the regulatory networks driving angiogenesis and lymphangiogenesis (angioma and lymphangioma) that are operative in CRC.

The magnitude of the challenges in this regard, but also the needs and opportunities associated with them, are reflected by the fact that CRC is the third most common malignancy worldwide. CRC represents approximately 15% of all human cancers and affects more than 1 million people each year, resulting in approximately 500,000 deaths (Parkin, 2001). Moreover, the disease recurs within 5 years in a significant percentage of treated patients, such that metastatic CRC becomes the main cause of death and a major source of unmet therapeutic needs (Ferlay et al., 2007). Since angiogenesis, lymphangiogenesis and metastasis represent, as argued earlier, a functional continuum in the pathogenesis of CRC, it is of interest to survey, at least some of the characteristics of the tumour vascular interface in this disease.

9.4.1 Angiogenesis in Primary CRC

A recent meta-analysis of published CRC-related databases documented a compelling increase in microvessel density (MVD) during the course of the disease progression, and the association of this property with poor prognosis (Des et al., 2006). Vascular growth is increased during CRC, with invasive lesions exhibiting more vessels compared to polyps. This increased vasculature is also directly correlated with a greater risk of metastasis and tumour recurrence (Des et al., 2006; Cao et al., 2009).

There are several known mechanisms of angiogenesis activation in CRC. For instance, the disease progression is often associated with the activation of pro-angiogenic hypoxia response pathways (Rasheed et al., 2008). In colorectal cancer, both HIF-1 alpha and HIF-2 alpha are upregulated, but only the former has a prognostic significance (Rasheed et al., 2009). This sensor of low oxygen concentration also exhibits a correlation with the elevated MVD, VEGF expression and lactate dehydrogenase (LDH) detected in tumours, as well as with high invasive and metastatic capacity (Koukourakis et al., 2005). As mentioned earlier, hypoxia is coupled with other angiogenesis-inducing stimuli, including oncogenic pathways (Rak et al., 1995), p53 mutations (Cassano et al., 2002), cyclooxygenase2 (Cox-2) expression (Tsujii et al., 1998), TF expression and thrombosis (Seto et al., 2000; Shigemori et al., 1998), and several other events, many of which converge and correlate with the up-regulation of VEGF. In contrast, the expression pattern of angiogenesis inhibitors, such as thrombospondin 1 and 2 (TSP-1 and -2) in specific lesions, is correlated with lower intratumoral vascular density, reduced metastatic potential and increased survival, even though the levels of these proteins do not necessarily exhibit a global decrease in CRC, as compared to normal tissues (Kaio et al., 2003; Maeda et al., 2001; Tokunaga et al., 1999; Rmali et al., 2007) (Fig. 9.3).

VEGF-A expression is increased in primary CRC lesions (Rmali et al., 2007), and it correlates with high MVD, poor prognosis (Des et al., 2006), metastasis (Takahashi et al., 1995) and a high risk of disease recurrence (Cascinu et al., 2000). This up-regulation occurs in tumour cells, as well as in adjacent stroma, and is often combined with upregulation of VEGFR1 and VEGFR2 (Brown et al., 1993). Similarly, VEGF-B expression is increased in adenoma compared to normal tissue, but in contrast to VEGF-A, it tends to decline in carcinomas. On the other hand, VEGF-C is not upregulated in adenomas, but increases in carcinomas and as compared to normal tissue, suggesting a function of this factor during the later stages of CRC progression, e.g. in the course of lymphatic metastasis (Hanrahan et al., 2003).

It is noteworthy that the interactions between VEGF-A and VEGF-B with their corresponding receptors may not only occur on the surface of endothelial cells, but also affect CRC cells directly, especially through binding to VEGFR1, which these cells often express and utilize as mechanisms promoting cellular invasion and migration (Lesslie et al., 2006). VEGFR1 also promotes colorectal cancer cell survival during epithelial-to-mesenchymal transition (Bates et al., 2003), and its expression seems to be correlated with higher tumour grade (Hanrahan et al., 2003). Another functional VEGF receptor, NRP1, is also expressed by colorectal cancer cells, and particularly in response to stimulation with epidermal growth factor (EGF) (Parikh et al., 2004).

In addition to 'professional' angiogenic factors, CRC progression leads also to the expression of more multifunctional polypeptides endowed with pro-angiogenic activities. This includes: insulin-like growth factors (IGF-1) and its receptors (IGF-IR) (Wu et al., 2002), platelet-derived endothelial cell growth factor (PD-ECGF or Thymidine phosphorylase), all of which are produced by CRC cells themselves, or by the infiltrating immune cells (Takahashi et al., 1996). These processes may also include several other elements of the CRC angiome (Carrer et al., 2008) that are surveyed in Table 9.2.

9.4.2 Angiogenesis and Metastasis in CRC

There is mounting evidence that angiogenesis may differ molecularly in cases of CRC with a good prognosis from that in tumours associated with a high probability of metastasis, as well as between the primary and metastatic tumour sites. Some progress in this area has been possible owing to microarray studies aimed at comparing transcriptional profiles in CRC patients affected, or not, by liver metastases (Nadal et al., 2007). While these comprehensive profiles are being mined and further refined, differences have also been observed in the case of known angiogenesis effectors.

Thus, in preclinical studies, VEGF expression was found to be essential for liver metastasis formation by CRC cells (Takahashi et al., 1995; Warren et al., 1995). However, these relationships are probably more complex, as no difference in VEGF mRNA expression has been detected between liver metastases and their corresponding primary tumours in one study (Kuramochi et al., 2006), while other groups have reported changes in the proportion of different VEGF isoforms, and the aberrant expression of VEGF189 in patients with liver metastases (Tokunaga et al., 1998). It is of considerable interest whether these mechanisms contribute to the metastatic pathways dependent on VEGFR1+ bone marrow derived cells (Kaplan et al., 2005) and to Id-1-expressing endothelial progenitor cells (Gao et al., 2008), or have a different meaning.

Due to its synergy with the VEGF pathway (Hanahan, 1997), the up-regulation of Ang-2 frequently observed in liver metastases of CRC is considered to be a pro-angiogenic change, and one that may contribute to the disease dissemination (Ochiumi et al., 2004; Ogawa et al., 2004). Similar linkages have been proposed for other angiogenic factors, including: PD-ECGF/thymidine phosphorylase, as well as some angiogenesis inhibitors, notably: angiostatin (Mi et al., 2006), endostatin and thrombospondin-1 (Maeda et al., 2001). As mentioned earlier, the latter class of inhibitors acts both locally and systemically, the latter effect being linked to metastasis inhibition in the presence of the primary tumour (Folkman and Kalluri, 2003). Indeed, removal of the primary CRC was associated with a decrease in plasma levels of angiostatin and endostatin (Peeters et al., 2006).

Table 9.2 Effectors of angiogenesis in CRC (see text)

Expression of angiogenic effectors	References
VEGF-A expression in CRC	
– more abundant in adenomas compared with normal tissues and in carcinomas compared with normal tissues	Hanrahan et al. (2003)
– in normal tissues distant from the primary tumour, significantly greater amount of mRNA in patients with Duke's B compared with Duke's A stage tumours	
– mRNA levels correlated significantly with tumour grade and tumour size, but not with patient age, sex, presence of infiltrative margin, lymphocytic response, vascular invasion, Duke's stage, or lymph node involvement	
– significantly increased in CRCs, but not in polyps	George et al. (2001)
– significantly higher levels in lymph node metastases compared with non-metastatic tumours	
– higher in tumours with liver metastasis than in those without	Kawakami et al. (2003)
– associated with progression, invasion and lymph node/liver metastasis of colorectal cancer	
VEGF-B expression in CRC	
– more abundant in adenomas compared with normal tissues	Hanrahan et al. (2003)
– decreased in carcinomas compared with adenomas	
– significantly higher in tumours with lymph node metastasis and lymphatic invasion	Kawakami et al. (2003)
VEGF-C expression in CRC	
– significantly increased in carcinomas compared with normal tissues, and in carcinomas compared with adenomas	Hanrahan et al. (2003)
– mRNA levels correlated significantly with tumour grade and tumour size, but not with patient age, sex, presence of infiltrative margin, lymphocytic response, vascular invasion, Duke's stage, or lymph node involvement	
– no significant difference between the expression levels for both VEGF-C and its receptor, VEGFR3 in cancer versus normal tissues	Parr and Jiang (2003)
– significantly elevated in CRCs, but not in polyps	George et al. (2001)
– no association between VEGF-C or VEGF-D and lymphatic spread	
– significantly higher in tumours with lymph node metastasis and lymphatic invasion	Kawakami et al. (2003)
– expression correlated with the depth of tumour invasion, lymphatic involvement, venous involvement, lymph node metastasis, and liver metastasis	Onogawa et al. (2004)
– expression was more frequently observed in tumours with nodal metastasis than in those without metastasis	Maeda et al. (2003)
– mRNA level in primary CRC correlated with VEGF-C protein expression, lymph node metastasis, and lymphatic invasion	Kawakami et al. (2003)
– rate of lymph node metastasis in VEGF-C positive patients was significantly higher than that in the negative group	Jia et al. (2004)
– expression correlated significantly with poorer histologic grade, depth of invasion, lymphatic invasion, lymph node metastasis, venous invasion, liver metastasis and Duke's stage	Furudoi et al. (2002)

(continued)

Table 9.2 (continued)

Expression of angiogenic effectors	References
VEGF-D expression in CRC	
– significantly more abundant in normal tissues than in adenomas and carcinomas	Hanrahan et al. (2003)
– significantly greater amount in normal tissues distant from the primary tumour, in patients with Duke's C compared with Duke's A stage tumours	
– significantly elevated in colorectal tumours	Parr and Jiang (2003)
– significantly lower in both polyps and CRCs compared with normal mucosa	George et al. (2001)
– no association between VEGF-C or VEGF-D and lymphatic spread	
– down-regulated in tumours with lymphatic involvement	Kawakami et al. (2003)
– expression correlated with the depth of tumour invasion, lymph node metastasis, and liver metastasis	Onogawa et al. (2004)
– significant relationship between the presence of VEGF-D protein and the incidence of lymph node metastasis	Funaki et al. (2003)
– high VEGF-D expression was not correlated with MVD, Duke's stage (A–C), or tumour differentiation, but was associated with lymphatic involvement and patient survival	
VEGFR1 expression in CRC	
– significantly correlated with tumour grade Duke's stage and lymph node involvement	Hanrahan et al. (2003)
VEGFR2 expression in CRC	
– correlated with lymph node involvement	Hanrahan et al. (2003)
– no significant difference between the expression levels of both VEGF-C and VEGFR2, in cancer tissues	Parr and Jiang (2003)
– similar levels in tumours and normal mucosae	George et al. (2001)
VEGFR3 expression in CRC	
– significantly higher in colon cancer than normal tissues	Parr and Jiang (2003)
– similar in tumour tissues and normal mucosae	George et al. (2001)

Indirect inhibition of angiogenesis in CRC can be accomplished through blocking various signalling pathways (Rak et al., 2000a), including Cox-2. The latter intervention inhibits VEGF expression and liver metastases (Yamauchi et al., 2003). Cox-2 and prostaglandins also regulate the expression of VEGF-C and may contribute to lymphatic metastasis of CRC (Soumaoro et al., 2006).

9.4.3 Tumour-Associated Lymphatic Circulation in CRC

Lymphatic microvessels are present around growing tumour nodules and likely provide conduits for regional dissemination of cancer cells to the lymph nodes (Padera et al., 2002; Alitalo et al., 2005; Achen and Stacker, 2008). Indeed the involvement of lymph nodes constitutes one of the main criteria in classification and staging of CRC (Royston and Jackson, 2009). Moreover, as in the case of 'angiocrine' effects associated with angiogenesis (Rak et al., 1994), there is also a reciprocal relationship between the paracrine activity of cancer cells stimulating lymphangiogenesis (Alitalo et al., 2005), and that of LECs, which may in turn impact the behaviour of adjacent cancer cells and inflammatory cells in a 'lymphocrine' manner (Schoppmann et al., 2006; Sundlisaeter et al., 2007).

Lymphatic vessel formation may occur via several mechanisms that, like angiogenesis, involve sprouting, incorporation of precursor cells and transdifferentiation of other cells into LECs (Fig. 9.2) (Sundlisaeter et al., 2007; Alitalo et al., 2005; Achen and Stacker, 2008). Indeed, some of the circulating endothelial precursors (CEP) co-express VEGFR3 and CD133, suggesting their role in lymphatic vasculogenesis, namely as LEC progenitors (Sundlisaeter et al., 2007; Alitalo et al., 2005; Achen and Stacker, 2008). However, these processes are relatively poorly understood, at the moment, as is the recruitment of LECs, their precursors and formation of lymphatic vessels in the course of CRC.

Pro-lymphangiogenic growth factors, their patterns of expression and their mode of action in CRC remain unclear. Thus, lymphangiogenic members of the VEGF family are expressed in CRC, albeit their levels vary during the disease progression (Sundlisaeter et al., 2007) (Table 9.2; Fig. 9.3). Although VEGF-C and VEGF-D may also provoke angiogenesis, their expression is coupled with an increase in lymphatic microcirculation and lymph node metastasis in experimental settings (Padera et al., 2002). On the other hand, the examination of clinical specimens led to a more complex picture, since in some studies, no VEGF-C increase was observed in parallel to lymphangiogenesis (Parr and Jiang, 2003), or lymph node involvement in CRC patients (Hanrahan et al., 2003; George et al., 2001), while such a link was detected by other groups (Jia et al., 2004; Furudoi et al., 2002; Kawakami et al., 2003; Onogawa et al., 2004; Maeda et al., 2003). The association between the increased expression of VEGF-D, lymphangiogenesis and lymph node metastasis (Parr and Jiang, 2003; Onogawa et al., 2004; Funaki et al., 2003) has also been reported by some, but not by other investigators (Kawakami et al., 2003; Hanrahan et al., 2003; George et al., 2001). It is possible that these results could be explained by functional redundancy and contribution of other lymphangiogenic activities, such as VEGF-A, PDGF-BB, FGF2, Ang-1, Ang-2, HGF, IGF-1, IGF-2 and other factors (Achen and Stacker, 2008; Sundlisaeter et al., 2007).

CRC progression is associated with metastasis to the liver and lung, but primarily to regional lymph nodes (Royston and Jackson, 2009). Even if some debate still exists in this area, several lines of evidence suggest that both regional and systemic dissemination of CRC involves lymphangiogenesis (Achen and Stacker, 2008; Kaneko et al., 2007), and its extent is therefore considered to be a prognostic indicator in CRC patients, including the likelihood of systemic metastasis (Royston and Jackson, 2009). The putative contribution of lymphatic vessels to distant metastasis is suggested by their structural properties, as thin-walled layers of LECs would facilitate entry of cancer cells into the lymphatic circulation and their transit to lymph nodes, whereupon they could access the circulating blood (Achen and Stacker, 2008; Royston and Jackson, 2009).

9.5 Targeting Vascular Processes in Metastatic Colorectal Disease

9.5.1 Anti-angiogenesis in CRC

Due to their essential role in growth and dissemination of CRC, vascular processes have become targets of new biological anticancer therapeutics, including agents with anti-angiogenic, vascular disruptive, anticoagulant and anti-lymphangiogenic mode of action. In recent years, some of these agents (bevacizumab) have made history and established CRC as a paradigm for the notion proposed by Folkman nearly four decades ago (Folkman, 1971), that blocking vascular mechanisms represents a viable strategy to treat human cancers (Ferrara et al., 2004). This is especially borne out in the clinical evidence, when such agents are combined with chemotherapeutic protocols (Ferrara et al., 2004; Hurwitz et al., 2004; Willett et al., 2004). This increase in efficacy is possibly due to simple synergy, due to combined effects on the vasculature (Denekamp, 1982; Teicher et al., 1992; Kerbel, 2008), or else a consequence of the postulated improvement of direct anticancer effects of chemotherapy via the process of 'vascular normalization' and better drug delivery (Jain, 2001).

It is also true, however, that since the approval of bevacizumab in 2004 for treatment of metastatic CRC, the clinical experience with this class of agents has revealed the absence of curative effects along with several other important therapeutic limitations (Kerbel, 2008). Notably, a recent randomized phase III clinical trial (CO-8) interrogating the possible role of bevacizumab in adjuvant long term treatment of CRC provided no conclusive evidence to this effect, suggesting that different agents, or paradigms must be sought to achieve this particular goal (Wolmark et al., 2009), and an overall further progress. These recent findings have re-written several previously held beliefs as to the effects of anti-angiogenesis (Kerbel, 1991; Folkman, 1971). Most notably, they unmasked the unsuspected limits, pitfalls, side effects and resistance mechanisms affecting the utility of anti-angiogenic agents. Some of these limitations were foreseen earlier (Rak and Kerbel, 1996), but others were only recently recognized and documented through translational studies in the course of the accumulating clinical experience (Bergers and Hanahan, 2008; Shojaei and Ferrara, 2008; Kerbel et al., 2001; Verheul and Pinedo, 2007; Jubb et al., 2006). As in any other field, these findings serve to guide the improvements in the efficacy and utility of anti-angiogenesis and may bring further progress in treatment of CRC.

In principle, targeting angiogenesis in CRC could be based on 'direct' approaches (Folkman and Kalluri, 2003) aimed at unique molecular features of tumour associated endothelial cells, either known, such as tumour endothelial markers (TEMs) (St. Croix et al., 2000), or unknown. This strategy could also involve usage of endogenous angiogenesis inhibitors (Folkman and Kalluri, 2003), or metronomic chemotherapy (Browder et al., 2000). For neither of these approaches the available clinical experience in CRC is particularly extensive, and the data consist of early (but promising) initial explorations (Bocci et al., 2008; Allegrini et al., 2008; Feldman et al., 2001). Alternative strategies may involve agents directed against angiogenic growth factor receptor tyrosine kinases (RTKs, e.g. VEGFR2), their ligands (VEGF), and mechanisms of their expression by cancer cells (e.g. RAS, EGFR or COX-2). These modalities are considered to be 'indirect' in nature (Folkman and Kalluri, 2003), but have been more extensively studied in patients with CRC (Table 9.3).

9.5.2 Anti-lymphangiogenesis

In addition to anti-angiogenic therapy, there is a growing interest in targeting lymphangiogenesis to prevent the metastatic spread of tumour cells through the lymphatics. Early explorations of this notion have begun in the earnest, but clinical trials are lacking to support the overt efficacy (Stacker and Achen, 2008). The linkage between the 'lymphangiogenic' switch and CRC progression is only beginning to emerge, and the expression profiles of the respective growth factors (e.g. VEGF-C) are somewhat controversial, if highly intriguing (Table 9.2).

In spite of these controversies, functional and therapeutic studies in this field are warranted and the opportunities in this area are forthcoming, owing to the generation of new anti-lymphangiogenic agents (Stacker and Achen, 2008). These efforts already led to the development of an antibody directed against VEGF-D, known as VD1, which exhibited promising experimental results in suppression of the metastatic spread (Stacker et al., 2001). A soluble VEGFR3 ectodomain (VEGFR3-Ig) was also used as a ligand-trap and inhibited tumour-associated lymphangiogenesis and metastasis (Karpanen et al., 2001). Similar properties were also observed in the case of the neutralizing antibody directed against VEGFR3, which also inhibits angiogenesis (Tammela et al., 2008), and with small RTK inhibitors blocking VEGFR3 activity (Underiner et al., 2004). In view of these promising developments, future clinical studies should be expected.

9.5.3 Future Directions in Targeting Tumour-Vascular Interface in Metastatic CRC

The visionary concept of angiogenesis as the 'organizing principle' in the understanding and treatment of cancer, as proposed and practiced by Judah Folkman for over 30 years (Folkman, 2007), has profoundly transformed the field and impacted the management of metastatic CRC (Hurwitz et al., 2004). At the same time, the presently available clinical experience with this and other types of human malignancy, as well as a plethora of new agents that have become available, gradually drive a revision of the traditional models of angiogenesis and anti-angiogenesis. New hopes will likely emerge out of learning from the previously suggested (Rak and Kerbel, 1996), or recently recognized (Kerbel, 2008; Bergers and Hanahan, 2008) pitfalls of therapeutic strategies, which were built on traditional concepts of angiogenesis regulation. The present limitations of anti-angiogenesis are likely

Table 9.3 Examples of the recent experience with anti-angiogenic agents in CRC

Drug	Trade name	Company	Mechanism	Results of clinical trials	References
Bevacizumab	Avastin	Genentech/Roche	Antibody against VEGF-A	Approval by the FDA in 2004	Hurwitz et al. (2004) and McCormack and Keam (2008)
PTK787 ZK222584	Vatalanib	Novartis	Inhibitor of VEGFR tyrosine kinase	Survival improvement in patients with high levels of lactate dehydrogenase	Drevs et al. (2002)
SU5416	Semaxanib	Pharmacia	Inhibitor of VEGFR tyrosine kinase	No improvement of CRC patients survival, high toxicity and thromboembolic events	Hoff et al. (2006)
Sorafenib BAY 43-9006	Nexavar	Bayer	Inhibitor of VEGFR and other tyrosine kinases including Raf	Effective in preclinical models	Kupsch et al. (2005) and Mross et al. (2007)
Cetuximab IMC-C225	Erbitux	ImClone	Antibody against EGFR	Approval by the FDA in 2004	Jean and Shah (2008)
AEE788		Novartis	Inhibitor of VEGFR and EGFR	Inhibition of tumour and metastases in preclinical studies	Traxler et al. (2004)

routed in explaining the angiogenesis process as being fundamentally local in nature, and driven by simple quantitative imbalances between angiogenesis stimulators and inhibitors (Hanahan and Folkman, 1996), and the uniform responses of endothelial cells to them.

Indeed, new developments suggest that targeting a particular angiogenic growth factor must encounter multiple limitations, even if directed at a molecule as central to angiogenesis as VEGF. It is becoming increasingly clear that, for instance, high levels of VEGF are not always consistent with more angiogenic and more aggressive tumour growth (Stockmann et al., 2008), and that VEGF-driven angiogenesis can also be non-productive (Thurston et al., 2007), as well as tumour type-, site- and stage-specific (Bergers et al., 1999; Gao et al., 2008; Seaman et al., 2007). Moreover, angiogenesis inhibition can in some cases be ineffective (Viloria-Petit et al., 2003), provoke cancer cell invasion (Ebos et al., 2009; Paez-Ribes et al., 2009) or lead to selective (Yu et al., 2002b) or instructive (Shahrzad et al., 2008) acquisition of a more malignant phenotype by cancer cells, while possibly impacting their stem cell subset (Gilbertson and Rich, 2007). It is becoming increasingly clear that instead of being local in nature, angiogenic processes emerge as systemic regulatory networks involving soluble mediators (Folkman and Kalluri, 2003), circulating bone marrow-derived cells (De Palma and Naldini, 2006), platelets (Italiano et al., 2008) and microvesicles (Gesierich et al., 2006). These processes also appear to be affected by age-specific changes and vascular co-morbidities, such as atherosclerosis (Klement et al., 2007). Linkages come to light between angiogenesis, lymphangiogenesis and metastasis (Achen and Stacker, 2008), and these various facets are interwoven with their inducing oncogenic, inflammatory and microenvironmental pathways (Kerbel, 2008).

These networks, rather than balance mechanisms, are poorly understood in the context of CRC, and little is known about their operation in individual patients. With further progress in dissecting these relationships and with developing a new understanding of their modus operandi and the corresponding biomarkers (Sessa et al., 2008; Kerbel, 2008), it may be possible, in a not too distant future, to offer the opportunity to apply a personalized anti-angiogenesis and a more effective overall therapy to patients with metastatic CRC.

Acknowledgments This work was supported by operating grants to J.R. from the Canadian Cancer Society (CCS) and Team Grant from Canadian Institutes of Health Research. JR is a recipient of the Jack Cole Chair in Pediatric Oncology at McGill University. Infrastructure funds were contributed by Fonds de la recherche en santé du Québec (FRSQ). We thank our families, especially Françoise Garnier, Jean-Pierre Garnier, Anna Rak and Danuta Rak for their support and patience.

Abbreviations and Acronyms

Ang-2	Angiopoietin-2
APC	Adenomatous polyposis coli
ARNT	Aryl hydrocarbon nuclear translocator
BECs	Blood vessel endothelial cells
bFGF	Basic fibroblast growth factor
BM	Bone marrow
BMDCs	Bone marrow-derived cells

CEPs	Circulating endothelial progenitors
CNS	Central nervous system
COX-2	Cyclooxygenase2
CRC	Colorectal cancer
CSCs	Cancer stem cells
CSFs	Colony stimulating factors
CXCR4	Chemokine C-X-C motif receptor 4
Dll4-4	Notch ligand, delta-like 4 (Dll-4)
EGF	Epidermal growth factor
ECM	Extracellular matrix
EPCs	Endothelial progenitor cells
EPCR	Endothelial protein C receptor
FGF	Fibroblast growth factor
Flk-1	Fetal liver kinase 1
Flt-1	fms-related tyrosine kinase 1
Foxc2	Forkhead box C2
GI	Gastrointestinal
HGF	Hepatocyte growth factor
HER-2	Human epidermal growth factor receptor-2
HIF	Hypoxia inducible factor
HPCs	Hematopoietic progenitor cells
HSCs	Hematopoietic stem cells
Id1	DNA-binding protein inhibitor 1
IGF-1	Insulin-like growth factor-1
IGF-1R	Insulin-like growth factor-1 receptor
HRE	Hypoxia responsive element
KDR	Kinase insert domain-containing receptor
LDH	Lactate dehydrogenase
LECs	Lymphatic endothelial cells
LYVE-1	Lymphatic vessel endothelial hyaluronan receptor 1
MMP	Matrix metalloproteinase
MVD	Microvessel density
NRP1	Neuropilin 1
PARs	Protease activated receptors
PDGF-B	Platelet-derived growth factor B (PDGF-B)
PEDF	Pigment epithelium-derived factor
PF4	Platelet factor 4
PI3K	Phosphatidyl inositol kinase 3
PLGF	Placental growth factor
Prox-1	Prospero homeobox transcription factor
SDF1	Stromal-derived factor 1
sVEGFR	Soluble splice isoforms of vascular endothelial growth factor receptor
TF	Tissue factor
TICs	Tumour initiating cells
Tie2/TEK	Tyrosine kinase with immunoglobulin-like and EGF-like domains 2

TM	Thrombomodulin
TSP	Thrombospondin
TVI	Tumour-vascular interface
UTR	3' untranslated region
VEGF	Vascular endothelial growth factor
VEGFR2	Vascular endothelial growth factor receptor 2
VHL	Von Hippel Lindau

References

Abe K, Shoji M, Chen J, Bierhaus A, Danave I, Micko C et al. (1999). Regulation of vascular endothelial growth factor production and angiogenesis by the cytoplasmic tail of tissue factor. *Proc Natl Acad Sci USA* **96**: 8663–68.

Abtahian F, Guerriero A, Sebzda E, Lu MM, Zhou R, Mocsai A et al. (2003). Regulation of blood and lymphatic vascular separation by signaling proteins SLP-76 and Syk. *Science* **299**: 247–51.

Achen MG, Stacker SA (2008). Molecular control of lymphatic metastasis. *Ann N Y Acad Sci* **1131**: 225–34.

Albrektsen T, Sorensen BB, Hjorto GM, Fleckner J, Rao LV, Petersen LC (2007). Transcriptional program induced by factor VIIa-tissue factor, PAR1 and PAR2 in MDA-MB-231 cells. *J Thromb Haemost* **5**: 1588–97.

Alitalo K, Carmeliet P (2002). Molecular mechanisms of lymphangiogenesis in health and disease. *Cancer Cell* **1**: 219–27.

Alitalo K, Tammela T, Petrova TV (2005). Lymphangiogenesis in development and human disease. *Nature* **438**: 946–53.

Allegrini G, Falcone A, Fioravanti A, Barletta MT, Orlandi P, Loupakis F et al. (2008). A pharmacokinetic and pharmacodynamic study on metronomic irinotecan in metastatic colorectal cancer patients. *Br J Cancer* **98**: 1312–19.

Al-Nedawi K, Meehan B, Kerbel RS, Allison AC, Rak J (2009a). Endothelial expression of autocrine VEGF upon the uptake of tumor-derived microvesicles containing oncogenic EGFR. *Proc Natl Acad Sci USA* **106**: 3794–99.

Al-Nedawi K, Meehan B, Micallef J, Lhotak V, May L, Guha A et al. (2008). Intercellular transfer of the oncogenic receptor EGFRvIII by microvesicles derived from tumour cells. *Nat Cell Biol* **10**: 619–24.

Al-Nedawi K, Meehan B, Rak J (2009b). Microvesicles: messengers and mediators of tumor progression. *Cell Cycle* **8**: 2014–18.

Altinbas M, Coskun HS, Er O, Ozkan M, Eser B, Unal A et al. (2004). A randomized clinical trial of combination chemotherapy with and without low-molecular-weight heparin in small cell lung cancer. *J Thromb Haemost* **2**: 1266–71.

Ancrile B, Lim KH, Counter CM (2007). Oncogenic Ras-induced secretion of IL6 is required for tumorigenesis. *Genes Dev* **21**: 1714–19.

Asahara T, Murohara T, Sullivan A, Silver M, van der Zee R, Li T et al. (1997). Isolation of putative progenitor endothelial cells for angiogenesis. *Science* **275**: 964–67.

Asahara T, Takahashi T, Masuda H, Kalka C, Chen D, Iwaguro H et al. (1999). VEGF contributes to postnatal neovascularization by mobilizing bone marrow-derived endothelial progenitor cells. *EMBO J* **18**: 3964–72.

Augustin HG, Koh GY, Thurston G, Alitalo K (2009). Control of vascular morphogenesis and homeostasis through the angiopoietin-Tie system. *Nat Rev Mol Cell Biol* **10**: 165–77.

Avraamides CJ, Garmy-Susini B, Varner JA (2008). Integrins in angiogenesis and lymphangiogenesis. *Nat Rev Cancer* **8**: 604–17.

Bao S, Wu Q, Sathornsumetee S, Hao Y, Li Z, Hjelmeland AB et al. (2006). Stem Cell-like Glioma Cells Promote Tumor Angiogenesis through Vascular Endothelial Growth Factor. *Cancer Res* **66**: 7843–48.
Bates RC, Goldsmith JD, Bachelder RE, Brown C, Shibuya M, Oettgen P et al. (2003). Flt-1-dependent survival characterizes the epithelial-mesenchymal transition of colonic organoids. *Curr Biol* **13**: 1721–27.
Belting M, Ahamed J, Ruf W (2005). Signaling of the tissue factor coagulation pathway in angiogenesis and cancer. *Arterioscler Thromb Vasc Biol* **25**: 1545–50.
Bergers G, Brekken R, McMahon G, Vu TH, Itoh T, Tamaki K et al. (2000). Matrix metalloproteinase-9 triggers the angiogenic switch during carcinogenesis. *Nat Cell Biol* **2**: 737–44.
Bergers G, Hanahan D (2008). Modes of resistance to anti-angiogenic therapy. *Nat Rev Cancer* **8**: 592–603.
Bergers G, Javaherian K, Lo KM, Folkman J, Hanahan D (1999). Effects of angiogenesis inhibitors on multistage carcinogenesis in mice. *Science* **284**: 808–12.
Berra E, Pages G, Pouyssegur J (2000). MAP kinases and hypoxia in the control of VEGF expression. *Cancer Metastasis Rev* **19**: 139–45.
Bertolini F, Shaked Y, Mancuso P, Kerbel RS (2006). The multifaceted circulating endothelial cell in cancer: towards marker and target identification. *Nat Rev Cancer* **6**: 835–45.
Bocci G, Falcone A, Fioravanti A, Orlandi P, Di PA, Fanelli G et al. (2008). Antiangiogenic and anticolorectal cancer effects of metronomic irinotecan chemotherapy alone and in combination with semaxinib. *Br J Cancer* **98**: 1619–29.
Bouck N, Stellmach V, Hsu SC (1996). How tumors become angiogenic. *Adv Cancer Res* **69**: 135–74.
Boutin AT, Weidemann A, Fu Z, Mesropian L, Gradin K, Jamora C et al. (2008). Epidermal sensing of oxygen is essential for systemic hypoxic response. *Cell* **133**: 223–34.
Browder T, Butterfield CE, Kraling BM, Shi B, Marshall B, O'Reilly MS et al. (2000). Antiangiogenic scheduling of chemotherapy improves efficacy against experimental drug-resistant cancer. *Cancer Res* **60**: 1878–86.
Brown LF, Berse B, Jackman RW, Tognazzi K, Manseau EJ, Senger DR et al. (1993). Expression of vascular permeability factor (vascular endothelial growth factor) and its receptors in adenocarcinomas of the gastrointestinal tract. *Cancer Res* **53**: 4727–35.
Broxterman HJ, Lankelma J, Hoekman K (2003). Resistance to cytotoxic and anti-angiogenic anticancer agents: similarities and differences. *Drug Resist Updat* **6**: 111–27.
Buller HR, van Doormaal FF, van Sluis GL, Kamphuisen PW (2007). Cancer and thrombosis: from molecular mechanisms to clinical presentations. *J Thromb Haemost* **5**(**Suppl 1**): 246–54.
Burri PH (1991). Intussusceptive microvascular growth, a new mechanism of capillary network expansion. *Angiogenesis, International Symposium*, St Gallen, March 13–15, 1991. Abstract: 88.
Calabrese C, Poppleton H, Kocak M, Hogg TL, Fuller C, Hamner B et al. (2007). A perivascular niche for brain tumor stem cells. *Cancer Cell* **11**: 69–82.
Camerer E, Gjernes E, Wiiger M, Pringle S, Prydz H (2000). Binding of factor VIIa to tissue factor on keratinocytes induces gene expression. *J Biol Chem* **275**: 6580–85.
Cao Y, Tan A, Gao F, Liu L, Liao C, Mo Z (2009). A meta-analysis of randomized controlled trials comparing chemotherapy plus bevacizumab with chemotherapy alone in metastatic colorectal cancer. *Int J Colorectal Dis* **24**: 677–85.
Carmeliet P (2000). Mechanisms of angiogenesis and arteriogenesis. *Nat Med* **6**: 389–95.
Carmeliet P (2001). Biomedicine. Clotting factors build blood vessels. *Science* **293**: 1602–4.
Carmeliet P (2005). Angiogenesis in life, disease and medicine. *Nature* **438**: 932–36.
Carmeliet P, Jain RK (2000). Angiogenesis in cancer and other diseases. *Nature* **407**: 249–57.
Carmeliet P, Moons L, Luttun A, Vincenti V, Compernolle V, De Mol M et al. (2001). Synergism between vascular endothelial growth factor and placental growth factor contributes to angiogenesis and plasma extravasation in pathological conditions. *Nat Med* **7**: 575–83.

Carrer A, Zacchigna S, Balani A, Pistan V, Adami A, Porcelli F et al. (2008). Expression profiling of angiogenic genes for the characterisation of colorectal carcinoma. *Eur J Cancer* **44**: 1761–69.

Casanovas O, Hicklin DJ, Bergers G, Hanahan D (2005). Drug resistance by evasion of antiangiogenic targeting of VEGF signaling in late-stage pancreatic islet tumors. *Cancer Cell* **8**: 299–309.

Cascinu S, Staccioli MP, Gasparini G, Giordani P, Catalano V, Ghiselli R et al. (2000). Expression of vascular endothelial growth factor can predict event-free survival in stage II colon cancer. *Clin Cancer Res* **6**: 2803–7.

Cassano A, Bagala C, Battelli C, Schinzari G, Quirino M, Ratto C et al. (2002). Expression of vascular endothelial growth factor, mitogen-activated protein kinase and p53 in human colorectal cancer. *Anticancer Res* **22**: 2179–84.

Choi DS, Lee JM, Park GW, Lim HW, Bang JY, Kim YK et al. (2007). Proteomic analysis of microvesicles derived from human colorectal cancer cells. *J Proteome Res* **6**: 4646–55.

Coughlin SR (2000). Thrombin signalling and protease-activated receptors. *Nature* **407**: 258–64.

Coultas L, Chawengsaksophak K, Rossant J (2005). Endothelial cells and VEGF in vascular development. *Nature* **438**: 937–45.

Coussens LM, Werb Z (2002). Inflammation and cancer. *Nature* **420**: 860–67.

Cueni LN, Detmar M (2008). The lymphatic system in health and disease. *Lymphat Res Biol* **6**: 109–22.

Dameron KM, Volpert OV, Tainsky MA, Bouck N (1994). Control of angiogenesis in fibroblasts by p53 regulation of thrombospondin-1. *Science* **265**: 1582–84.

Das S, Skobe M (2008). Lymphatic vessel activation in cancer. *Ann N Y Acad Sci* **1131**: 235–41.

De PM, Naldini L (2006). Role of haematopoietic cells and endothelial progenitors in tumour angiogenesis. *Biochim Biophys Acta* **1766**: 159–66.

Dejana E (2004). Endothelial cell-cell junctions: happy together. *Nat Rev Mol Cell Biol* **5**: 261–70.

del Conde, I, Shrimpton CN, Thiagarajan P, Lopez JA (2005). Tissue-factor-bearing microvesicles arise from lipid rafts and fuse with activated platelets to initiate coagulation. *Blood* **106**: 1604–11.

Denekamp J (1982). Endothelial cell proliferation as a novel approach to targeting tumor therapy. *Br J Cancer* **45**: 136–39.

Des GG, Uzzan B, Nicolas P, Cucherat M, Morere JF, Benamouzig R et al. (2006). Microvessel density and VEGF expression are prognostic factors in colorectal cancer. Meta-analysis of the literature. *Br J Cancer* **94**: 1823–32.

Dews M, Homayouni A, Yu D, Murphy D, Sevignani C, Wentzel E et al. (2006). Augmentation of tumor angiogenesis by a Myc-activated microRNA cluster. *Nat Genet* **38**: 1060–65.

Di VD, Kim J, Hager MH, Morello M, Yang W, Lafargue CJ et al. (2009). Oncosome formation in prostate cancer: association with a region of frequent chromosomal deletion in metastatic disease. *Cancer Res* **69**: 5601–9.

Dick JE (2009). Looking ahead in cancer stem cell research. *Nat Biotechnol* **27**: 44–46.

Dolo V, D'Ascenzo S, Giusti I, Millimaggi D, Taraboletti G, Pavan A (2005). Shedding of membrane vesicles by tumor and endothelial cells. *Ital J Anat Embryol* **110**: 127–33.

Drevs J, Muller-Driver R, Wittig C, Fuxius S, Esser N, Hugenschmidt H et al. (2002). PTK787/ZK 222584, a specific vascular endothelial growth factor-receptor tyrosine kinase inhibitor, affects the anatomy of the tumor vascular bed and the functional vascular properties as detected by dynamic enhanced magnetic resonance imaging. *Cancer Res* **62**: 4015–22.

Dumont DJ, Yamaguchi TP, Conlon RA, Rossant J, Breitman ML (1992). *tek*, a novel tyrosine kinase gene located on mouse chromosome 4, is expressed in endothelial cells and their presumptive precursors. *Oncogene* **7**: 1471–80.

Dvorak HF (2002). Vascular permeability factor/vascular endothelial growth factor: a critical cytokine in tumor angiogenesis and a potential target for diagnosis and therapy. *J Clin Oncol* **20**: 4368–80.

Dvorak HF, Nagy JA, Dvorak AM (1991). Structure of solid tumors and their vasculature:implications for therapy with monoclonal antibodies. *Cancer Cells* **3**: 77–85.
Dvorak FH, Rickles FR. (2006). Malignancy and hemostasis. In: Coleman RB, Marder VJ, Clowes AW, George JN, Goldhaber SZ (eds.) *Hemostasis and Thrombosis, Basic Principles and Clinical Practice*. Lippincott Company Williams & Wilkins: Philadelphia, PA, pp. 851–73.
Ebos JM, Lee CR, Cruz-Munoz W, Bjarnason GA, Christensen JG, Kerbel RS (2009). Accelerated metastasis after short-term treatment with a potent inhibitor of tumor angiogenesis. *Cancer Cell* **15**: 232–39.
Eliceiri BP, Cheresh DA (2001). Adhesion events in angiogenesis. *Curr Opin Cell Biol* **13**: 563–68.
Ellis LM (2004). Angiogenesis and its role in colorectal tumor and metastasis formation. *Semin Oncol* **31**: 3–9.
Ema M, Rossant J (2003). Cell fate decisions in early blood vessel formation. *Trends Cardiovasc Med* **13**: 254–59.
Escudier B, Eisen T, Stadler WM, Szczylik C, Oudard S, Siebels M et al. (2007). Sorafenib in advanced clear-cell renal-cell carcinoma. *N Engl J Med* **356**: 125–34.
Falanga A (2005). Thrombophilia in cancer. *Semin Thromb Hemost* **31**: 104–10.
Fan F, Wey JS, McCarty MF, Belcheva A, Liu W, Bauer TW et al. (2005). Expression and function of vascular endothelial growth factor receptor-1 on human colorectal cancer cells. *Oncogene* **24**: 2647–53.
Fearon ER, Vogelstein B (1990). A genetic model for colorectal tumorigenesis. *Cell* **61**: 759–67.
Feldman AL, Alexander HR Jr, Bartlett DL, Kranda KC, Miller MS, Costouros NG et al. (2001). A prospective analysis of plasma endostatin levels in colorectal cancer patients with liver metastases. *Ann Surg Oncol* **8**: 741–45.
Ferlay J, Autier P, Boniol M, Heanue M, Colombet M, Boyle P (2007). Estimates of the cancer incidence and mortality in Europe in 2006. *Ann Oncol* **18**: 581–92.
Ferrara N (2002). VEGF and the quest for tumour angiogenesis factors. *Nat Rev Cancer* **2**: 795–803.
Ferrara N (2005). VEGF as a therapeutic target in cancer. *Oncology* **69**(Suppl 3): 11–16.
Ferrara N, Hillan KJ, Gerber HP, Novotny W (2004). Discovery and development of bevacizumab, an anti-VEGF antibody for treating cancer. *Nat Rev Drug Discov* **3**: 391–400.
Fidler IJ (2003). The pathogenesis of cancer metastasis: the 'seed and soil' hypothesis revisited. *Nat Rev Cancer* **3**: 453–58.
Fischer C, Mazzone M, Jonckx B, Carmeliet P (2008). FLT1 and its ligands VEGFB and PlGF: drug targets for anti-angiogenic therapy? *Nat Rev Cancer* **8**: 942–56.
Folkman J (1971). Tumor angiogenesis: therapeutic implications. *N Engl J Med* **285**: 1182–86.
Folkman J (1985). Tumor angiogenesis. *Adv Cancer Res* **43**: 175–203.
Folkman J (2007). Angiogenesis: an organizing principle for drug discovery? *Nat Rev Drug Discov* **6**: 273–86.
Folkman J, Kalluri R. (2003). Tumor angiogenesis. In: Kufe DW, Pollock RE, Weichselbaum RR, Bast RC Jr, Gansler TS, Holland JF, Frei E III (eds.) *Cancer Medicine*. BC Decker Inc.: Hamilton, London, pp. 161–94.
Fotopoulou C, duBois A, Karavas AN, Trappe R, Aminossadati B, Schmalfeldt B et al. (2008). Incidence of venous thromboembolism in patients with ovarian cancer undergoing platinum/paclitaxel-containing first-line chemotherapy: an exploratory analysis by the Arbeitsgemeinschaft Gynaekologische Onkologie Ovarian Cancer Study Group. *J Clin Oncol* **26**: 2683–89.
Fraisl P, Mazzone M, Schmidt T, Carmeliet P (2009). Regulation of angiogenesis by oxygen and metabolism. *Dev Cell* **16**: 167–79.
Francis JL, Amirkhosravi A (2002). Effect of antihemostatic agents on experimental tumor dissemination. *Semin Thromb Hemost* **28**: 29–38.
Funaki H, Nishimura G, Harada S, Ninomiya I, Terada I, Fushida S et al. (2003). Expression of vascular endothelial growth factor D is associated with lymph node metastasis in human colorectal carcinoma. *Oncology* **64**: 416–22.

Furudoi A, Tanaka S, Haruma K, Kitadai Y, Yoshihara M, Chayama K et al. (2002). Clinical significance of vascular endothelial growth factor C expression and angiogenesis at the deepest invasive site of advanced colorectal carcinoma. *Oncology* **62**: 157–66.

Gale NW, Thurston G, Hackett SF, Renard R, Wang Q, McClain J et al. (2002). Angiopoietin-2 is required for postnatal angiogenesis and lymphatic patterning, and only the latter role is rescued by Angiopoietin-1. *Dev Cell* **3**: 411–23.

Gao D, Nolan DJ, Mellick AS, Bambino K, McDonnell K, Mittal V (2008). Endothelial progenitor cells control the angiogenic switch in mouse lung metastasis. *Science* **319**: 195–98.

George ML, Tutton MG, Janssen F, Arnaout A, Abulafi AM, Eccles SA et al. (2001). VEGF-A, VEGF-C, and VEGF-D in colorectal cancer progression. *Neoplasia* **3**: 420–27.

Gerhardt H, Golding M, Fruttiger M, Ruhrberg C, Lundkvist A, Abramsson A et al. (2003). VEGF guides angiogenic sprouting utilizing endothelial tip cell filopodia. *J Cell Biol* **161**: 1163–77.

Gesierich S, Berezovskiy I, Ryschich E, Zoller M (2006). Systemic induction of the angiogenesis switch by the tetraspanin D6.1A/CO-029. *Cancer Res* **66**: 7083–94.

Giaccia A. (2003). Genetic basis of altered responsiveness of cancer cells to their microenvironment. In: Rak J (ed.) *Oncogene-Directed Therapies*. Humana Press: Totowa, pp. 113–32.

Gilbertson RJ, Rich JN (2007). Making a tumour's bed: glioblastoma stem cells and the vascular niche. *Nat Rev Cancer* **7**: 733–36.

Gimbrone M, Leapman S, Cotran R, Folkman J (1972). Tumor dormancy in vivo by prevention of neovascularization. *J Exp Med* **136**: 261–76.

Griffin CT, Srinivasan Y, Zheng YW, Huang W, Coughlin SR (2001). A role for thrombin receptor signaling in endothelial cells during embryonic development. *Science* **293**: 1666–70.

Grothey A, Ellis LM (2008). Targeting angiogenesis driven by vascular endothelial growth factors using antibody-based therapies. *Cancer J* **14**: 170–77.

Grunstein J, Masbad JJ, Hickey R, Giordano F, Johnson RS (2000). Isoforms of vascular endothelial growth factor act in a coordinate fashion to recruit and expand tumor vasculature. *Mol Cell Biol* **20**: 7282–91.

Hanahan D (1997). Signaling vascular morphogenesis and maintenance. *Science* **277**: 48–50.

Hanahan D, Folkman J (1996). Patterns and emerging mechanisms of the angiogenic switch during tumorigenesis. *Cell* **86**: 353–64.

Hanahan D, Weinberg RA (2000). The hallmarks of cancer. *Cell* **100**: 57–70.

Hanrahan V, Currie MJ, Gunningham SP, Morrin HR, Scott PA, Robinson BA et al. (2003). The angiogenic switch for vascular endothelial growth factor (VEGF)-A, VEGF-B, VEGF-C, and VEGF-D in the adenoma-carcinoma sequence during colorectal cancer progression. *J Pathol* **200**: 183–94.

Harris AL (2002). Hypoxia–a key regulatory factor in tumour growth. *Nat Rev Cancer* **2**: 38–47.

Hembrough TA, Swartz GM, Papathanassiu A, Vlasuk GP, Rote WE, Green SJ et al. (2003). Tissue factor/factor VIIa inhibitors block angiogenesis and tumor growth through a nonhemostatic mechanism. *Cancer Res* **63**: 2997–3000.

Hendrix MJ, Seftor EA, Hess AR, Seftor RE (2003). Vasculogenic mimicry and tumour-cell plasticity: lessons from melanoma. *Nat Rev Cancer* **3**: 411–21.

Hirakawa S, Hong YK, Harvey N, Schacht V, Matsuda K, Libermann T et al. (2003). Identification of vascular lineage-specific genes by transcriptional profiling of isolated blood vascular and lymphatic endothelial cells. *Am J Pathol* **162**: 575–86.

Hoff PM, Wolff RA, Bogaard K, Waldrum S, Abbruzzese JL (2006). A Phase I study of escalating doses of the tyrosine kinase inhibitor semaxanib (SU5416) in combination with irinotecan in patients with advanced colorectal carcinoma. *Jpn J Clin Oncol* **36**: 100–3.

Holash J, Maisonpierre PC, Compton D, Boland P, Alexander CR, Zagzag D et al. (1999). Vessel cooption, regression, and growth in tumors mediated by angiopoietins and VEGF. *Science* **284**: 1994–98.

Holmgren L, O'Reilly MS, Folkman J (1995). Dormancy of micrometastases: balanced proliferation and apoptosis in the presence of angiogenesis suppression. *Nature Med* **1**: 149–53.

Hurwitz H, Fehrenbacher L, Novotny W, Cartwright T, Hainsworth J, Heim W et al. (2004). Bevacizumab plus irinotecan, fluorouracil, and leucovorin for metastatic colorectal cancer. *N Engl J Med* **350**: 2335–42.

Italiano JE Jr, Richardson JL, Patel-Hett S, Battinelli E, Zaslavsky A, Short S et al. (2008). Angiogenesis is regulated by a novel mechanism: pro- and antiangiogenic proteins are organized into separate platelet alpha granules and differentially released. *Blood* **111**: 1227–33.

Itzkowitz SH, Yio X (2004). Inflammation and cancer IV. Colorectal cancer in inflammatory bowel disease: the role of inflammation. *Am J Physiol Gastrointest Liver Physiol* **287**: G7–17.

Iversen LH, Thorlacius-Ussing O (2003). Systemic coagulation reactivation in recurrence of colorectal cancer. *Thromb Haemost* **89**: 726–34.

Jackson DG (2004). Biology of the lymphatic marker LYVE-1 and applications in research into lymphatic trafficking and lymphangiogenesis. *APMIS* **112**: 526–38.

Jain RK (1990). Vascular and interstitial barriers to delivery of therapeutic agents in tumors. *Cancer Metastasis Rev* **9**: 253–66.

Jain RK (2001). Normalizing tumor vaculature with anti-angiogenic therapy: a new paradigm for combination therapy. *Nature Med* **7**: 987–89.

Jain RK, Duda DG, Clark JW, Loeffler JS (2006). Lessons from phase III clinical trials on anti-VEGF therapy for cancer. *Nat Clin Pract Oncol* **3**: 24–40.

Jain RK, Padera TP (2002). Prevention and treatment of lymphatic metastasis by antilymphangiogenic therapy. *J Natl Cancer Inst* **94**: 785–87.

Jean GW, Shah SR (2008). Epidermal growth factor receptor monoclonal antibodies for the treatment of metastatic colorectal cancer. *Pharmacotherapy* **28**: 742–54.

Jia YT, Li ZX, He YT, Liang W, Yang HC, Ma HJ (2004). Expression of vascular endothelial growth factor-C and the relationship between lymphangiogenesis and lymphatic metastasis in colorectal cancer. *World J Gastroenterol* **10**: 3261–63.

Jimeno A, Daw NC, Amador ML, Cusatis G, Kulesza P, Krailo M et al. (2007). Analysis of biologic surrogate markers from a Children's Oncology Group Phase I trial of gefitinib in pediatric patients with solid tumors. *Pediatr Blood Cancer* **49**: 352–57.

Jubb AM, Oates AJ, Holden S, Koeppen H (2006). Predicting benefit from anti-angiogenic agents in malignancy. *Nat Rev Cancer* **6**: 626–35.

Kaelin WG Jr (2008). The von Hippel-Lindau tumour suppressor protein: O_2 sensing and cancer. *Nat Rev Cancer* **8**: 865–73.

Kaio E, Tanaka S, Kitadai Y, Sumii M, Yoshihara M, Haruma K et al. (2003). Clinical significance of angiogenic factor expression at the deepest invasive site of advanced colorectal carcinoma. *Oncology* **64**: 61–73.

Kakkar AK, DeRuvo N, Chinswangwatanakul V, Tebbutt S, Williamson RC (1995). Extrinsic-pathway activation in cancer with high factor VIIa and tissue factor. *Lancet* **346**: 1004–5.

Kakkar AK, Levine MN, Kadziola Z, Lemoine NR, Low V, Patel HK et al. (2004). Low molecular weight heparin, therapy with dalteparin, and survival in advanced cancer: the fragmin advanced malignancy outcome study (FAMOUS). *J Clin Oncol* **22**: 1944–48.

Kalas W, Yu JL, Milsom C, Rosenfeld J, Benezra R, Bornstein P et al. (2005). Oncogenes and Angiogenesis: down-regulation of thrombospondin-1 in normal fibroblasts exposed to factors from cancer cells harboring mutant ras. *Cancer Res* **65**: 8878–86.

Kalluri R (2003). Basement membranes: structure assembly and role in tumor angiogenesis. *Nature Reviews Cancer* **3**: 422–33.

Kamei M, Saunders WB, Bayless KJ, Dye L, Davis GE, Weinstein BM (2006). Endothelial tubes assemble from intracellular vacuoles in vivo. *Nature* **442**: 453–56.

Kaneko I, Tanaka S, Oka S, Kawamura T, Hiyama T, Ito M et al. (2007). Lymphatic vessel density at the site of deepest penetration as a predictor of lymph node metastasis in submucosal colorectal cancer. *Dis Colon Rectum* **50**: 13–21.

Kaplan RN, Riba RD, Zacharoulis S, Bramley AH, Vincent L, Costa C et al. (2005). VEGFR1-positive haematopoietic bone marrow progenitors initiate the pre-metastatic niche. *Nature* **438**: 820–27.

Karin M (2005). Inflammation and cancer: the long reach of Ras. *Nat Med* **11**: 20–21.

Karpanen T, Alitalo K (2008). Molecular biology and pathology of lymphangiogenesis. *Annu Rev Pathol* **3**: 367–97.

Karpanen T, Egeblad M, Karkkainen MJ, Kubo H, Yla-Herttuala S, Jaattela M et al. (2001). Vascular endothelial growth factor C promotes tumor lymphangiogenesis and intralymphatic tumor growth. *Cancer Res* **61**: 1786–90.

Kawakami M, Furuhata T, Kimura Y, Yamaguchi K, Hata F, Sasaki K et al. (2003). Expression analysis of vascular endothelial growth factors and their relationships to lymph node metastasis in human colorectal cancer. *J Exp Clin Cancer Res* **22**: 229–37.

Kerbel RS (1991). Inhibition of tumor angiogenesis as a strategy to circumvent acquired resistance to anti-cancer therapeutic agents. *BioEssays* **13**: 31–36.

Kerbel RS (2008). Tumor angiogenesis. *N Engl J Med* **358**: 2039–49.

Kerbel RS, Folkman J (2002). Clinical translation of angiogenesis inhibitors. *Nature Reviews Cancer* **2**: 727–39.

Kerbel RS, Yu J, Tran J, Man S, Viloria-Petit A, Klement G et al. (2001). Possible mechanisms of acquired resistance to anti-angiogenic drugs: implications for the use of combination therapy approaches. *Cancer Metastasis Rev* **20**: 79–86.

Kevil CG, De Benedetti A, Payne DK, Coe LL, Laroux FS, Alexander JS (1996). Translational regulation of vascular permeability factor by eukaryotic initiation factor 4E: implications for tumor angiogenesis. *Int J Cancer* **65**: 785–90.

Khorana AA, Ahrendt SA, Ryan CK, Francis CW, Hruban RH, Hu YC et al. (2007). Tissue factor expression, angiogenesis, and thrombosis in pancreatic cancer. *Clin Cancer Res* **13**: 2870–75.

Klement H, St CB, Milsom C, May L, Guo Q, Yu JL et al. (2007). Atherosclerosis and Vascular Aging as Modifiers of Tumor Progression, Angiogenesis, and Responsiveness to Therapy. *Am J Pathol* **171**: 1342–51.

Klement GL, Yip TT, Cassiola F, Kikuchi L, Cervi D, Podust V et al. (2009). Platelets actively sequester angiogenesis regulators. *Blood* **113**: 2835–42.

Klerk CP, Smorenburg SM, Otten HM, Lensing AW, Prins MH, Piovella F et al. (2005). The effect of low molecular weight heparin on survival in patients with advanced malignancy. *J Clin Oncol* **23**: 2130–35.

Konerding MA, Fait E, Gaumann A (2001). 3D microvascular architecture of pre-cancerous lesions and invasive carcinomas of the colon. *Br J Cancer* **84**: 1354–62.

Koukourakis MI, Giatromanolaki A, Simopoulos C, Polychronidis A, Sivridis E (2005). Lactate dehydrogenase 5 (LDH5) relates to up-regulated hypoxia inducible factor pathway and metastasis in colorectal cancer. *Clin Exp Metastasis* **22**: 25–30.

Kupsch P, Henning BF, Passarge K, Richly H, Wiesemann K, Hilger RA et al. (2005). Results of a phase I trial of sorafenib (BAY 43-9006) in combination with oxaliplatin in patients with refractory solid tumors, including colorectal cancer. *Clin Colorectal Cancer* **5**: 188–96.

Kuramochi H, Hayashi K, Uchida K, Miyakura S, Shimizu D, Vallbohmer D et al. (2006). Vascular endothelial growth factor messenger RNA expression level is preserved in liver metastases compared with corresponding primary colorectal cancer. *Clin Cancer Res* **12**: 29–33.

Ladomery MR, Harper SJ, Bates DO (2007). Alternative splicing in angiogenesis: the vascular endothelial growth factor paradigm. *Cancer Lett* **249**: 133–42.

Lazarus RA, Olivero AG, Eigenbrot C, Kirchhofer D (2004). Inhibitors of Tissue Factor.Factor VIIa for anticoagulant therapy. *Curr Med Chem* **11**: 2275–90.

Lee AY, Rickles FR, Julian JA, Gent M, Baker RI, Bowden C et al. (2005). Randomized comparison of low molecular weight heparin and coumarin derivatives on the survival of patients with cancer and venous thromboembolism. *J Clin Oncol* **23**: 2123–29.

Lesslie DP, Summy JM, Parikh NU, Fan F, Trevino JG, Sawyer TK et al. (2006). Vascular endothelial growth factor receptor-1 mediates migration of human colorectal carcinoma cells by activation of Src family kinases. *Br J Cancer* **94**: 1710–17.

Lohela M, Bry M, Tammela T, Alitalo K (2009). VEGFs and receptors involved in angiogenesis versus lymphangiogenesis. *Curr Opin Cell Biol* **21**: 154–65.

Lyden D, Hattori K, Dias S, Costa C, Blaikie P, Butros L et al. (2001). Impaired recruitment of bone-marrow-derived endothelial and hematopoietic precursor cells blocks tumor angiogenesis and growth. *Nat Med* **7**: 1194–201.

Lykke J, Nielsen HJ (2004). Haemostatic alterations in colorectal cancer: perspectives for future treatment. *J Surg Oncol* **88**: 269–75.

Mack M, Kleinschmidt A, Bruhl H, Klier C, Nelson PJ, Cihak J et al. (2000). Transfer of the chemokine receptor CCR5 between cells by membrane-derived microparticles: a mechanism for cellular human immunodeficiency virus 1 infection. *Nat Med* **6**: 769–75.

Maeda K, Nishiguchi Y, Kang SM, Yashiro M, Onoda N, Sawada T et al. (2001). Expression of thrombospondin-1 inversely correlated with tumor vascularity and hematogenous metastasis in colon cancer. *Oncol Rep* **8**: 763–66.

Maeda K, Yashiro M, Nishihara T, Nishiguchi Y, Sawai M, Uchima K et al. (2003). Correlation between vascular endothelial growth factor C expression and lymph node metastasis in T1 carcinoma of the colon and rectum. *Surg Today* **33**: 736–39.

Makinen T, Alitalo K (2007). Lymphangiogenesis in development and disease. *Novartis Found Symp* **283**: 87–98.

Mantovani A, Allavena P, Sica A, Balkwill F (2008). Cancer-related inflammation. *Nature* **454**: 436–444.

Mazure NM, Chen EY, Laderoute KR, Giaccia AJ (1997). Induction of vascular endothelial growth factor by hypoxia is modulated by a phosphatidylinositol 3-kinase/Akt signaling pathway in Ha-ras- transformed cells through a hypoxia inducible factor-1 transcriptional element. *Blood* **90**: 3322–31.

McCormack PL, Keam SJ (2008). Bevacizumab: a review of its use in metastatic colorectal cancer. *Drugs* **68**: 487–506.

McDonald DM, Choyke PL (2003). Imaging of angiogenesis: from microscope to clinic. *Nat Med* **9**: 713–25.

Mi J, Sarraf-Yazdi S, Zhang X, Cao Y, Dewhirst MW, Kontos CD et al. (2006). A comparison of antiangiogenic therapies for the prevention of liver metastases. *J Surg Res* **131**: 97–104.

Milsom C, Anderson GM, Weitz JI, Rak J (2007). Elevated tissue factor procoagulant activity in CD133-positive cancer cells. *J Thromb Haemost* **5**: 2550–52.

Milsom CC, Yu JL, Mackman N, Micallef J, Anderson GM, Guha A et al. (2008). Tissue factor regulation by epidermal growth factor receptor and epithelial-to-mesenchymal transitions: effect on tumor initiation and angiogenesis. *Cancer Res* **68**: 10068–76.

Mizukami Y, Kohgo Y, Chung DC (2007). Hypoxia inducible factor-1 independent pathways in tumor angiogenesis. *Clin Cancer Res* **13**: 5670–74.

Morisada T, Oike Y, Yamada Y, Urano T, Akao M, Kubota Y et al. (2005). Angiopoietin-1 promotes LYVE-1-positive lymphatic vessel formation. *Blood* **105**: 4649–56.

Mross K, Steinbild S, Baas F, Gmehling D, Radtke M, Voliotis D et al. (2007). Results from an in vitro and a clinical/pharmacological phase I study with the combination irinotecan and sorafenib. *Eur J Cancer* **43**: 55–63.

Nadal C, Maurel J, Gascon P (2007). Is there a genetic signature for liver metastasis in colorectal cancer? *World J Gastroenterol* **13**: 5832–44.

Nakasaki T, Wada H, Shigemori C, Miki C, Gabazza EC, Nobori T et al. (2002). Expression of tissue factor and vascular endothelial growth factor is associated with angiogenesis in colorectal cancer. *Am J Hematol* **69**: 247–54.

Naumov GN, MacDonald IC, Chambers AF, Groom AC (2001). Solitary cancer cells as a possible source of tumor dormancy? *Sem Cancer Biol* **11**: 271–76.

Ngo CV, Picha K, McCabe F, Millar H, Tawadros R, Tam SH et al. (2007). CNTO 859, a humanized anti-tissue factor monoclonal antibody, is a potent inhibitor of breast cancer metastasis and tumor growth in xenograft models. *Int J Cancer* **120**: 1261–67.

Nierodzik ML, Karpatkin S (2006). Thrombin induces tumor growth, metastasis, and angiogenesis: evidence for a thrombin-regulated dormant tumor phenotype. *Cancer Cell* **10**: 355–62.

Noguera-Troise I, Daly C, Papadopoulos NJ, Coetzee S, Boland P, Gale NW et al. (2006). Blockade of Dll4 inhibits tumour growth by promoting non-productive angiogenesis. *Nature* **444**: 1032–37.

Ochiumi T, Tanaka S, Oka S, Hiyama T, Ito M, Kitadai Y et al. (2004). Clinical significance of angiopoietin-2 expression at the deepest invasive tumor site of advanced colorectal carcinoma. *Int J Oncol* **24**: 539–47.

Ogawa M, Yamamoto H, Nagano H, Miyake Y, Sugita Y, Hata T et al. (2004). Hepatic expression of ANG2 RNA in metastatic colorectal cancer. *Hepatology* **39**: 528–39.

Onogawa S, Kitadai Y, Tanaka S, Kuwai T, Kuroda T, Chayama K (2004). Regulation of vascular endothelial growth factor (VEGF)-C and VEGF-D expression by the organ microenvironment in human colon carcinoma. *Eur J Cancer* **40**: 1604–9.

Pacilli A, Pasquinelli G (2009). Vascular wall resident progenitor cells: a review. *Exp Cell Res* **315**: 901–14.

Padera TP, Kadambi A, di Tomaso E, Carreira CM, Brown EB, Boucher Y et al. (2002). Lymphatic metastasis in the absence of functional intratumor lymphatics. *Science* **296**: 1883–86.

Paez-Ribes M, Allen E, Hudock J, Takeda T, Okuyama H, Vinals F et al. (2009). Antiangiogenic therapy elicits malignant progression of tumors to increased local invasion and distant metastasis. *Cancer Cell* **15**: 220–31.

Paku S, Paweletz N (1991). First steps of tumor-related angiogenesis. *Lab Invest* **65**: 334–46.

Palumbo JS, Talmage KE, Massari JV, La Jeunesse CM, Flick MJ, Kombrinck KW et al. (2007). Tumor cell-associated tissue factor and circulating hemostatic factors cooperate to increase metastatic potential through natural killer cell-dependent and -independent mechanisms. *Blood* **110**: 133–41.

Parikh AA, Fan F, Liu WB, Ahmad SA, Stoeltzing O, Reinmuth N et al. (2004). Neuropilin-1 in human colon cancer: expression, regulation, and role in induction of angiogenesis. *Am J Pathol* **164**: 2139–51.

Parkin DM (2001). Global cancer statistics in the year 2000. *Lancet Oncol* **2**: 533–43.

Parr C, Jiang WG (2003). Quantitative analysis of lymphangiogenic markers in human colorectal cancer. *Int J Oncol* **23**: 533–39.

Patan S, Munn LL, Jain RK (1996). Intussusceptive microvascular growth in a human colon adenocarcinoma xenograft: a novel mechanism of tumor angiogenesis. *Microvasc Res* **51**: 260–72.

Paweletz N, Knierim M. (1989). *Tumor Related Angiogenesis*. Academic Press: Orlando, FL, pp. 197–42.

Peeters CF, de Waal RM, Wobbes T, Westphal JR, Ruers TJ (2006). Outgrowth of human liver metastases after resection of the primary colorectal tumor: a shift in the balance between apoptosis and proliferation. *Int J Cancer* **119**: 1249–53.

Peters BA, Diaz LA, Polyak K, Meszler L, Romans K, Guinan EC et al. (2005). Contribution of bone marrow-derived endothelial cells to human tumor vasculature. *Nat Med* **11**: 261–62.

Petrova TV, Makinen T, Makela TP, Saarela J, Virtanen I, Ferrell RE et al. (2002). Lymphatic endothelial reprogramming of vascular endothelial cells by the Prox-1 homeobox transcription factor. *EMBO J* **21**: 4593–99.

Pettersson A, Nagy JA, Brown LF, Sundberg C, Morgan E, Jungles S et al. (2000). Heterogeneity of the angiogenic response induced in different normal adult tissues by vascular permeability factor/vascular endothelial growth factor. *Lab Invest* **80**: 99–115.

Pinedo HM, Verheul HM, D'Amato RJ, Folkman J (1998). Involvement of platelets in tumour angiogenesis? *Lancet* **352**: 1775–77.

Rafii S, Lyden D, Benezra R, Hattori K, Heissig B (2002). Vascular and haematopoietic stem cells: novel targets for anti-angiogenesis therapy? *Nat Rev Cancer* **2**: 826–35.

Rak J. (2009). *Ras oncogenes and tumour vascular interface. Cancer Genome and Tumor Microenvironment.* Springer: New York. pp. 133–65.

Rak J, Filmus J, Kerbel RS (1996). Reciprocal paracrine interactions between tumor cells and endothelial cells. The "angiogenesis progression" hypothesis. *Eur J Cancer* **32A**: 2438–50.

Rak JW, Hegmann EJ, Lu C, Kerbel RS (1994). Progressive loss of sensitivity to endothelium-derived growth inhibitors expressed by human melanoma cells during disease progression. *J Cell Physiol* **159**: 245–55.

Rak J, Kerbel RS (1996). Treating cancer by inhibiting angiogenesis: new hopes and potential pitfalls. *Cancer Metastasis Rev* **15**: 231–36.

Rak J, Kerbel RS (2003). Oncogenes and tumor angiogenesis. In: Rak J (ed.) *Oncogene-Directed Therapies*. Humana Press: Totowa, NJ, pp. 171–18.

Rak J, Milsom C, Yu J (2008). Tissue factor in cancer. *Curr Opin Hematol* **15**: 522–28.

Rak J, Mitsuhashi Y, Bayko L, Filmus J, Sasazuki T, Kerbel RS (1995). Mutant *ras* oncogenes upregulate VEGF/VPF expression: implications for induction and inhibition of tumor angiogenesis. *Cancer Res* **55**: 4575–80.

Rak J, Mitsuhashi Y, Sheehan C, Tamir A, Viloria-Petit A, Filmus J et al. (2000a). Oncogenes and tumor angiogenesis: differential modes of vascular endothelial growth factor up-regulation in ras-transformed epithelial cells and fibroblasts. *Cancer Res* **60**: 490–98.

Rak J, Yu JL (2004). Oncogenes and tumor angiogenesis: the question of vascular "supply" and vascular "demand". *Semin Cancer Biol* **14**: 93–104.

Rak JW, Yu JL, Kerbel RS, Coomber BL (2002). What do oncogenic mutations have to do with angiogenesis/vascular dependence of tumors. *Cancer Res* **62**: 1931–34.

Rak J, Yu JL, Klement G, Kerbel RS (2000b). Oncogenes and angiogenesis: signaling three-dimensional tumor growth. *J Investig Dermatol Symp Proc* **5**: 24–33.

Rak J, Yu JL, Luyendyk J, Mackman N (2006). Oncogenes, trousseau syndrome, and cancer-related changes in the coagulome of mice and humans. *Cancer Res* **66**: 10643–46.

Rasheed S, Harris AL, Tekkis PP, Turley H, Silver A, McDonald PJ et al. (2009). Hypoxia-inducible factor-1alpha and -2alpha are expressed in most rectal cancers but only hypoxia-inducible factor-1alpha is associated with prognosis. *Br J Cancer* **100**: 1666–73.

Rasheed S, McDonald PJ, Northover JM, Guenther T (2008). Angiogenesis and hypoxic factors in colorectal cancer. *Pathol Res Pract* **204**: 501–10.

Rastinejad F, Polverini PJ, Bouck N (1989). Regulation of the activity of a new inhibitor by angiogenesis by a cancer suppressor gene. *Cell* **56**: 345–55.

Ratajczak J, Wysoczynski M, Hayek F, Janowska-Wieczorek A, Ratajczak MZ (2006). Membrane-derived microvesicles: important and underappreciated mediators of cell-to-cell communication. *Leukemia* **20**: 1487–95.

Relf M, LeJeune S, Scott PA, Fox S, Smith K, Leek R et al. (1997). Expression of the angiogenic factors vascular endothelial cell growth factor, acidic and basic fibroblast growth factor, tumor growth factor beta-1, platelet-derived endothelial cell growth factor, placenta growth factor, and pleiotrophin in human primary breast cancer and its relation to angiogenesis. *Cancer Res* **57**: 963–69.

Reya T, Morrison SJ, Clarke MF, Weissman IL (2001). Stem cells, cancer, and cancer stem cells. *Nature* **414**: 105–11.

Reynolds LE, Wyder L, Lively JC, Taverna D, Robinson SD, Huang X et al. (2002). Enhanced pathological angiogenesis in mice lacking beta3 integrin or beta3 and beta5 integrins. *Nat Med* **8**: 27–34.

Rickles FR (2006). Mechanisms of cancer-induced thrombosis in cancer. *Pathophysiol Haemost Thromb* **35**: 103–10.

Rickles FR (2009). Cancer and thrombosis in women – molecular mechanisms. *Thromb Res* **123 Suppl 2**: S16–20.

Risau W (1997). Mechanisms of angiogenesis. *Nature* **386**: 671–74.

Rivoltini L, Gambacorti-Passerini C, Supino R, Parmiani G (1989). Generation and partial characterization of melanoma sublines resistant to lymphokine activated killer (LAK) cells. Relevance to doxorubicin resistance. *Int J Cancer* **43**: 880–85.

Rmali KA, Puntis MC, Jiang WG (2007). Tumour-associated angiogenesis in human colorectal cancer. *Colorectal Dis* **9**: 3–14.

Royston D, Jackson DG (2009). Mechanisms of lymphatic metastasis in human colorectal adenocarcinoma. *J Pathol* **217**: 608–19.

Ruf W (2007). Redundant signaling of tissue factor and thrombin in cancer progression? *J Thromb Haemost* **5**: 1584–87.

Schacht V, Ramirez MI, Hong YK, Hirakawa S, Feng D, Harvey N et al. (2003). T1alpha/ podoplanin deficiency disrupts normal lymphatic vasculature formation and causes lymphedema. *EMBO J* **22**: 3546–56.

Schoppmann SF, Fenzl A, Nagy K, Unger S, Bayer G, Geleff S et al. (2006). VEGF-C expressing tumor-associated macrophages in lymph node positive breast cancer: impact on lymphangiogenesis and survival. *Surgery* **139**: 839–46.

Seaman S, Stevens J, Yang MY, Logsdon D, Graff-Cherry C, St CB (2007). Genes that distinguish physiological and pathological angiogenesis. *Cancer Cell* **11**: 539–54.

Semenza GL (2003). Targeting HIF-1 for cancer therapy. *Nat Rev Cancer* **3**: 721–32.

Sessa C, Guibal A, Del CG, Ruegg C (2008). Biomarkers of angiogenesis for the development of antiangiogenic therapies in oncology: tools or decorations? *Nat Clin Pract Oncol* **5**: 378–91.

Seto S, Onodera H, Kaido T, Yoshikawa A, Ishigami S, Arii S et al. (2000). Tissue factor expression in human colorectal carcinoma: correlation with hepatic metastasis and impact on prognosis. *Cancer* **88**: 295–301.

Shahrzad S, Quayle L, Stone C, Plumb C, Shirasawa S, Rak JW et al. (2005). Ischemia-induced K-ras mutations in human colorectal cancer cells: role of microenvironmental regulation of MSH2 expression. *Cancer Res* **65**: 8134–41.

Shahrzad S, Shirasawa S, Sasazuki T, Rak JW, Coomber BL (2008). Low-dose metronomic cyclophosphamide treatment mediates ischemia-dependent K-ras mutation in colorectal carcinoma xenografts. *Oncogene* **27**: 3729–38.

Shaked Y, Ciarrocchi A, Franco M, Lee CR, Man S, Cheung AM et al. (2006). Therapy-induced acute recruitment of circulating endothelial progenitor cells to tumors. *Science* **313**: 1785–87.

Shantsila E, Watson T, Lip GY (2007). Endothelial progenitor cells in cardiovascular disorders. *J Am Coll Cardiol* **49**: 741–52.

Shibuya M (2006). Differential roles of vascular endothelial growth factor receptor-1 and receptor-2 in angiogenesis. *J Biochem Mol Biol* **39**: 469–78.

Shigemori C, Wada H, Matsumoto K, Shiku H, Nakamura S, Suzuki H (1998). Tissue factor expression and metastatic potential of colorectal cancer. *Thromb Haemost* **80**: 894–98.

Shojaei F, Ferrara N (2008). Refractoriness to antivascular endothelial growth factor treatment: role of myeloid cells. *Cancer Res* **68**: 5501–4.

Shojaei F, Singh M, Thompson JD, Ferrara N (2008). Role of Bv8 in neutrophil-dependent angiogenesis in a transgenic model of cancer progression. *Proc Natl Acad Sci USA* **105**: 2640–45.

Shweiki D, Itin A, Soffer D, Keshet E (1992). Vascular endothelial growth factor induced by hypoxia may mediate hypoxia-initated angiogenesis. *Nature* **359**: 843–45.

Silva R, D'Amico G, Hodivala-Dilke KM, Reynolds LE (2008). Integrins: the keys to unlocking angiogenesis. *Arterioscler Thromb Vasc Biol* **28**: 1703–13.

Skobe M, Hawighorst T, Jackson DG, Prevo R, Janes L, Velasco P et al. (2001). Induction of tumor lymphangiogenesis by VEGF-C promotes breast cancer metastasis. *Nat Med* **7**: 192–98.

Skobe M, Rockwell P, Goldstein N, Vosseler S, Fusenig NE (1997). Halting angiogenesis suppresses carcinoma cell invasion. *Nature Med* **3**: 1222–27.

Skog J, Wurdinger T, van RS, Meijer DH, Gainche L, Curry WT Jr et al. (2008). Glioblastoma microvesicles transport RNA and proteins that promote tumour growth and provide diagnostic biomarkers. *Nat Cell Biol* **10**: 1470–76.

Soker S, Takashima S, Miao HQ, Neufeld G, Klagsbrun M (1998). Neuropilin-1 is expressed by endothelial and tumor cells as an isoform- specific receptor for vascular endothelial growth factor. *Cell* **92**: 735–45.

Soumaoro LT, Uetake H, Takagi Y, Iida S, Higuchi T, Yasuno M et al. (2006). Coexpression of VEGF-C and Cox-2 in human colorectal cancer and its association with lymph node metastasis. *Dis Colon Rectum* **49**: 392–98.

Sparmann A, Bar-Sagi D (2004). Ras-induced interleukin-8 expression plays a critical role in tumor growth and angiogenesis. *Cancer Cell* **6**: 447–58.

Stacker SA, Achen MG (2008). From anti-angiogenesis to anti-lymphangiogenesis: emerging trends in cancer therapy. *Lymphat Res Biol* **6**: 165–72.

Stacker SA, Caesar C, Baldwin ME, Thornton GE, Williams RA, Prevo R et al. (2001). VEGF-D promotes the metastatic spread of tumor cells via the lymphatics. *Nat Med* **7**: 186–91.

Stalmans I, Ng YS, Rohan R, Fruttiger M, Bouche A, Yuce A et al. (2002). Arteriolar and venular patterning in retinas of mice selectively expressing VEGF isoforms. *J Clin Invest* **109**: 327–36.

Staton CA, Chetwood AS, Cameron IC, Cross SS, Brown NJ, Reed MW (2007). The angiogenic switch occurs at the adenoma stage of the adenoma carcinoma sequence in colorectal cancer. *Gut* **56**: 1426–32.

St. Croix B, Rago C, Velculescu V, Traverso G, Romans KE, Montgomery E et al. (2000). Genes expressed in human tumor endothelium. *Science* **289**: 1197–202.

Stockmann C, Doedens A, Weidemann A, Zhang N, Takeda N, Greenberg JI et al. (2008). Deletion of vascular endothelial growth factor in myeloid cells accelerates tumorigenesis. *Nature* **456**: 814–18.

Sundlisaeter E, Dicko A, Sakariassen PO, Sondenaa K, Enger PO, Bjerkvig R (2007). Lymphangiogenesis in colorectal cancer–prognostic and therapeutic aspects. *Int J Cancer* **121**: 1401–9.

Swift MR, Weinstein BM (2009). Arterial-venous specification during development. *Circ Res* **104**: 576–88.

Takahashi Y, Bucana CD, Liu W, Yoneda J, Kitadai Y, Cleary KR et al. (1996). Platelet-derived endothelial cell growth factor in human colon cancer angiogenesis: role of infiltrating cells. *J Natl Cancer Inst* **88**: 1146–51.

Takahashi Y, Kitadai Y, Bucana CD, Cleary KR, Ellis LM (1995). Expression of vascular endothelial growth factor and its receptor, KDR, correlates with vascularity, metastasis, and proliferation of human colon cancer. *Cancer Res* **55**: 3964–68.

Tammela T, Zarkada G, Wallgard E, Murtomaki A, Suchting S, Wirzenius M et al. (2008). Blocking VEGFR-3 suppresses angiogenic sprouting and vascular network formation. *Nature* **454**: 656–60.

Tang N, Wang L, Esko J, Giordano FJ, Huang Y, Gerber HP et al. (2004). Loss of HIF-1alpha in endothelial cells disrupts a hypoxia-driven VEGF autocrine loop necessary for tumorigenesis. *Cancer Cell* **6**: 485–95.

Taraboletti G, D'Ascenzo S, Giusti I, Marchetti D, Borsotti P, Millimaggi D et al. (2006). Bioavailability of VEGF in tumor-shed vesicles depends on vesicle burst induced by acidic pH. *Neoplasia* **8**: 96–103.

Teicher BA, Sotomayor EA, Huang ZD (1992). Antiangiogenic agents potentiate cytotoxic cancer therapies against primary and metastatic disease. *Cancer Res* **52**: 6702–4.

Teodoro JG, Parker AE, Zhu X, Green MR (2006). p53-mediated inhibition of angiogenesis through up-regulation of a collagen prolyl hydroxylase. *Science* **313**: 968–71.

Thurston G, Noguera-Troise I, Yancopoulos GD (2007). The Delta paradox: DLL4 blockade leads to more tumour vessels but less tumour growth. *Nat Rev Cancer* **7**: 327–31.

Tischer E, Mitchell R, Hartman T, Silva M, Gospodarowicz D, Fiddes JC et al. (1991). The human gene for vascular endothelial growth factor. Multiple protein forms are encoded through alternative exon splicing. *J Biol Chem* **266**: 11947–54.

Tokunaga T, Nakamura M, Oshika Y, Abe Y, Ozeki Y, Fukushima Y et al. (1999). Thrombospondin 2 expression is correlated with inhibition of angiogenesis and metastasis of colon cancer. *Br J Cancer* **79**: 354–59.

Tokunaga T, Oshika Y, Abe Y, Ozeki Y, Sadahiro S, Kijima H et al. (1998). Vascular endothelial growth factor (VEGF) mRNA isoform expression pattern is correlated with liver metastasis and poor prognosis in colon cancer. *Br J Cancer* **77**: 998–1002.

Tomita T (2008). Immunocytochemical localization of lymphatic and venous vessels in colonic polyps and adenomas. *Dig Dis Sci* **53**: 1880–85.

Traxler P, Allegrini PR, Brandt R, Brueggen J, Cozens R, Fabbro D et al. (2004). AEE788: a dual family epidermal growth factor receptor/ErbB2 and vascular endothelial growth factor receptor tyrosine kinase inhibitor with antitumor and antiangiogenic activity. *Cancer Res* **64**: 4931–41.

Tsopanoglou NE, Maragoudakis ME (2004). Role of thrombin in angiogenesis and tumor progression. *Semin Thromb Hemost* **30**: 63–69.

Tsujii M, Kawano S, Tsuji S, Sawaoka H, Hori M, DuBois RN (1998). Cyclooxygenase regulates angiogenesis induced by colon cancer cells. *Cell* **93**: 705–16.

Underiner TL, Ruggeri B, Gingrich DE (2004). Development of vascular endothelial growth factor receptor (VEGFR) kinase inhibitors as anti-angiogenic agents in cancer therapy. *Curr Med Chem* **11**: 731–45.

Uyttendaele H, Marazzi G, Wu G, Yan Q, Sassoon D, Kitajewski J (1996). Notch4/int-3, a mammary proto-oncogene, is an endothelial cell-specific mammalian Notch gene. *Development* **122**: 2251–59.

Valenti R, Huber V, Iero M, Filipazzi P, Parmiani G, Rivoltini L (2007). Tumor-released microvesicles as vehicles of immunosuppression. *Cancer Res* **67**: 2912–15.

Varki A (2007). Trousseau's syndrome: multiple definitions and multiple mechanisms. *Blood* **110**: 1723–29.

Verheul HM, Pinedo HM (2007). Possible molecular mechanisms involved in the toxicity of angiogenesis inhibition. *Nat Rev Cancer* **7**: 475–85.

Versteeg HH, Schaffner F, Kerver M, Petersen HH, Ahamed J, Felding-Habermann B et al. (2008). Inhibition of tissue factor signaling suppresses tumor growth. *Blood* **111**: 190–99.

Viloria-Petit A, Miquerol L, Yu JL, Gertsenstein M, Sheehan C, May L et al. (2003). Contrasting effects of VEGF gene disruption in embryonic stem cell-derived versus oncogene-induced tumors. *EMBO J* **22**: 4091–102.

Viloria-Petit AM, Rak J, Hung M-C, Rockwell P, Goldstein N, Kerbel RS (1997). Neutralizing antibodies against EGF and ErbB-2/*neu* receptor tyrosine kinases down-regulate VEGF production by tumor cells in vitro and in vivo: angiogenic implications for signal transduction therapy of solid tumors. *Am J Pathol* **151**: 1523–30.

Vlahakis NE, Young BA, Atakilit A, Sheppard D (2005). The lymphangiogenic vascular endothelial growth factors VEGF-C and -D are ligands for the integrin alpha9beta1. *J Biol Chem* **280**: 4544–52.

Wang HU, Chen ZF, Anderson DJ (1998). Molecular distinction and angiogenic interaction between embryonic arteries and veins revealed by ephrin-B2 and its receptor Eph-B4. *Cell* **93**: 741–53.

Warren RS, Yuan H, Mati MR, Gillett NA, Ferrara N (1995). Regulation by vascular endothelial growth factor of human colon cancer tumorigenesis in a mouse model of experimental liver metastasis. *J Clin Invest* **95**: 1789–97.

Wigle JT, Harvey N, Detmar M, Lagutina I, Grosveld G, Gunn MD et al. (2002). An essential role for Prox1 in the induction of the lymphatic endothelial cell phenotype. *EMBO J* **21**: 1505–13.

Willett CG, Boucher Y, di Tomaso E, Duda DG, Munn LL, Tong RT et al. (2004). Direct evidence that the VEGF-specific antibody bevacizumab has antivascular effects in human rectal cancer. *Nat Med* **10**: 145–47.

Wolmark N, Yothers G, O'Connell J, Sharif S, Atkins JN, Seay TA, Fehrenbacher L, O'Reilly S, Allegra CJ (2009). A phase III trial comparing mFOLFOX6 to mFOLFOX6 plus bevacizumab in stage II or III carcinoma of the colon: results of NSABP protocol C-08. *J Clin Oncol* **27**: 18 s, Abstract, ASCO, LBA4.

Woolard J, Wang WY, Bevan HS, Qiu Y, Morbidelli L, Pritchard-Jones RO et al. (2004). VEGF165b, an inhibitory vascular endothelial growth factor splice variant: mechanism of action, in vivo effect on angiogenesis and endogenous protein expression. *Cancer Res* **64**: 7822–35.

Wu Y, Yakar S, Zhao L, Hennighausen L, LeRoith D (2002). Circulating insulin-like growth factor-I levels regulate colon cancer growth and metastasis. *Cancer Res* **62**: 1030–35.

Yamauchi T, Watanabe M, Hasegawa H, Nishibori H, Ishii Y, Tatematsu H et al. (2003). The potential for a selective cyclooxygenase-2 inhibitor in the prevention of liver metastasis in human colorectal cancer. *Anticancer Res* **23**: 245–49.

Yancopoulos GD, Davis S, Gale NW, Rudge JS, Wiegand SJ, Holash J (2000). Vascular-specific growth factors and blood vessel formation. *Nature* **407**: 242–48.

Yu JL, May L, Lhotak V, Shahrzad S, Shirasawa S, Weitz JI et al. (2005). Oncogenic events regulate tissue factor expression in colorectal cancer cells: implications for tumor progression and angiogenesis. *Blood* **105**: 1734–41.

Yu J, May L, Milsom C, Anderson GM, Weitz JI, Luyendyk JP et al. (2008). Contribution of host-derived tissue factor to tumor neovascularization. *Arterioscler Thromb Vasc Biol* **28**: 1975–81.

Yu JL, Rak JW (2003). Host microenvironment in breast cancer development: inflammatory and immune cells in tumour angiogenesis and arteriogenesis. *Breast Cancer Res* **5**: 83–88.

Yu JL, Rak JW (2004). Shedding of tissue factor (TF)-containing microparticles rather than alternatively spliced TF is the main source of TF activity released from human cancer cells. *J Thromb Haemost* **2**: 2065–67.

Yu JL, Rak JW, Carmeliet P, Nagy A, Kerbel RS, Coomber BL (2001). Heterogeneous vascular dependence of tumor cell populations. *Am J Pathol* **158**: 1325–34.

Yu JL, Rak JW, Coomber BL, Hicklin DJ, Kerbel RS (2002b). Effect of p53 status on tumor response to antiangiogenic therapy. *Science* **295**: 1526–28.

Yu J, Rak JW, Klement G, Kerbel RS (2002a). VEGF isoform expression as a determinant of blood vessel patterning in human melanoma xenografts. *Cancer Res* **62**: 1838–46.

Zerbib P, Grimonprez A, Corseaux D, Mouquet F, Nunes B, Petersen LC et al. (2009). Inhibition of tissue factor-factor VIIa proteolytic activity blunts hepatic metastasis in colorectal cancer. *J Surg Res* **153**: 239–45.

Zhang Y, Deng Y, Luther T, Muller M, Ziegler R, Waldherr R et al. (1994). Tissue factor controls the balance of angiogenic and antiangiogenic properties of tumor cells in mice. *J Clin Invest* **94**: 1320–27.

Zhao J, Aguilar G, Palencia S, Newton E, Abo A (2009). rNAPc2 inhibits colorectal cancer in mice through tissue factor. *Clin Cancer Res* **15**: 208–16.

Zhu L, Gibson P, Currle DS, Tong Y, Richardson RJ, Bayazitov IT et al. (2009). Prominin 1 marks intestinal stem cells that are susceptible to neoplastic transformation. *Nature* **457**: 603–7.

Zumsteg A, Christofori G (2009). Corrupt policemen: inflammatory cells promote tumor angiogenesis. *Curr Opin Oncol* **21**: 60–70.

van Beijnum JR, Griffioen AW (2005). In silico analysis of angiogenesis associated gene expression identifies angiogenic stage related profiles. *Biochim Biophys Acta* **1755**: 121–34.

Chapter 10
ROLE OF THE HOST INFLAMMATORY RESPONSE IN COLON CARCINOMA INITIATION, PROGRESSION AND LIVER METASTASIS

Pnina Brodt

Department of Surgery, Medicine and Oncology, McGill University and the McGill University Health Center, Royal Victoria Hospital, Montreal, QC, Canada, e-mail: pnina.brodt@mcgill.ca

Abstract: The host innate immune response can play a dual role in cancer progression. On one hand, it can mount an anti-tumourigenic host defense response that brings about the elimination of transformed/malignant cells. On the other hand, it can promote the initiation and progression of the malignant process through a network of chemokines and cytokines that facilitate tumour cell survival, migration and invasion, tumour–induced angiogenesis and metastasis. Here, I review a compelling body of evidence that implicates inflammation in the etiology, progression and metastasis of colon cancer. Experimental and clinical findings linking inflammatory bowel diseases such as ulcerative colitis to colon cancer development at one end of the process and data implicating inflammatory chemokines and cytokines in liver metastasis are reviewed. Conflicting evidence on the role of tumour infiltrating inflammatory cells in the progression of the primary tumours are discussed. Collectively, the data provide a strong rationale for the use of anti-inflammatory drugs not only for prevention of disease onset, but also for limiting liver metastasis.

Key words: Colon cancer · Inflammation · Liver metastasis · Cytokines · Chemokines

10.1 General Introduction

Cancers of the colon and rectum rank third in overall incidence in Canada behind lung and breast cancer (Boring et al., 1994). Up to 30% of the Western population is expected to develop some form of colorectal neoplasm, from a benign polyp to invasive adenocarcinoma, by the age of 70. As life expectancy increases, the problem is expected to become more prevalent. While 85% of colorectal carcinoma (CRC) patients can undergo potentially curative surgery, up to 50% of these will succumb to their disease within 5 years, mainly because of distant metastases to the liver (Cohen, 1989). At present, surgical resection is the only curative option for hepatic metastases; however, only 25–30% of liver resection patients survive 5 years disease-free (Cohen, 1989). While improvements in surgical techniques and a more aggressive approach to resection of CRC liver metastases have expanded the options for this subset of patients, most patients with liver metastases still die of their disease. Clinical variables such as number of metastases, size of metastases and unilobar versus bilobar disease are of significance in predicting the outcome of liver resection (Wei et al., 2006). However, more sophisticated and patient-specific markers are needed in order to improve selection and management of patients with liver metastases. The identification and validation of these markers depends, in turn, on a better understanding of the biology of CRC progression and liver metastasis, particularly the early stages of the process that determine tumour cell arrest, extravasation and survival in the hepatic microenvironment. Here, the contribution of the host response to CRC progression and liver metastases is reviewed with a focus on the role of inflammation during the various stages of the disease.

10.2 Role of Inflammation in Cancer Progression: Focus on CRC

The tumour microenvironment plays an important role in tumour development and progression both at the primary site and at sites of metastasis. The microenvironment consists of the tumour-associated stroma that includes resident fibroblasts, adipocytes and blood and lymph vessel-lining endothelial cells and their respective extracellular matrix (ECM) proteins, as well as resident or infiltrating host inflammatory and immune cells. The malignant cells can communicate with this dynamically changing microenvironment through the release of, and response to, soluble mediators such as growth factors and cytokines. The tumour cells also interact through cell-cell and cell-matrix adhesion, mediated by receptors and counter-receptors that can themselves evolve as the tumour progresses. This inter-cellular communication also entails the release of proteolytic enzymes by tumour or host inflammatory cells that remodel tissue barriers around the expanding tumours and contribute to neo-vascularization and tumour migration and invasion (Bissell et al., 2005; Coussens and Werb, 2002; Robinson and Coussens, 2005; Witz and Levy-Nissenbaum, 2006). It has become clear in recent years that inflammatory cells and the various soluble mediators that they elaborate play a central role in cancer progression, by sustaining an inflammatory environment prior to tumour development that, in turn, promotes the appearance of malignant cells or by providing a fertile ground for tumour expansion once malignant cells emerge. Inflammation can promote tumour development and progression through various mechanisms including a direct effect on tumour cell proliferation and survival mediated through the release of growth enhancing cytokines, by contributing to the processes of angiogenesis and metastasis through recruitment of endothelial cells and their progenitors, through the release of chemokines that promote tumour cell motility and by downregulating the activity of tumour-suppressive host immune cells. In addition, the host inflammatory response can also alter tumour cell responses to treatment with agents such as hormones and chemotherapeutic drugs (reviewed in (Germano et al., 2008; Mantovani et al., 2008)).

There is a large and compelling body of literature that implicates the host inflammatory response in the development and spread of colon carcinoma (Ahmadi et al., 2009; Feagins et al., 2009; Johnson and Lund, 2007; Klampfer, 2008; Rhodes and Campbell, 2002). Recent clinical evidence points to a strong causative link between Inflammatory Bowel Diseases (IBD) – a group of chronic inflammatory disorders of the gastrointestinal tract that includes Crohn's disease (CD) and ulcerative colitis (UC) and the early stages of colon cancer. For example, patients with ulcerative colitis and Crohn's disease are at a five-fold higher risk of developing colon cancer than the general population (Rhodes and Campbell, 2002). In fact, the regular use of the anti-inflammatory 5-aminosalicylates was shown to reduce the incidence of colon cancer amongst patients with ulcerative colitis (Eaden et al., 2000) and a recent randomized controlled trial demonstrated that aspirin was effective in preventing sporadic adenomas (Baron et al., 2003). While a background of inflammation could promote colonic neoplasia, there is also evidence that the neoplastic epithelium can, in turn, elaborate soluble factors into the immediate microenvironment that modify the stroma and could induce or sustain an inflammatory response (Mantovani et al., 2008).

Macrophages are the major effector cells of the host innate immune response. These cells are released from the bone marrow as immature monocytes and undergo terminal differentiation in their tissues of residence (e.g. Kupffer cells in the liver). There, they provide the first line of defense against invading pathogens and participate in tissue remodelling and repair. Mucosal macrophages and their cytokines play an important role in the development of IBDs. An increase in the number of newly recruited monocytes and activated macrophages has been noted in the inflamed gut of IBD patients. These activated macrophages are a major source of inflammatory cytokines in the gut, and the imbalance of cytokines in the gut can contribute to, and exacerbate IBD pathogenesis, among others by regulating the differentiation and function of infiltrating T cells. Among the cytokines that have been implicated in the development and maintenance of IBD and the progression to colon cancer are macrophage-derived tumor necrosis factor (TNF-α), interleukin (IL-1) and IL-6 [(Yang et al., 1997; Zhao et al., 2001; Rose-John et al., 2007) and reviewed in Rhodes and Campbell, 2002]. A recent study using a mouse model of induced ulcerative colitis has shown that mice lacking the TNF receptor TNFR1 had reduced infiltration of macrophages and neutrophils, decreased mucosal damage and reduced tumour incidence relative to wild-type controls. When wild-type mice were transplanted with bone marrow from TNFR1-deficient mice, they developed significantly fewer tumours. These data identified TNF-α/TNFR interactions as essential for the initiation and progression of colitis-associated colon cancer (Popivanova,

2008) and provided additional support for targeting TNF-α and other cytokines as a strategy for inhibiting colon cancer (Wilson, 2008).

10.2.1 Role of Tumour-Infiltrating Macrophages in Tumour Progression and in CRC

In response to a growing tumour, the resident macrophages can be rapidly activated and additional monocytes can be recruited from the bone marrow in response to chemotactic factors (Yang et al., 1997). These macrophages infiltrate the tumour site and become part of the tumour microenvironment. Once at the tumour site, however, macrophages can play diverse and even opposing roles in tumour development. Activated macrophages can limit tumour growth through the release of tumouricidal and apoptotic factors such as TNF-α and nitric oxide (Bingle et al., 2002), and by recruiting T lymphocytes and NK cells through the release of cytokines such as IL-12 and IL-18 (Bingle et al., 2002). In contrast to these host protective effects, macrophages can promote tumour progression and metastasis by contributing to ECM remodeling, tumour invasion, neo-vascularization and growth through the release of ECM-degrading proteinases (e.g. matrix metalloproteinase MMP-9), angiogenic factors (e.g. vascular endothelial growth factor (VEGF)) and growth promoting factors such as colony stimulating factor (CSF-1), insulin-related growth factor (IGF-I) and epidermal growth factor (EGF) (Bingle et al., 2002; Condeelis and Pollard, 2006; Wynes et al., 2004; Wynes and Riches, 2003). Macrophages are versatile cells with an inherent plasticity that allows them to respond to diverse environmental stimuli by activating distinct molecular/functional programs. They have been shown to differentiate into two main subtypes, classified as M1 and M2. M1 macrophages are activated by microbial stimuli (e.g. lipopolysaccharide (LPS)) and interferon gamma (INFγ) whereas anti-inflammatory molecules such as IL-4, IL-13 and IL-10 induce a distinct activation program leading to acquisition of an M2 phenotype. While M1 macrophages engage mainly in classical macrophage functions such as killing microorganisms and producing reactive oxygen and nitrogen species, M2 macrophages, characterized by their IL-12^{low}/IL-10^{high} phenotype, can fine-tune the inflammatory response, induce an adaptive immune response, produce growth factors and promote angiogenesis and tissue remodeling and repair. Tumour-associated macrophages (TAMs) are generally of the M2 subset, but recent studies have shown that they may represent a uniquely 'educated' subtype of the M2 macrophages (Biswas et al., 2006; Mantovani et al., 2005; Mantovani et al., 2004; Sica et al., 2006). Using functionalized nanoparticle-based imaging techniques, these cells were recently shown to cluster in discrete foci within tumours and extend cytoplasmic protrusions that can facilitate physical interactions with neighboring tumour cells (Leimgruber et al., 2009). The recruitment of macrophages into the tumour site and/or their activation is mediated through a complex network of chemotactic cytokines (chemokines) that can determine both the type and magnitude of the leukocyte infiltrate (Balkwill, 2004). Among the chemokines implicated in the recruitment and activation of macrophages into tumour sites are monocyte chemotactic protein (MCP)-1/(CCL-2), macrophage colony stimulating factor (CSF-1), VEGF and CXCL8 (IL-8) (Bingle et al., 2002). MCP-1 production has been observed in colon carcinomas, and its expression levels within the tumour tissue, in the stroma, or in the serum, have been shown to correlate with tumour progression (Baier et al., 2005; Bailey et al., 2007; Bingle et al., 2002; Dehqanzada et al., 2006; Ueno et al., 2002). VEGF is a potent pro-angiogenic cytokine that is produced by tumour cells, as well as by infiltrating leukocytes such as macrophages and T cells (Bingle et al., 2002; Leek et al., 2000). The macrophage inflammatory proteins MIP-1α (CCL3) and MIP-1β (CCL4) have also been identified in various malignancies including colon and hepatocellular carcinomas and their expression correlated with invasiveness and metastasis. These factors can induce angiogenesis and tumour motility, recruit immune NK and T cells into the tumours, regulate the release of macrophage inflammatory cytokine and regulate the tumouricidal potential of resident and recruited macrophages (Baier et al., 2005; Muller et al., 2001; Nath et al., 2006; Wolf et al., 2003; Yang et al., 2005; Zlotnik, 2004).

Clinical and experimental studies have collectively shown that colon carcinomas are infiltrated with macrophages (Bacman et al., 2007) and the number of TAMs was shown to increase with tumour volume (Higgins et al., 1996). The recruitment of macrophages into the tumour stroma appears to be mediated by monocyte/macrophage chemokines CCL4 and CCL5 because a recent study has shown that these chemokines predominate among the chemokines highly upregulated in the microenvironment of colon cancer (Erreni et al., 2009).

However, the ultimate effect of these TAMs on disease progression and outcome may be complex and multi-factorial. Clinical studies suggest that their presence is inhibitory to tumour progression. For example, immunohistochemistry performed on colon cancer tissue microarrays showed increased numbers of macrophages at the tumour site relative to the normal mucosa, but the numbers decreased in higher stage tumours, suggesting that while macrophages were initially attracted to the tumour site, this attraction actually decreased with tumour progression (Sickert et al., 2005). Moreover, a recent analysis of 446 colorectal cancer specimens by immunohistochemistry using antibodies to the monocyte/macrophage marker CD68 revealed that a dense macrophage infiltration at the tumour front was a favourable prognostic factor, suggesting that the TAMs exerted anti-tumourigenic effects. This study also suggested that tumour cell-macrophage contact was important for this effect (Forssell et al., 2007). Similar conclusions were obtained in another study where TAM infiltration into the tumours was quantified by immunohistochemistry. This study concluded that the 5-year survival rate was significantly poorer in patients with lower numbers relative to those with a high TAM count (Tan et al., 2005). Similarly, an analysis of vessel density and TAMs in colon cancer specimens concluded that low TAM numbers (as measured using anti-CD68 antibodies) and high numbers of microvessels were associated with an unfavourable prognosis (Lackner et al., 2004). Intriguingly, a similar analysis of 131 stage II and III colon cancer specimens revealed that, while TAM infiltration alone was not significantly associated with outcome, the presence of CD68$^+$/VEGF$^+$ but not CD68$^+$/VEGF$^-$ TAM in the tumour stroma was predictive of improved survival, suggesting that different macrophage subtypes may influence tumour progression differently. Taken together, these clinical data are consistent with the conclusion that TAM infiltration provides a line of defense against proliferating tumour cells rather than promotes tumour progression.

This conclusion is at variance with some experimental studies using human or murine tumour cell lines. For example in a recent study, Jedinak et al. have shown that conditioned medium harvested from activated macrophages induced proliferation, migration and VEGF production in human colon cancer cells. These effects were attributed to TNF-α, IL-1β and IL-6 present in the conditioned medium (Jedinak et al., 2010). Similarly, Li et al. have shown that macrophage-derived IL-6 can stimulate IL-6 production in colon cancer cells. This study also demonstrated co-localization of macrophages and IL-6 in 126 colon cancer specimens analyzed. Increased IL-6 production was accompanied by the activation of STAT-3, a tumour survival factor (Li et al., 2009). A study by Zins et al. using human SW620 colon cancer cells revealed that colon cancer cell-derived TNF-α induced TNF-α and CSF-1 production in co-cultured murine macrophages, and this led to increased VEGF-A and MMP-2 production in the macrophages, identifying a potential tumour – promoting cross-talk between the tumour cells and macrophages. Moreover, selective depletion of peritoneal or liver macrophages prior to injection of rat colon cancer cells resulted in more differentiated tumours, implicating macrophages in the acquisition of a more malignant phenotype. Interestingly, however, in the same study the macrophage-depleted rats bearing highly differentiated tumours, had a worse prognosis, as they displayed a higher tumour burden and poorer survival (Oosterling et al., 2005).

This apparent contradiction between the clinical findings and results of experimental studies may be due, at least in part, to the involvement of other arms of the innate and adaptive immune response in vivo during colon cancer growth. Namely, during the clinical course of the disease, TAMs may contribute to a tumour-inhibitory response through the recruitment over time of cytotoxic T-cells and NK cells, a process that is absent in some of the animal models or in vitro systems analyzed. It should also be noted that in addition to TAMs, other bone-marrow (BM)-derived cells also contribute to colon carcinogenesis. For example, Taketo recently reported that in colon adenomas that develop in the *cis-Apc/Smad4* mouse model, immature $CD34^+/CD31^-$ BM-derived myeloid cells that produce MMP-2 and MMP-9 are recruited into the growing polyps by the epithelially-derived chemokine CCL9 and these cells contribute to the acquisition of a malignant/invasive phenotype (Taketo, 2009). Readers are encouraged to consult Chapter 5 by A. Kreso et al., in this book for more information on this issue.

10.2.2 Review of Macrophage-Derived Cytokines that Play a Role in CRC and Liver Metastasis

As discussed above, macrophages can mediate their pleiotropic effects through the release of various cytokines. Among the cytokines implicated in colon cancer tumourigenesis and metastasis, IL-1, IL-6, TNF-α and IL-23 play a major role. Brief overviews of the biology, signaling mechanisms and functions of these cytokines are therefore provided here as the background to a more detailed discussion of their role in colon cancer progression and metastasis later in the chapter.

10.2.2.1 Role of IL-6

IL-6 belongs to a family of cytokines with overlapping activities that signal through receptor complexes containing the signal-transducing protein gp130 (Taga and Kishimoto, 1997). It is produced by different cell types including lymphocytes, macrophages and epithelial cells and can play diverse roles both as a regulator of the acute inflammatory response and the transition between innate and acquired immunity. It is also a survival and growth-promoting factor for hematopoietic and epithelial cells.

Two modes of signalling have been identified for IL-6. Classical IL-6 signalling involves binding of this cytokine to its cellular receptor IL-6Rα (CD126), an event that triggers the recruitment of gp130 (CD130) into the complex and results in Janus kinase (JAK) activation and the phosphorylation of transcription factors of the signal transducer and activator of transcription (STAT) family, particularly STAT3. Once phosporylated, STAT3 dimerizes and translocates to the nucleus where it binds to DNA and activates transcription of different genes including oncogenes (e.g. c-*Myc*), cell survival genes (e.g. *Bcl-x*), caspases and cell cycle regulators such as p21 and CyclinD1 (Hirano et al., 2000). An alternative signalling mechanism (trans-signalling) does not require the participation of a membrane anchored IL-6Rα, but involves a soluble form of this receptor (sIL-6R) that is produced either through alternative splicing or through proteolytic cleavage of the membrane protein by metalloproteinases. This soluble form of the receptor is shed by the cells and binds IL-6 extra-cellularly. The complex can then activate gp130 to initiate signalling even in the absence of the membrane bound IL-6 receptor. The majority of cells in the body express gp130, but IL-6Rα is expressed mainly on hematopoietic cells (i.e. lymphocytes, neutrophils and macrophages) and hepatocytes. Hence, trans-signalling increases the number of cell types that can be stimulated by IL-6 and broadens the scope of IL-6 activities.

The involvement of IL-6 in the etiology and progression of IBD has been confirmed by numerous studies. In IBD patients, circulating as well as intestinal IL-6 and sIL-6R levels are increased and the levels were shown to correlate with disease severity. Their expression levels also increase in patients with active disease. In addition, mucosal T cells of IBD patients, a large proportion of which express gp130, but not the IL-6R were shown to be highly resistant to apoptosis, implicating T-cell-mediated IL-6 trans-signalling in the etiology and maintenance of IBD (Mitsuyama et al., 2006). Support for the causative role of IL-6 in IBD also comes from mouse models of dextran sulfate sodium-induced colitis. In IL-6-deficient mice, only limited disease was observed (Suzuki et al., 2001) and this was more recently extended to a colitis-induced cancer model (Grivennikov et al., 2009). In addition, anti-IL-6R antibodies can attenuate the disease in a mouse model of Th1 cell-mediated colitis (Yamamoto et al., 2000).

10.2.2.2 Role of TNF-α and the TNF Receptors

Another factor that plays a major role in colitis-induced colon cancer and in the progression and metastasis of the disease is tumour necrosis factor (TNF)-α (Wilson, 2008). TNF-α is a pleiotropic pro-inflammatory cytokine, the prototype and best studied of a superfamily of 19 related pro-inflammatory, type II transmembrane proteins that bind to a total of 29 cell surface receptors. First described by Carswell et al. in 1975 as a macrophage-derived, endotoxin-induced serum factor that causes murine tumour necrosis in vivo (Carswell et al., 1975), it has since become clear that this cytokine can have multiple and diametrically opposing effects on tumour cell survival and malignant progression. While at high concentrations, it can cause hemorrhagic necrosis, induce apoptosis and stimulate anti-tumour immunity, it can also have positive effects on tumour initiation and progression (Balkwill, 2002). For example, $TNFalpha^{-/-}$ mice were resistant to skin carcinogenesis (Arnott et al., 2004; Moore et al., 1999) and $TNFR1^{-/-}$ mice were resistant to both chemical carcinogenesis (Knight et al., 2000) and the growth of colon cancer metastases in the liver (Kitakata et al., 2002). Clinical data support the critical role of TNF-α in tumour progression in general, and colon carcinoma in particular. TNF-α expression was associated with poor prognosis in various malignancies (Balkwill et al., 2005), although the molecular mechanisms underlying this tumour-promoting effect are not always fully understood (Galban et al., 2003; Lewis and Pollard, 2006).

The human TNF-α is synthesized as a plasma membrane 26-kDa pro-protein that is processed by matrix metalloproteinases to release the mature, soluble 17-kDa protein. While both the cell-associated and secreted forms are biologically active, they may have distinct biological effects (reviewed in Palladino et al., 2003). TNF-α is produced by various cells of the innate and acquired immune response including neutrophils, macrophages, T and B lymphocytes, NK cells as well as by non-immune cells such as stromal fibroblasts and various cancer cells. It mediates host responses in acute and chronic inflammatory conditions and can provide protection from infection and malignancy. TNF-α is biologically active as a self-assembling, non-covalently-associated trimer that can bind to two cell surface receptors to mediate its diverse biological activities; the p55/p60 TNFR1 and the p75/p80 TNFR2. These receptors are part of a superfamily of type I transmembrane proteins characterized by cysteine-rich domains that form intra-chain disulphide bonds through highly conserved cysteine residues. The binding of the trimeric TNF-α to TNFRI triggers the release of the silencer of death domain (SODD) and recruitment of the adaptor TNFR-associated death domain (TRADD). TRADD recruitment can serve as a platform to assemble alternative signalling complexes leading on one hand to the activation of the transcription factors NFκB and JNK. On the other hand, it directs the recruitment of Fas-associated death domain-containing protein (FADD) and caspase-8 that results in TNF-induced apoptosis. Activation of NFκB and JNK induces the expression of diverse molecules that are collectively responsible for the pleiotropic effects of TNF-α (Chen and Goeddel, 2002; Hehlgans and Pfeffer, 2005; Locksley et al., 2001). Nuclear factor kappa-light-chain-enhancer of activated B cells (NFκB), the major conveyer of TNFR-induced survival signals mediates this effect by inducing the expression of several anti-apoptotic proteins including caspase inhibitor of apoptosis proteins (cIAPs), caspase 8 homologue FLICE-inhibitory protein (c-FLIP), A1, A20, TNF receptor-associated factor-2 (TRAF2), and B-cell lymphoma-extra large protein (Bcl-x_L) which block the activity of either death receptors or the mitochondrial pathway (Karin and Lin, 2002). Other NFκB-regulated genes encode TNF-α itself, IL-1, IL-6, and CXCL8 (IL-8) cytokines that have been implicated in tumour initiation and progression in humans and mice (Luo et al., 2005). Recently, it was suggested that NFκB also functions by attenuating TNF-α-induced JNK activation (De Smaele et al., 2001; Tang et al., 2001). This ability to recruit multiple signalling complexes is the basis for the duality in the biological effects of TNF-α namely, its ability to induce cell death in some conditions but act as a survival factor in others.

The relative roles of TNFR1 and TNFR2 in mediating TNF-α-induced cellular responses are not fully understood. It has been suggested that TNFR1 is activated by soluble ligand while TNFR2 binds primarily transmembrane TNF. The TNF receptors can also be shed and act as soluble TNF-binding proteins (decoys), thereby competing with cell surface receptors for free ligand and reducing TNF bioavailability and bioactivity. The transmembrane TNF can also bind to the soluble TNF receptors and generate reverse signalling (Hehlgans and Pfeffer, 2005). In contrast to TNFR1, TNFR2 lacks a death domain and its role in apoptosis is therefore likely limited. Its expression can be induced by cytokines such as TNF-α and IL-1. Recent evidence suggests that one of its functions may be to modulate and enhance the activities of TNFR1 on immune and endothelial cells (Chan et al., 2003; Leeuwenberg et al., 1995; Moynagh, 2005; Weiss et al., 1997). TNFR2 can also cooperate with other receptor systems and was shown to regulate extracellular matrix remodelling and cell growth in concert with the IGF-1 receptor (Theiss et al., 2005). The relative importance of the two TNF receptors in intracellular signalling may be cell- and tissue-specific. TNFR1 is widely expressed on most mammalian cells while the expression of TNFR2 appears to be more tissue- and cell-restricted and it is expressed primarily on hematopoietic cells (Marino and Cardier, 2003; Mukhopadhyay et al., 2001).

10.2.2.3 Role of IL-1

The IL-1 family of ligands comprises 11 members, of which the prototypical IL-1α and IL-1β as well as the IL-1 receptor antagonist (IL-1Ra) are the most extensively studied (Arend et al., 2008; Dinarello, 1996; Dinarello, 2009b). IL-1α and IL-1β are synthesized by many cells including monocytes, resident macrophages, neutrophils and hepatocytes. Both ligands lack signal peptides and require enzymatic processing to be secreted. The pro-IL-1α is synthesized as a 31 kDa precursor that is biologically active. Although it may be cleaved by the cysteine protease calpain to release the mature 17 kDa protein, cleavage is not essential for IL-1α activity and the bulk of IL-1α remains bound to the plasma membrane or is intracellular. IL-1β is also synthesized as a 31-kDa molecule but it is active only as a processed, mature 17 kDa peptide that is released from cells. IL-1β processing is catalyzed by the IL-1β-converting enzyme (ICE) or caspase-1. The IL-1 receptor has two forms. IL-1RI has a long cytoplasmic tail and can activate signalling. IL-1RII has only a short intracellular domain and is biologically inert. However, IL-1RII may act as a decoy receptor to compete for ligand binding with IL-1RI on the cell membrane or in a secreted form extracellularly, thereby reducing IL-1 bioavailability and attenuating its activity. Following ligand binding, the receptor recruits the interacting protein IL-1RAcP and this complex can recruit several adaptor proteins including myeloid differentiation factor 88 (MyD88), IL-1R-associated kinase (IRAK) and tumour necrosis factor receptor-associated factor 6 (TRAF6) to initiate downstream signalling. This leads to activation of NFκB, JNK and the p38 MAPK. The activities of IL-1α and IL-1β can be antagonized by IL-1Ra, a third ligand, closely related structurally to the other IL-1 ligands. IL-1Ra cannot interact with IL-1RAcP, but can bind to the receptors and thereby inhibits IL-1 binding. This system of ligands, receptors and natural inhibitors for both ensures that under normal physiological conditions, the biological activity of this potent pro-inflammatory system is tightly controlled (Arend et al., 2008).

IL-1β contributes to inflammation in various ways. It can induce gene expression and synthesis of cyclooxygenase type 2 (COX-2) and inducible nitric oxide synthase (iNOS), thereby increasing the production of prostaglandin-E2 (PGE2) and nitric oxide (NO), two major mediators of inflammation in IBD that also play a role in liver metastasis (see below). In addition, IL-1β can induce expression of adhesion molecules such as intercellular adhesion molecule-1 (ICAM-1) on mesenchymal cells and vascular cell adhesion molecule-1 (VCAM-1) on endothelial cells (see Chapter 7, in this book, for complementary reading). In addition, IL-1β stimulates chemokine production and triggers the infiltration of inflammatory and immunocompetent cells from the circulation into extravascular spaces and tissues (reviewed in (Dinarello, 2009a)). IL-1β is also a pro-angiogenic factor (Ueno et al., 2002) and plays a role in blood vessel formation and metastasis.

Tumour cells engineered to express IL-1α were shown to induce anti-tumour immunity and have a reduced tumourigenicity, while tumour cells expressing IL-1β had increased invasiveness and tumour-associated angiogenesis. IL-1β also induces immune suppression in the host (Song et al., 2003). Moreover, IL-1β-, but not IL-1α-deficient mice do not develop tumours upon tumour cell implantations, and this could be attributed to a failure to induce angiogenesis (Voronov et al., 2003). It is also of relevance to note that IL-1β regulates IL-6 production (Dinarello, 2009a) and can thereby indirectly activate the JAK/STAT signalling pathways.

IL-18, another member of the larger IL-1 family, has also been implicated in malignancy (as will also be discussed below). Similarly to IL-1β, it is synthesized as a biologically inactive (23 kDa) precursor that is also cleaved by caspase-1 (Palladino et al., 2003). It is expressed in a variety of immune cells including macrophages, dendritic cells and Kupffer cells as well as in non-immune cells such as keratinocytes, chondrocytes, synovial fibroblasts and osteoblasts. Unlike IL-1β, inflammatory stimuli do not impact on IL-18 precursor production and its biological activity is regulated through processing of the pool of precursors by caspase-1. The IL-18 receptor forms a complex that is structurally and functionally similar to the

IL-1R receptor complex. IL-18 binds to IL-18Ra and this recruits IL-18Rb to form a high-affinity heterotrimeric complex that recruits MyD88, IRAK, and TRAF6, resulting in similar responses to those engendered by IL-1. The receptor is expressed on immune and non-immune cells including T cells, NK cells, macrophages, B cells, neutrophils, basophils and mast cells as well as on endothelial cells, smooth muscle cells, synovial fibroblasts, chondrocytes, and epithelial cells. Expression of the IL-18R complex, in particular of IL-18Rb, is modulated by various cytokines (reviewed in (Arend et al., 2008)).

10.2.2.4 Role of IL-23

IL-23 is a pro-inflammatory cytokine closely related to IL-12, but with distinct effects on local inflammatory responses, on the tumour microenvironment and on intra-tumoural lymphocytic infiltration. Both cytokines share a common p40 subunit that is covalently linked to a p35 subunit (IL-12) or a p19 subunit (IL-23) (Oppmann et al., 2000). IL-23 is produced by activated M1 macrophages and dendritic cells and has been implicated in several chronic inflammatory conditions, including IBD. In the inflammatory microenvironment, this cytokine can have several pro-tumourigenic effects including the upregulation of the matrix metalloproteinase MMP-9, increased angiogenesis and inhibition of cytotoxic $CD8^+$ T-cell infiltration that provides protection from T-cell mediated immune rejection of nascent tumours. Genetic deletion or antibody-mediated depletion of IL-23 were shown to increase cytotoxic T cells infiltration into sites of carcinogen-induced tumour formation. As well, transplanted tumours were growth-restricted in IL-23 or IL-23-receptor-deficient mice, identifying this cytokine as a facilitator of the inflammation/tumourigenesis interface through subversion of a T-cell mediated immune rejection ((Langowski et al., 2006) as reviewed in (Tan et al., 2009)).

10.3 Role of Inflammatory Cytokines and Chemokines in Colon Cancer Cell Invasion and Migration

As discussed above, macrophages and their secreted cytokines play a central role in the development of inflammation-associated colon cancer and are an integral part of the tumour microenvironment at the primary site, where they can facilitate tumour invasion and tumour-induced neo-vascularization through the release of cytokines such as TNF-α, IL-1 and IL-6 and pro-angiogenic factors such as VEGF and IL-8 (Mantovani et al., 2008). These factors can regulate the invasive potential of the cells in several ways including the induction of NFκB-regulated extracellular matrix-degrading metalloproteinases (such as MMP-9) (Fukuyama et al., 2007) and the transcriptional activation of chemokine receptors such as CXCR4 that mediate tumour cell chemotaxis in response to stromal-derived chemokines such as CXCL12 (Hagemann et al., 2005; Kulbe et al., 2005). The chemokines comprise a superfamily of at least 46 cytokines that bind and activate G protein-coupled receptors to induce directed migration (chemotaxis). First described in the context of leukocyte migration to sites of inflammation or injury, this family of mediators has received much attention recently as critical mediators of tumour cell migration to sites of metastasis. Up-regulated expression of various chemokine receptors has been documented in different tumours and they have frequently been identified as 'metastasis genes' in gene profiling studies of metastatic tumours. For example, CXCR4 was identified as a marker of tumour progression and aggressive phenotype in tissue microarrays of breast carcinoma specimens (Muller et al., 2001; Salvucci et al., 2006) and implicated in breast carcinoma cell migration and metastasis to regional lymph nodes and the lung (Muller et al., 2001). CCR7 was implicated in autocrine-mediated directional movement of tumour cells to the lymphatics via interstitial flow and found to be upregulated in metastatic breast carcinoma and melanoma (Muller et al., 2001; Shields et al., 2007).

Several chemokine/chemokine receptor pairs were also implicated in colon cancer cell metastasis to lymph nodes and the liver. For example, a microarray-based analysis of CXCR4 expression found that expression of this receptor is significantly increased in liver metastases relative to primary CRC tumours. The levels of CXCR4 expression in primary tumours was associated with increased incidence of liver metastasis and poor prognosis, suggesting that CXCR4/CXCL12 signalling is relevant to progression and liver metastasis in this disease (Kim et al., 2005). These findings were supported by other studies. For example, an analysis of chemokine receptors CXCR1-4 in colorectal adenomas, CRC and respective hepatic metastasis by a combination of quantitative real-time PCR, immuno-histochemistry and Western blotting revealed a significant increase in CXC receptors 1, 2 and 4 in all CRC specimens. In this study, CXCR4 levels correlated with tumour grade, whereas CXCR3 levels were significantly over-expressed in liver metastases (Rubie et al., 2008). Moreover, a concomitant high expression of CXCR4 and VEGF was found to be a strong and independent predictor of early distant relapse in colorectal cancer and this was attributed to the ability of CXCR4 to stimulate clonogenic growth, induce the release of VEGF and up-regulate ICAM-1 expression, as revealed in analyses of colon cancer cell lines (Ottaiano et al., 2006). Other studies using human and murine cell lines also implicated CXCR4 and CXCR3 in metastasis of colon cancer cells; however, it appears that, while CXCR3/CXCL10 promote invasion in colon cancer cells (Zipin-Roitman et al., 2007), CXCR4 may promote mainly tumour expansion in the colonized site (Zeelenberg et al., 2003). At variance with some of these findings is a recent study based on the use of human and murine CRC cell lines and a CXCR3-specific inhibitor AMG487. Blockade of CXCR3 selectively inhibited experimental lung, but not liver metastasis of the tumour cells (Cambien et al., 2009), leading the authors to conclude that this chemokine receptor may regulate site-selective lung metastasis of colon cancer cells (reviewed in (Fulton, 2009)). Interestingly, analysis of human specimens linked this receptor/ligand system to lymph node metastasis (Kawada et al., 2007), again highlighting the differences in results based on experimental models and analysis of human specimens.

Other chemokine/chemokine receptors have also been implicated in colon cancer liver metastasis. Ghadjar et al., using clinical specimens, documented a strong association between CCR6 staining intensity in primary CRC tumour specimens and the development of synchronous liver metastases, thereby implicating this receptor and its ligand CCL20 in CRC liver metastasis (Ghadjar et al., 2006). Rubie et al. reached a similar conclusion based on finding an increased expression of both CXCR4 and CXCR6 in hepatic metastasis of CRC patients. These authors also showed that only the expression of the CXCR6 ligands CCL20 and CCL21 was increased in the livers of CRC patients that developed liver metastases. This strongly supports an association between increased CCR6 expression in human CRC and the promotion of liver metastasis and implicates CCL20 as the recruiting chemokine (Rubie et al., 2006a; Rubie et al., 2006b). Finally, studies on the murine carcinoma CT-26 cells suggested that CXCR5 expression on the tumour cells promotes the outgrowth of large tumours in the liver (Meijer et al., 2006). Taken together, the data provide compelling evidence for the involvement of several chemokine/chemokine receptor pairs in lymph node and liver metastasis of CRC. The findings also suggest that these chemokine receptors may contribute to metastasis in different ways namely, by mediating recruitment (e.g. CXCR6), invasion (e.g. CXCR3) and local expansion (e.g. CXCR4) of tumours. It should, however, be noted that while expression profiling provides strong but indirect support for the involvement of these receptors in colon cancer progression and liver metastasis, the functional data may not be as broadly applicable because it is based on the use of human and murine tumour cell lines. Cell lines can vary extensively in their repertoires of chemokine/chemokine receptor pairs, in the expression of these mediators in vitro versus in vivo and in their relative dependency on autocrine and paracrine chemokine signalling for chemotaxis and invasion.

10.4 Tumour Cells Entering the Liver Can Elicit a Rapid Host Inflammatory Response that Promotes Metastasis

10.4.1 Pre-extravasation Events

Much of the information available on the initial stages of liver colonization is, by necessity, based on the study of animal tumour models. These studies revealed that circulating tumour cells or tumour cell clusters that enter the hepatic microvasculature through the portal circulation normally arrest first in terminal portal venules that surround hepatic lobules (Vidal-Vanaclocha, 2008). Tumour cell entry into the sinusoidal vessels is followed by arrest and initially by massive cell destruction caused by physical factors such as deformation-associated trauma and mechanical stress. Cancer cells or clumps of cells can also obstruct the sinusoidal vessels, and this results in a blockade of the blood flow. The resulting transient ischemia/reperfusion triggers a pro-inflammatory response in the affected areas. This can result in further tumour cell damage and death due to the local release of nitric oxide (Qi et al., 2004) and reactive oxygen intermediates by hepatic sinusoidal cells and hepatocytes and to the production of toxic radicals (Wang et al., 2000; and reviewed in Yanagida et al. (2006)). Once in the sinusoids, the tumour cells can also be targeted and eliminated by tumouricidal or phagocytic Kupffer cells that reside in the sinusoids (Bayon et al., 1996; Kan et al., 1995). These resident macrophages can also activate other cells of the innate immune response such as NK cells and neutrophils through the release of cytokines such as INFγ and IL-1, adding to the local anti-tumourigenic arsenal (Bouwens et al., 1988; Gardner et al., 1991). In addition, the release of TNF-α in response to tumour infiltration can also directly cause tumour cell apoptosis in the sinusoidal vessels (Hehlgans and Pfeffer, 2005).

Tumour cells that survive these multiple assaults do so through different escape mechanisms. For example, tumour cells can escape the lethal effects of TNF-α by activating NFκB-mediated survival signalling and the subsequent release of survival factors such as IL-6 (Schneider et al., 2000). Indeed, a recent clinical study analyzing the role of IL-6 in the spread of colon cancer implicated this cytokine in lymph node and hepatic metastasis and concluded that serum IL-6 levels would be a useful predictive indicator for metastasis (Ashizawa et al., 2006), a conclusion also supported by other studies (Matzaraki et al., 2007). It is also possible that in cell clusters, the inner cells may be protected by the outer cells from attacks by Kupffer cells or neutrophils. Tumour-derived carcinoembryonic antigen (CEA) can provide another defense mechanism because it was shown to stimulate the production of the anti-inflammatory cytokine IL-10 and the pro-survival cytokine IL-6 by colon cancer cells, and thereby counter NO-dependent cancer cell death (Jessup et al., 2004a; Jessup et al., 2004b). Another protective mechanism for CRC cells may be the expression of MHC class I antigens. This was shown to protect rat colon carcinoma cells from hepatic NK cell-mediated apoptosis and cytolysis through blockade of the perforin/granzyme pathway (Luo et al., 2002).

While the innate immune response in the liver can mount an efficient first line of defense against some infiltrating tumour cells, it can also promote tumour cell adhesion to the vascular endothelial cells, transendothelial migration and escape from the tumoricidal effects of resident Kupffer cells and NK cells, thereby promoting metastasis. We and others have shown that, once they enter the hepatic microvasculature, some tumour cells including CRC cells can release or activate local cells such as resident Kupffer cells to secrete pro-inflammatory factors and reactive oxygen species leading to up-regulated expression of vascular endothelial cell adhesion receptors. Early studies from our group have shown that the liver-metastasizing potential of human colorectal carcinoma and murine lung carcinoma cells correlated with adhesion to hepatic sinusoidal endothelial cells in vitro. Cytokine-inducible E-selectin was subsequently identified as a mediator of this adhesion (Bresalier et al., 1998; Bresalier et al., 1996; Brodt et al., 1997) and it was shown to depend on sialyl-rich peripheral mucin carbohydrate structures (Bresalier et al., 1998). When mice were treated with anti-E-selectin antibodies following the intrasplenic/portal inoculation of metastatic tumour cells, liver metastasis was inhibited, providing the first line of evidence that this molecule was functionally involved in metastasis in vivo

10 Role of the Host Inflammatory Response   303

(Brodt et al., 1997). Subsequently, we have shown that the highly metastatic human colon CX-1 and murine lung H-59 tumour cells, but not their poorly metastatic counterparts MIP-101 and M-27 cells were able to up-regulate E-selectin expression upon entry into the liver. This followed the activation of a pro-inflammatory response involving Kupffer cell-mediated release of TNF-α and IL-1 in the sinusoidal micro-environment (Khatib et al., 2005) (see Fig. 10.1). For colon carcinoma

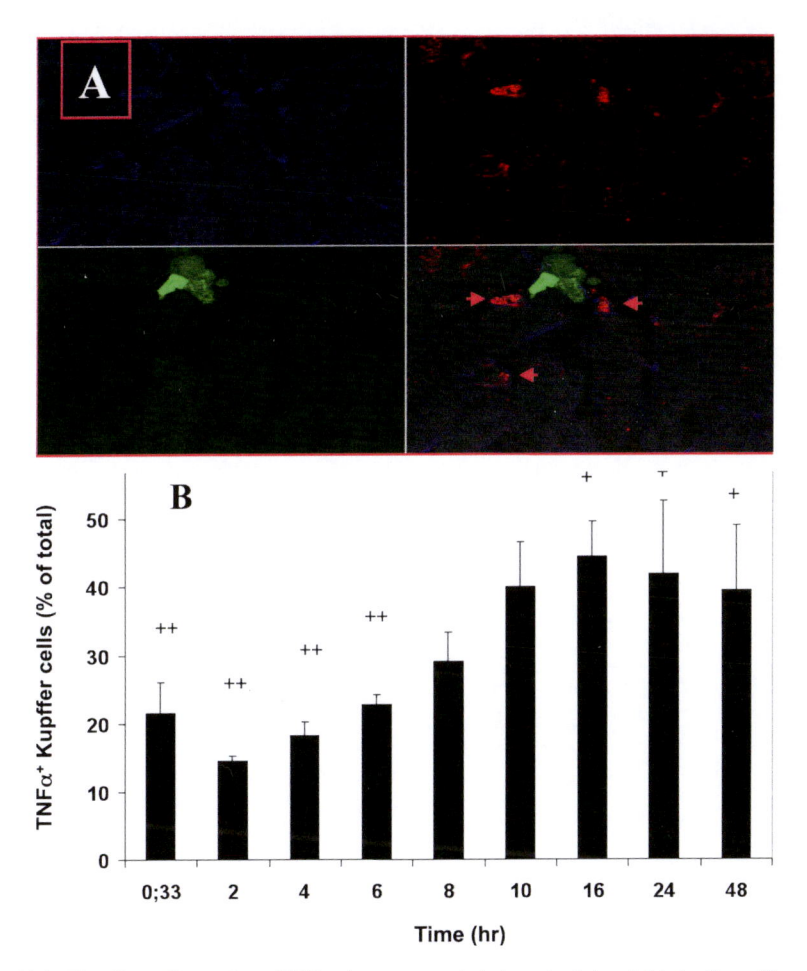

Fig. 10.1 Kupffer cells produce TNF-α in response to intrasplenic/portal injection of human colon carcinoma CX-1 cells. Cryostat sections were prepared following the injection of 10^6 tumour cells and immuno-labeled with the macrophage-specific mAb F4/80 and an anti-TNF-α antibody. Shown in (**a**) are representative images of Kupffer cells (*blue*), TNF-α (*red*), CX-1 cells (*green*), and a merged confocal image. *Arrowheads* show co-localization of TNF-α and Kupffer cells. Shown in (**b**) are the percentages of TNF-α$^+$ Kupffer cells at different time intervals after tumour injection. (+) $p < 0.05$ as compared to 20 min post tumour cell inoculation. (++) $p < 0.05$ as compared to percentage of TNF-α Kupffer cells at 16 h. Original magnifications, ×630. Reproduced with permission from Khatib et al. (2005)

cells, this process involved tumour-Kupffer cell association, as was evident from immuno-histochemistry and confocal microscopy (Khatib et al., 2005). This association could be mediated by tumour-derived CEA, as shown by others (Gangopadhyay et al., 1996; Gangopadhyay et al., 1998). However, tumour-Kupffer cell contact was not essential for this process, as seen with murine lung carcinoma H-59 cells, suggesting that it could be initiated by tumour-derived soluble factors or as a results of the ischemic insult triggered by tumour cell entry. Cytokine production was rapidly followed by sequential up-regulation of vascular endothelial cell adhesion molecules such as E- and P-selectin (maximal at 6–12 h post injection), VCAM-1 and ICAM-1 (12–48 h post injection). In addition, these adhesion molecules together with PECAM-1 led to tumour cell arrest and extravasation into the hepatic parenchyma (Auguste et al., 2007; Brodt et al., 1997; Khatib et al., 2005; Khatib et al., 1999) (see Figs. 10.2, 10.3 and 10.4). Interestingly, this effect was tumour-specific and correlated with the metastatic phenotype of the tumour cells. Furthermore, abrogation of the inflammatory response by antisense oligodeoxynucleotides that blocked TNFR-mediated ERK signalling and thereby E-selectin expression, significantly inhibited liver metastasis of human colorectal carcinoma CX-1 cells in athymic nude mice, identifying the inflammatory response as a potential target for anti-metastatic therapy (Khatib et al., 2002).

These findings were essentially confirmed by Kruskal et al. Using intravital microscopy for live imaging of the early steps in colon carcinoma liver colonization, they observed that both non-metastatic MIP-101 and metastatic CX-1 colon cancer cells initially adhered to periportal Kupffer cells upon entry into the liver. However, only the highly metastatic CX-1 cells activated the Kupffer cells leading

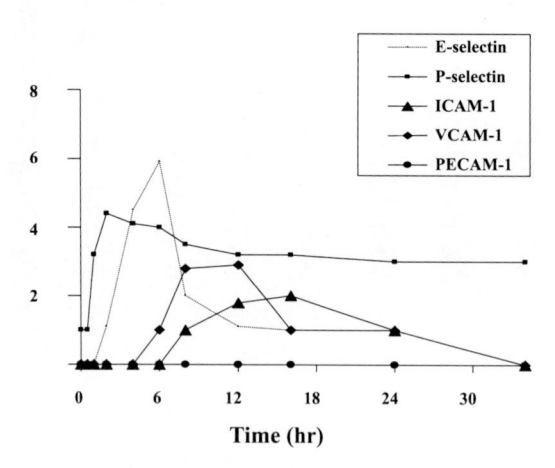

Fig. 10.2 Induction of multiple hepatic vascular cell adhesion molecules (CAMs) after tumour cell inoculation. Syngeneic C57BL/6 mice were injected with 10^6 H-59 cells by the intrasplenic/portal route, and their livers were removed at the time intervals indicated. Total RNA was extracted and analyzed by RT-PCR using specific primers for the murine CAMs indicated or for GAPDH. A summary of results of laser densitometry expressed as the ratio of CAM/GAPDH signal relative to the control (livers of non-injected mice) is shown. Reproduced with permission from Khatib et al. (2005)

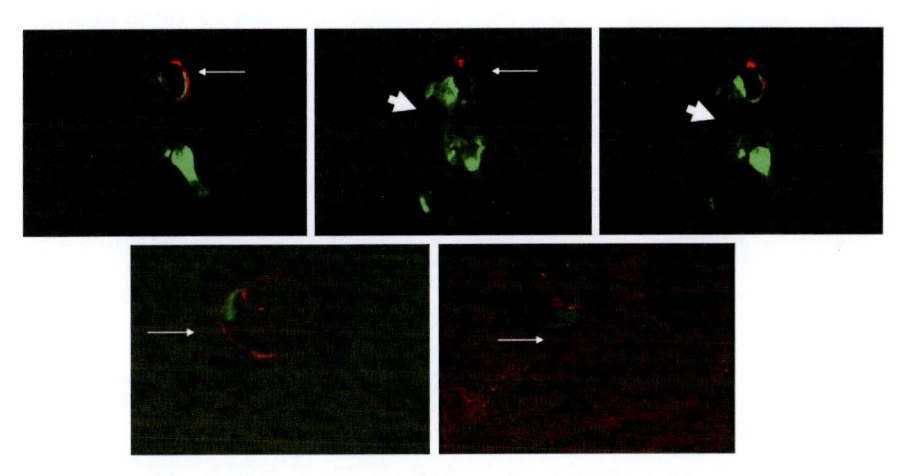

Fig. 10.3 Visualization of tumour cells in close contact with E-selectin⁺ hepatic sinusoidal endothelial cells by confocal microscopy. Cryostat sections were prepared from livers removed at different time intervals following the inoculation of H-59 (**a**) or CX-1 (**b**) cells and immunostained with anti E-selectin antibodies. Sections were analyzed with a Zeiss confocal microscope at a magnification of ×630. Tumour cells are shown in *green*. Arrows in **a** and **b** on merged images of *red* and *green* fluorescence indicate co-localized tumour cell/E-selectin signals indicating areas of contact. *Arrowheads* indicate cell transmigration as reconstructed from Z-stacks. Reproduced with permission from Auguste et al. (2007)

to activation of endothelial E-selectin and to tumour metastasis. In contrast, recruitment of systemic macrophages by MIP-101 led to regression of periportal MIP-101 tumour growth (Kruskal et al., 2007), suggesting that the tumour cells were targets of immune attack by these cells.

In a further extension to our studies, we also observed that non-metastatic lung carcinoma M-27 cells expressed high levels of the secretory leukocyte

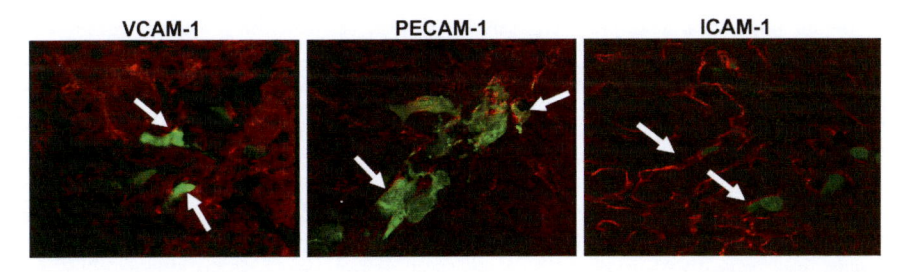

Fig. 10.4 Visualization of H-59 cell adhesion to hepatic sinusoidal endothelial cell CAM by confocal microscopy. Shown are representative images acquired with 100 μm cryostat sections that were obtained following inoculation of H-59 cells and stained with antibodies to VCAM-1, PECAM-1 or ICAM-1. A Zeiss confocal microscope was used for analysis at magnifications of ×630 (VCAM-1 and PECAM-1) or ×400 (ICAM-1). Tumour cells are in *green*. Arrows on the merged images of *red* and *green* fluorescence indicate co-localized tumour cell/CAM signals. Reproduced with permission from Auguste et al. (2007)

protease inhibitor (SLPI), a pleiotropic peptide with anti-inflammatory activity that can attenuate NFκB-mediated functions such as LPS-induced TNF-α production by macrophages (Jin et al., 1998; Jin et al., 1997). When this molecule was overexpressed in highly metastatic lung carcinoma H-59 cells, their ability to induce TNF-α production and E-selectin expression upon entry into the liver was attenuated. This resulted in a >80% reduction in their ability to form experimental hepatic metastases following intrasplenic/portal tumour injection (see Fig. 10.5), suggesting that the balance between tumour cell-derived pro- and anti-inflammatory factors may determine the host response to liver-invading tumour cells (Wang et al., 2006).

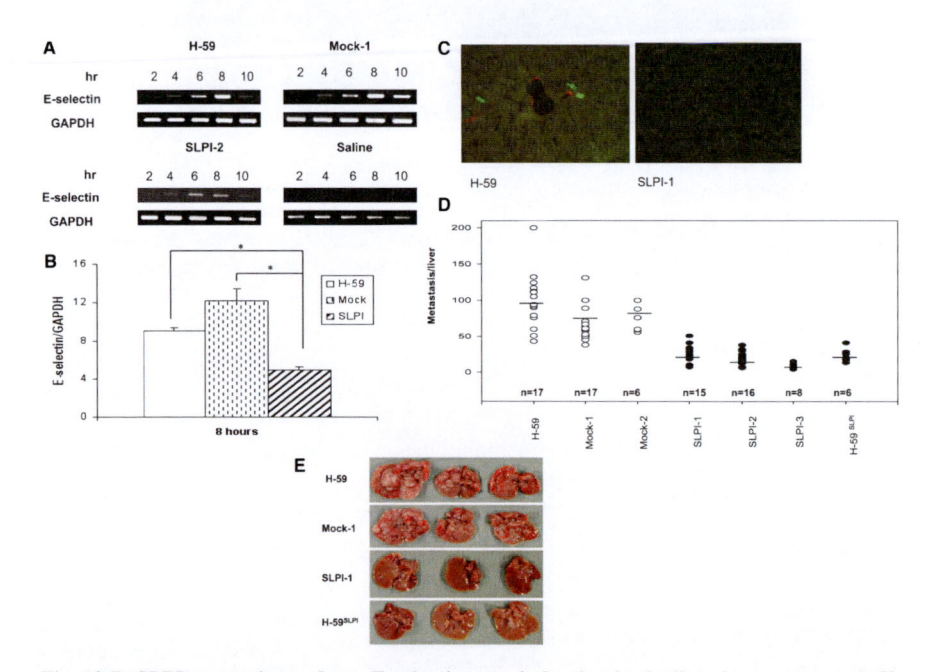

Fig. 10.5 SLPI expression reduces E-selectin gene induction in the liver in response to infiltrating tumour cells and inhibits metastasis. Mice were inoculated with 10^6 tumour cells by the intrasplenic/portal route and the livers were removed at the time intervals indicated. Total RNA was extracted and analyzed by RT-PCR. For each of the cell types, three livers were analyzed per each time point and each analysis was performed three times. Representative data are shown in (**a**). Results of laser densitometry are shown in the bar graph in (**b**). Shown are means and SD of the data obtained with H-59 ($n = 3$), Mock-1 and Mock-2 (Mock-transfected cells, $n = 6$) and three clones obtained from SLPI-transfected H-59 cells (SLPI-1, SLPI-2 and SLPI-3, $n = 9$). They are expressed as the ratios of E-selectin:GAPDH relative to the control group (livers of saline injected mice), that were assigned a value of 1 (**p < 0.01; Student's t test). Shown in (**c**) are results of immuno-histochemistry performed on cryostat sections of livers derived from the animals 8 h following the injection of GFP- expressing non-transfected (*left*) or SLPI-transfected (*right*) H-59 cells. The sections were stained with rat anti-murine E-selectin antibodies and an Alexa 568 goat anti-rat antibody (*red* staining). The images shown are representative of 60 fields analyzed using the 40× objective. (**d–e**) Liver metastases were enumerated 14 days after the intrasplenic/portal injection of 10^5 tumour cells. Results obtained with each individual cell type are shown in (**d**) and representative livers are shown in (**e**). Reproduced with permission from Wang et al. (2006)

The importance of TNF-α in promoting early events in liver metastasis was also demonstrated in TNFR1-deficient mice. These mice developed fewer hepatic metastases and this was attributed to a significantly reduced VCAM-1 induction in these, as compared to wild-type mice (Kitakata et al., 2002). Interestingly however, in a recent study of fourteen clinical CRC specimens implanted orthotopically in the cecal wall of nude mice, TNF-α production by the colon cancer cells was found to correlate with a reduced liver-metastasizing potential (Soma et al., 1998), highlighting the dual role that this cytokine can play in the process of metastasis.

Cells can attach to E-selectin via oligosaccharide and sulfo-polysaccharide ligands present on glycoproteins and glycolipids. Among these are sialylated Lewis-a (sLew^a) and Lewis-x (sLew^x) groups that have been identified as markers of progression for several human malignancies of the GI tract (Magnani, 2004). As well, glycoproteins such as PSGL-1, ESL-1, death receptor-3 (DR3), MAdCAM-1, lysosomal membrane glycoproteins LAMP-1 and LAMP-2 and CD44 variant isoforms have been identified as selectin ligands (reviewed in (Witz, 2008)) (see Chapter 7, in this book, for more information). These counter-receptors have terminal fucosyl and sialyl groups that bind to the lectin domain of E-selectin. Expression of these ligands is modified by fucosyltransferases such as FUT4 and FUT7, that are also frequently up-regulated in malignant cells (Ogawa et al., 1996). The attachment to endothelial E-selectin in turn, initiates a signalling cascade that promotes endothelial cell retraction and tumour cell migration. Huot and associates have investigated this process in some detail. In a series of studies, they have shown that CRC cell attachment to human umbilical vein endothelial cells (HUVEC) is mediated via E-selectin and triggers the activation of stress-activated protein kinase-2/p38 signalling in the tumour cells that is essential for their transendothelial migration. The same group also identified DR3, a member of the TNFR superfamily, as an E-selectin ligand on CRC cells and showed that E-selectin-mediated DR3 activation induced p38 and ERK activation, conferring motility signals on the CRC cells. In addition, E-selectin-mediated DR3 activation induced the formation of gaps between endothelial cells through Src kinase activation and the dissociation of the VE-cadherin/β-catenin complex (Houle and Huot, 2006; Tremblay et al., 2006). DR3 expression was detected in primary human CRC, but not in normal colon tissue, suggesting that it is relevant to tumour progression in this disease (Tremblay et al., 2006). In further dissecting the cell–cell interactions that follow CRC cell attachment to E-selectin, under conditions of flow in vitro, this group identified three critical steps that appear to be necessary for tumour cells diapedesis across an endothelial monolayer: 1. formation of a mosaic between cancer cells and endothelial cells. 2. paracellular diapedesis at the junction of three endothelial cells and 3. trans-cellular diapedesis. The evidence suggested that extravasation, at least in vitro, was ICAM-1- and VCAM-1-independent and required ERK activation downstream of E-selectin (Tremblay et al., 2008).

In line with some of these findings are results reported by Aychek et al. This group has shown that adhesion to E-selectin altered gene expression in the attached cells and that these changes were more pronounced in highly metastatic than in poorly metastatic CRC cells. This suggested that metastatic cells may be more responsive to signals transmitted through this adhesion molecule (Aychek et al., 2008).

Vidal-Vanalocha and associates studied the process of tumour transendothelial migration in vivo using the highly metastatic B16F10 melanoma cells. In a series of studies, they have shown that within 24 h of tumour cell entry into the liver, VCAM-1 expression levels on hepatic sinusoidal endothelial cells significantly increased. They further demonstrated that VCAM-1 played a role in liver colonization by these tumour cells because its blockade with specific antibodies decreased the microvascular retention of luciferase-tagged tumour cells and significantly reduced metastasis. These findings are in agreement with our own findings and those of others (Wang et al., 2002) and reveal a common pattern of endothelial cell adhesion molecule expression during the early stages of liver colonization that is reproducible with different tumour types. Further studies by this group implicated sequential IL-1β- and TNF-α-induced IL-18 production in sinusoidal endothelial VCAM-1 induction. They also suggested that it was mediated via hydrogen peroxide and could be recapitulated by VEGF (Carrascal et al., 2003; Vidal-Vanaclocha, 2008; Vidal-Vanaclocha et al., 2000).

While the findings described above are based mainly on animal models of metastasis and in vitro studies, they are strongly supported by clinical data. These data provide compelling evidence that the host inflammatory response can promote CRC liver-metastasis, in part through activation of endothelial cell adhesion receptors. For example, increased expression of cytokine-inducible vascular endothelial E-selectin was noted in and around hepatic metastases of CRC (Ye et al., 1995). Furthermore, elevated serum levels of soluble E-selectin, ICAM-1 and VCAM-1 were detected in patients with primary CRC or locally recurring tumours and these levels correlated with disease outcome (Alexiou et al., 2001; Wittig et al., 1996). Moreover, increased expression of the E-selectin carbohydrate ligands SLe^x and SLe^a was noted on metastatic CRC cells and in CRC liver metastases (Hoff et al., 1989; Matsushita et al., 1998; Sato et al., 1997), as well as on other liver-metastasizing malignancies and their levels were found to correlate with the metastatic phenotype (reviewed in Krause and Turner, 1999). In addition, increased COX-2 expression was noted in CRC specimens in comparison to normal mucosa and a still greater expression was seen in hepatic metastases (Chen et al., 2001). Similarly, high expression of TGF-β1, a modulator of the stromal/inflammatory response, was noted in hepatic metastases of CRC (Picon et al., 1998) and an association was documented between TGF-β1 expression levels and recurrence of the disease (Friedman et al., 1995), suggesting that inflammatory mediators affect disease outcome and may provide clinical biomarkers for this malignancy.

10.4.2 Post-extravasation Events

Once tumour cells extravasate from the sinusoidal vessels into the space of Disse, they may follow one of several possible scenarios. They may begin a process of proliferation or migrate further into preferred sites of growth, possibly in response to chemotactic or growth factors, to proliferate and establish macrometastases. Alternatively, they may initiate a short-lived process of proliferation that is aborted before metastases are established or enter a state of dormancy as solitary cells, never to produce a metastasis (Groom et al., 1999; Vidal-Vanaclocha, 2008). The factors that determine the fate of the tumour cells are not, as yet, fully understood, but different studies suggest that various liver cells including stellate cells, hepatocytes, portal tract fibroblasts and macrophages can be recruited into emerging metastases and contribute to the process of liver colonization in various ways. For example, recent studies with colon carcinoma CT-26 cells revealed that these tumour cells produced the chemokine CCL2 in vivo and this coincided with the recruitment of macrophages and hepatic stellate cells into the tumours. In CCR2-deficient mice, a reduction in macrophage and hepatic stellate cell accumulation in the tumours was observed, and this corresponded to reduced MMP-2 levels and decreased neo-vascularization and resulted in reduced numbers of hepatic metastases. These findings suggest that the recruitment of stellate cells and macrophages into the tumours promoted MMP-2 production and contributed to tumour induced-neo-vascularization (Xiaoqin Yang et al., 2006) and metastases. Stellate cells recruited into metastases differentiate into myofibroblasts and are a source of various soluble factors including VEGF, PDGF, HGF and TGF-β, factors that can contribute to recruitment of endothelial cells, angiogenesis, tumour cell proliferation and inflammation. Portal tract fibroblasts generate an inflammatory microenvironment in the tumours through the release of the pro-angiogenic factor IL-8, in response to local TNF-α production (Mueller et al., 2007). Hepatocytes can also contribute to tumour progression by producing growth factors such as IGF-I and IGF-II that stimulate tumour cell growth (Long et al., 1994; Long et al., 1995; Yakar et al., 2005). Finally, infiltrating macrophages can contribute to the local expansion of metastases through the release of extracellular matrix degrading proteinases such as MMP-2 and MMP-9. These infiltrating macrophages also promote angiogenesis through the release of IL-8 and the induction of VEGF production and increase the expression of vascular endothelial cell adhesion molecules for further dissemination [reviewed in (Rhodes and Campbell, 2002) and (Vidal-Vanaclocha, 2008)]. Clearly, various cellular components of the hepatic stroma can participate in, and contribute to colon cancer metastasis by promoting different steps required for the successful colonization of the liver.

10.5 Summary and Future Directions

Collectively, the work described herein provides compelling evidence that the host inflammatory response contributes actively to colon cancer progression by promoting tumour initiation, altering the local microenvironment of the primary tumours and promoting metastasis through the release of an array of chemokines and cytokines. While the use of anti-inflammatory drugs for CRC prevention in high-risk groups has become part of the clinical management of IBD, experimental evidence is emerging in support of the use of anti-inflammatory drugs to prevent hepatic metastasis. We have shown that anti-E-selectin antibodies and antisense oligonucleotides that inhibit E-selectin expression can inhibit experimental liver metastasis of murine and human tumour cells (Brodt et al., 1997; Khatib et al., 2002). Others have targeted E-selectin or E-selectin ligands as means of inhibiting metastases using anti-selectin antibodies, anti-selectin counter-receptor antibodies, and selectin antagonists such as soluble ligands (reviewed in (Kneuer et al., 2006)). For example, the carbohydrate groups sLew^x and sLew^a or their mimics have been used to inhibit E-selectin functions and could be used as potential inhibitors of metastasis (Magnani, 2004). Lovastatin was shown to reduce TNF-α-induced E-selectin expression, colon carcinoma cell adhesion to HUVEC and tumour cell migration and was proposed as a potential E-selectin inhibitor in vivo (Nubel et al., 2004). The histamine receptor-2 antagonist cimetidine, known to have survival benefits for colon cancer patients, was also identified as a blocker of E-selectin expression and shown to inhibit CRC cell adhesion to endothelial cell monolayers in vitro and inhibit metastasis in vivo (Kobayashi et al., 2000). In a few reported small trials, cimetidine has, in fact, been administered clinically to patients with advanced disease and was found to have a modest beneficial effect but overall patient survival did not increase (Burtin et al., 1988; Yoshimatsu et al., 2006). Other strategies employing anti-inflammatory agents were also shown to be effective in inhibiting metastasis. For example, Egberts et al. recently reported on the successful inhibition of the growth and metastasis of three different human pancreatic carcinomas growing orthotopically in immuno-deficient mice with the anti-TNF antibody infliximab. Furthermore, both infliximab and the TNF-trap Etanercept significantly reduced the number of liver metastases in a tumour resection model, suggesting that these drugs could be highly effective for prevention of metastasis in an adjuvant setting (Egberts et al., 2008). In a similar vein, pre-clinical data identified IL-6 and IL-6 signalling antagonists (Becker et al., 2005; Grivennikov and Karin, 2008), as well as IL-1 inhibitors (Matsuo et al., 2009; Melisi et al., 2009) as potential drugs for the prevention of liver metastasis from different malignancies including colorectal carcinoma. With a growing understanding of the complex interaction between the innate immune response and disseminating cancer cells, the arsenal of potential drugs is likely to grow and be further refined for optimal, specific and non-toxic targeting of early steps in the process of CRC liver metastasis.

Abbreviations and Acronyms

Bcl-x_L	B-cell lymphoma-extra large protein
CD	Crohn's disease
CEA	Carcinoembryonic antigen
c-FLIP	caspase 8 homologue FLICE-inhibitory protein
cIAPs	caspase inhibitor of apoptosis proteins
CRC	Colorectal carcinoma
CSF-1	Colony stimulating factor
COX-2	Cyclooxygenase type 2
DR3	Death receptor 3

ECM	Extracellular matrix
ERK	Extracellular signal-regulated kinase
ESL-1	E-selectin ligand-1
FADD	Fas-associated death domain-containing protein
IBD	Inflammatory bowel diseases
ICAM-1	Intercellular adhesion molecule-1
ICE	IL-1β-converting enzyme
IL-1	Interleukin-1
INFγ	Interferon gamma
iNOS	Inducible nitric oxide synthase
IRAK	IL-1R associated kinase
JNK	Jun N-terminal kinase
LAMP-1	Lysosomal membrane glycoprotein-1
LPS	Lipopolysaccharide
MAdCAM-1	Mucosal addressin cell adhesion molecule-1
MCP	Monocyte chemotactic protein
MIP	Macrophage inflammatory proteins
MMP	Matrix metalloproteinase
NFκB	Nuclear factor kappa-light-chain-enhancer of activated B cells
NK cells	Natural killer cells
PSGL-1	P-selectin glycoprotein ligand-1
SLPI	Secretory leukocyte protease inhibitor
SODD	Silencer of death domain
STAT	Signal transducer and activator of transcription
TAMs	Tumour-associated macrophages
TNF-α	Tumour necrosis factor-α
TNFR	Tumour necrosis factor receptor
TRADD	TNFR-associated death domain
TRAF	Tumour necrosis factor receptor-associated factor
UC	Ulcerative colitis
VCAM-1	Vascular cell adhesion molecule-1
VEGF	Vascular endothelial growth factor

Acknowledgments The studies by Brodt and associates described in this chapter were supported by grant MOP-81201 from the Canadian Institutes for Health Research.

References

Ahmadi A, Polyak S, Draganov PV (2009). Colorectal cancer surveillance in inflammatory bowel disease: the search continues. *World J Gastroenterol* **15**: 61–66.

Alexiou D, Karayiannakis AJ, Syrigos KN, Zbar A, Kremmyda A, Bramis I et al. (2001). Serum levels of E-selectin, ICAM-1 and VCAM-1 in colorectal cancer patients: correlations with clinicopathological features, patient survival and tumour surgery. *Eur J Cancer* **37**: 2392–97.

Arend WP, Palmer G, Gabay C (2008). IL-1, IL-18, and IL-33 families of cytokines. *Immunol Rev* **223**: 20–38.

Arnott CH, Scott KA, Moore RJ, Robinson SC, Thompson RG, Balkwill FR (2004). Expression of both TNF-alpha receptor subtypes is essential for optimal skin tumour development. *Oncogene* **23**: 1902–10.

Ashizawa T, Okada R, Suzuki Y, Tagaki M, Yamazaki T, Sumi T et al. (2006). Study of interleukin-6 in the spread of colorectal cancer: the diagnostic significance of IL-6. *Acta Med Okayama* **60**: 325–30.

Auguste A, Fallavollita L, Wang N, Bikfalvi A, Brodt P (2007). The host inflammatory response promotes liver metastasis by increasing tumor cell arrest and extravasation. *Am J Pathol* **170**: 1781–92.

Aychek T, Miller K, Sagi-Assif O, Levy-Nissenbaum O, Israeli-Amit M, Pasmanik-Chor M et al. (2008). E-selectin regulates gene expression in metastatic colorectal carcinoma cells and enhances HMGB1 release. *Int J Cancer* **123**: 1741–50.

Bacman D, Merkel S, Croner R, Papadopoulos T, Brueckl W, Dimmler A (2007). TGF-beta receptor 2 downregulation in tumour-associated stroma worsens prognosis and high-grade tumours show more tumour-associated macrophages and lower TGF-beta1 expression in colon carcinoma: a retrospective study. *BMC Cancer* **7**: 156.

Baier PK, Wolff-Vorbeck G, Eggstein S, Baumgartner U, Hopt UT (2005). Cytokine expression in colon carcinoma. *Anticancer Res* **25**: 2135–39.

Bailey C, Negus R, Morris A, Ziprin P, Goldin R, Allavena P et al. (2007). Chemokine expression is associated with the accumulation of tumour associated macrophages (TAMs) and progression in human colorectal cancer. *Clin Exp Metastasis* **24**: 121–30.

Balkwill F (2002). Tumor necrosis factor or tumor promoting factor? *Cytokine Growth Factor Rev* **13**: 135–41.

Balkwill F (2004). The significance of cancer cell expression of the chemokine receptor CXCR4. *Semin Cancer Biol* **14**: 171–79.

Balkwill F, Charles KA, Mantovani A (2005). Smoldering and polarized inflammation in the initiation and promotion of malignant disease. *Cancer Cell* **7**: 211–17.

Baron JA, Cole BF, Sandler RS, Haile RW, Ahnen D, Bresalier R et al. (2003). A randomized trial of aspirin to prevent colorectal adenomas. *N Engl J Med* **348**: 891–99.

Bayon LG, Izquierdo MA, Sirovich I, van Rooijen N, Beelen RH, Meijer S (1996). Role of Kupffer cells in arresting circulating tumor cells and controlling metastatic growth in the liver. *Hepatology* **23**: 1224–31.

Becker C, Fantini MC, Wirtz S, Nikolaev A, Lehr HA, Galle PR et al. (2005). IL-6 signaling promotes tumor growth in colorectal cancer. *Cell Cycle* **4**: 217–20.

Bingle L, Brown NJ, Lewis CE (2002). The role of tumour-associated macrophages in tumour progression: implications for new anticancer therapies. *J Pathol* **196**: 254–65.

Bissell MJ, Kenny PA, Radisky DC (2005). Microenvironmental regulators of tissue structure and function also regulate tumor induction and progression: the role of extracellular matrix and its degrading enzymes. *Cold Spring Harb Symp Quant Biol* **70**: 1–14.

Biswas SK, Gangi L, Paul S, Schioppa T, Saccani A, Sironi M et al. (2006). A distinct and unique transcriptional program expressed by tumor-associated macrophages (defective NF-kappaB and enhanced IRF-3/STAT1 activation). *Blood* **107**: 2112–22.

Boring CC, Squires TS, Tong T, Montgomery S (1994). Cancer statistics, 1994. *CA Cancer J Clin* **44**: 7–26.

Bouwens L, Jacobs R, Remels L, Wisse E (1988). Natural cytotoxicity of rat hepatic natural killer cells and macrophages against a syngeneic colon adenocarcinoma. *Cancer Immunol Immunother* **27**: 137–41.

Bresalier RS, Byrd JC, Brodt P, Ogata S, Itzkowitz SH, Yunker CK (1998). Liver metastasis and adhesion to the sinusoidal endothelium by human colon cancer cells is related to mucin carbohydrate chain length. *Int J Cancer* **76**: 556–62.

Bresalier RS, Ho SB, Schoeppner HL, Kim YS, Sleisenger MH, Brodt P et al. (1996). Enhanced sialylation of mucin-associated carbohydrate structures in human colon cancer metastasis. *Gastroenterology* **110**: 1354–67.

Brodt P, Fallavollita L, Bresalier RS, Meterissian S, Norton CR, Wolitzky BA (1997). Liver endothelial E-selectin mediates carcinoma cell adhesion and promotes liver metastasis. *Int J Cancer* **71**: 612–19.

Burtin C, Noirot C, Scheinmann P, Galoppin L, Sabolovic D, Bernard P (1988). Clinical improvement in advanced cancer disease after treatment combining histamine and H2-antihistaminics (ranitidine or cimetidine). *Eur J Cancer Clin Oncol* **24**: 161–67.

Cambien B, Karimdjee BF, Richard-Fiardo P, Bziouech H, Barthel R, Millet MA et al. (2009). Organ-specific inhibition of metastatic colon carcinoma by CXCR3 antagonism. *Br J Cancer* **100**: 1755–64.

Carrascal MT, Mendoza L, Valcarcel M, Salado C, Egilegor E, Telleria N et al. (2003). Interleukin-18 binding protein reduces b16 melanoma hepatic metastasis by neutralizing adhesiveness and growth factors of sinusoidal endothelium. *Cancer Res* **63**: 491–97.

Carswell EA, Old LJ, Kassel RL, Green S, Fiore N, Williamson B (1975). An endotoxin-induced serum factor that causes necrosis of tumors. *Proc Natl Acad Sci USA* **72**: 3666–70.

Chan FK, Shisler J, Bixby JG, Felices M, Zheng L, Appel M et al. (2003). A role for tumor necrosis factor receptor-2 and receptor-interacting protein in programmed necrosis and antiviral responses. *J Biol Chem* **278**: 51613–21.

Chen G, Goeddel DV (2002). TNF-R1 signaling: a beautiful pathway. *Science* **296**: 1634–35.

Chen WS, Wei SJ, Liu JM, Hsiao M, Kou-Lin J, Yang WK (2001). Tumor invasiveness and liver metastasis of colon cancer cells correlated with cyclooxygenase-2 (COX-2) expression and inhibited by a COX-2-selective inhibitor, etodolac. *Int J Cancer* **91**: 894–99.

Cohen AM (1989). *Colorectal Cancer*. J. B. Lippincott Company: Philadelphia, PA, 907 pp.

Condeelis J, Pollard JW (2006). Macrophages: obligate partners for tumor cell migration, invasion, and metastasis. *Cell* **124**: 263–66.

Coussens LM, Werb Z (2002). Inflammation and cancer. *Nature* **420**: 860–67.

De Smaele E, Zazzeroni F, Papa S, Nguyen DU, Jin R, Jones J et al. (2001). Induction of gadd45[beta] by NF-[kappa]B downregulates pro-apoptotic JNK signalling. *Nature* **414**: 308–13.

Dehqanzada ZA, Storrer CE, Hueman MT, Foley RJ, Harris KA, Jama YH et al. (2006). Correlations between serum monocyte chemotactic protein-1 levels, clinical prognostic factors, and HER-2/neu vaccine-related immunity in breast cancer patients. *Clin Cancer Res* **12**: 478–86.

Dinarello CA (1996). Biologic basis for interleukin-1 in disease. *Blood* **87**: 2095–147.

Dinarello CA (2009a). Immunological and inflammatory functions of the interleukin-1 family. *Annu Rev Immunol* **27**: 519–50.

Dinarello CA (2009b). Immunological and Inflammatory Functions of the Interleukin-1 Family. *Ann Rev Immunol* **27**: 519–50.

Eaden J, Abrams K, Ekbom A, Jackson E, Mayberry J (2000). Colorectal cancer prevention in ulcerative colitis: a case-control study. *Aliment Pharmacol Ther* **14**: 145–53.

Egberts J-H, Cloosters V, Noack A, Schniewind B, Thon L, Klose S et al. (2008). Anti-Tumor Necrosis Factor Therapy Inhibits Pancreatic Tumor Growth and Metastasis. *Cancer Res* **68**: 1443–50.

Erreni M, Bianchi P, Laghi L, Mirolo M, Fabbri M, Locati M et al. (2009). Chapter 5 Expression of chemokines and chemokine receptors in human colon cancer. In *Methods in Enzymology*. Academic Press: San Diego, CA, pp. 105–121.

Feagins LA, Souza RF, Spechler SJ (2009). Carcinogenesis in IBD: potential targets for the prevention of colorectal cancer. *Nat Rev Gastroenterol Hepatol* **6**: 297–305.

Forssell J, Oberg A, Henriksson ML, Stenling R, Jung A, Palmqvist R (2007). High macrophage infiltration along the tumor front correlates with improved survival in colon cancer. *Clin Cancer Res* **13**: 1472–79.

Friedman E, Gold LI, Klimstra D, Zeng ZS, Winawer S, Cohen A (1995). High levels of transforming growth factor beta 1 correlate with disease progression in human colon cancer. *Cancer Epidemiol Biomarkers Prev* **4**: 549–54.

Fukuyama R, Ng KP, Cicek M, Kelleher C, Niculaita R, Casey G et al. (2007). Role of IKK and oscillatory NFkappaB kinetics in MMP-9 gene expression and chemoresistance to 5-fluorouracil in RKO colorectal cancer cells. *Mol Carcinogen* **46**: 402–13.

Fulton AM (2009). The chemokine receptors CXCR4 and CXCR3 in cancer. *Curr Oncol Rep* **11**: 125–31.

Galban S, Fan J, Martindale JL, Cheadle C, Hoffman B, Woods MP et al. (2003). von Hippel-Lindau protein-mediated repression of tumor necrosis factor alpha translation revealed through use of cDNA arrays. *Mol Cell Biol* **23**: 2316–28.

Gangopadhyay A, Lazure DA, Kelly TM, Thomas P (1996). Purification and analysis of an 80-kDa carcinoembryonic antigen-binding protein from Kupffer cells. *Arch Biochem Biophys* **328**: 151–57.

Gangopadhyay A, Lazure DA, Thomas P (1998). Adhesion of colorectal carcinoma cells to the endothelium is mediated by cytokines from CEA stimulated Kupffer cells. *Clin Exp Metastasis* **16**: 703–12.

Gardner CR, Wasserman AJ, Laskin DL (1991). Liver macrophage-mediated cytotoxicity toward mastocytoma cells involves phagocytosis of tumor targets. *Hepatology* **14**: 318–24.

Germano G, Allavena P, Mantovani A (2008). Cytokines as a key component of cancer-related inflammation. *Cytokine* **43**: 374–79.

Ghadjar P, Coupland SE, Na IK, Noutsias M, Letsch A, Stroux A et al. (2006). Chemokine receptor CCR6 expression level and liver metastases in colorectal cancer. *J Clin Oncol* **24**: 1910–16.

Grivennikov S, Karin E, Terzic J, Mucida D, Yu G-Y, Vallabhapurapu S et al. (2009). IL-6 and Stat3 Are Required for Survival of Intestinal Epithelial Cells and Development of Colitis-Associated Cancer. *Cancer Cell* **15**: 241–241.

Grivennikov S, Karin M (2008). Autocrine IL-6 signaling: a key event in tumorigenesis? *Cancer Cell* **13**: 7–9.

Groom AC, MacDonald IC, Schmidt EE, Morris VL, Chambers AF (1999). Tumour metastasis to the liver, and the roles of proteinases and adhesion molecules: new concepts from in vivo videomicroscopy. *Can J Gastroenterol* **13**: 733–43.

Hagemann T, Wilson J, Kulbe H, Li NF, Leinster DA, Charles K et al. (2005). Macrophages induce invasiveness of epithelial cancer cells via NF-kappa B and JNK. *J Immunol* **175**: 1197–205.

Hehlgans T, Pfeffer K (2005). The intriguing biology of the tumour necrosis factor/tumour necrosis factor receptor superfamily: players, rules and the games. *Immunology* **115**: 1–20.

Higgins CA, Hatton WJ, McKerr G, Harvey D, Carson J, Hannigan BM (1996). Macrophages and apoptotic cells in human colorectal tumours. *Biologicals* **24**: 329–32.

Hirano T, Ishihara K, Hibi M (2000). Roles of STAT3 in mediating the cell growth, differentiation and survival signals relayed through the IL-6 family of cytokine receptors. *Oncogene* **19**: 2548–56.

Hoff SD, Matsushita Y, Ota DM, Cleary KR, Yamori T, Hakomori S et al. (1989). Increased expression of sialyl-dimeric LeX antigen in liver metastases of human colorectal carcinoma. *Cancer Res* **49**: 6883–88.

Houle F, Huot J (2006). Dysregulation of the endothelial cellular response to oxidative stress in cancer. *Mol Carcinog* **45**: 362–67.

Johnson IT, Lund EK (2007). Review article: nutrition, obesity and colorectal cancer. *Aliment Pharmacol Therap* **26**: 161–81.

Jedinak A, Dudhgaonkar S, Sliva D (2010). Activated macrophages induce metastatic behavior of colon cancer cells. *Immunobiology* **215**: 242–9.

Jessup JM, Laguinge L, Lin S, Samara R, Aufman K, Battle P et al. (2004a). Carcinoembryonic antigen induction of IL-10 and IL-6 inhibits hepatic ischemic/reperfusion injury to colorectal carcinoma cells. *Int J Cancer* **111**: 332–37.

Jessup JM, Samara R, Battle P, Laguinge LM (2004b). Carcinoembryonic antigen promotes tumor cell survival in liver through an IL-10-dependent pathway. *Clin Exp Metastasis* **21**: 709–17.

Jin F, Nathan CF, Radzioch D, Ding A (1998). Lipopolysaccharide-related stimuli induce expression of the secretory leukocyte protease inhibitor, a macrophage-derived lipopolysaccharide inhibitor. *Infect Immun* **66**: 2447–52.

Jin FY, Nathan C, Radzioch D, Ding A (1997). Secretory leukocyte protease inhibitor: a macrophage product induced by and antagonistic to bacterial lipopolysaccharide. *Cell* **88**: 417–26.

Kan Z, Ivancev K, Lunderquist A, McCuskey PA, McCuskey RS, Wallace S (1995). In vivo microscopy of hepatic metastases: dynamic observation of tumor cell invasion and interaction with Kupffer cells. *Hepatology* **21**: 487–94.

Karin M, Lin A (2002). NF-kappaB at the crossroads of life and death. *Nat Immunol* **3**: 221–27.

Kawada K, Hosogi H, Sonoshita M, Sakashita H, Manabe T, Shimahara Y et al. (2007). Chemokine receptor CXCR3 promotes colon cancer metastasis to lymph nodes. *Oncogene* **26**: 4679–88.

Khatib AM, Auguste P, Fallavollita L, Wang N, Samani A, Kontogiannea M et al. (2005). Characterization of the host proinflammatory response to tumor cells during the initial stages of liver metastasis. *Am J Pathol* **167**: 749–59.

Khatib AM, Fallavollita L, Wancewicz EV, Monia BP, Brodt P (2002). Inhibition of hepatic endothelial E-selectin expression by C-raf antisense oligonucleotides blocks colorectal carcinoma liver metastasis. *Cancer Res* **62**: 5393–98.

Khatib AM, Kontogiannea M, Fallavollita L, Jamison B, Meterissian S, Brodt P (1999). Rapid induction of cytokine and E-selectin expression in the liver in response to metastatic tumor cells. *Cancer Res* **59**: 1356–61.

Kim J, Takeuchi H, Lam ST, Turner RR, Wang HJ, Kuo C et al. (2005). Chemokine receptor CXCR4 expression in colorectal cancer patients increases the risk for recurrence and for poor survival. *J Clin Oncol* **23**: 2744–53.

Kitakata H, Nemoto-Sasaki Y, Takahashi Y, Kondo T, Mai M, Mukaida N (2002). Essential roles of tumor necrosis factor receptor p55 in liver metastasis of intrasplenic administration of colon 26 cells. *Cancer Res* **62**: 6682–87.

Klampfer L (2008). The role of signal transducers and activators of transcription in colon cancer. *Front Biosci* **13**: 2888–99.

Kneuer C, Ehrhardt C, Radomski MW, Bakowsky U (2006). Selectins – potential pharmacological targets? *Drug Discov Today* **11**: 1034–40.

Knight B, Yeoh GC, Husk KL, Ly T, Abraham LJ, Yu C et al. (2000). Impaired preneoplastic changes and liver tumor formation in tumor necrosis factor receptor type 1 knockout mice. *J Exp Med* **192**: 1809–18.

Kobayashi K, Matsumoto S, Morishima T, Kawabe T, Okamoto T (2000). Cimetidine inhibits cancer cell adhesion to endothelial cells and prevents metastasis by blocking E-selectin expression. *Cancer Res* **60**: 3978–84.

Krause T, Turner GA (1999). Are selectins involved in metastasis? *Clin Exp Metastasis* **17**: 183–92.

Kruskal JB, Azouz A, Korideck H, El-Hallak M, Robson SC, Thomas P et al. (2007). Hepatic colorectal cancer metastases: imaging initial steps of formation in mice. *Radiology* **243**: 703–11.

Kulbe H, Hagemann T, Szlosarek PW, Balkwill FR, Wilson JL (2005). The inflammatory cytokine tumor necrosis factor-alpha regulates chemokine receptor expression on ovarian cancer cells. *Cancer Res* **65**: 10355–62.

Lackner C, Jukic Z, Tsybrovskyy O, Jatzko G, Wette V, Hoefler G et al. (2004). Prognostic relevance of tumour-associated macrophages and von Willebrand factor-positive microvessels in colorectal cancer. *Virchows Arch* **445**: 160–67.

Langowski JL, Zhang X, Wu L, Mattson JD, Chen T, Smith K et al. (2006). IL-23 promotes tumour incidence and growth. *Nature* **442**: 461–65.

Leek RD, Hunt NC, Landers RJ, Lewis CE, Royds JA, Harris AL (2000). Macrophage infiltration is associated with VEGF and EGFR expression in breast cancer. *J Pathol* **190**: 430–36.

Leeuwenberg JF, van Tits LJ, Jeunhomme TM, Buurman WA (1995). Evidence for exclusive role in signalling of tumour necrosis factor p55 receptor and a potentiating function of p75 receptor on human endothelial cells. *Cytokine* **7**: 457–62.

Leimgruber A, Berger C, Cortez-Retamozo V, Etzrodt M, Newton AP, Waterman P et al. (2009). Behavior of endogenous tumor-associated macrophages assessed in vivo using a functionalized nanoparticle. *Neoplasia* **11**: 459–68.

Lewis CE, Pollard JW (2006). Distinct role of macrophages in different tumor microenvironments. *Cancer Res* **66**: 605–12.

Li Y-Y, Hsieh L-L, Tang R-P, Liao S-K, Yeh K-Y (2009). Interleukin-6 (IL-6) released by macrophages induces IL-6 secretion in the human colon cancer HT-29 cell line. *Human Immunology* **70**: 151–58.

Locksley RM, Killeen N, Lenardo MJ (2001). The TNF and TNF receptor superfamilies: integrating mammalian biology. *Cell* **104**: 487–501.

Long L, Nip J, Brodt P (1994). Paracrine growth stimulation by hepatocyte-derived insulin-like growth factor-1: a regulatory mechanism for carcinoma cells metastatic to the liver. *Cancer Res* **54**: 3732–37.

Long L, Rubin R, Baserga R, Brodt P (1995). Loss of the metastatic phenotype in murine carcinoma cells expressing an antisense RNA to the insulin-like growth factor receptor. *Cancer Res* **55**: 1006–9.

Luo D, Vermijlen D, Kuppen PJ, Wisse E (2002). MHC class I expression protects rat colon carcinoma cells from hepatic natural killer cell-mediated apoptosis and cytolysis, by blocking the perforin/granzyme pathway. *Comp Hepatol* **1**: 2.

Luo JL, Kamata H, Karin M (2005). IKK/NF-kappaB signaling: balancing life and death – a new approach to cancer therapy. *J Clin Invest* **115**: 2625–32.

Magnani JL (2004). The discovery, biology, and drug development of sialyl Lea and sialyl Lex. *Arch Biochem Biophys* **426**: 122–31.

Mantovani A, Allavena P, Sica A, Balkwill F (2008). Cancer-related inflammation. *Nature* **454**: 436–44.

Mantovani A, Sica A, Locati M (2005). Macrophage polarization comes of age. *Immunity* **23**: 344–46.

Mantovani A, Sica A, Sozzani S, Allavena P, Vecchi A, Locati M (2004). The chemokine system in diverse forms of macrophage activation and polarization. *Trends Immunol* **25**: 677–86.

Marino E, Cardier JE (2003). Differential effect of IL-18 on endothelial cell apoptosis mediated by TNF-alpha and Fas (CD95). *Cytokine* **22**: 142–48.

Matsuo Y, Sawai H, Ma J, Xu D, Ochi N, Yasuda A et al. (2009). IL-1alpha secreted by colon cancer cells enhances angiogenesis: the relationship between IL-1alpha release and tumor cells' potential for liver metastasis. *J Surg Oncol* **99**: 361–67.

Matsushita Y, Kitajima S, Goto M, Tezuka Y, Sagara M, Imamura H et al. (1998). Selectins induced by interleukin-1beta on the human liver endothelial cells act as ligands for sialyl Lewis X-expressing human colon cancer cell metastasis. *Cancer Lett* **133**: 151–60.

Matzaraki V, Alexandraki KI, Venetsanou K, Piperi C, Myrianthefs P, Malamos N et al. (2007). Evaluation of serum procalcitonin and interleukin-6 levels as markers of liver metastasis. *Clin Biochem* **40**: 336–42.

Meijer J, Zeelenberg IS, Sipos B, Roos E (2006). The CXCR5 chemokine receptor is expressed by carcinoma cells and promotes growth of colon carcinoma in the liver. *Cancer Res* **66**: 9576–82.

Melisi D, Niu J, Chang Z, Xia Q, Peng B, Ishiyama S et al. (2009). Secreted Interleukin-1β Induces a Metastatic Phenotype in Pancreatic Cancer by Sustaining a Constitutive Activation of Nuclear Factor-β. *Mol Cancer Res* **7**: 624–33.

Mitsuyama K, Sata M, Rose-John S (2006). Interleukin-6 trans-signaling in inflammatory bowel disease. *Cytokine Growth Factor Rev* **17**: 451–61.

Moore RJ, Owens DM, Stamp G, Arnott C, Burke F, East N et al. (1999). Mice deficient in tumor necrosis factor-alpha are resistant to skin carcinogenesis. *Nat Med* **5**: 828–31.

Moynagh PN (2005). The NF-kappaB pathway. *J Cell Sci* **118**: 4589–92.

Mueller L, Goumas FA, Affeldt M, Sandtner S, Gehling UM, Brilloff S et al. (2007). Stromal fibroblasts in colorectal liver metastases originate from resident fibroblasts and generate an inflammatory microenvironment. *Am J Pathol* **171**: 1608–18.

Mukhopadhyay A, Suttles J, Stout RD, Aggarwal BB (2001). Genetic deletion of the tumor necrosis factor receptor p60 or p80 abrogates ligand-mediated activation of nuclear factor-kappa B and of mitogen-activated protein kinases in macrophages. *J Biol Chem* **276**: 31906–12.

Muller A, Homey B, Soto H, Ge N, Catron D, Buchanan ME et al. (2001). Involvement of chemokine receptors in breast cancer metastasis. *Nature* **410**: 50–56.

Nath A, Chattopadhya S, Chattopadhyay U, Sharma NK (2006). Macrophage inflammatory protein (MIP)1alpha and MIP1beta differentially regulate release of inflammatory cytokines and generation of tumoricidal monocytes in malignancy. *Cancer Immunol Immunother* **55**: 1534–41.

Nubel T, Dippold W, Kleinert H, Kaina B, Fritz G (2004). Lovastatin inhibits Rho-regulated expression of E-selectin by TNFalpha and attenuates tumor cell adhesion. *Faseb J* **18**: 140–42.

Ogawa J, Inoue H, Koide S (1996). Expression of alpha-1,3-fucosyltransferase type IV and VII genes is related to poor prognosis in lung cancer. *Cancer Res* **56**: 325–29.

Oosterling S, van der Bij GJ, Meijer GA, Tuk CW, van Garderen E, van Rooijen N et al. (2005). Macrophages direct tumour histology and clinical outcome in a colon cancer model. *J Pathol* **207**: 147–55.

Oppmann B, Lesley R, Blom B, Timans JC, Xu Y, Hunte B et al. (2000). Novel p19 protein engages IL-12p40 to form a cytokine, IL-23, with biological activities similar as well as distinct from IL-12. *Immunity* **13**: 715–25.

Ottaiano A, Franco R, Aiello Talamanca A, Liguori G, Tatangelo F, Delrio P et al. (2006). Overexpression of both CXC chemokine receptor 4 and vascular endothelial growth factor proteins predicts early distant relapse in stage II–III colorectal cancer patients. *Clin Cancer Res* **12**: 2795–803.

Palladino MA, Bahjat FR, Theodorakis EA, Moldawer LL (2003). Anti-TNF-[alpha] therapies: the next generation. *Nat Rev Drug Discov* **2**: 736–46.

Picon A, Gold LI, Wang J, Cohen A, Friedman E (1998). A subset of metastatic human colon cancers expresses elevated levels of transforming growth factor beta1. *Cancer Epidemiol Biomarkers Prev* **7**: 497–504.

Popivanova BK (2008). Blocking TNF-α in mice reduces colorectal carcinogenesis associated with chronic colitis. *J Clin Investig* **118**: 560–70.

Qi K, Qiu H, Rutherford J, Zhao Y, Nance DM, Orr FW (2004). Direct visualization of nitric oxide release by liver cells after the arrest of metastatic tumor cells in the hepatic microvasculature. *J Surg Res* **119**: 29–35.

Rhodes JM, Campbell BJ (2002). Inflammation and colorectal cancer: IBD-associated and sporadic cancer compared. *Trends Mol Med* **8**: 10–16.

Robinson SC, Coussens LM (2005). Soluble mediators of inflammation during tumor development. *Adv Cancer Res* **93**: 159–87.

Rose-John S, Waetzig GH, Scheller Jr, Gratzinger J, Seegert D (2007). The IL-6/sIL-6R complex as a novel target for therapeutic approaches. *Expert Opin Ther Targets* **11**: 613–24.

Rubie C, Kollmar O, Frick VO, Wagner M, Brittner B, Graber S et al. (2008). Differential CXC receptor expression in colorectal carcinomas. *Scand J Immunol* **68**: 635–44.

Rubie C, Oliveira V, Kempf K, Wagner M, Tilton B, Rau B et al. (2006a). Involvement of chemokine receptor CCR6 in colorectal cancer metastasis. *Tumour Biol* **27**: 166–74.

Rubie C, Oliveira-Frick V, Rau B, Schilling M, Wagner M (2006b). Chemokine receptor CCR6 expression in colorectal liver metastasis. *J Clin Oncol* **24**: 5173–74. Author reply 5174.

Salvucci O, Bouchard A, Baccarelli A, Deschenes J, Sauter G, Simon R et al. (2006). The role of CXCR4 receptor expression in breast cancer: a large tissue microarray study. *Breast Cancer Res Treat* **97**: 275–83.

Sato M, Narita T, Kimura N, Zenita K, Hashimoto T, Manabe T et al. (1997). The association of sialyl Lewis(a) antigen with the metastatic potential of human colon cancer cells. *Anticancer Res* **17**: 3505–11.

Schneider MR, Hoeflich A, Fischer JR, Wolf E, Sordat B, Lahm H (2000). Interleukin-6 stimulates clonogenic growth of primary and metastatic human colon carcinoma cells. *Cancer Lett* **151**: 31–38.

Shields JD, Fleury ME, Yong C, Tomei AA, Randolph GJ, Swartz MA (2007). Autologous chemotaxis as a mechanism of tumor cell homing to lymphatics via interstitial flow and autocrine CCR7 signaling. *Cancer Cell* **11**: 526–38.

Sica A, Schioppa T, Mantovani A, Allavena P (2006). Tumour-associated macrophages are a distinct M2 polarised population promoting tumour progression: potential targets of anti-cancer therapy. *Eur J Cancer* **42**: 717–27.

Sickert D, Aust DE, Langer S, Haupt I, Baretton GB, Dieter P (2005). Characterization of macrophage subpopulations in colon cancer using tissue microarrays. *Histopathology* **46**: 515–21.

Soma G, Inagawa H, Fukushima Y, Kanou J, Tomita K, Takano M et al. (1998). Preservation of metastatic ability of colorectal tumor cells stratified by inducibility of endogenous tumor necrosis factor after orthotopic transplantation in nude mice. *Anticancer Res* **18**: 3427–32.

Song X, Voronov E, Dvorkin T, Fima E, Cagnano E, Benharroch D et al. (2003). Differential effects of IL-1 alpha and IL-1 beta on tumorigenicity patterns and invasiveness. *J Immunol* **171**: 6448–56.

Suzuki A, Hanada T, Mitsuyama K, Yoshida T, Kamizono S, Hoshino T et al. (2001). CIS3/SOCS3/SSI3 plays a negative regulatory role in STAT3 activation and intestinal inflammation. *J Exp Med* **193**: 471–81.

Taga T, Kishimoto T (1997). gp130 and the interleukin-6 family of cytokines. *Ann Rev Immunol* **15**: 797–819.

Taketo MM (2009). Role of bone marrow-derived cells in colon cancer: lessons from mouse model studies. *J Gastroenterol* **44**: 93–102.

Tan SY, Fan Y, Luo HS, Shen ZX, Guo Y, Zhao LJ (2005). Prognostic significance of cell infiltrations of immunosurveillance in colorectal cancer. *World J Gastroenterol* **11**: 1210–14.

Tan ZY, Bealgey KW, Fang Y, Gong YM, Bao S (2009). Interleukin-23: Immunological roles and clinical implications. *Int J Biochem Cell Biol* **41**: 733–35.

Tang G, Minemoto Y, Dibling B, Purcell NH, Li Z, Karin M et al. (2001). Inhibition of JNK activation through NF-[kappa]B target genes. *Nature* **414**: 313–17.

Theiss AL, Simmons JG, Jobin C, Lund PK (2005). Tumor necrosis factor (TNF) alpha increases collagen accumulation and proliferation in intestinal myofibroblasts via TNF receptor 2. *J Biol Chem* **280**: 36099–109.

Tremblay PL, Auger FA, Huot J (2006). Regulation of transendothelial migration of colon cancer cells by E-selectin-mediated activation of p38 and ERK MAP kinases. *Oncogene* **25**: 6563–73.

Tremblay PL, Huot J, Auger FA (2008). Mechanisms by which E-selectin regulates diapedesis of colon cancer cells under flow conditions. *Cancer Res* **68**: 5167–76.

Ueno H, Murphy J, Jass JR, Mochizuki H, Talbot IC (2002). Tumour 'budding' as an index to estimate the potential of aggressiveness in rectal cancer. *Histopathol* **40**: 127–32.

Vidal-Vanaclocha F (2008). The prometastatic microenvironment of the liver. *Cancer Microenviron* **1**: 113–29.

Vidal-Vanaclocha F, Fantuzzi G, Mendoza L, Fuentes AM, Anasagasti MJ, Martin J et al. (2000). IL-18 regulates IL-1beta-dependent hepatic melanoma metastasis via vascular cell adhesion molecule-1. *Proc Natl Acad Sci USA* **97**: 734–39.

Voronov E, Shouval DS, Krelin Y, Cagnano E, Benharroch D, Iwakura Y et al. (2003). IL-1 is required for tumor invasiveness and angiogenesis. *Proc Natl Acad Sci USA* **100**: 2645–50.

Wang HH, McIntosh AR, Hasinoff BB, MacNeil B, Rector E, Nance DM et al. (2002). Regulation of B16F1 melanoma cell metastasis by inducible functions of the hepatic microvasculature. *Eur J Cancer* **38**: 1261–70.

Wang HH, McIntosh AR, Hasinoff BB, Rector ES, Ahmed N, Nance DM et al. (2000). B16 melanoma cell arrest in the mouse liver induces nitric oxide release and sinusoidal cytotoxicity: a natural hepatic defense against metastasis. *Cancer Res* **60**: 5862–69.

Wang N, Thuraisingam T, Fallavollita L, Ding A, Radzioch D, Brodt P (2006). The secretory leukocyte protease inhibitor is a type 1 insulin-like growth factor receptor-regulated protein that protects against liver metastasis by attenuating the host proinflammatory response. *Cancer Res* **66**: 3062–70.

Wei AC, Greig PD, Grant D, Taylor B, Langer B, Gallinger S (2006). Survival after hepatic resection for colorectal metastases: a 10-year experience. *Ann Surg Oncol* **13**: 668–76.

Weiss T, Grell M, Hessabi B, Bourteele S, Muller G, Scheurich P et al. (1997). Enhancement of TNF receptor p60-mediated cytotoxicity by TNF receptor p80: requirement of the TNF receptor-associated factor-2 binding site. *J Immunol* **158**: 2398–404.

Wilson JAP (2008). Tumor Necrosis Factor {alpha} and Colitis-Associated Colon Cancer. *N Engl J Med* **358**: 2733–2734.

Wittig BM, Kaulen H, Thees R, Schmitt C, Knolle P, Stock J et al. (1996). Elevated serum E-selectin in patients with liver metastases of colorectal cancer. *Eur J Cancer* **32A**: 1215–18.

Witz I (2008). The selectin–selectin ligand axis in tumor progression. *Cancer Metast Rev* **27**: 19–30.

Witz IP, Levy-Nissenbaum O (2006). The tumor microenvironment in the post-PAGET era. *Cancer Lett* **242**: 1–10.

Wolf M, Clark-Lewis I, Buri C, Langen H, Lis M, Mazzucchelli L (2003). Cathepsin D specifically cleaves the chemokines macrophage inflammatory protein-1 alpha, macrophage inflammatory protein-1 beta, and SLC that are expressed in human breast cancer. *Am J Pathol* **162**: 1183–90.

Wynes MW, Frankel SK, Riches DW (2004). IL-4-induced macrophage-derived IGF-I protects myofibroblasts from apoptosis following growth factor withdrawal. *J Leukoc Biol* **76**: 1019–27.

Wynes MW, Riches DW (2003). Induction of macrophage insulin-like growth factor-I expression by the Th2 cytokines IL-4 and IL-13. *J Immunol* **171**: 3550–59.

Yang X, Lu P, Ishida Y, Kuziel WA, Fujii C, Mukaida N (2006). Attenuated liver tumor formation in the absence of CCR2 with a concomitant reduction in the accumulation of hepatic stellate cells, macrophages and neovascularization. *Int J Cancer* **118**: 335–45.

Yakar S, Leroith D, Brodt P (2005). The role of the growth hormone/insulin-like growth factor axis in tumor growth and progression: lessons from animal models. *Cytokine Growth Factor Rev* **16**: 407–20.

Yamamoto M, Yoshizaki K, Kishimoto T, Ito H (2000). IL-6 Is Required for the Development of Th1 Cell-Mediated Murine Colitis. *J Immunol* **164**: 4878–82.

Yanagida H, Kaibori M, Yoshida H, Habara K, Yamada M, Kamiyama Y et al. (2006). Hepatic Ischemia/Reperfusion Upregulates the Susceptibility of Hepatocytes To Confer the Induction of Inducible Nitric Oxide Synthase Gene Expression. *Shock* **26**: 162–68.

Yang SK, Eckmann L, Panja A, Kagnoff MF (1997). Differential and regulated expression of C-X-C, C-C, and C-chemokines by human colon epithelial cells. *Gastroenterology* **113**: 1214–23.

Yang X, Lu P, Fujii C, Nakamoto Y, Gao JL, Kaneko S et al. (2005). Essential contribution of a chemokine, CCL3, and its receptor, CCR1, to hepatocellular carcinoma progression. *Int J Cancer* **118**: 1869–76.

Ye C, Kiriyama K, Mistuoka C, Kannagi R, Ito K, Watanabe T et al. (1995). Expression of E-selectin on endothelial cells of small veins in human colorectal cancer. *Int J Cancer* **61**: 455–60.

Yoshimatsu K, Ishibashi K, Yokomizo H, Umehara A, Yoshida K, Fujimoto T et al. (2006). Can the survival of patients with recurrent disease after curative resection of colorectal cancer be prolonged by the administration of cimetidine? *Gan To Kagaku Ryoho* **33**: 1730–32.

Zeelenberg IS, Ruuls-Van Stalle L, Roos E (2003). The chemokine receptor CXCR4 is required for outgrowth of colon carcinoma micrometastases. *Cancer Res* **63**: 3833–39.

Zhao D, Keates AC, Kuhnt-Moore S, Moyer MP, Kelly CP, Pothoulakis C (2001). Signal transduction pathways mediating neurotensin-stimulated interleukin-8 expression in human colonocytes. *J Biol Chem* **276**: 44464–71.

Zipin-Roitman A, Meshel T, Sagi-Assif O, Shalmon B, Avivi C, Pfeffer RM et al. (2007). CXCL10 promotes invasion-related properties in human colorectal carcinoma cells. *Cancer Res* **67**: 3396–405.

Zlotnik A (2004). Chemokines in neoplastic progression. *Semin Cancer Biol* **14**: 181–85.

Chapter 11

MOLECULAR PROGNOSTIC MARKERS IN COLON CANCER

Thomas Winder[1,3] and Heinz-Josef Lenz[1,2]

[1] Division of Medical Oncology, Keck School of Medicine, University of Southern California/Norris Comprehensive Cancer Center, Los Angeles, CA 90033, USA
[2] Department of Preventive Medicine, Keck School of Medicine, University of Southern California/Norris Comprehensive Cancer Center, Los Angeles, CA 90033, USA, e-mail: lenz_h@ccnt.usc.edu
[3] Department for Internal Medicine, Academic Teaching Hospital Feldkirch, Feldkirch 6800, Austria

Abstract: Colorectal cancer arises as a consequence of the accumulation of genetic and epigenetic alterations. Significant progress has been made to identify the different biomarkers associated with the biological and clinical behaviour of colorectal tumours. Several new molecular predictive and prognostic markers have been identified and are now being translated into routine clinical practice. One of the challenges is that most biomarker studies that are carried out retrospectively need to be validated prospectively with molecular markers as a secondary objective according to level II evidence. Establishing associations between molecular fingerprints, disease-free survival/overall survival and response will result in more successful and less toxic therapeutic regimens for cancer patients. This book chapter aims to summarize the most currently available markers in colorectal cancer that provide prognostic or predictive information, including clinicopathologic prognostic markers, genomic instability, genetic markers and epigenetic markers.

Key words: Colorectal carcinoma · Prognostic markers · Predictive markers · Genomic instability · Methylation

11.1 Introduction

Colorectal cancer is a result of an accumulation of genetic and epigenetic alterations that lead to the transformation of normal colonic epithelium to colon adenocarcinoma. The sequential process of benign adenomas to malignant adenocarcinomas is well characterized (Fig. 11.1). Several molecular events affect signalling pathways creating a clonal growth advantage that leads to outgrowth of malignant cells, which manifests itself as invasive adenocarcinoma. Vogelstein et al. postulated a seminal model of colorectal tumourigenesis in which the steps required for the development of cancer often involve the mutational activation of oncogenes (K-Ras) coupled with the loss of several genes that normally suppress tumourigenesis (*APC, DCC, p53*) (Vogelstein et al., 1988). Moreover, it has been estimated that a minimum of four to five mutational events must accumulate during carcinogenesis to develop an invasive colorectal cancer (Fujiwara et al., 1998). This stepwise accumulation of molecular alterations occurs concomitantly with a stepwise change in morphology; beginning with a small adenomatous polyp, followed by formation of a larger polyp with dysplasia, which ultimately leads to the development of invasive carcinoma. This adenoma-carcinoma molecular pathway applies predominantly to sporadic colorectal cancers, but it also characterizes familial adenomatous polyposis (FAP). Alternatively, this pathway may be referred to as the chromosomal instability pathway because colorectal tumours arising from this pathway are characterized by gross chromosomal abnormalities including deletions, insertions, and loss of heterozygosity (Noffsinger, 2009).

Subsequently, another pathway leading from adenomatous polyps to colorectal cancer, the DNA mismatch repair pathway, was described by Aaltonen et al. (Aaltonen et al., 1993). This pathway is associated with colorectal cancers arising from hereditary non-polyposis colon cancer (HNPCC). The key elements of this pathway are dysfunction of DNA mismatch repair enzymes resulting from germline mutation in one of several DNA mismatch repair genes, most commonly *MLH1* or *MSH2*. The result is the development of microsatellite instability (MSI) in the tumours derived through this genetic pathway (Noffsinger, 2009).

Evidence that adenomas might not represent the only colorectal cancer precursor began to emerge around the 1990s (Longacre and Fenoglio-Preiser, 1990). Lesions formerly classified as hyperplastic polyps were recognized as a heterogeneous group

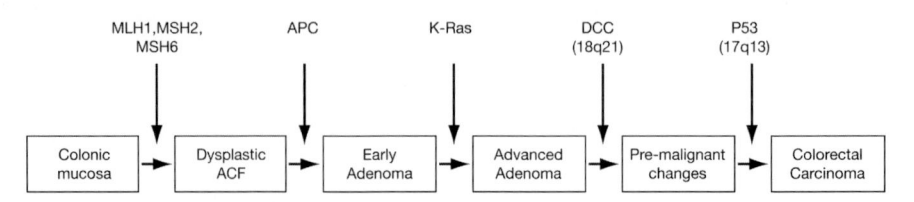

Fig. 11.1 Pathway of mutations in colorectal cancer development. Abbreviations: MLH (mutL homolog); MSH (mutS homolog); APC (adenomatosis polyposis coli); ACF (aberrant crypt focus); DCC (deleted in colon cancer)

Table 11.1 Molecular classification of colorectal carcinoma

	Chromosomal instability pathway	Mismatch repair pathway	Serrated pathway	
Heredity	Hereditary and sporadic	Hereditary	Hereditary and sporadic	
CIMP status	Negative	Negative	High	
MSI status	MSS	MSI-H	MSI-H	MSI-L
Chromosomal instability	Present	Absent	Absent	Absent
KRAS mutation	+++	+/–	—	—
BRAF mutation	—	—	+++	+++
MLH1 status	Normal	Mutation	Methylated	Partial methylation

Abbreviations: CIMP (CpG island methylator phenotype); MSI (microsatellite instability); MSI-H (high-level microsatellite instability); MSI-L (low-level microsatellite instability); MSS (microsatellite stability).
Adapted from Noffsinger et al. (2009)

of polyps, some of which have a significant risk for neoplastic transformation. These findings suggested that an alternate serrated pathway to colorectal carcinoma might exist (Noffsinger, 2009) (see Table 11.1).

The aim of this chapter is to provide an update of the most recent data on predictive and prognostic markers in colon cancer. The development of individualized therapeutic strategies requires a profound understanding of the molecular mechanisms in tumour development and of action of chemotherapeutic and targeting agents.

11.2 Pathologic Prognostic Markers

The Union Internationale Contre le Cancer/American Joint Cancer Committeee (UICC/AJCC) tumour node metastasis (TNM) stage remains the gold standard of prognostic factors in CRC. The TNM staging system was initially developed to predict prognosis, but its function has expanded to aid in the choice of treatment. While adjuvant treatment is widely accepted in the treatment of stage III disease, patients with stage II are not yet recommended for this treatment protocol (Zlobec and Lugli, 2008). Tumour grade is recognized as an important prognostic factor in CRC, and its grading system is based on the percentage of gland formation. However, different grading systems complicate an appropriate determination of the prognostic significance in CRC. The College of American Pathologists has recommended a two-tier system, whereas the WHO has recommended a four-tier system (Turner et al., 2007).

Tumour budding, also known as dedifferentiation, is a recently recognized feature that represents a high-grade, undifferentiated component of a tumour at the leading invasive edge. Tumour budding may predict high risk of recurrence after curative surgery and the survival rate in stage II patients may not be significantly different than that in all stage III patients (Park et al., 2005). However, this feature needs to be better defined because the frequency of tumour budding varies widely in the literature (Turner et al., 2007).

The presence and the number of lymph node involvement is undoubtedly the most essential prognostic factor in CRC. Therefore, accurate analysis of regional lymph nodes is one of the most important issues for an optimal pathological staging and for decision-making regarding adjuvant chemotherapy in CRC. The College of American Pathologists has established guidelines for the pathologic evaluation of colorectal cancer resection specimens. These guidelines include the recommendation that, if fewer than 12 lymph nodes are found, additional techniques for visual enhancement should be considered (Compton, 2000). The most compelling evidence for a therapeutic benefit of increased lymph node recovery comes from the Intergroup 0089 trial. After stratification for stage and adjustment for covariates, including the number of positive lymph nodes, both overall survival and cause-specific survival were related to the number of lymph nodes recovered in both node-positive and node-negative diseases (Le Voyer et al., 2003). Readers may consult chapter 12 in this book for more information.

11.3 Genomic Instability

11.3.1 Loss of Heterozygosity of 17p and 18q (LOH)

Colorectal cancer is characterized by the sequential inactivation of tumour suppressor genes (*p53*, *DCC*, *Smad2*, *Smad4*) and genetic alterations involving oncogenes (e.g. K-*Ras*). Tumours generate, through the inactivation of tumour suppressor genes, chromosomal instability with frequent allelic losses. The short arm of chromosome 17 (17p) and the long arm of chromosome 18 (18q) are frequently lost and are observed in up to 70% of colorectal carcinomas. To that effect, *DCC*, *Smad2* and *Smad4* genes located on chromosome 18q and *p53* located on chromosome 17p, have been shown to play a role in the pathogenesis of colorectal cancer (Baker et al., 1989; Fearon et al., 1990). Moreover, Watanabe et al. showed a prognostic influence for 18qLOH in stage III colon cancer (Watanabe et al., 2001). However, the Pan-European Trials in Adjuvant Colon Cancer 3 (PETACC 3) trial did not show 18q LOH to be an independent prognostic factor in stage II + III colon cancer (Roth et al., 2009).

Loss of heterozygosity (LOH) has been implicated as an important mechanism of tumour suppressor gene inactivation. One of the most promising markers studied to date is chromosome 18q loss, observed in up to 70% of CRC and in almost 50% of late adenomas (Vogelstein et al., 1988). This loss involves a candidate tumour suppressor gene, termed *DCC* (deleted in colon cancer gene), which encodes a protein with significant homology to the cell adhesion molecule and is mapped to chromosome 18q21. DCC is thought to play a key role in colorectal carcinogenesis

(Fearon et al., 1990). The DCC protein was identified as a transmembrane receptor for netrins, a key factor in axon guidance in the developing nervous system (Keino-Masu et al., 1996). The highest levels of DCC expression appear to be present in the nervous system. Loss of DCC as a result of 18q deletion impairs adequate levels of programmed cell death, and provides the malignant cells with selective growth advantage (Mehlen and Fearon, 2004). Chromosomal loss of 18q leads to haplo-insufficiency at DCC and thus decreased protein expression. Chromosome 18q LOH and decreased mRNA expression of DCC have been associated with poor survival in colorectal cancer stage II as well as stage III (Fearon et al., 1990; Shibata et al., 1996). Moreover, patients with locally advanced stage II or stage III disease appear to demonstrate a significantly poorer prognosis with loss of 18q (Sun et al., 1999). Popat et al. summarized in a large meta-analysis that the evaluation of chromosome 18q loss and DCC status may define patients who are more likely to benefit from adjuvant chemotherapy (Popat and Houlston, 2005). Nevertheless, these findings need further validation in prospective clinical trials using consistent methodology.

The *Smad* tumour suppressor genes located on chromosome 18q encode proteins that play an essential role as downstream regulators in the transforming growth factor ß (TGF-beta) signalling pathways. The Smad4 protein acts as a trimer and forms complexes with the receptor-phosphorylated Smad2 and Smad3. These complexes then translocate from the cytoplasm to the nucleus where association with DNA binding factors facilitates the transcription of target genes. Abrogation of Smad4 function may cause a breakdown in this signalling pathway and loss of transcription of genes critical to cell-cycle control (Woodford-Richens et al., 2001). Smad4 is structurally altered in colorectal carcinomas where it has been associated with late stage or metastatic colorectal cancer. Moreover, the level of Smad4 mRNA expression has been associated with a 5-year probability of recurrence of 30% (high Smad4 mRNA expression) and 80% (low Smad4 mRNA expression) in Dukes C patients after 5-FU-based adjuvant chemotherapy (Alhopuro et al., 2005). Recently, Roth et al. showed an independent prognostic value of Smad4 loss in Stage III colon cancer patients (Roth et al., 2009).

The tumour suppressor gene *p53* is mutated in approximately 50% of CRC and is located on chromosome 17p. p53 acts as a checkpoint monitoring the integrity of the genome. If DNA is damaged, p53 accumulates and switches off replication to allow extra time for its repair. Tumour cells in which p53 is inactivated or lost will be genetically less stable leading to rapid selection of malignant clones (Lane, 1992). p53 abnormalities have been studied extensively for their role in prognosis and response to therapy in colorectal cancer. However, the results are heterogeneous and conflicting because p53 abnormalities are usually detected through various methodologies that do not directly address the functional status of the two alleles of the gene. Therefore, Munro et al. concluded in a review that with current methods of assessment, p53 is a poor guide to both prognosis and response or resistance to therapy in CRC (Munro et al., 2005).

11.3.2 DNA – Ploidy

Chromosomal instability (CIN) is found in 60–70% of cases and is characterized by aneuploid cell populations, multiple losses of heterozygosity events (LOH) and a higher frequency in tumours localized in the left colon or rectum. Ploidy analysis is performed on a sample of the tumour to determine how many of the cells have the normal amount of DNA and how many have more or less than the normal amount (called aneuploid). Cancerous cells are rapidly dividing cells. Tumours with higher proportions of aneuploid cells are considered to be more aggressive. DNA ploidy can be determined by morphometric and image cytometry, but the flow cytometric approach, permitting a fast, automated and highly sensitive determination, is by far the most widely used method (Silvestrini, 2000). Unfortunately, there is no laboratory standardization in terms of type of material or quality control programs. Therefore, studies on DNA ploidy are discordant and must be interpreted with caution.

The American Society of Clinical Oncology (ASCO) Tumour Marker Expert Panel reviewed the literature for the use of ploidy as prognostic factor in CRC. Of the 14 series, eight found that patients with a DNA aneuploid tumour or elevated DNA index had significantly worse survival after surgery than those patients with DNA diploid or lower DNA index tumours. However, the authors concluded that the inconsistent results do not support the use of flow cytometrically-derived DNA ploidy to determine prognosis of operable colorectal cancer (Locker et al., 2006).

11.3.3 Microsatellite Instability (MSI)

Microsatellite instability (MSI) is a measure of the inability of the DNA nucleotide mismatch repair system (MMR) to correct errors that commonly occur during the replication of DNA. It is characterized by the accumulation of single nucleotide mutations and length alterations in repetitive microsatellite nucleotide sequences common throughout the genome. Initially, MSI was linked to the hereditary non-polyposis colorectal cancer (HNPCC) but 15–20% of the sporadic CRC demonstrated high levels of MSI (MSI-H) as well (Peltomaki, 2003). In most sporadic cases, MSI occurs when the promoter region of the mismatch repair genes (*MLH1*, *MSH2* and *MSH6*) is silenced by CpG island hypermethylation (Cunningham et al., 1998). Identification of MSI requires DNA extraction from tumour and normal tissue.

MSI-H tumours are associated with ages < 60, higher T stage, lower N stage, right-sided tumour location and often display unusual histopathologic characteristics (mucinous and poorly-differentiated). Another important difference between tumours with MSI-H and MSI-stable (MSS) status concerns their predictive and prognostic significance. In a review including 32 studies with 7,642 patients, Popat et al. demonstrated that MSI-H was associated with significantly improved prognosis compared with MSS tumours (Popat et al., 2005a). Accordingly, the data of the PETAC III trial presented recently at the ASCO 2009 meeting by Tejpar et al. showed MSI-H as a strong prognostic factor for relapse-free and overall survival in Stage II and III colorectal cancer. However, the subgroup analysis suggested a stronger effect in Stage II than in Stage III, which might be explained by stage-specific biological effects of MSI (Tejpar et al., 2009).

MSI status has also been reported as a predictive marker for lack of response to 5-fluorouracil (FU)-based chemotherapy (Ribic et al., 2003). Furthermore, Sargent et al. showed in an independent dataset from randomized clinical trials that MSI-H tumours receiving 5-FU-based chemotherapy were associated with significantly shorter overall survival (HR = 3.15, p = 0.03) (Sargent et al., 2008). The retrospective National Cancer Institute/National Surgical Adjuvant Breast and Bowel Project (NCI-NSABP) analysis, which focused on the role of MSI-H as a predictive marker for the benefit of adjuvant chemotherapy, failed to identify an interaction between adjuvant chemotherapy and MSI status. They suggest that the improved prognosis for MSI-H CRC patients is explained by the specific tumour biology and that it is not necessarily a treatment effect (Kim et al., 2007). At ASCO 2009, Tejpar showed an improved 5-year DFS for MSI-H versus MSS patients treated with 5-FU (83 and 66%, respectively; p = 0.0077). Recently, Bertagnolli et al. showed in the randomly-assigned CALGB-89803 study that MSI-H predicts improved outcome in patients with stage III CRC treated with irinotecan, FU, and leucovorin as compared with those receiving FU/leucovorin (Bertagnolli et al., 2009). However, the PETACC 3 data presented by Tejpar at the 2009 ASCO meeting did not confirm an effect of the addition of irinotecan in patients with MSI-H (Tejpar et al., 2009).

Due to the conflicting data, the use of MSI status in the prediction of benefit from 5-FU or irinotecan in colorectal cancer cannot be recommended at this time. This marker should be more extensively investigated in large prospective series, especially in patients being considered for treatment with 5-FU alone (i.e. stage II patients).

11.4 Genetic Markers

11.4.1 Metabolic Genes

11.4.1.1 Thymidylate Synthase (TS)

Since its introduction in 1957 by Heidelberger et al. (Heidelberger et al., 1957), the fluoropyrimidine 5-FU still remains the basis of CRC treatment, both in adjuvant and palliative settings. Moreover, the fluoropyrimidines remain a major component of many standard regimens for numerous cancer types (e.g. breast cancer and epithelial tumours of the upper aerodigestive tract) and a baseline component in many experimental regimens. The single agent response rates of 5-FU vary from 20 to 25% of patients with advanced stage CRC (Gill et al., 2004). 5-FU, an anolog of uracil, is an anticancer pro-drug that is converted intracellularly into three main active metabolites: 5-fluoro-2-deoxyuridine monophosphate (FdUMP), fluorodeoxyuridine triphosphate (FdUTP), and fluouridine triphosphate (FUTP). The main toxicities under 5-FU treatment are leucopenia, stomatitis and diarrhea. The efficacy of 5-FU-based chemotherapy has been associated with expression levels of several genes including thymidylate synthase (*TS*), thymidine phosphorylase (*TP*), and dihydropyrimidine dehydrogenase (*DPD*).

Thymidylate synthase (TS) is the primary target of the active metabolite of 5-FU, 5-fluorodeoxyuridine monophosphate (FdUMP). FdUMP forms an extremely stable ternary complex with TS, FdUMP and the cofactor 5,10-methylenetetrahydrofolate (CH2FH4) blocking the conversion of deoxyuridine monophosphate (dUMP) to deoxythymidine monophosphate (dTMP). Thus, TS is the sole de novo source of thymidine in the cell. Inhibition of TS blocks dTMP production, and therefore rapidly shuts off DNA synthesis and repair and triggers apoptosis (Danenberg, 1977; Spears et al., 1988).

Although conflicting results on TS protein and mRNA expression have been reported, several independent studies consistently agreed that low levels of intratumoural TS protein and mRNA expression are strong prognostic markers for response to 5-FU-based chemotherapy regimens in CRC (Popat et al., 2004). Additionally, tumours expressing high levels of TS appeared to have poorer overall survival (OS) compared with tumours expressing low levels. *TS* gene expression levels, polymorphisms and protein expression levels can be assessed in tumour tissue and blood samples using PCR and immunohistochemistry (IHC) techniques. Both techniques show a strong association, especially in low TS levels. Although IHC is most accessible, both in terms of cost and labor intensiveness, the assignment of TS protein expression is semi-quantitative, observer-dependent and is assessed by a number of differing scoring systems. So far, the PCR technique of deriving *TS* gene expression allows quantitative estimates and therefore should be the benchmark (Popat et al., 2004, 2005b). Development of laser capture micro-dissection decreases the level of significant normal tissue contamination that when present, can affect gene expression.

TS gene expression is in part regulated by the *TS* promoter enhancer region (TSER). The variable number of tandem repeat polymorphic copies in this region mainly leads to double or triple (2R or 3R) tandem repeats of a 28-bp sequence present in the 5'-untranslated region of the gene. Two polymorphisms have been associated with altered *TS* gene expression. The first and most frequent polymorphism consists of a double (2R) or a triple (3R) tandem repeat. Polymorphisms within the tandem repeats have been postulated to affect transcriptional and/or translational efficacy of the *TS* gene (Pullarkat et al., 2001). The frequency of polymorphisms differs between ethnicities.

Pullarkat et al. (Pullarkat et al., 2001) showed in metastatic CRC (mCRC) patients, homozygous for the 3R variant (3R/3R), a 3.6-fold increase in *TS* mRNA levels in comparison to patients homozygous for the 2R (2R/2R) *TS* variant. Moreover, patients with 3R/3R genotypes benefit less from 5-FU-based chemotherapy than those with 2R/2R and 2R/3R genotypes. In addition, a multicenter prospective study in mCRC patients treated with 5-FU-based chemotherapy demonstrated that TS activity measured in primary tumour was a significant survival predictor. The 2R/2R TS genotype is associated with favorable median survival compared to the 2R/3R and 3R/3R genotype (19 month versus 10.3 month versus 14 month) (Etienne et al., 2002). However, carriers of the 3R/3R genotype experience less toxic side effects of a 5-FU-based regimen when compared to patients expressing the 2R/3R or 2R/2R *TS* genotype. A systematic review and meta-analysis revealed in 3,497 patients with CRC that high levels of TS in patients at any stage of their disease are predictive of outcome (Popat et al., 2004).

The mentioned relation of *TS* gene expression levels and distinct *TS* gene polymorphisms applies to the majority of patients. However, approximately 25% of patients homozygous for the 3R/3R TS genotype were identified to have low TS expression levels. A single nucleotide polymorphism (SNP) resulting in a G → C change has been observed within the 3R variant of the *TS* gene (3RC polymorphism). Whereas the G allele of this SNP has been linked to increased gene expression and protein levels, the 3RC polymorphism was found to lead to significantly decreased TS expression compared to the 3RG variant (Mandola et al., 2003). These findings may explain the observation that patients with the 3R/3R polymorphism may have low *TS* gene expression levels and might benefit from 5-FU-based chemotherapy.

It must be noted that the TS genotype analysis is affected by the material (blood or tumour tissue). In human colon cancer, the TS locus at the short arm of chromosome 18 is frequently altered. Loss of heterozygosity (LOH) at this locus leads to different genotypes in tumours than in peripheral blood. Therefore, evaluation of TS polymorphisms should include the search for LOH of the short arm of chromosome 18 in order to predict the clinical response to 5-FU-based chemotherapy.

Large prospective clinical trials are needed to validate the role of TS before implementing TS genotyping and intratumoural TS protein and mRNA expression into routine clinical practice.

11.4.1.2 Dihydropyrimidine Dehydrogenase (DPD)

Patients with dihydropyrimidine dehydrogenase (DPD) levels within the normal range rapidly inactivate 80% of the administered 5-FU as 2-fluoro-ß-alanine by the liver. Patients deficient in DPD retain 5-FU over a much longer half-life and excrete mostly unchanged 5-FU in the urine. In such patients, however, deficiency in DPD activity leads to severe toxicity in the context of 5-FU (e.g. diarrhea, neutropenia, hand foot syndrome), which may even be fatal. DPD activity is highly variable in normal tissues and thus, could affect the pharmacokinetics, toxicity, and antitumour activity of 5-FU (Salonga et al., 2000). Recently, a clinical test (TheraGuide 5-FU^{TM}) for assessing the risk of toxicity due to 5-FU-based chemotherapy has become available. TheraGuide-5-testing by Myriad offers full sequencing of the *DPD* gene as well as analysis of the *TS* gene.

Several clinical studies demonstrated an association between low DPD expression and better outcome in patients treated with a 5-FU-based chemotherapy (Soong et al., 2008). Moreover, Hoffmann et al. identified that *DPD* mRNA expression levels in peripheral blood of rectal cancer patients are associated with residual tumour categories. Hence, DPD expression levels might serve as a molecular marker for complete tumour resection (Hoffmann et al., 2009). The range of *DPD* mRNA expression among the responding tumours is relatively narrow (0.60×10^{-3} to 2.5×10^{-3}, 4.2 fold) compared with that of the non-responders (0.2×10^{-3} to 16×10^{-3}, 80 fold). Therefore, DPD expression $< 2.5 \times 10^{-3}$ is associated with a corresponding response rate of 50% (Salonga et al., 2000).

11.4.1.3 *Methylenetetrahydrofolate Reductase (MTHFR)*

Methylenetetrahydrofolate reductase (MTHFR) is an important enzyme in the folate pathway converting 5,10-MTHF to 5-methyltetrahydrofolate. Reduced enzyme activity has been associated with increased levels of 5,10-MTHF available for inhibiting TS, and therefore increased efficacy of 5-FU. Two SNPs within the *MTHFR* gene (C677T and A1298C) have been associated with altered enzyme activity. Notably, the amino acid change of alanine to valine (C677T) leads to reduced enzyme activity of the T allele and subsequently to an increased response rate to 5-FU-based regimens. The number of T alleles seems to correlate with response to 5-FU treatment (Funke et al., 2008).

11.4.2 EGFR Pathway and Potential Markers

11.4.2.1 K-Ras

Activating mutations in the K-Ras oncogene on the short arm of chromosome 12 are commonly associated with progression from a benign adenoma to a dysplastic adenocarcinoma and have been reported to occur in 30–40% of CRC (Vogelstein et al., 1988). Proteins of the Ras family are small G proteins that act as GDP/GTP-regulated switches to convey extracellular signals that influence cell proliferation and apoptosis. Mutations affecting any of these proteins at amino acids 12, 13 or 61 lock the enzyme in the GTP-bound, activated form (Haigis et al., 2008). Because of the K-Ras significance in EGFR signalling and in carcinogenesis, K-Ras mutational status is a promising predictive marker in EGFR targeted therapy (see Chapter 8 for more information).

After a series of non-randomized studies reporting little or no benefit from anti-EGFR therapy in *K-Ras* mutant subjects, evidence arising from randomized studies has become available. Lievre et al. showed for the first time that *K-Ras* mutations in metastatic CRC patients are a predictor of resistance to cetuximab therapy and are associated with a worse prognosis (Lievre et al., 2006). Moreover, *K-Ras* mutations are associated with a shorter survival in this patient cohort. The association of *K-Ras* mutations and resistance to anti-EGFR treatment, either cetuximab or panitumumab, was confirmed in large, retrospectively evaluated phase III studies (Amado et al., 2008; Karapetis et al., 2008).

In summary, these clinical studies highlight a strong predictive value of *K-Ras* mutations on EGFR targeted therapy in metastatic CRC patients. Therefore, the

National Comprehensive Cancer Network has revised its CRC practice guideline and recommends that CRC patients with known *K-Ras* mutation should not be treated with anti EGFR-antibody alone or in combination with other anticancer agents. The European Medicine Agency restricted the use of anti-EGFR antibody in metastatic CRC patients only with wild-type *K-Ras* status. Based on systematic review of the literature, the American Society of Clinical Oncology recommended testing of *K-Ras* mutation status before treatment with anti-EGFR antibodies in metastatic CRC (Allegra et al., 2009).

11.4.2.2 B-Raf

Genes of the *Raf* family mediate cellular response to growth signals. Genetic and biochemical evidence indicates that B-Raf is the principal downstream effector of K-Ras (see Chapter 8 for more details). Activating mutations in the *B-Raf* gene occur only in colorectal tumours that do not carry mutations in the *K-Ras* gene. Various studies have revealed that an activating mutation of B-Raf kinase (B-Raf-V600E) occurs in approximately 70% of sporadic MSI-H CRCs and approximately 10% of unselected CRCs. More specifically, *B-Raf* mutations are frequently associated with MLH1 inactivation due to promoter methylation but not to germline mutation (Minoo et al., 2007). Thus, mismatch repair-deficient tumours have a very high incidence of *B-Raf* mutations and a lower incidence of *K-Ras* mutations compared with MMR-proficient colorectal cancers (Rajagopalan et al., 2002).

A recent restrospective trial of 113 patients indicated that occurrence of oncogenic *B-Raf* alleles negatively interferes with the clinical response to monoclonal antibodies targeting EGFR (cetuximab and panitumumab). In addition, the data suggest that the role of *B-Raf* mutations in patients treated with EGFR-targeted drugs is similar to that played by mutated *K-Ras*. Moreover, individuals with *B-Raf* mutated tumours had a shorter PFS and OS than patients with *B-Raf* wild-type tumours (log-rank $p = 0.01$ and $p < 0.001$, respectively) (Di Nicolantonio et al., 2008). However, the latest data from the Crystal trial, presented at ASCO 2009, did not confirm B-Raf as a predictor for resistance to anti-EGFR monoclonal antibody treatment (Kohne et al., 2009). Therefore, further studies are needed to fully evaluate this marker in a prospective randomized clinical trial.

11.4.2.3 Germline Polymorphisms Within the EGFR Signalling Pathway

Cyclooxygenase-2 (COX-2) converts arachidonic acid to prostaglandins and promotes inflammation and cell proliferation. COX-2 is over-expressed in the majority of human colon cancers and is involved in cellular processes including tumour onset, metastases, angiogenesis, and resistance to chemotherapy. Supporting the importance of COX-2 in colorectal carcinogenesis, randomized trials have shown that aspirin and COX-2 selective inhibitors reduce risk of recurrent adenoma among high-risk patients (Flossmann and Rothwell, 2007; Ogino et al., 2008). The association of skin toxicity and favorable therapeutic response in EGFR-targeted therapy has stimulated the search for different polymorphisms that might have a functional impact on the EGFR pathway.

COX-2 G765C is a frequent single nucleotide polymorphism and the C-allele was shown to be associated with significantly lower *COX-2* promoter activity compared with the G-variant. Lurje et al. showed for the first time in a retrospective phase II clinical trial that polymorphisms in *COX-2* seem to be useful molecular markers to predict clinical outcome in patients with mCRC treated with single agent cetuximab. In addition, patients with the COX-2-765 C/C homozygous genotype had a favorable progression-free survival (PFS) (5.9 months) compared to homozygous and heterozygous G allele (1.3 months) (Lurje et al., 2008a).

The chimeric IgG1 monoclonal antibody cetuximab might also be able to induce antibody-dependent cell-mediated cytotoxicity. The killing function of immune cells is affected by two functional FC gamma receptor (*FCGR*) gene polymorphisms, FCGR2A-H131R and FCGR3A-V158F. Evidence now exists showing that these two polymorphisms may be useful molecular markers to predict clinical outcome in metastatic CRC patients treated with cetuximab (Zhang et al., 2007). However, larger, biomarker-embedded clinical trials are needed to confirm and validate these preliminary findings.

11.4.3 Angiogenesis

11.4.3.1 VEGF-Dependent Regulation of Angiogenesis

Vascular endothelial growth factor (VEGF) and its receptors VEGFR1, VEGFR2 and VEGFR3 are intimately involved in cell migration and proliferation and enhance endothelial cell survival and protection against endothelial cell apoptosis and senescence. The VEGF family is comprised of the five VEGF glycoproteins (VEGF-A, VEGF-B, VEGF-C, VEGF-D, VEGF-E) and PlGF-1 and PlGF-2. The best characterized of the VEGF family members, VEGF-A (commonly referred to as VEGF) and its receptor VEGFR2 are currently the key targets for anti-angiogenetic agents (Grothey and Galanis, 2009) (see Chapter 9, in this book for more details).

Bevacizumab is a recombinant humanized monoclonal IgG1 antibody targeting vascular endothelial growth factor-A (VEGF-A) reducing the availability of free circulating VEGF-A and thereby preventing receptor activation. Hurwitz et al. showed for the first time that bevacizumab significantly improved overall survival in patients with mCRC (Hurwitz et al., 2004). These data led to the FDA approval for the treatment of metastatic colorectal cancer in February 2004.

DNA sequence variations within the *VEGF* gene lead to altered VEGF production and/or activity. Lurje et al. indicated in patients with locally advanced colon cancer, that high expression variants of VEGF C+936T (VEGF +936 C/C) were significantly associated with time to recurrence (Lurje et al., 2008b). These findings demonstrate that VEGF C+936T may be an important prognostic factor for stage III CRC suggesting a potential role of tumour-associated angiogenesis in the development of CRC tumour relapse.

VEGF exerts its angiogenic effects via two different receptors, VEGFR1 and VEGFR2. Recently, our group showed that *VEGFR1* gene expression levels might predict risk for tumour recurrence in adjuvant colon cancer patients. Patients with lower *VEGFR1* gene expression levels had significantly longer time to tumour recurrence compared to those with higher *VEGFR1* gene expression (Ning et al., 2009). Moreover, we were able to show in patients with metastatic colorectal cancer treated with first line 5-FU or capecitabine with oxaliplatin and bevacizumab that high *VEGFR2* gene expression is associated with longer PFS than low *VEGFR2* gene expression levels (median PFS of 13.9 versus 7.2 months, respectively) (El-Khoueiry et al., 2009). However, our exploratory data warrant future confirmatory trials.

11.4.3.2 VEGF-Independent Regulation of Angiogenesis

The VEGF-independent regulation of angiogenesis stimulates vasculogenesis and angiogenesis in a complicated network. The EphrinB2-EphB4 pathway plays an important role in a variety of processes including angiogenesis, vascular remodeling, maturation and directed growth (Tickle and Altabef, 1999). The Delta-Notch pathway is shown not only to regulate artery-vein differentiation but also to stimulate blood vessel formation. An inhibitor of Delta-like 4 ligand (Dll4) such as a neutralizing antibody may have an anti-angiogenic effect by increasing non-functional endothelial sprouting and branching (Noguera-Troise et al., 2006).

Recently, interleukin-8 (IL-8), a member of the CXC chemokine family, has been reported to play a major role in VEGF-independent tumour angiogenesis. Induction of IL-8 preserved the angiogenic response in hypoxia-inducible factor 1 (HIF1)-α-deficient colon cancer cells, suggesting that IL-8 mediates angiogenesis independently of VEGF. Lurje et al. showed in stage III CRC patients that high expression variants of IL-8 T251A polymorphism (A/A genotype) were at higher risk of developing tumour recurrence (Lurje et al., 2008b). Furthermore, high expression variants of IL-1ß C+3954T polymorphism (T/T genotype) in stage II colon cancer patients indicated higher risk of developing tumour recurrence (Lurje et al., 2009). However, these findings require further confirmation in prospective clinical trials.

11.5 Epigenetic Markers

11.5.1 CpG Island Methylator Phenotype (CIMP)

CpG islands are short sequences in the CpG dinucleotide and can be found in the 5' region of about half of all human genes. Methylation of cytosine within 5' CpG islands is associated with loss of gene expression and has been seen in physiological conditions such as X chromosome inactivation and genomic imprinting. The CpG island methylator phenotype (CIMP) with widespread promoter methylation and tumour suppressor inactivation is a distinct epigenetic phenotype thought to be an important mechanism in colon cancer carcinogenesis. Methylation triggers the binding of methylated DNA-specific binding proteins to CpG sites, attracting histone-modifying enzymes that, in turn, focally establish a silenced chromatin state. Therefore, tumour suppressor gene methylation in cancer is usually associated with lack of gene transcription and absence of coding region mutation. Thus, CIMP is regarded as an alternative mechanism of gene inactivation in cancer (Issa, 2004; Lurje et al., 2007; Toyota et al., 1999).

CIMP-high CRC appear to have a distinct clinico-pathological and molecular profiles compared with CIMP-low tumours, which is associated with older age, proximal tumour location, poor differentiation, lower *TP53* mutation, MSI-H, and *BRAF* V600E mutation (Samowitz et al., 2005; van Rijnsoever et al., 2002). Aberrant CpG island hypermethylation (CIMP-high) does not occur in nonmalignant, normally differentiated cells. Methylated DNA derived from primary colorectal cancers cannot only be detected in the tumour tissue itself, but also in the serum and stool of corresponding patients. Therefore, Wallner et al. suggested that the methylation status of specific genes in the serum of patients with colorectal cancer could possibly be used as a pre-therapeutic predictor of outcome. The multivariate analysis in this study showed methylated serum DNA to be independently associated with poor outcome and a relative risk of death of 3.4 (95% CI, 1.4–8.1) (Wallner et al., 2006). However, a standardization of sample collection, DNA isolation and preparation as well as the usage of standardized assays need to be established before these markers can be introduced into routine clinical practice.

11.6 Ongoing Trials

11.6.1 E5202

This randomized phase III trial by the Eastern Cooperative Oncology Group is prospectively evaluating the prognostic value of MSI and 18q status in patients who have undergone surgery for stage II colon cancer. Patients are stratified into low-risk and high-risk categories based on 18q LOH and MSI status. Patients considered low risk (no 18q LOH) are being observed, and those considered high risk (i.e. 18q LOH, low frequency MSI or MSS) are randomly allocated to adjuvant treatment with 5-fluorouracil (5-FU), leucovorin, and oxaliplatin (FOLFOX) versus FOLFOX/bevacizumab (ECOG, 2005).

11.6.2 CALGB-C80405

The C80405 randomized phase III trial, conducted by the Cancer and Leukemia Group B (CALGB), is studying the efficacy of cetuximab and/or bevacizumab in combination with chemotherapy in patients with metastatic colorectal cancer. Patients are stratified according to physician-selected chemotherapy (oxaliplatin, leucovorin calcium, and fluorouracil [FOLFOX] *vs* irinotecan hydrochloride, leucovorin calcium, or fluorouracil [FOLFIRI]), prior adjuvant chemotherapy (yes *vs* no), and prior pelvic radiotherapy (yes *vs* no). Patients are randomly allocated to; 1. oxaliplatin or irinotecan with leucovorin, 5-FU and bevacizumab. 2. oxaliplatin or irinotecan with leucovorin, 5-FU and cetuximab or 3. oxaliplatin or irinotecan with leucovorin, 5-FU, bevacizumab and cetuximab (SWOG, 2005).

11.6.3 PETACC-8

The randomized phase III PETACC-8 trial conducted by the Fédération Francophone de Cancérologie Digestive is studying cetuximab in combination with oxaliplatin, leucovorin and 5-FU *vs* oxaliplatin/leucovorin/5-FU alone. In this open-label, randomized, controlled, multicenter study, patients are stratified according to obstruction/perforation status (no obstruction and no perforation *vs* obstruction and/or perforation), N stage (N1 versus N2), and T stage (T1-3 versus T4) (FFCD, 2005).

11.7 Conclusions

Several prognostic and predictive molecular markers for colorectal cancer have been identified in the past few years (Table 11.2). However, the implementation of these biomarkers into routine clinical use remains a challenge. Only a small fraction (K-Ras) of these promising molecular markers has reached access into routine clinical practice. To recommend the application of new molecular markers in routine clinical practice, a level II (at least) evidence is required. However, the currently available data on molecular markers in CRC have solely reached the level III evidence. Thus, prospectively performed clinical trials that study molecular markers as a secondary objective are required.

By identifying and understanding molecular markers, it is becoming increasingly apparent that disease progression is largely driven by complex pathways and analysis of one single marker is unlikely to predict progression of disease with a high degree of accuracy and reproducibility. Therefore, parameters need to be agreed upon in order to validate and standardize testing as a biomarker before they are tested in prospective clinical trials. Moreover, the rapid progress in molecular technologies also requires new study designs to translate the promising molecular markers efficiently and safely to the clinic.

With the development of new effective anticancer drugs and the integration of novel-targeted therapies, it is critical to gain a better understanding of the metabolism of these new agents and their mechanisms of resistance. Recently, new technologies have emerged, such as DNA microarray and proteomics, furthering the discovery of novel biomarkers and pathways in colon cancer progression. The introduction of new therapeutic agents and the discovery and validation of predictive and prognostic markers will enable oncologists to individualize therapeutic strategies by maximizing drug efficacy and minimizing adverse side effects in colon cancer patients. As of June 6th 2009, the two established molecular markers in colorectal cancer are MSI for prognosis and K-Ras for prediction.

Table 11.2 Molecular markers and their clinical consequences in colorectal cancer

Marker	Location	Function	Consequence
Genomic instability			
DCC	Chromoseome 18q LOH	Apoptosis ↓	Survival ↓
Microsatellite Instability	MSI-high	MMR function ↓	Prognosis ↑
Genetic markers			
K-Ras	Chromosome 12, mutations at codons 12 + 13	GTPase activity ↓ Constitutive actication of downstream pathways	Resistance to anti-EGFR MoAb treatment (Panitumumab or Cetuximab)
B-Raf	V600E mutation	Constitutive activation of downstream pathways	Resistance to anti-EGFR MoAb treatment (Panitumumab or Cetuximab)
Thymidylate-Synthase (TS)	1. TSER 28-bp (2R)/(3R) tandem repeat 5UTR 2. TSER 3R G>C SNP	1. TS expression ↑ 2. TS expression ↓	1. 5-FU response ↓ 2. 5-FU response ↑
Dihydropyrimidin-Dehydrogenase (DPD)	G>A SNP exon 14	DPD activity ↓	5-FU toxicity ↑↑ 5-FU response
Methylentetrahydrofolat-Reductase (MTHFR)	SNP (C677T und A1298C)	TS expression ↓	5-FU response ↑
COX2 Gene	G-765C polymorphism	Promoter activity ↑	Cetuximab PFS ↑
IL-8 VEGF	IL-8 T-251A (A/A) VEGF C+936T (C/C)	VEGF expression ↑	Recurrence ↑
Epigenetic markers			
CIMP	CIMP-high	Gene transcription ↓	Relative risk of death ↑

Abbreviations: DCC (deleted in colon cancer); LOH (Loss of heterozygosity); MSI-H (high-level of microsatellite instability); MMR (mismatch repair); MoAb (monoclonal antibody); TSER (TS enhancer region); UTR (untranslated region); SNP (single nucleotide polymorphism).

Abbreviations and Acronyms

APC	Adenomatous polyposis coli
ASCO	American Society of Clinical Oncology
CALGB	Cancer and Leukemia Group B
CIMP	CpG Island Methylator Phenotype
CIN	Chromosomal instability

CH2FH4	5,10-methylenetetrahydrofolate
CpG	Cytosine-phosphate-guanine
CRC	Colorectal cancer
COX	Cyclooxygenase
DCC	Deleted of colon cancer gene
Dll4	Delta-like ligand 4
DPD	Dihydropyrimidine dehydrogenase
EGFR	Epidermal growth factor receptor
FOLFIRI	5-FU/leucovorin/irinotecan
FOLFOX	5-FU/leucovorin/oxaliplatin
dTMP	deoxythymidine monophosphate
dUMP	deoxyuridine monophosphate
FAP	Familial adenomatous polyposis
FCGR	FC gamma receptor
FdUMP	5-fluoro-2-deoxyuridine monophosphate
FdUTP	Fluorodeoxyuridine triphosphate
5-FU	5-fluorouracil
FUTP	Fluouridine triphosphate
HIF1	Hypoxia-inducible factor 1
HNPCC	Hereditary non-polyposis colon cancer
IHC	Immunohistochemistry
IL-8	Interleukin-8
LOH	Loss of heterozygosity
mCRC	Metastatic CRC
MMR	Mismatch repair system
MSI	Microsatellite instability
MTHFR	Methylenetetrahydrofolate reductase
NCI/NSABP	National Surgical Adjuvant Breast and Bowel Project
OS	Overall survival
PETACC	Pan-European Trials in Adjuvant Colon Cancer
PFS	Progression-free survival
SNP	Single nucleotide polymorphism
TGFβ	Transforming growth factor ß
TNM	Tumour node metastasis
TP	Thumidine phosphorylase
TS	Thymidylate synthase
UICC/AJCC	Union Internationale Contre le Cancer/American Joint Cancer Committee
VEGF	Vascular endothelial growth factor
VEGFR	Vascular endothelial growth factor receptor

Acknowledgments Supported in part by a Research Grant of the Austrian Society of Hematology and Oncology and the 'Kurt und Senta-Herrmann Stiftung'.

References

Aaltonen LA, Peltomaki P, Leach FS, Sistonen P, Pylkkanen L, Mecklin JP et al. (1993). Clues to the pathogenesis of familial colorectal cancer. *Science* **260**: 812–16.

Alhopuro P, Alazzouzi H, Sammalkorpi H, Davalos V, Salovaara R, Hemminki A et al. (2005). SMAD4 levels and response to 5-fluorouracil in colorectal cancer. *Clin Cancer Res* **11**: 6311–16.

Allegra CJ, Jessup JM, Somerfield MR, Hamilton SR, Hammond EH, Hayes DF et al. (2009). American Society of Clinical Oncology provisional clinical opinion: testing for KRAS gene mutations in patients with metastatic colorectal carcinoma to predict response to anti-epidermal growth factor receptor monoclonal antibody therapy. *J Clin Oncol* **27**: 2091–96.

Amado RG, Wolf M, Peeters M, Van Cutsem E, Siena S, Freeman DJ et al. (2008). Wild-type KRAS is required for panitumumab efficacy in patients with metastatic colorectal cancer. *J Clin Oncol* **26**: 1626–34.

Baker SJ, Fearon ER, Nigro JM, Hamilton SR, Preisinger AC, Jessup JM et al. (1989). Chromosome 17 deletions and p53 gene mutations in colorectal carcinomas. *Science* **244**: 217–21.

Bertagnolli MM, Niedzwiecki D, Compton CC, Hahn HP, Hall M, Damas B et al. (2009). Microsatellite instability predicts improved response to adjuvant therapy with irinotecan, fluorouracil, and leucovorin in stage III colon cancer: cancer and leukemia group B protocol 89803. *J Clin Oncol* **27**: 1814–21.

Compton CC (2000). Updated protocol for the examination of specimens from patients with carcinomas of the colon and rectum, excluding carcinoid tumors, lymphomas, sarcomas, and tumors of the vermiform appendix: a basis for checklists. Cancer Committee. *Arch Pathol Lab Med* **124**: 1016–25.

Cunningham JM, Christensen ER, Tester DJ, Kim CY, Roche PC, Burgart LJ et al. (1998). Hypermethylation of the hMLH1 promoter in colon cancer with microsatellite instability. *Cancer Res* **58**: 3455–60.

Danenberg PV (1977). Thymidylate synthetase – a target enzyme in cancer chemotherapy. *Biochim Biophys Acta* **473**: 73–92.

Di Nicolantonio F, Martini M, Molinari F, Sartore-Bianchi A, Arena S, Saletti P et al. (2008). Wild-type BRAF is required for response to panitumumab or cetuximab in metastatic colorectal cancer. *J Clin Oncol* **26**: 5705–12.

ECOG (2005). Oxaliplatin, leucovorin, and fluorouracil with or without bevacizumab in treating patients who have undergone surgery for stage II colon cancer. Available from: http://clinicaltrials.gov/ct2/show/NCT00217737?term=E5202&rank=1. National Cancer Institute.

El-Khoueiry A, Pohl A, Danenberg K, Cooc J, Zhang W, Yang D, Singh H, Shriki J, Iqbal S, Lenz HJ (2009). ASCO meeting. *J Clin Oncol* **27**: 15 s (suppl; abstr 4056).

Etienne MC, Chazal M, Laurent-Puig P, Magne N, Rosty C, Formento JL et al. (2002). Prognostic value of tumoral thymidylate synthase and p53 in metastatic colorectal cancer patients receiving fluorouracil-based chemotherapy: phenotypic and genotypic analyses. *J Clin Oncol* **20**: 2832–43.

Fearon ER, Cho KR, Nigro JM, Kern SE, Simons JW, Ruppert JM et al. (1990). Identification of a chromosome 18q gene that is altered in colorectal cancers. *Science* **247**: 49–56.

FFCD (2005). Combination chemotherapy with or without cetuximab in treating patients with stage III colon cancer that was completely removed by surgery. Digestive FFdC (ed.). Available from: http://clinicaltrials.gov/ct2/show/NCT00265811?term=PETACC-8&rank=1. National Cancer Institute (NCI).

Flossmann E, Rothwell PM (2007). Effect of aspirin on long-term risk of colorectal cancer: consistent evidence from randomised and observational studies. *Lancet* **369**: 1603–13.

Fujiwara T, Stolker JM, Watanabe T, Rashid A, Longo P, Eshleman JR et al. (1998). Accumulated clonal genetic alterations in familial and sporadic colorectal carcinomas with widespread instability in microsatellite sequences. *Am J Pathol* **153**: 1063–78.

Funke S, Brenner H, Chang-Claude J (2008). Pharmacogenetics in colorectal cancer: a systematic review. *Pharmacogenomics* **9**: 1079–99.

Gill S, Loprinzi CL, Sargent DJ, Thome SD, Alberts SR, Haller DG et al. (2004). Pooled analysis of fluorouracil-based adjuvant therapy for stage II and III colon cancer: who benefits and by how much? *J Clin Oncol* **22**: 1797–806.

Grothey A, Galanis E (2009). Targeting angiogenesis: progress with anti-VEGF treatment with large molecules. *Nat Rev Clin Oncol* **6**: 507–18.

Haigis KM, Kendall KR, Wang Y, Cheung A, Haigis MC, Glickman JN et al. (2008). Differential effects of oncogenic K-Ras and N-Ras on proliferation, differentiation and tumor progression in the colon. *Nat Genet* **40**: 600–8.

Heidelberger C, Chaudhuri NK, Danneberg P, Mooren D, Griesbach L, Duschinsky R et al. (1957). Fluorinated pyrimidines, a new class of tumour-inhibitory compounds. *Nature* **179**: 663–66.

Hoffmann AC, Brabender J, Metzger R, Ling F, Warnecke-Eberz U, Lurje G et al. (2009). Dihydropyrimidine dehydrogenase mRNA expression in peripheral blood of rectal cancer patients is significantly associated with residual tumor and distant metastases following resection. *J Surg Oncol* **99**: 296–301.

Hurwitz H, Fehrenbacher L, Novotny W, Cartwright T, Hainsworth J, Heim W et al. (2004). Bevacizumab plus irinotecan, fluorouracil, and leucovorin for metastatic colorectal cancer. *N Engl J Med* **350**: 2335–42.

Issa JP (2004). CpG island methylator phenotype in cancer. *Nat Rev Cancer* **4**: 988–93.

Karapetis CS, Khambata-Ford S, Jonker DJ, O'Callaghan CJ, Tu D, Tebbutt NC et al. (2008). K-ras mutations and benefit from cetuximab in advanced colorectal cancer. *N Engl J Med* **359**: 1757–65.

Keino-Masu K, Masu M, Hinck L, Leonardo ED, Chan SS, Culotti JG et al. (1996). Deleted in Colorectal Cancer (DCC) encodes a netrin receptor. *Cell* **87**: 175–85.

Kim GP, Colangelo LH, Wieand HS, Paik S, Kirsch IR, Wolmark N et al. (2007). Prognostic and predictive roles of high-degree microsatellite instability in colon cancer: a National Cancer Institute-National Surgical Adjuvant Breast and Bowel Project Collaborative Study. *J Clin Oncol* **25**: 767–72.

Kohne C, Stroiakovski D, Chang-Chien C, Lim R, Pintér T, Bodoky G et al. (2009). Predictive biomarkers to improve treatment of metastatic colorectal cancer (mCRC); Outcomes with cetuximab plus FOLFIRI in the CRYSTAL trial. *J Clin Oncol* **27**: 15s (suppl; abstr 4068).

Lane DP (1992). Cancer. p53, guardian of the genome. *Nature* **358**: 15–16.

Le Voyer TE, Sigurdson ER, Hanlon AL, Mayer RJ, Macdonald JS, Catalano PJ et al. (2003). Colon cancer survival is associated with increasing number of lymph nodes analyzed: a secondary survey of intergroup trial INT-0089. *J Clin Oncol* **21**: 2912–19.

Lievre A, Bachet JB, Le Corre D, Boige V, Landi B, Emile JF et al. (2006). KRAS mutation status is predictive of response to cetuximab therapy in colorectal cancer. *Cancer Res* **66**: 3992–95.

Locker GY, Hamilton S, Harris J, Jessup JM, Kemeny N, Macdonald JS et al. (2006). ASCO 2006 update of recommendations for the use of tumor markers in gastrointestinal cancer. *J Clin Oncol* **24**: 5313–27.

Longacre TA, Fenoglio-Preiser CM (1990). Mixed hyperplastic adenomatous polyps/serrated adenomas. A distinct form of colorectal neoplasia. *Am J Surg Pathol* **14**: 524–37.

Lurje G, Hendifar AE, Schultheis AM, Pohl A, Husain H, Yang D et al. (2009). Polymorphisms in interleukin 1 beta and interleukin 1 receptor antagonist associated with tumor recurrence in stage II colon cancer. *Pharmacogenet Genomics* **19**: 95–102.

Lurje G, Nagashima F, Zhang W, Yang D, Chang HM, Gordon MA et al. (2008a). Polymorphisms in cyclooxygenase-2 and epidermal growth factor receptor are associated with progression-free survival independent of K-ras in metastatic colorectal cancer patients treated with single-agent cetuximab. *Clin Cancer Res* **14**: 7884–95.

Lurje G, Zhang W, Lenz HJ (2007). Molecular prognostic markers in locally advanced colon cancer. *Clin Colorectal Cancer* **6**: 683–90.

Lurje G, Zhang W, Schultheis AM, Yang D, Groshen S, Hendifar AE et al. (2008b). Polymorphisms in VEGF and IL-8 predict tumor recurrence in stage III colon cancer. *Ann Oncol* **19**: 1734–41.

Mandola MV, Stoehlmacher J, Muller-Weeks S, Cesarone G, Yu MC, Lenz HJ et al. (2003). A novel single nucleotide polymorphism within the 5′ tandem repeat polymorphism of the thymidylate synthase gene abolishes USF-1 binding and alters transcriptional activity. *Cancer Res* **63**: 2898–904.

Mehlen P, Fearon ER (2004). Role of the dependence receptor DCC in colorectal cancer pathogenesis. *J Clin Oncol* **22**: 3420–28.

Minoo P, Moyer MP, Jass JR (2007). Role of BRAF-V600E in the serrated pathway of colorectal tumourigenesis. *J Pathol* **212**: 124–33.

Munro AJ, Lain S, Lane DP (2005). P53 abnormalities and outcomes in colorectal cancer: a systematic review. *Br J Cancer* **92**: 434–44.

Ning Y, Lurje, G., Danenberg, K., Cooc, J., Yang, D., Pohl, A., Zhang, W., Lenz, H. (2009). ASCO Annual Meeting. *J Clin Oncol* **27**: 15s (suppl; abstr 4040), Orlando.

Noffsinger AE (2009). Serrated polyps and colorectal cancer: new pathway to malignancy. *Ann Rev Pathol* **4**: 343–64.

Noguera-Troise I, Daly C, Papadopoulos NJ, Coetzee S, Boland P, Gale NW et al. (2006). Blockade of Dll4 inhibits tumour growth by promoting non-productive angiogenesis. *Nature* **444**: 1032–37.

Ogino S, Kirkner GJ, Nosho K, Irahara N, Kure S, Shima K et al. (2008). Cyclooxygenase-2 expression is an independent predictor of poor prognosis in colon cancer. *Clin Cancer Res* **14**: 8221–27.

Park KJ, Choi HJ, Roh MS, Kwon HC, Kim C (2005). Intensity of tumor budding and its prognostic implications in invasive colon carcinoma. *Dis Colon Rectum* **48**: 1597–602.

Peltomaki P (2003). Role of DNA mismatch repair defects in the pathogenesis of human cancer. *J Clin Oncol* **21**: 1174–79.

Popat S, Houlston RS (2005). A systematic review and meta-analysis of the relationship between chromosome 18q genotype, DCC status and colorectal cancer prognosis. *Eur J Cancer* **41**: 2060–70.

Popat S, Hubner R, Houlston RS (2005a). Systematic review of microsatellite instability and colorectal cancer prognosis. *J Clin Oncol* **23**: 609–18.

Popat S, Matakidou A, Houlston RS (2004). Thymidylate synthase expression and prognosis in colorectal cancer: a systematic review and meta-analysis. *J Clin Oncol* **22**: 529–36.

Popat S, Wort R, Houlston RS (2005b). Relationship between thymidylate synthase (TS) genotype and TS expression: a tissue microarray analysis of colorectal cancers. *Int J Surg Pathol* **13**: 127–33.

Pullarkat ST, Stoehlmacher J, Ghaderi V, Xiong YP, Ingles SA, Sherrod A et al. (2001). Thymidylate synthase gene polymorphism determines response and toxicity of 5-FU chemotherapy. *Pharmacogenomics J* **1**: 65–70.

Rajagopalan H, Bardelli A, Lengauer C, Kinzler KW, Vogelstein B, Velculescu VE (2002). Tumorigenesis: RAF/RAS oncogenes and mismatch-repair status. *Nature* **418**: 934.

Ribic CM, Sargent DJ, Moore MJ, Thibodeau SN, French AJ, Goldberg RM et al. (2003). Tumor microsatellite-instability status as a predictor of benefit from fluorouracil-based adjuvant chemotherapy for colon cancer. *N Engl J Med* **349**: 247–57.

Roth A, Tejpar S, Yan P, Fiocca R, Dietrich D, Delorenzi M et al. (2009). 2009 ASCO Meeting. *J Clin Oncol* **27**: 15 s (suppl; abstr 4002).

Salonga D, Danenberg KD, Johnson M, Metzger R, Groshen S, Tsao-Wei DD et al. (2000). Colorectal tumors responding to 5-fluorouracil have low gene expression levels of dihydropyrimidine dehydrogenase, thymidylate synthase, and thymidine phosphorylase. *Clin Cancer Res* **6**: 1322–27.

Samowitz WS, Albertsen H, Herrick J, Levin TR, Sweeney C, Murtaugh MA et al. (2005). Evaluation of a large, population-based sample supports a CpG island methylator phenotype in colon cancer. *Gastroenterology* **129**: 837–45.

Sargent DJ, Marsoni S, Thibodeau SN, Labianca R, Hamilton S, Torri V et al. (2008) ASCO Meeting. *J Clin Oncol* **26** (suppl; abstr 4008).

Shibata D, Reale MA, Lavin P, Silverman M, Fearon ER, Steele G Jr et al. (1996). The DCC protein and prognosis in colorectal cancer. *N Engl J Med* **335**: 1727–32.

Silvestrini R (2000). Relevance of DNA-ploidy as a prognostic instrument for solid tumors. *Ann Oncol* **11**: 259–61.

Soong R, Shah N, Salto-Tellez M, Tai BC, Soo RA, Han HC et al. (2008). Prognostic significance of thymidylate synthase, dihydropyrimidine dehydrogenase and thymidine phosphorylase protein expression in colorectal cancer patients treated with or without 5-fluorouracil-based chemotherapy. *Ann Oncol* **19**: 915–19.

Spears CP, Gustavsson BG, Berne M, Frosing R, Bernstein L, Hayes AA (1988). Mechanisms of innate resistance to thymidylate synthase inhibition after 5-fluorouracil. *Cancer Res* **48**: 5894–900.

Sun XF, Rutten S, Zhang H, Nordenskjold B (1999). Expression of the deleted in colorectal cancer gene is related to prognosis in DNA diploid and low proliferative colorectal adenocarcinoma. *J Clin Oncol* **17**: 1745–50.

SWOG (2005). Cetuximab and/or bevacizumab combined with combination chemotherapy in treating patients with metastatic colorectal cancer. Available from: http://clinicaltrials.gov/ct2/show/NCT00265850?term=CALGB-C80405&rank=1. National Cancer Institute.

Tejpar S, Bosman F, Delorenzi M, Fiocca R, Yan P, Klingbiel D et al. (2009). ASCO Meeting. *J Clin Oncol* **27**: 15 s (suppl; abstr 4001).

Tickle C, Altabef M (1999). Epithelial cell movements and interactions in limb, neural crest and vasculature. *Curr Opin Genet Dev* **9**: 455–60.

Toyota M, Ahuja N, Ohe-Toyota M, Herman JG, Baylin SB, Issa JP (1999). CpG island methylator phenotype in colorectal cancer. *Proc Natl Acad Sci USA* **96**: 8681–86.

Turner RR, Li C, Compton CC (2007). Newer pathologic assessment techniques for colorectal carcinoma. *Clin Cancer Res* **13**: 6871s–76s.

Vogelstein B, Fearon ER, Hamilton SR, Kern SE, Preisinger AC, Leppert M et al. (1988). Genetic alterations during colorectal-tumor development. *N Engl J Med* **319**: 525–32.

Wallner M, Herbst A, Behrens A, Crispin A, Stieber P, Goke B et al. (2006). Methylation of serum DNA is an independent prognostic marker in colorectal cancer. *Clin Cancer Res* **12**: 7347–52.

Watanabe T, Wu TT, Catalano PJ, Ueki T, Satriano R, Haller DG et al. (2001). Molecular predictors of survival after adjuvant chemotherapy for colon cancer. *N Engl J Med* **344**: 1196–206.

Woodford-Richens KL, Rowan AJ, Gorman P, Halford S, Bicknell DC, Wasan HS et al. (2001). SMAD4 mutations in colorectal cancer probably occur before chromosomal instability, but after divergence of the microsatellite instability pathway. *Proc Natl Acad Sci USA* **98**: 9719–23.

Zhang W, Gordon M, Schultheis AM, Yang DY, Nagashima F, Azuma M et al. (2007). FCGR2A and FCGR3A polymorphisms associated with clinical outcome of epidermal growth factor receptor expressing metastatic colorectal cancer patients treated with single-agent cetuximab. *J Clin Oncol* **25**: 3712–18.

Zlobec I, Lugli A (2008). Prognostic and predictive factors in colorectal cancer. *J Clin Pathol* **61**: 561–69.

van Rijnsoever M, Grieu F, Elsaleh H, Joseph D, Iacopetta B (2002). Characterisation of colorectal cancers showing hypermethylation at multiple CpG islands. *Gut* **51**: 797–802.

Chapter 12

THE SENTINEL LYMPH NODE AND STAGING OF COLORECTAL CANCER

Gaetan des Guetz[1] and Bernard Uzzan[2]

[1] Department of Oncology, APHP, hôpital Avicenne, Bobigny 93009, France,
e-mail: gaetan.des-guetz@avc.aphp.fr
[2] Department of Pharmacology, APHP, hôpital Avicenne, Bobigny 93009, France

Abstract: The use of sentinel lymph node (SLN) biopsy (SLNB) for staging of colorectal cancer (CRC) is a controversial issue. To clarify the usefulness of this technique with its different modalities of detection and various protocols for the histopathological work-up of the SLN, we performed a meta-analysis (MA) about the feasibility of this approach. We compared this new method of lymph node staging in colorectal cancer to standard evaluation of lymph node involvement. In our MA, the global sensitivity of sentinel lymph node mapping (SLNM) was 70% with an 81% level of specificity. The pooled DAOR (Diagnostic Accuracy Odds Ratio) was 10.7 (95% CI: 7–16.5). This means that a patient whose SLN is invaded has 10.7 times more risk to be node-positive than an SLN-negative patient. SLN mapping in CRC seems feasible but a learning curve is necessary. Saha et al. has gained a considerable experience with this technique, attested by their numerous publications. In their hands, SLN mapping had a better sensitivity (90%) than in other studies. The SLNM technique should be better standardized in future studies. On the other hand, we know that SLNB is successfully applied in breast cancer since it offers esthetical advantage by avoiding large biopsy. In this regard, CRC differs from breast cancer. Nevertheless, a major benefit may be obtained in CRC since SLNB permits upstaging of some cancer and better evaluation of lymph node involvement, thanks to thin slicing of SLN. Although this issue is still under debate, there is growing evidence that, if at least RT-PCR-techniques were used, the detection of small tumour deposits in the SLN might be of prognostic and thus of clinical value. Future studies should focus on two aspects. First, careful patient selection may allow determining whether an improvement of the sensitivity to detect macrometastases is feasible. Second, large prospective trials using a standardized histopathological lymph node assessment should compare SLN and Non-SLN for their incidence to bear small tumour deposits. If SLNB proves to be a sensitive technique, its prognostic and predictive value should be evaluated.

Key words: Neoplasm staging · Colonic neoplasms/pathology · Colonic neoplasms/surgery · Lymph nodes/pathology · Lymph nodes/surgery

12.1 Introduction

The most important indicator of prognosis in potentially curable colon cancer is the presence of metastatic disease within regional lymph nodes (LN). Sentinel lymph node (SLN) staging is based on the assumption that lymphatic flow drains sequentially from peripheral to central tissue locations, with limited functional collaterals outside of the dominant vascular supply.

Consequently, tracer substances injected at a tumour site should follow the same pathway by which metastatic tumour cells traverse lymphatic channels. If these conditions are met, the first LN encountered, termed the sentinel node (SN), is a reliable indicator of the tumour status of the entire nodal basin (Fig. 12.1).

Patients whose regional LNs contain metastatic tumour cells are at high risk of disease recurrence and are therefore most likely to benefit from adjuvant chemotherapy. Unfortunately, more than 25% of patients whose regional LNs show no evidence of disease by conventional histopathological staging will develop recurrent disease within 5 years of surgery. A substantial effort is underway in the scientific community to develop methods that will identify these high-risk individuals at the time of their initial treatment, primarily with the intent of considering them for adjuvant therapies. A large body of research indicates that a more thorough investigation of regional LNs can detect the presence of tumour cells or products that are not identified by conventional histopathological staging.

Fig. 12.1 Method to localize the first sentinel node. *Blue dye* is injected around the tumour to visualize the lymphatic tract. The first lymph node (sentinel lymph node, SN) can then be easily removed and analyzed

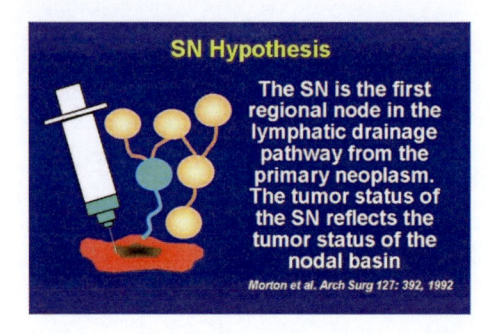

SN Hypothesis

The SN is the first regional node in the lymphatic drainage pathway from the primary neoplasm. The tumor status of the SN reflects the tumor status of the nodal basin

Morton et al. Arch Surg 127: 392, 1992

12.2 Feasibility of Sentinel Lymph Node Mapping

A number of studies have sought to determine the feasibility of using SLN sampling to colon cancer staging. Several of these studies suggest that SLN sampling can be applied to colon cancer with a high level of accuracy for characterization of overall nodal status.

Three years ago, we performed a MA on the diagnostic accuracy of SLN in CRC, since the diagnostic value of SLNM in patients with colorectal cancer was controversial (Des Guetz et al., 2007). A PubMed query (key words: colorectal cancer, sentinel node) provided 182 studies that associated sentinel lymph node (SLN) with CRC, the abstracts of which were reviewed. Altogether, 48 studies dealing with the diagnostic value of SLNM were selected from PubMed, and 6 other studies were retrieved from reviews. The results of this MA are discussed in the next sections. Since then, a few additional studies have been published, but they do not invalidate the conclusions of our study.

12.3 Techniques of Sentinel Lymph Node Diagnosis

In our MA, we detailed the different techniques of SLN described in the literature for CRC. Two methods were employed for diagnosis of SLN: blue dyes or radiolabelled tracers (Figs. 12.2 and 12.3). Two blue dyes were used by many groups: patent blue dye V in Europe and isosulfan blue 1% (Lymphazurin) in North America (Bendavid

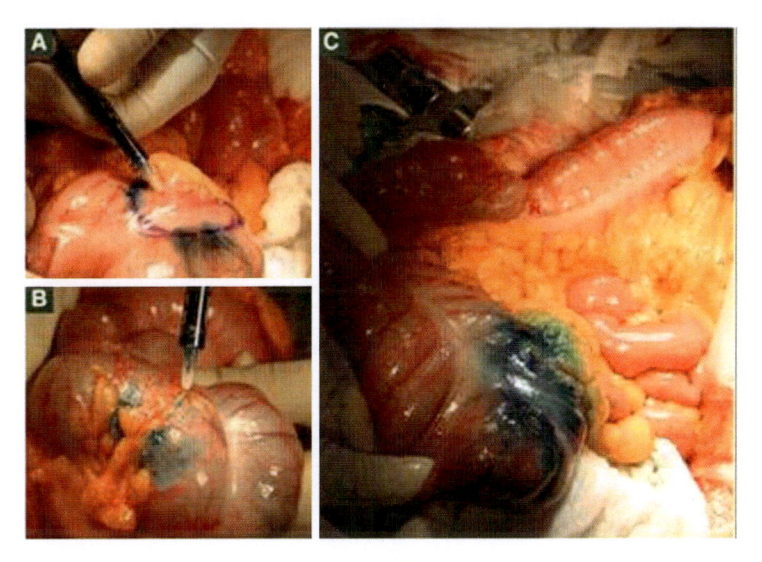

Fig. 12.2 Injection of dye around the tumour. The first sequences of the SLN (sentinel lymph nodes) technique are shown with injection during surgery of lymphazurin around the tumour (from S. Saha with permission)

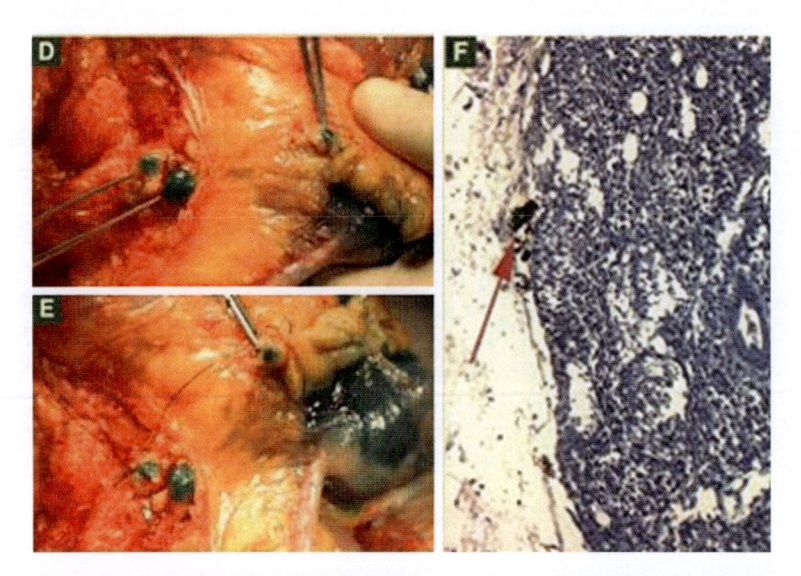

Fig. 12.3 Detection of sentinel lymph nodes. After injection of the blue dye, the first three blue SLNs are seen. In *panel* **f**, some metastatic cells are identified in the lymph node. It is simple to evaluate lymph node involvement

et al., 2002; Broderick-Villa et al., 2004; Medina-Franco et al., 2005; Paramo et al., 2002; Read et al., 2005; Redston et al., 2006; Saha et al., 2006; Smith et al., 2005; Waters et al., 2000). Radioactive technetium labelling was rarely performed (Kitagawa et al., 2002; Patten et al., 2004). The three studies using radioactive tracers only showed FN rates of 8–20% (Bembenek et al., 2004; Kitagawa et al., 2002; Merrie et al., 2001). One study (Saha et al., 2004a) compared lymphazurin 1% and ^{99m}Tc sulfur colloid for SLNM in CRC. No significant difference in feasibility or accuracy was found between the two methods, but the detection yield of metastases was significantly higher when SLNM was performed using both techniques simultaneously. The use of a radioactive tracer requires additional equipment, such as a gamma probe to detect the radioactivity level of the lymph nodes. It is simple to use blue dye techniques, usually in four injections peri-tumourally. The volume of blue dye used ranged from 0.5 to 4×4 ml in four studies (Bembenek et al., 2005; Patten et al., 2004; Lasser et al., 2003; Viehl et al., 2003), (see Table 12.1). The injections were usually done in vivo although ten ex vivo studies were performed (Baton et al., 2005; Bell et al., 2005; Bembenek et al., 2004; Broderick-Villa et al., 2004; Cserni et al., 1999; Demirbas et al., 2004; Lasser et al., 2003; Smith et al., 2005; Fitzgerald et al., 2002; Wong et al., 2004). The site of injection was mostly sub-serosally and sometimes sub-mucosally during an endoscopic procedure, mainly for rectal cancer (Bilchik and Trocha, 2003; Evangelista et al., 2002; Joosten et al., 1999; Kitagawa et al., 2002). In a few studies, the two techniques (in vivo and ex vivo) were used and did not show different sensitivities (Medina-Franco et al., 2005; Roseano et al., 2003). In all but one study using blue dye (Gandy et al., 2002), the identification time between injection of the tracer and labelling of SNs ranged from 1 to 60 min.

12 The Sentinel Lymph Node and Staging of Colorectal Cancer

Table 12.1 Main characteristics of the studies included in the meta-analysis (from Des Guetz et al., 2007)

First author year of issue (references)	N (M/F)	Colon (n)	Rectum (n)	Technical procedure	Mode of injection	Stage (T_{0-1-2}/T_{3-4})	Nb of lymph nodes	Nb of SLN	Nb of failures (%)	IHC	TP	TN	FN	FP	Patients assessed
Saha 2006 (Saha et al., 2006)	500	ND	ND	In vivo	0.5–3 ml L	100/268	ND	1–4	11 (2)	CK$_{AE-1/AE-3}$	186	157	21	54	418
Bilchik 2002 (Bilchik et al., 2002)	30 (12/18)	30	0	In vivo	0.5–1 ml L	24/6	14 (2–21)	1.8 (1–3)	0	CK$_{AE-1/AE-3}$	4	24	2	4	34
Redston 2006 (Redston et al., 2006)	72	72	0	In vivo	1 ml L	ND	17	2.1	6 (8)	CK$_{AE-1/AE-3}$-CEA	14	23	10	14	61
Baton 2005 (Baton et al., 2005)	31 (21/10)	0	31	Ex vivo	4 × 1–2 ml PB	12/18	21 (7–38)	2 (0–3)	1 (3)	CK$_{AE-1/AE-3}$-CK-20	4	20	3	3	30
Lasser 2003 (Lasser et al., 2003)	32 (16/17)	32	0	Ex vivo	4 × 2 ml PB	9/23	23 (10–55)	2 (1–4)	0	CK$_{AE-1/AE-3}$-CK-20	5	18	4	3	30
Bell 2005 (Bell et al., 2005)	57	45	12	Ex vivo	4 × 0.5 ml PB	ND	30	2.9 (0–8)	2 (3)	CK	6	31	9	2	48
Bembenek 2005 (Bembenek et al., 2005)	55 (28/27)	55	0	In vivo	4 × 2–4 ml PB	ND	26 (10–59)	2	8 (15)	CK	13	20	1	12	46

(continued)

Table 12.1 (continued)

First author year of issue (references)	N (M/F)	Colon (n)	Rectum (n)	Technical procedure	Mode of injection	Stage (T_{0-1-2}/T_{3-4})	Nb of lymph nodes	Nb of SLN	Nb of failures (%)	IHC	TP	TN	FN	FP	Patients assessed
Bembenek 2004 (Bembenek et al., 2004)	48 (34/14)	0	48	Ex vivo	1 ml Sulfur colloidal Tc 99m	26/22	18 (9–69)	3	2 (4)	MNF-16	7	29	9	1	46
Codignola 2005 (Codignola et al., 2005)	56 (20/36)	52	4	In vivo	1–2 ml PB	13/43	21 (6–47)	2 (1–5)	0	CK	16	13	6	21	56
Dahl 2005 (Dahl et al., 2005)	30 (17/13)	30	0	In vivo	1 ml PB	ND	17 (4–35)	6 (1–8)	2 (7)	ND	10	18	2	0	30
Medina-Franco (Medina-Franco et al., 2005) 2005	10 (3/7)	7	3	In and Ex vivo	1 ml L	4/6	16 (5–42)	2.5 (1–7)	0	IHC	3	6	0	1	10
Bertoglio 2004 (Bertoglio et al., 2004)	26 (14/12)	20	6	In vivo	4 × 1–2 ml PB	ND	ND	2.9	2 (8)	ND	7	15	2	0	24
Braat 2005 (Braat et al., 2005)	91 (50/41)	57	34	Ex vivo and In vivo	1–2 ml PB	26/65		1.7 (0–4)	9 (10)	$CK_{7/8}$	23	45	8	6	82
Read 2005 (Read et al., 2005)	41	41	0	In vivo	1–2 ml L	ND	14 (7–45)	2 (1–3)	8 (20)	ND	2	26	9	1	38

(continued)

12 The Sentinel Lymph Node and Staging of Colorectal Cancer

Table 12.1 (continued)

First author year of issue (references)	N (M/F)	Colon (n)	Rectum (n)	Technical procedure	Mode of injection	Stage (T_{0-1-2}/T_{3-4})	Nb of lymph nodes	Nb of SLN	Nb of failures (%)	IHC	TP	TN	FN	FP	Patients assessed
Smith 2005 (Smith et al., 2005)	37 (23/17)	29	8	Ex vivo	1–1.5 ml L	ND	16.9 (7–37)	4 (1–8)	1 (3)	CK READ	14	15	2	6	37
Broderick 2004 (Broderick-Villa et al., 2004)	40 (25/15)	32	10	Ex vivo	1 ml L	14/26	8 (1–41)	1.9 (0–5)	4 (10)		9	21	7	2	39
Demirbas 2004 (Demirbas et al., 2004)	41 (23/18)	25	16	Ex vivo	1 ml PB	ND	5.5	3	4 (10)	$CK_{AE-1/AE-3}$-Cam5.2	18	15	2	2	37
Patten 2004 (Patten et al., 2004)	57	57	0	In vivo	Sulfur colloidal Tc 99m then 3–5 ml L (1%)	21/36	14.4	3.5 (0–11)	1 (2)	CK	11	29	11	5	56
Wong 2004 (Wong et al., 2004)	124 (64/60)	112	12	Ex vivo	4 × 0.125 ml L (1%)	ND	ND	3.8	4 (3)	$CK_{AE-1/AE-3}$	27	53	24	13	117
Roseano 2003 (Roseano et al., 2003)	23 (12/11)	14	9	Ex vivo and In vivo	PB	ND	14.6	2.5	0	$CK_{AE-1/AE-3}$		19	2	0	23

(continued)

Table 12.1 (continued)

First author year of issue (references)	N (M/F)	Colon (n)	Rectum (n)	Technical procedure	Mode of injection	Stage (T_{0-1-2}/T_{3-4})	Nb of lymph nodes	Nb of SLN	Nb of failures (%)	IHC	TP	TN	FN	FP	Patients assessed
Cox 2002 (Cox et al., 2002)	17 (6/11)	17	0	Ex vivo and In vivo	1 ml L	7/10	12 (1–29)	5.5 (2–11)	0	IHC	2	10	1	4	17
Viehl 2003 (Viehl et al., 2003)	31 (23/8)	31	0	In vivo	+ 1 ml L	5/26	ND	ND	4 (13)	CK22	4	15	6	2	27
Bendavid 2002 (Bendavid et al., 2002)	20	20	0	In vivo	1 ml L (1%)	ND	ND	3.9	2 (10)	CK$_{AE-1/AE-3}$	6	6	1	5	18
Fitzgerald 2002 (Fitzgerald et al., 2002)	26	16	10	Ex vivo	1 ml L	13/13	14.8	2.5	3 (12)	Cam 5.2	1	18	2	2	23
Gandy 2002 (Gandy et al., 2002)	19 (10/9)	12	7	In vivo	2 ml PB (2.5%)	ND	17 (7–27)	ND	7 (37)	ND	5	6	1	0	12
Kitagawa 2002 (Kitagawa et al., 2002)	56 (40/16)	19	37	In vivo	99m Tc labeled tin colloid	29/27	23.9	3.5	5 (9)	ND	18	29	4	0	51
Nastro 2002 (Nastro et al., 2002)	8 (5–3)	ND	ND	In vivo	2 ml PB 2 ml colloidal Tc 99m	ND	ND	ND	2 (25)	CK/CEA	2	2	0	2	6

(continued)

Table 12.1 (continued)

First author year of issue (references)	N (M/F)	Colon (n)	Rectum (n)	Technical procedure	Mode of injection	Stage (T_{0-1-2}/T_{3-4})	Nb of lymph nodes	Nb of SLN	Nb of failures (%)	IHC	TP	TN	FN	FP	Patients assessed
Paramo 2002 (Paramo et al., 2002)	55 (28/27)	55	0	In vivo	1 ml L	14/41	12	1–4	10 (18)	Cam 5.2	5	30	1	9	45
Esser 2001 (Esser et al., 2001)	38 (7/31)	26	5	In vivo	1–2 ml L	ND	15	ND	13 (34)	ND	2	15	1	0	18
Merrie 2001 (Merrie et al., 2001)	25	25	0	Ex vivo	Antimony colloidal Tc 99m	ND	17 (4–52)	ND	3 (12)	CK 20	4	12	3	4	23
Waters 2000 (Waters et al., 2000)	22 (8/14)	22	0	In vivo	1 × 4 ml L	ND	11.6	ND	2 (9)	CK/CEA	6	13	0	1	20
Cserni 1999 (Cserni et al., 1999)	25 (11/14)	ND	ND	Ex vivo	2 ml PB	2/23	15 (2–34)	4 (0–12)	1 (4)	ND	6	12	4	2	24
Joosten 1999 (Joosten et al., 1999)	50	44	6	In vivo	PB	ND	14	3 (1–16)	15 (30)	CK19	8	13	12	2	35

M, male; F, female; SLN, Sentinel Lymph Node; IHC, Immunohistochemistry; PB, Patent blue dye V; L, Lymphazurin; TP, TN, FN, FP are defined as true positive, true negative, false negative, false positive; ND, Not Determined.

12.4 Comparaison Between Sentinel Lymph Node Mapping and Standard Methods

In our MA, we compared the diagnostic value of SLNM with that of conventional histopathologic examination. We used the diagnostic accuracy odds ratio (DAOR) method. Because of the significant heterogeneity, we chose the random effect model (Der Simonian and Laird). Statistics were performed on 33 studies, including 1,794 patients (1,201 colon and 332 rectum cancers) (Fig. 12.4). The mean SLNM failure rate was 10%. The global sensitivity and specificity of the SLNM were 70 and

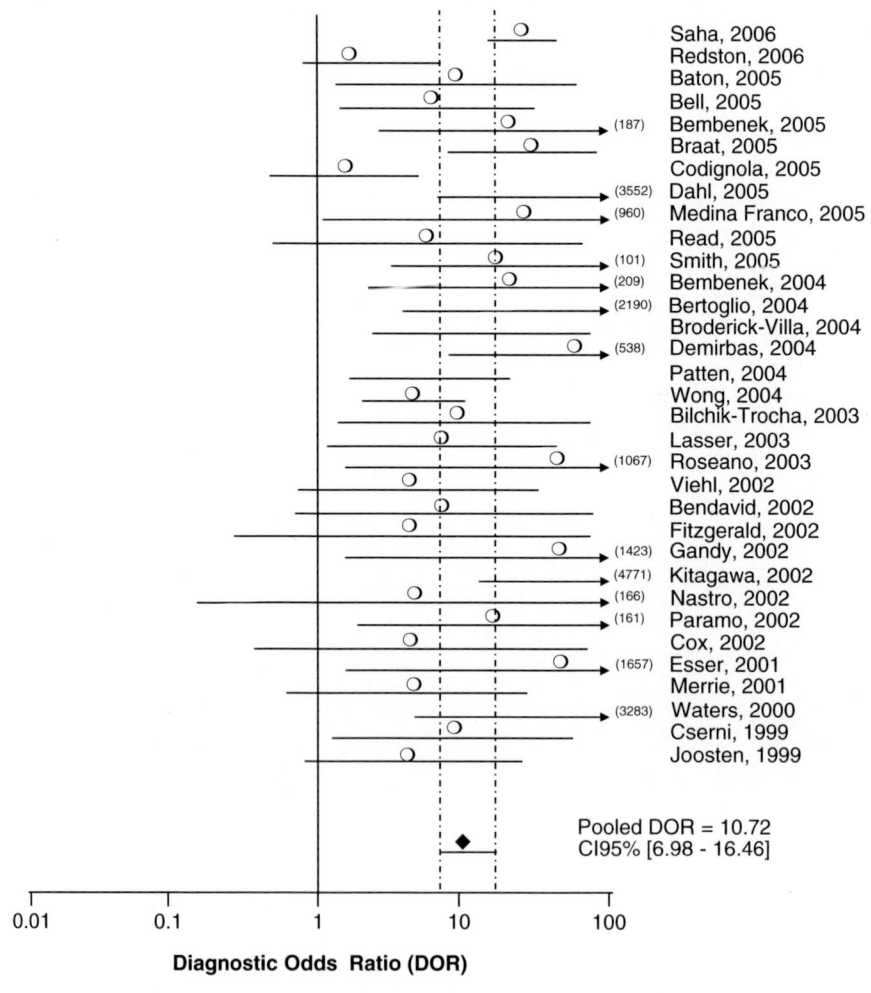

Fig. 12.4 Forest plot of all studies included in the meta-analysis. Each horizontal line represents the 95% confidence interval of the diagnostic odds ratio (DAOR) for the corresponding study (from des Guetz et al., 2007)

81%, respectively. The pooled DAOR was 10.7 (95% confidence interval 7.0–16.5). This means that a patient whose SLN is invaded is 10.7 times more at risk to be node-positive than an SLN-negative patient. This suggests that lymphatic mapping appears to be readily applicable to CRC. However, the prognostic implication of micrometastases found in SLNs requires further evaluation.

The large series by Saha et al. is a major contribution to the heterogeneity between studies since its DAOR was 25.8 (95% CI 14.9–44.5) contrasting with a global DAOR of 10.7. This reflects Dr. Saha's 10-year experience as the promoter of the method of SLNM in CRC. When meta-analysing the 33 independent studies with the fixed-effect model (Mantel-Haenszel procedure), the test of heterogeneity was statistically significant, leading us to perform the calculation with the random effect model (Der Simonian and Laird procedure) in order to take into account the heterogeneity between studies. However, we explored the possible causes of heterogeneity by excluding the Saha study, and then found that the statistical heterogeneity was no longer present, thus allowing us to apply the fixed effect model, which led to a DAOR of 8.72, 95% CI [6.55; 11.60], very close to the one obtained by the random effect model.

12.5 Prognostic Relevance of Occult Tumour Cells in Lymph Nodes

In colorectal cancer especially, we need to evaluate more precisely the extent of the disease. It is not acceptable to miss nodal extension because there is no other prognostic factor that should be used to justify an adjuvant treatment. Our MA showed a median risk of False Negative (FN) of 9% using the SLNM technique. If we consider all studies published in breast cancer, where SLNM has been extensively studied, we also have the same figure of 8.4% FN rate (Lyman et al., 2005). Considering the disease stage, it is important to interpret these data. In general, in breast cancer, SLN mapping is proposed for T1-2 tumours (Lyman et al., 2005). In the series of CRC, we often found more than half of the patients with T3-4 tumours (Braat et al., 2005; Broderick-Villa et al., 2004; Codignola et al., 2005; Lasser et al., 2003; Paramo et al., 2002; Saha et al., 2006). The pooling of T0-2 and T3-4 tumours within studies and the frequent absence of information on T stage prevented us from relating T stage and SLN positivity. In CRC, it has previously been shown that massive lymph node involvement was the cause of high rate of FN of SLNM (Doekhie et al., 2005). So, in future studies of CRC, it would be necessary to stratify patients according to their T stage. A large study (Saha et al., 2004b) found a higher success rate of SLNM for colon versus rectum cancers, but nodal upstaging, skip metastases and occult metastases were similar for both types of neoplasms. Moreover in breast cancer studies, different characteristics of the published studies were highlighted to decrease FN rate (Lyman et al., 2005). For trials that included more than 100 patients, the FN rate was 6.7% versus 9% for trials including less than 100 patients. This technique seems to be operator-dependent. Thus, a learning curve is probably necessary to obtain good results for SLNM. A study by Paramo and colleagues reported that minimum number of cases (8 cases) required to be sure to obtain reproducible results in CRC (Paramo et al., 2002), but this conclusion seems too optimistic. This could explain the difference between the results of Saha et al. and the prospective multicentre study reported by Bertagnolli that was performed in many centres with sometimes less experienced surgeons (Redston et al., 2006). So, for a surgeon motivated to use this technique, SLNM in CRC is technically feasible (Lasser et al., 2003). Another characteristic of the studies that predicted low FNs was a rate of successful mapping higher than 90%. Obviously, the Saha study was more relevant with 5% of FN (Saha et al., 2006) than many others that contained less than forty patients. However, two recent studies contradict this finding. First, the study by Faerden et al. performed in two centres, including 200 patients, identified SLN in 93% but found limited sensitivity of SLN (32/60, 53%) and no upstaging (Faerden et al., 2008). The second one from MD Anderson Cancer Center, a prospective study, with 120 patients, found a sensitivity of 29/49 (59%), and 7% patients were upstaged (Lim et al., 2008).

The main issue is the prognostic significance for stage II CRC. In stage III CRCs, the remission rate is approximately 70%. In stage II CRCs, it reaches 80%, with 20% of patients experiencing relapse. Adjuvant chemotherapy with 5-FU/leucovorin/oxaliplatin (FOLFOX), the present standard treatment in gastrointestinal oncology, is mandatory for stage III CRCs (Andre et al., 2004). The issue of indication of adjuvant chemotherapy is still pending for stage II CRCs. Indeed, some clinical signs such as perforation or occlusion or histopathological signs such as lymphatic invasion or peri-neural invasion are considered by some authors as enticing to perform chemotherapy (Compton et al., 2000). Similarly, the presence of micrometastases could be an indication for chemotherapy. These latter histopathological elements may correspond to an ill-staged disease. Furthermore, an involvement of the first lymph nodes, better characterized by a detailed analysis of these first nodes, could allow a better staging. Two reviews have been published dealing with the prognostic value of micrometastases (Doekhie et al., 2006; Iddings et al., 2006). The issue of the involvement of SLN is even more relevant. More precisely, the issue is whether an upstaging of SLN allows a better prognostic evaluation of a disease artificially set at stage II. In addition, an interim analysis from the first multicentre prospective study was published 2 years ago. The rate of micrometastases detected using immunohistochemistry (IHC) techniques was 29.7%. One hundred and fifty two patients with resectable colorectal cancer were enrolled for 5 years in this trial. Results were correlated with disease-free survival. The sensitivity of lymphatic mapping was significantly better in colon cancer (75%) than in rectal cancer (36%), $p < 0.05$. Of 92 node-negative colon cancer patients, seven (8%) were upstaged to N1 and 18 (22%) had micrometastases revealed by IHC. The authors reported that 4/92 patients classified as N0 after routine histopathological work-up developed systemic recurrence. All of them had positive findings in the SLN after RT-PCR-ultrastaging, whereas none of the 26 patients with a negative SLN recurred after ultrastaging. The correlation was significant only for positive molecular markers by RT-PCR, whereas IHC-findings failed to reach prognostic relevance. Thus, although very limited in the number of patients, this study is a promising approach to further determine the prognostic and predictive impact of micrometastases in colon cancer. Before using this technique in a prospective study, however, the predictive value of the SLN for molecular ultrastaging and the false–negative rate for RT-PCR-positive patients should be determined by examining SLNs and non-SLNs in a significant number of patients with the same (molecular) method (Bilchik et al., 2007).

12.6 Perspectives

The main drawback of precise analysis of SLN histology is the time-consuming need for numerous slides of first lymph nodes. However, it is also time-consuming to analyze more than 12 nodes (Morris et al., 2007; Wong et al., 1999). The main advantage of SLNM technique in breast cancer or in malignant melanoma is the aesthetic gain. Indeed, avoiding a lymphedema is important for a woman. Of course, this does not apply to CRC in which lymph node ablation is easily performed from an anatomical point of view. A major difference between the application of the SLNM technique to melanoma and breast cancer on one hand and to CRC on the other hand is that, in CRC, this technique cannot fully replace classical histopathological examination, but can only be used as a complementary method to upstage some tumours (about 10%) (Liberale et al., 2007).

Moreover, a recent interesting prospective randomized study, posterior of our MA, compared SLN evaluation in addition to standard histopathology to the latter one. They found a major significant nodal upstaging with SLN ultrastaging (control versus SLN: 39% versus 57%) but exclusion of micrometastases abolished the difference between ultrastaging and standard histopathology. Among the Node (-) patients evaluated with conventional histopathology, 11% were upstaged when step sections with hematoxylin/eosin (HE) were performed (Stojadinovic et al., 2007).

12.7 Conclusion

To conclude, we believe that the predictive value of SLNM should be studied more precisely in prospective studies and especially the prognostic value of ultra-staging is presently required. This new evaluation of lymph node involvement could be taken into account to evaluate the appropriateness of chemotherapy and/or targeted therapies, now considered as the future of cancer treatment in an adjuvant setting.

Abbreviations and Acronyms

CRC   Colorectal cancer
DAOR   Diagnostic Accuracy Odds Ratio

FN	False negative
FP	False positive
FOLFOX	5-FU/leucovorin/oxaliplatin
HE	Hematoxylin/eosin
IHC	Immunohistochemistry
LN	Lymph node
MA	Meta-analysis
SLN	Sentinel lymph node
SLNB	Sentinel lymph node biopsy
SLNM	Sentinel lymph node mapping
SN	Sentinel node
TN	True negative
TP	True positive

References

Andre T, Boni C, Mounedji-Boudiaf L, Navarro M, Tabernero J, Hickish T et al. (2004). Oxaliplatin, fluorouracil, and leucovorin as adjuvant treatment for colon cancer. *N Engl J Med* **350**: 2343–51.

Baton O, Lasser P, Sabourin JC, Boige V, Duvillard P, Elias D et al. (2005). Ex vivo sentinel lymph node study for rectal adenocarcinoma: preliminary study. *World J Surg* **29**: 1166–70; discussion 1171.

Bell SW, Mourra N, Flejou JF, Parc R, Tiret E (2005). Ex vivo sentinel lymph node mapping in colorectal cancer. *Dis Colon Rectum* **48**: 74–79.

Bembenek A, Rau B, Moesta T, Markwardt J, Ulmer C, Gretschel S et al. (2004). Sentinel lymph node biopsy in rectal cancer – not yet ready for routine clinical use. *Surgery* **135**: 498–505; discussion 506–7.

Bembenek A, Schneider U, Gretschel S, Fischer J, Schlag PM (2005). Detection of lymph node micrometastases and isolated tumor cells in sentinel and nonsentinel lymph nodes of colon cancer patients. *World J Surg* **29**: 1172–75.

Bendavid Y, Latulippe JF, Younan RJ, Leclerc YE, Dube S, Heyen F et al. (2002). Phase I study on sentinel lymph node mapping in colon cancer: a preliminary report. *J Surg Oncol* **79**: 81–84; discussion 85.

Bertoglio S, Sandrucci S, Percivale P, Goss M, Gipponi M, Moresco L et al. (2004). Prognostic value of sentinel lymph node biopsy in the pathologic staging of colorectal cancer patients. *J Surg Oncol* **85**: 166–70.

Bilchik AJ, Hoon DSB, Saha S, Turner RR, Wiese D, DiNome M et al. (2007). Prognostic impact of micrometastases in colon cancer: interim results of a prospective multicenter trial. *Ann Surg* **246**: 568–77.

Bilchik AJ, Nora D, Tollenaar RA, van de Velde CJ, Wood T, Turner R et al. (2002). Ultrastaging of early colon cancer using lymphatic mapping and molecular analysis. *Eur J Cancer* **38**: 977–85.

Bilchik AJ, Trocha SD (2003). Lymphatic mapping and sentinel node analysis to optimize laparoscopic resection and staging of colorectal cancer: an update. *Cancer Control* **10**: 219–23.

Braat AE, Oosterhuis JW, Moll FC, de Vries JE, Wiggers T (2005). Sentinel node detection after preoperative short-course radiotherapy in rectal carcinoma is not reliable. *Br J Surg* **92**: 1533–38.

Broderick-Villa G, Amr D, Haigh PI, O'Connell TX, Danial T, Difronzo LA (2004). Ex vivo lymphatic mapping: a technique to improve pathologic staging in colorectal cancer. *Am Surg* **70**: 937–41.

Compton C, Fenoglio-Preiser CM, Pettigrew N Fielding LP (2000). American joint committee on cancer prognostic factors consensus conference. *Cancer* **88**: 1739–57.

Codignola C, Zorzi F, Zaniboni A, Mutti S, Rizzi A, Padolecchia E et al. (2005). Is there any role for sentinel node mapping in colorectal cancer staging? Personal experience and review of the literature. *Jpn J Clin Oncol* **35**: 645–50.

Cox ED, Kellicut D, Adair C, Marley K, Otchy DP, Peoples GE (2002). Sentinel lymph node evaluation is technically feasible and may improve staging in colorectal cancer. *Curr Surg* **59**: 301–6.

Cserni G, Vajda K, Tarjan M, Bori R, Svebis M, Baltas B (1999). Nodal staging of colorectal carcinomas from quantitative and qualitative aspects. Can lymphatic mapping help staging? *Pathol Oncol Res* **5**: 291–96.

Dahl K, Westlin J, Kraaz W, Winqvist O, Bergkvist L, Thorn M (2005). Identification of sentinel nodes in patients with colon cancer. *Eur J Surg Oncol* **31**: 381–85.

Demirbas S, Ince M, Baloglu H, Celenk T (2004). Should sentinel lymph node mapping be performed for colorectal cancer? *Turk J Gastroenterol* **15**: 39–44.

Des Guetz G, Uzzan B, Nicolas P, Cucherat M, de Mestier P, Morere JF et al. (2007). Is Sentinel Lymph Node Mapping in Colorectal Cancer a Future Prognostic Factor? A Meta-analysis. *World J Surg* **31**: 1304–12.

Doekhie FS, Kuppen PJ, Peeters KC, Mesker WE, van Soest RA, Morreau H et al. (2006). Prognostic relevance of occult tumour cells in lymph nodes in colorectal cancer. *Eur J Surg Oncol* **32**: 253–58.

Doekhie FS, Peeters KC, Kuppen PJ, Mesker WE, Tanke HJ, Morreau H et al. (2005). The feasibility and reliability of sentinel node mapping in colorectal cancer. *Eur J Surg Oncol* **31**: 854–62.

Esser S, Reilly WT, Riley LB, Eyvazzadeh C, Arcona S (2001). The role of sentinel lymph node mapping in staging of colon and rectal cancer. *Dis Colon Rectum* **44**: 850–54; discussion 854–6.

Evangelista W, Satolli MA, Malossi A, Mussa B, Sandrucci S (2002). Sentinel lymph node mapping in colorectal cancer: a feasibility study. *Tumori* **88**: 37–40.

Faerden A, Sjo O, Andersen S, Hauglann B, Nazir N, Gravedaug B et al. (2008). Sentinel node mapping does not improve staging of lymph node metastasis in colonic cancer. *Dis Colon Rectum* **51**: 891–96.

Gandy CP, Biddlestone LR, Roe AM, O'Leary DP (2002). Intra-operative injection of Patent Blue V dye to facilitate nodal staging in colorectal cancer. *Colorectal Dis* **4**: 447–49.

Iddings D, Ahmad A, Elashoff D, Bilchik A (2006). The prognostic effect of micrometastases in previously staged lymph node negative (N0) colorectal carcinoma: a meta-analysis. *Ann Surg Oncol* **13**: 1386–92.

Joosten JJ, Strobbe LJ, Wauters CA, Pruszczynski M, Wobbes T, Ruers TJ (1999). Intraoperative lymphatic mapping and the sentinel node concept in colorectal carcinoma. *Br J Surg* **86**: 482–86.

Kitagawa Y, Watanabe M, Hasegawa H, Yamamoto S, Fujii H, Yamamoto K et al. (2002). Sentinel node mapping for colorectal cancer with radioactive tracer. *Dis Colon Rectum* **45**: 1476–80.

Patten LC, Berger DH, Rodriguez-Bigas M et al. (2004). A prospective evaluation of radiocolloid and immunohistochemical staining in colon carcinoma lymphatic mapping. *Cancer* **100**: 2104–9.

Lasser P, Cote JF, Sabourin JC, Boige V, Elias D, Duvillard P et al. (2003). [Is sentinel lymph node mapping relevant for colon cancer: a feasibility study]. *Ann Chir* **128**: 433–37.

Liberale G, Lasser P, Sabourin JC, Malka D, Duvillard P, Elias D et al. (2007). Sentinel lymph nodes of colorectal carcinoma: reappraisal of 123 cases. *Gastroenterol Clin Biol* **31**: 281–85.

Lim S, Feig B, Wang H, Hunt K, Rodriguez-Bigas M, Skibber J et al. (2008). Sentinel lymph node evaluation does not improve staging accuracy in colon cancer. *Ann Surg Oncol* **15**: 46–51.

Lyman GH, Giuliano AE, Somerfield MR, Benson AB, III, Bodurka DC, Burstein HJ et al. (2005). American society of clinical oncology guideline recommendations for sentinel lymph node biopsy in early-stage breast cancer. *J Clin Oncol* **23**: 7703–20.

Medina-Franco H, Takahashi T, Gonzalez-Ruiz GF, De-Anda J, Velazco L (2005). Sentinel lymph node biopsy in colorectal cancer: a pilot study. *Rev Invest Clin* **57**: 49–54.

Merrie AE, van Rij AM, Phillips LV, Rossaak JI, Yun K, McCall JL (2001). Diagnostic use of the sentinel node in colon cancer. *Dis Colon Rectum* **44**: 410–17.

Morris EJA, Maughan NJ, Forman D, Quirke P (2007). Identifying stage III colorectal cancer patients: the influence of the patient, surgeon, and pathologist. *J Clin Oncol* **25**: 2573–79.

Nastro P, Sodo M, Dodaro CA, Gargiulo S, Acampa W, Bracale U et al. (2002). Intraoperative radiochromoguided mapping of sentinel lymph node in colon cancer. *Tumori* **88**: 352–53.

Paramo JC, Summerall J, Poppiti R, Mesko TW (2002). Validation of sentinel node mapping in patients with colon cancer. *Ann Surg Oncol* **9**: 550–54.

Read TE, Fleshman JW, Caushaj PF (2005). Sentinel lymph node mapping for adenocarcinoma of the colon does not improve staging accuracy. *Dis Colon Rectum* **48**: 80–85.

Redston M, Compton CC, Miedema BW, Niedzwiecki D, Dowell JM, Jewell SD et al. (2006). Analysis of micrometastatic disease in sentinel lymph nodes from resectable colon cancer: results of Cancer and Leukemia Group B Trial 80001. *J Clin Oncol* **24**: 878–83.

Roseano M, Scaramucci M, Ciutto T, Balani A, Turoldo A, Zanconati F et al. (2003). Sentinel lymph node mapping in the management of colorectal cancer: preliminary report. *Tumori* **89**: 412–16.

Saha S, Dan AG, Berman B, Wiese D, Schochet E, Barber K et al. (2004a). Lymphazurin 1% versus ^{99m}Tc sulfur colloid for lymphatic mapping in colorectal tumors: a comparative analysis. *Ann Surg Oncol* **11**: 21–26.

Saha S, Monson KM, Bilchik A, Beutler T, Dan AG, Schochet E et al. (2004b). Comparative analysis of nodal upstaging between colon and rectal cancers by sentinel lymph node mapping: a prospective trial. *Dis Colon Rectum* **47**: 1767–72.

Saha S, Seghal R, Patel M, Doan K, Dan A, Bilchik A et al. (2006). A multicenter trial of sentinel lymph node mapping in colorectal cancer: prognostic implications for nodal staging and recurrence. *Am J Surg* **191**: 305–10.

Smith FM, Coffey JC, Khasri NM, Walsh MF, Parfrey N, Gaffney E et al. (2005). Sentinel nodes are identifiable in formalin-fixed specimens after surgeon-performed ex vivo sentinel lymph node mapping in colorectal cancer. *Ann Surg Oncol* **12**: 504–9.

Stojadinovic A, Nissan A, Protic M, Adair CF, Prus D, Usaj S et al. (2007). Prospective randomized study comparing sentinel lymph node evaluation with standard pathologic evaluation for the staging of colon carcinoma: results from the United States Military Cancer Institute Clinical Trials Group Study GI-01. *Ann Surg* **245**: 846–57.

Fitzgerald TL, Khalifa MA, Al Zahrani M et al. (2002). Ex vivo sentinel lymph node biopsy in colorectal cancer: a feasibility study. *J Surg Oncol* **80**: 27–32.

Viehl CT, Hamel CT, Marti WR, Guller U, Eisner L, Stammberger U et al. (2003). Identification of sentinel lymph nodes in colon cancer depends on the amount of dye injected relative to tumor size. *World J Surg* **27**: 1285–90.

Waters GS, Geisinger KR, Garske DD, Loggie BW, Levine EA (2000). Sentinel lymph node mapping for carcinoma of the colon: a pilot study. *Am Surg* **66**: 943–45; discussion 945–6.

Wong JH, Johnson DS, Namiki T, Tauchi-Nishi P (2004). Validation of ex vivo lymphatic mapping in hematoxylin-eosin node-negative carcinoma of the colon and rectum. *Ann Surg Oncol* **11**: 772–77.

Wong JH, Severino R, Honnebier MB, Tom P, Namiki TS (1999). Number of Nodes Examined and Staging Accuracy in Colorectal Carcinoma. *J Clin Oncol* **17**: 2896–900.

Chapter 13

TREATMENT OF COLORECTAL CANCER

Eisar Al-Sukhni[1] and Steven Gallinger[2]

[1] *Ontario Cancer Institute, Toronto General Hospital, University Health Network, Toronto, ON, Canada*
[2] *Ontario Cancer Institute, Toronto General Hospital, University Health Network, Toronto, ON, Canada, e-mail: steven.gallinger@uhn.on.ca*

Abstract: Treatment of colorectal cancer is multidisciplinary and has evolved substantially over the past few decades due to advances in surgical techniques and chemotherapeutics. A better understanding of surgical anatomy has enhanced outcomes, especially after rectal cancer surgery. Long term survival rates of patients with metastatic disease are higher due to expanded indications for curative resection of liver metastases and the recent addition of a number of cytotoxic and biologic agents. Further progress is likely with the introduction of novel agents and novel combinations.

Key words: Colorectal neoplasms · Surgery · Radiation therapy · Adjuvant chemotherapy · Surveillance

13.1 Surgical Anatomy

The colon and rectum form a hollow epithelial tube about 150 cm long, extending from the caecum in the right lower abdomen to the anorectal junction at the level of the pelvic floor. The most distal portion of the small bowel, the terminal ileum, empties into the caecum, the widest and most proximal portion of the right colon. This continues up along the right side of the abdomen as the ascending colon before turning to form the hepatic flexure. The transverse colon runs leftward from the hepatic flexure toward the spleen with which it becomes closely associated at the splenic flexure. The splenic flexure curves into the descending colon, running along the left abdominal wall down to the pelvic brim where it transitions into the sigmoid colon. This tortuous, mobile segment of large bowel narrows at the level of the sacral promontory to become the rectum, which then extends about 12–15 cm to end at the proximal border of the anal sphincter complex. This complex maintains continence and consists of the internal anal sphincter, a continuation of the smooth muscle of the rectum; the external anal sphincter, composed of skeletal muscle; and the puborectalis portion of the levator ani muscles.

The arterial supply to the colon and rectum is derived from the superior and inferior mesenteric arteries (SMA and IMA), with the junction of the transverse and descending colon marking the boundary of the two vascular territories (Fig. 13.1). The SMA gives off the ileocolic artery, supplying the terminal ileum, caecum, and appendix; the right colic artery, supplying the ascending colon and hepatic flexure; and the middle colic artery, which further divides into right and left branches to

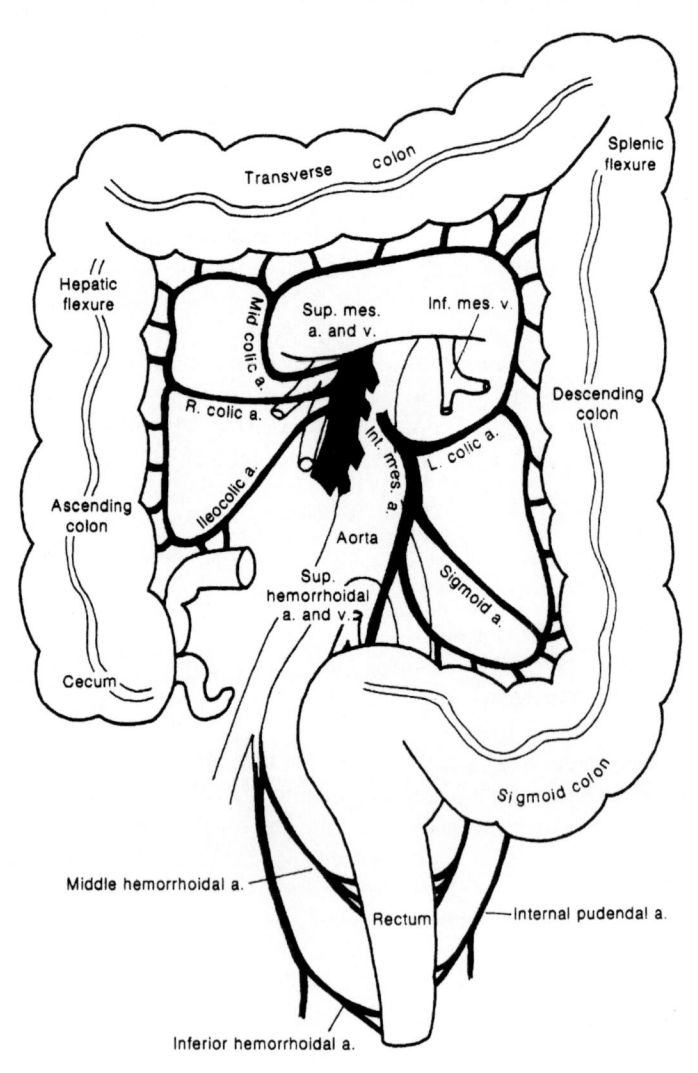

Fig. 13.1 Vascular anatomy of the colon and rectum. Branches of the superior and inferior mesenteric arteries supply the *right* and *left* portions of the colon respectively. The rectum also receives supply from branches of the internal iliac artery

supply the proximal and distal segments of the transverse colon, respectively. The IMA supplies the distal transverse colon, splenic flexure, and descending colon via its left colic branch, the sigmoid colon via its sigmoid branches, and the superior part of the rectum via its terminal branch, the superior rectal artery. The middle and inferior rectum are supplied by the middle and inferior rectal arteries, respectively, as branches of the internal iliac artery. Anastomoses between the main branches, termed marginal arteries, run along the bowel wall and provide collateral supply from one vascular territory to the next. Some individual variations exist, but for the most part this vascular anatomy is consistent.

The venous and lymphatic drainage of the large bowel largely parallels its arterial supply. Regions supplied by the SMA drain into the superior mesenteric vein (SMV), whereas those supplied by the IMA drain into the inferior mesenteric vein (IMV). The IMV drains into the splenic vein which then joins the SMV to form the portal vein, delivering blood to the liver instead of draining directly into the systemic circulation. The distal portion of the rectum is drained into the inferior vena cava via the middle and inferior rectal veins. The venous drainage of the colon and rectum determines patterns of metastases. Metastases from lesions in the colon and upper rectum predominate in the liver, while metastases to the lung are more likely to come from lower rectal tumours.

Lymphatics drain into lymph nodes at various levels along the bowel and its arteries. The primary sites of nodal metastasis are the epicolic nodes, found along the bowel wall, and the paracolic nodes, which lie along the marginal arteries. Downstream drainage continues along the main colic vessels via the intermediate nodes to terminate at the principal nodes, situated at the origins of the SMA and IMA. Readers are encouraged to consult Chapter 2 by C. Ferrario and M. Basik, in this book, to obtain further details on the physiopathology of colorectal cancer.

13.2 Surgical Options

13.2.1 Colon Cancer

Surgery is the mainstay of therapy for colorectal cancer (CRC) and is considered curative for localized disease. The routine principles of oncologic surgery dictate removal of the entire tumour with tumour-free margins and adequate lymphadenectomy. This is achieved by ligation of the main vascular pedicle to the tumour along with all the epicolic and paracolic lymph nodes that parallel it. The extent of resection is therefore determined by the vascular supply to the region of colon bearing the tumour.

A number of segmental colonic resection options are available (Fig. 13.2). A right hemicolectomy is appropriate for tumours of the caecum and ascending colon and involves removal of a portion of the distal ileum, caecum, ascending colon, and transverse colon just proximal to the middle colic artery (Fig. 13.2A). Tumours of the hepatic flexure and proximal transverse colon require removal of the middle

362   E. Al-Sukhni and S. Gallinger

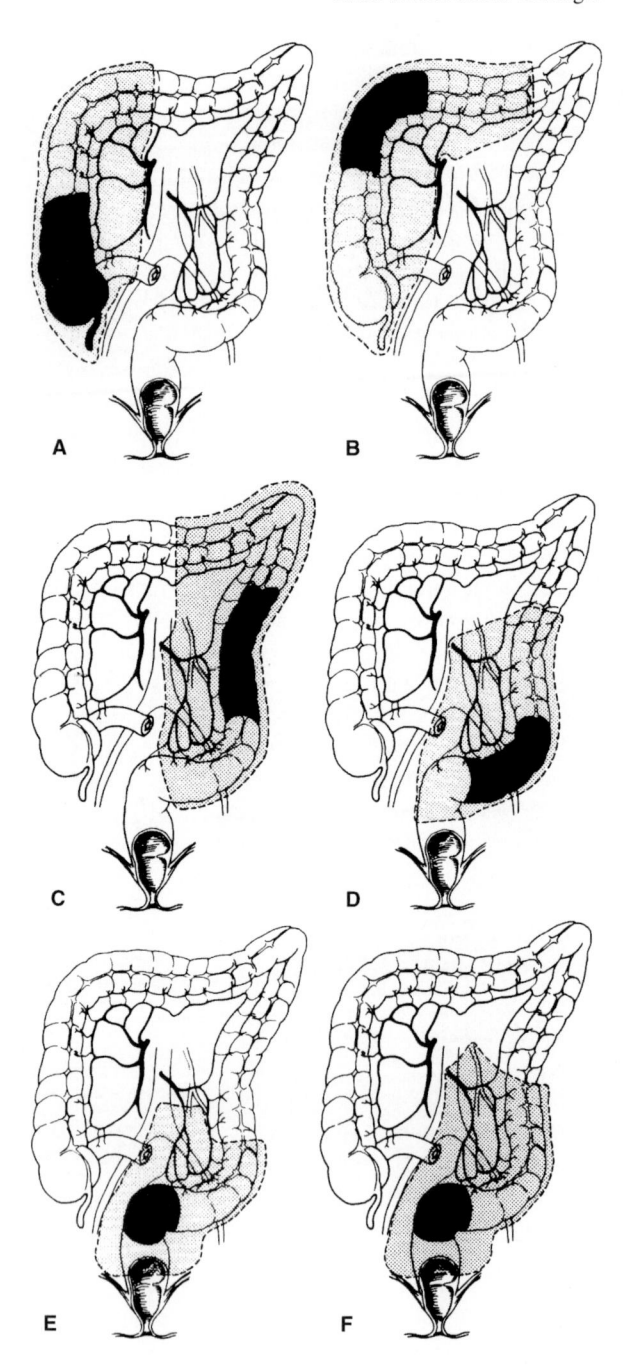

Fig. 13.2 Surgical resection options for colorectal tumours. For each tumour location (depicted in *black*), the *grey* zone represents the segment of colon resected along with its mesentery

colic artery at its origin in addition to the territory covered by a right hemicolectomy; this is referred to as an extended right hemicolectomy (Fig. 13.2B). For tumours of the mid-transverse colon, a transverse colectomy is required to remove the entire territory of the middle colic artery. A left hemicolectomy removes the transverse colon distal to the right branch of the middle colic artery as well as the descending colon, ending just proximal to the rectum (Fig. 13.2C). This is indicated for tumours of the distal transverse and descending colon. Finally, an anterior resection down to 2 cm below the tumour is used for lesions of the sigmoid colon or rectum thus removing the sigmoid colon and involved rectum, with ligation of the superior rectal vessels or IMA at their origins (Fig. 13.2D–F).

Removal of the entire colon may be necessary in the presence of multiple synchronous tumours or in patients deemed at high risk of metachronous colonic tumour development e.g. patients with familial adenomatous polyposis (FAP) or hereditary nonpolyposis colorectal cancer (HNPCC). If the rectum is uninvolved, a subtotal colectomy is performed, including removal of the entire colon with an ileorectal anastomosis. If the rectum requires resection as well, as in the case of some FAP patients with profuse rectal polyps, a proctocolectomy is performed with the option of either end ileostomy or creation of an ileal pouch-anal anastomosis.

Laparoscopic surgery for colon cancer has received increasing attention over the past decade. It offers the advantages of faster recovery and a reduction in postoperative pain, ileus, and pulmonary complications. Earlier concerns regarding the oncologic adequacy of laparoscopy have been tempered with the publication of multiple randomized controlled trials demonstrating no differences in long-term survival or recurrence rates (either at the primary site or at the port/incisional site) in comparison with conventional resection (Kuhry et al., 2008; Araujo et al., 2003; Braga et al., 2005; COSTSG, 2004; Curet et al., 2000; Jayne et al., 2007; Kaiser et al., 2004; Lacy et al., 2002; Leung et al., 2004; Liang et al., 2007; Milsom et al., 1998; Winslow et al., 2002; Zhou et al., 2004).

13.2.2 Rectal Cancer

While the primary goals of oncologic resection remain the same as for colon cancer, surgical decision-making in rectal cancer is complicated by a number of anatomical and functional considerations. The narrow and bony framework of the pelvis can restrict the ability to achieve adequate mobilization of the specimen from an abdominal approach, limiting margins and the potential for restoration of bowel continuity. A second issue is the proximity of the rectum to the anal sphincter, which at times places the goals of adequate margins and preservation of the sphincter complex in conflict. Patient body habitus may also be a factor, as mobilization of the rectum deep in the pelvis is more difficult in the large or overweight patient. The surgeon must take into account a number of factors, both tumour- and patient-related, to determine the appropriate procedure in each case.

Current options for removal of rectal tumours include traditional radical procedures (anterior resection and abdominoperineal resection (APR)) as well as more local approaches that have expanded the cases eligible for sphincter preservation. APR uses a combined abdominal and perineal approach to remove the rectum and anus completely, including the anal sphincter, levator muscles, and ischiorectal fat bilaterally. The patient is then left with a permanent end colostomy. While historically the procedure of choice for rectal cancer (Miles, 1908), its frequency has declined over time with the development of advanced stapling and local excision techniques (Fain et al., 1975; Miller and Moritz, 1996; Kim and Madoff, 1998; Bleday et al., 1997). However, APR remains appropriate for tumours involving the sphincter, for patients with poor preoperative sphincter function, and for low rectal tumours that do not meet the criteria for local resection (Chessin and Guillem, 2005) (see below).

Anterior resection as described previously (variably referred to as low anterior resection (LAR), or ultra-low anterior resection, depending on the level of division relative to the pelvic floor) can remove tumours as low as two centimetres above the anal verge and allows restoration of bowel continuity with colorectal or coloanal anastomosis (Dixon, 1939). Given the higher risk of anastomotic leak in rectal compared with colon surgery – a risk that increases with lower anastomoses – a loop ileostomy may be created as a temporary measure to 'protect' the anastomosis. While an ileostomy will not reduce the rate of anastomotic leak, it diverts fecal flow proximal to the anastomosis, thus decreasing the risk of peritoneal contamination (Tan et al., 2009).

Whether anterior resection or APR is performed, the success of surgery in locally controlling the disease is critically dependent on the ability to achieve clear margins, not only distal to the tumour but also circumferential to it. Multiple studies have shown that intramural spread of cancer cells is typically limited to two cm beyond the distal margin of the tumour (Pollett and Nicholls, 1983; Black and Waugh, 1948; Grinnell, 1954; Williams et al., 1983; Quer et al., 1953); consequently, a distal resection margin of two cm is now generally accepted as adequate to minimize the risk of local recurrence. The circumferential (or radial) resection margin is an independent predictor of local recurrence and survival (Gunderson and Sosin, 1974; Pilipshen et al., 1984; Minsky et al., 1988) and is dependent on complete removal of the rectal mesentery en bloc with the rectum using sharp dissection – a technique termed total mesorectal excision (TME) (Heald et al. 1982). Prior to the introduction of TME by Heald in 1982, traditional rectal surgery involved blunt dissection which frequently breached the mesorectum and resulted in high rates of local failure. With the application of TME, local recurrence rates following surgery for rectal cancer have been reduced from 15 to 35% to less than 7% (Heald et al. 1982; Heald and Ryall, 1986 Merchant et al., 1999; Leo et al., 1996).

While radical surgery with TME has become the new standard of treatment for rectal cancer, it is not without risks and drawbacks. In addition to the morbidity and mortality risks associated with the physiologic stresses of a major operation, it carries the potential for anastomotic leak, poor functional sphincter outcome, permanent stoma, and bladder and sexual dysfunction secondary to injury to sympathetic nerves (Enker et al., 1999; Pakkastie et al., 1994; Mealy et al., 1992; Averbach et al., 1996; Lee and Park, 1998; Williamson et al., 1995; Petrelli et al., 1993;

Rothenberger and Wong, 1992). Such risks may make it an unacceptable option for certain patients. Traditionally, local excision was reserved for patients who were not medically fit for radical resection or who refused, as it was associated with high rates of local recurrence. More recently, however, there has been increasing interest in the potential for local excision, with or without neo-adjuvant or adjuvant therapy, to achieve local control while minimizing risks associated with pelvic dissection. Local resection (in the form of trans-anal excision or the more newly developed trans-anal endoscopic microsurgery) removes the full thickness of the rectum wall but does not include lymphadenectomy (Meredith et al., 2009; Middleton et al., 2005; Murra and Stahl, 1993; Neary et al., 2003). Therefore, the primary issue in determining eligibility for local resection becomes the risk of lymph node metastases. Studies have variably related this to tumour T stage, depth of submucosal invasion, degree of histological differentiation, location in the rectum, and the presence of lymphovascular or perineural invasion (Blumberg et al., 1999; Rasheed et al., 2008; Brodsky et al., 1992; Nascimbeni et al., 2002; Yamamoto et al., 2004; Choi et al., 2008). Specifically, the rate of positive lymph nodes in patients with T1 disease ranges from 6 to 14%, rising to 17–23% in T2 and 49–66% in T3 disease (Blumberg et al., 1999; Nascimbeni et al., 2002; Choi et al., 2008; Ricciardi et al., 2006; Fang et al., 2005; Sitzler et al., 1997). Closely related to the risk of lymph node positivity is the risk of local recurrence following curative resection for early rectal cancer, which is generally under 10% following LAR or APR but as high as 28% following local excision and rises with rising T stage (Endreseth et al., 2005; Mellgren et al., 2000; Bentrem et al., 2005; Paty et al., 2002). A similar association exists with degree of histological differentiation, where poorly-differentiated tumours are associated with higher rates of lymph node positivity and greater risk of local failure (Ricciardi et al., 2006; Zenni et al., 1998). On this basis, most surgeons will consider curative local excision only for patients with T1 tumours that are well-to moderately-differentiated. For technical reasons, they also require that the tumour is less than 3–4 cm in size, that it occupies less than one third of the rectal lumen, and that it lies within ten cm of the anal verge (Meredith et al., 2009; Perretta et al., 2006; Moore and Guillem, 2002; Sengupta and Tjandra, 2001). Patients with T2 or T3 disease who show significant clinical response to neo-adjuvant chemo-radiation may also be candidates, although this remains controversial (Nair et al., 2008; Kim et al., 2001; Greenberg et al., 2008; Steele et al., 1999; Thomas et al., 2008). In all cases, patients may require the addition of adjuvant chemotherapy, radiation or radical surgery following local excision if their tumour shows features considered to be poor prognostic indicators. These include lymphovascular invasion, positive or unclear margins, poor histologic differentiation, or final pathologic T stage greater than T1.

In contrast to the volume of evidence supporting the use of laparoscopic surgery for colon cancer, there is scarce data available regarding long-term outcomes following laparoscopic rectal cancer surgery (Araujo et al., 2003; Zhou et al., 2004). Currently, minimally invasive rectal cancer surgery is used primarily in the context of high anterior resection for tumours of the upper rectum, although its indications may be expanded subject to the results of ongoing clinical trials.

13.3 Neo-Adjuvant and Adjuvant Therapy

Following curative resection, as many as 25 and 60% of patients with stage II and stage III CRC, respectively, will relapse with disease secondary to local recurrence or undetected distant metastases (Desch et al., 2005). Neo-adjuvant and/or adjuvant treatment in the form of chemotherapy, radiation, or both are often added in an attempt to reduce this risk. Neo-adjuvant treatment is administered pre-operatively for the purpose of improving the success of surgery, whereas adjuvant treatment is administered post-operatively to eradicate residual microscopic disease. The options differ for colon versus rectal cancer, and can be further modified by a number of factors including location of the tumour, presence and extent of known metastases, and medical fitness of the patient.

13.3.1 Fluoropyrimidines

The role of 5-fluorouracil (5-FU) in the adjuvant treatment of CRC has been established for over 20 years, and it remains the primary agent used in any chemotherapeutic treatment protocol. This fluorinated pyrimidine, once metabolized in the cell, interferes with DNA synthesis by inhibiting thymidylate synthetase-driven production of dTTP. The earliest randomized controlled trials (RCTs) of adjuvant therapy for CRC, performed in the 1970s and 1980s, used 5-FU either alone or in combination with semustine (MeCCNU), an alkylating agent (Panettiere et al., 1988; Abdi et al., 1989). These failed to show a survival benefit, and in fact there was evidence of increased leukemia rates in the group treated with semustine. In 1988, however, a meta-analysis of these RCT's showed a small benefit for adjuvant chemotherapeutic regimens which included 5-FU (Buyse et al., 1988), and this spurred further investigation with larger trials. That same year, results of the National Surgical Adjuvant Breast and Bowel Project (NSABP) C-01 trial became available (Wolmark et al., 1988). This protocol compared adjuvant therapy consisting of semustine, vincristine, and 5-FU (MOF) with surgery alone in patients with stage II and III colon cancer and found improved disease-free and overall survival in the group treated with chemotherapy. Although this survival advantage was no longer apparent on subsequent long-term analysis (Smith et al., 2004), additional trials supported the use of 5-FU as adjuvant therapy, albeit in combination with other agents. The first of these was the North Central Cancer Treatment Group (NCCTG) study, published in 1989, which randomized patients with stage II and III CRC to receive surgery alone, surgery followed by levamisole, or surgery followed by a combination of 5-FU and levamisole (Laurie et al., 1989). Patients in both adjuvant treatment arms had better disease-free survival at 5 years than those who received surgery alone, with a greater effect seen in the 5-FU/levamisole group. A similar, larger study published the following year by the National Cancer Institute showed similar results (Moertel et al., 1995). In both studies, the benefits appeared to be limited to stage III patients, although a non-statistically significant trend towards better survival was noted in those with stage II disease. More recently, results from the Netherlands Adjuvant

Colon Cancer Project (NACCP) and the Norwegian Gastrointestinal Cancer Group have confirmed this benefit in stage III colon cancer, but found no benefit for the adjuvant regimen in rectal cancer (Taal et al., 2001; Dahl et al., 2009).

The anti-tumour mechanism of action of levamisole, an anti-helminthic agent, remained unclear in the aforementioned studies but was hypothesized to be related to its immuno-modulatory effect on T cells. Its role as an adjuvant agent in CRC was subsequently questioned, however, as it was found that monotherapy with levamisole offered no survival advantage over surgery alone (O'Connell et al., 1998; Wolmark et al., 1999), and a meta-analysis of trials utilizing the 5-FU/levamisole regimen correlated survival with the dose of 5-FU rather than the addition of levamisole (Zalcberg et al., 1996). In the 1990s, interest shifted to leucovorin (LV, folinic acid), a reduced folate that was demonstrated to enhance the action of 5-FU in metastatic CRC by stabilizing the 5-FU thymidylate synthetase complex and prolonging its cytotoxic action. A number of large RCTs have since shown significant prolongation in disease-free and overall survival with the addition of 5-FU/LV following resection in patients with stage III colon cancer (Wolmark et al., 1999; Francini et al., 1994; O'Connell et al., 1997; Zaniboni et al., 1998; Wolmark et al., 1993; IMPACT, 1995; Yamamoto et al., 1998; Scheithauer et al., 1995). Furthermore, this combination was found to be superior to other chemotherapeutic regimens, including MOF and 5-FU/levamisole, with respect to its effect on survival in this group of patients. No added benefit was seen with the addition of levamisole to 5-FU/LV, although there was an increase in toxicity (Wolmark et al., 1999). As with previous studies, the benefit of adjuvant chemotherapy was not seen in patients with stage II colon cancer, nor did it apply to patients with rectal cancer, who were excluded from most trials.

Most investigators have administered 5-FU via the intravenous route in a variety of doses in either bolus or continuous infusion schedules. While survival outcomes are essentially the same with any schedule, each is associated with a different toxicity profile including gastrointestinal, hematologic, and dermatologic side effects. Efforts to improve the efficacy and tolerability of 5-FU led to the development of oral fluoropyrimidines which have the theoretical advantage of greater convenience than continuous infusion and more steady therapeutic levels than bolus-administered 5-FU. Following initial studies that found oral fluorouracil less predictably absorbed and consequently less effective than intravenous 5-FU with respect to degree and duration of tumour response (Hahn et al., 1975), new drugs have been formulated with improved absorption and bioavailability. Capecitabine, an oral prodrug of fluorouracil, is not catabolized at the level of the gastrointestinal mucosa but instead is absorbed intact then converted to 5-FU (Ishikawa et al., 1998). Tegafur uracil combines an oral fluoropyrimidine with an inhibitor of dihydropyrimidine dehydrogenase, the enzyme responsible for the catabolism of fluoropyrimidines in the intestine, to enhance mucosal absorption (Ho et al., 1998; Unemi and Takeda, 1981). Both drugs have been shown to be equally effective to intravenous 5-FU, with fewer adverse side effects noted in the case of capecitabine (Sastre et al., 2009; Comella et al., 2009; Rothenberg et al., 2008; Cassidy et al., 2008; Diaz-Rubio et al., 2007; Martoni et al., 2006; Pfeiffer et al., 2006; Twelves et al., 2005; Van Cutsem et al.,

2004; Cassidy et al., 2002; Van Cutsem et al., 2001; Hoff et al., 2001; de la Torre et al., 2008; Lembersky et al., 2006; Nogue et al., 2005).

13.3.2 Oxaliplatin

Oxaliplatin is a platinum-based alkylating agent that inhibits DNA synthesis through covalent cross-linking of DNA molecules. While not effective as monotherapy for CRC, its benefit in combination with 5-FU/LV in the adjuvant treatment of CRC has been proven in two large randomized trials. The Multicenter International Study of Oxaliplatin/5-FU/LV in the Adjuvant Treatment of Colon Cancer (MOSAIC) compared outcomes in patients with resected stage II or III colon cancer who were randomized to receive 6 months of 5-FU/LV with or without oxaliplatin (Andre et al., 2009; 2004). Disease-free survival was significantly improved in stage III (but not stage II) patients who received oxaliplatin. The NSABP C-07 trial randomized a similar group of patients to the same treatment arms and found the same results (Kuebler et al., 2007). Oxaliplatin-related adverse events in the form of neutropenia and neurotoxicity were seen in both trials. Although neither study was able to demonstrate improvement in overall survival, oxaliplatin has been approved in North America for the adjuvant treatment of colon cancer.

13.3.3 Monoclonal Antibodies

In the past few years, attention has focused on the anti-neoplastic potential of monoclonal antibodies to treat CRC. The most prominent of these have been antibodies directed against the epidermal growth factor receptor (EGFR) as well as antiangiogenic antibodies directed against vascular endothelial growth factor (VEGF). In the first category, the chimeric antibody cetuximab and the humanized antibody panitumumab are among the most extensively studied for CRC (Van Cutsem et al., 2009a; Sobrero et al., 2008; Saltz et al., 2007a; Tol et al., 2009; Bokemeyer et al., 2009; Jonker et al., 2007; Gibson et al., 2006; Cunningham et al., 2004). They function by binding to the extracellular domain of EGFR, inhibiting its function in tumour proliferation and metastasis (Baselga, 2001). Bevacizumab is an antibody targeted against VEGF which acts by inhibiting the proliferation of new blood vessels to the tumour (Adams and Weiner, 2005). All three of these agents have shown promise in the treatment of metastatic CRC and their roles in the adjuvant setting are currently under investigation in a number of multicentre RCT's in North America and Europe.

13.3.4 Other Agents

A number of other therapies have been studied for their possible benefit in the adjuvant treatment of CRC. These include irinotecan, mitomycin C as well various forms of non-specific immunotherapy such as BCG, histamine type 2 (H2) receptor antagonists, interferon-alpha (IFN-α), and interleukin-2 (IL-2). Irinotecan, a semisynthetic analogue of the plant alkaloid camptothecin, interferes with DNA replication and transcription through inhibition of topoisomerase I (Iyer and Ratain, 1998). It has proven useful in the treatment of metastatic CRC (Bidard et al., 2009; Saltz et al., 2000; Douillard et al., 2000; Cunningham et al., 1998), but multiple randomized trials combining it with 5-FU/leucovorin failed to demonstrate a similar benefit in the adjuvant setting (Van Cutsem et al., 2009b; Ychou et al., 2009; Saltz et al., 2007b). Mitomycin C is an anti-neoplastic antibiotic which inhibits DNA synthesis by alkylating and crosslinking DNA strands. Neither mitomycin C nor any of the non-specific immunotherapy agents investigated in randomized clinical trials have demonstrated a survival advantage to date (Kuhry et al., 2008).

13.3.5 Radiotherapy

Adjuvant radiotherapy may have a role in the loco-regional control of locally advanced colon cancer, particularly for tumours involving the posterior wall of the retroperitoneal portions of the colon, but this is controversial. Reduced loco-regional recurrence and improved survival in patients treated with radiotherapy following complete resection of colon cancer have been reported in small case series, primarily in patients with T4 disease or positive lymph nodes (Willett et al., 1993; Amos et al., 1996). Strong evidence is lacking, however, and both early and late radiotherapy-associated complications have been reported, including small bowel obstruction, enteritis, and stricture. At this time, radiotherapy is not part of the routine treatment of colon cancer.

The use of radiation in the management of rectal cancer is supported by strong evidence. Several multicentre trials of either pre- or post-operative radiotherapy in resectable rectal cancer have demonstrated reduced local recurrence rates compared with surgery alone (GITSG, 1985; Thomas and Lindblad, 1988; Fisher et al., 1988; Krook et al., 1991; CCCG, 2001). This difference is present even after the optimization of rectal surgery, as demonstrated in the Dutch TME trial in which all patients underwent rectal resection with TME (Kapiteijn et al., 2001). In this study, the relative reduction in local failure with radiotherapy was in fact even greater than seen in studies utilizing standard rectal cancer surgery.

Neo-adjuvant radiotherapy has been shown to be superior to that given post-operatively, for several reasons. First, while radiotherapy given at either point will reduce the risk of local failure following curative resection, the relative risk reduction appears to be greater with pre-operative treatment (Frykholm et al., 1993; Sauer et al., 2004). Second, the efficiency of radiation per dose is higher when administered in the pre-operative rather than the post-operative setting, probably because of better oxygen delivery to tissues before surgical dissection (Frykholm et al., 1993). Third, pre-operative radiation offers a slight improvement in overall survival which is not seen with post-operative radiation (unless combined with chemotherapy) (Colorectal Cancer Collaborative Group, 2001). Finally, post-operative radiotherapy results in higher toxicity than pre-operative treatment (Frykholm et al., 1993); this is likely related to the use of higher doses and the exposure of more residual tissue to radiation when given postoperatively. Furthermore, trials of pre-operative rectal irradiation have shown significant down-staging of tumours at all stages (Colorectal Cancer Collaborative Group, 2001). This offers the potential for less extensive resection and may increase the chances of sphincter-preservation or allow the resection of tumours initially deemed unresectable.

Combining chemotherapy with radiation confers an even greater advantage than achieved by either modality alone. A review of all randomized trials comparing pre-operative radiotherapy to pre-operative chemo-radiotherapy in stage II and III rectal cancer found a significant decrease in local recurrence and significant increase in pathological complete response with chemo-radiotherapy, although there was no difference in rates of sphincter preservation or overall survival at 5 years (Ceelen et al., 2009). Rates of post-operative morbidity, including anastomotic leaks, were the same in both groups.

A drawback of neo-adjuvant therapy is the potential to over-treat some patients. Rectal cancer staging using endorectal ultrasound or MRI retains some degree of inaccuracy, and a significant proportion of patients with pre-operatively staged T3 tumours or node-positive disease will ultimately be found to have stage I disease (Sauer et al., 2004). Such patients may be unnecessarily exposed to the toxic effects of chemo-radiation without added benefit. Readers are encouraged to consult Chapter 14 by T. Vuong et al., in this book, for more information on these topics.

13.3.6 *Summary of Recommendations for Colon Cancer*

The current standard of therapy for stage III colon cancer is complete resection followed by 6 months of fluoropyrimidine-based chemotherapy, either oral or infusional, combined with leucovorin (NCCN Clinical Practice Guidelines in Oncology, 2009). For patients with stage II disease, the value of chemotherapy is controversial. While no individual study has demonstrated a significant benefit, meta-analyses to address this issue, including the International Multi-center Pooled Analysis of Colon cancer Trials (IMPACT) study, have shown that the relative survival benefit of adjuvant chemotherapy in stage II patients parallels its benefit in stage III patients; however, because the actual risk of recurrence or death is lower in stage II disease, absolute improvement in overall survival is very small and not statistically significant (IMPACT B2, 1995; Gill et al., 2004; Figueredo et al., 2004). Subgroup analyses have suggested that the greatest benefit is seen in patients with high risk features such as lymphovascular invasion, stage T4, obstruction, or poor differentiation. Consequently, adjuvant chemotherapy in stage II disease is generally reserved for patients with these features.

Oxaliplatin should be added to the chemotherapy regimen for stage III disease (referred to as FOLFOX: 5-FU/LV plus oxaliplatin), but is not currently supported for use in stage II disease.

13.3.7 Summary of Recommendations for Rectal Cancer

The National Comprehensive Cancer Network (NCCN) guidelines recommend that patients with stage II or III (T3/T4 or lymph node positive) disease who are able to tolerate combined modality therapy undergo neo-adjuvant fluoropyrimidine-based chemo-radiotherapy followed by curative resection. Evidence supporting the use of adjuvant chemotherapy is less robust for rectal cancer than for colon cancer; however, based on data extrapolated from colon cancer studies, experts recommend that all patients treated with neo-adjuvant chemo-radiation should receive 6 months of fluoropyrimidine-based chemotherapy, regardless of the final pathologic stage (NCCN Clinical Practice Guidelines in Oncology, 2009). For patients who do not receive neo-adjuvant therapy, adjuvant treatment consisting of fluoropyrimidine-based chemotherapy and radiation is recommended for pT3 or lymph node-positive disease. This recommendation also applies to patients who undergo local excision and are found to have pT2 disease or high risk features on final pathology.

13.4 Surveillance

While the addition of chemotherapy and radiotherapy significantly improves outcomes following curative resection, about half of patients will ultimately develop recurrence of their disease. The majority of these recurrences arise in the first 2–3 years after surgery and most frequently take the form of metastases to the liver, lung, or peritoneum. In the case of rectal cancer, loco-regional recurrences form a substantial proportion of cases as well (Galandiuk et al., 1992). Furthermore, patients who develop one tumour are at increased risk of developing a second cancer (Enblad et al., 1990; Bulow et al., 1990; Cali et al., 1993). Randomized trials have demonstrated that follow up which is targeted to detect recurrent or metachronous disease allows early intervention and prolongs survival (Rodriguez-Moranta et al., 2005; Pietra et al., 1998). While the heterogeneity of surveillance schedules in the surgical literature precludes the recommendation of any particular scheme, meta-analyses have demonstrated that more intense follow-up employing a greater number of investigations decreases the time to identification of recurrence, increases the rate of curative surgery, and results in significantly improved overall survival (Renehan et al., 2002; Jeffery et al., 2007). Recently published follow-up data from a multi-centre RCT indicates that this benefit applies equally to early stage as well as late stage CRC (Tsikitis et al., 2009).

Various surgical groups have assimilated the available evidence into practice guidelines for CRC surveillance following initial resection (Figueredo et al., 2003; NCCN Clinical Practice Guidelines in Oncology, 2009). As no single imaging or laboratory test can identify recurrence at all sites, a combined approach comprising clinical assessment, serum carcinoembryonic antigen (CEA), abdominal imaging, chest imaging and colonoscopy is generally recommended. Baseline investigations are usually obtained pre-operatively and repeated at regular intervals post-operatively. A rising serum CEA can be the earliest sign of recurrence in patients with elevated pre-operative levels that normalize immediately after resection. Most guidelines agree on focusing surveillance during the first 3 years following resection, when the likelihood of recurrence is highest, then prolonging intervals of follow-up thereafter. Patients who remain disease-free after 5 years are typically considered 'cured' and may not require ongoing investigations unless symptomatic.

13.5 Management of Metastatic Disease

Metastatic disease eventually develops in up to half of CRC patients after curative surgery and is present in about one-quarter of patients at initial presentation. As described previously, sites most commonly involved are the liver, lungs, and peritoneum; spread to bones, ovaries, and the brain is less common. Traditionally, the systemic dissemination of cancer rendered such patients incurable. However, the development in recent years of better chemotherapeutic agents and an increasingly aggressive surgical approach to metastasectomy has led to a shift in this paradigm, so that a growing number of these patients are now assessed with the possibility of cure in mind. This applies specifically to patients with limited metastases to the liver or lung, where survival rates 5 years following resection in recent reports surpass 40 and 50%, respectively (Wei et al., 2006; Fernandez et al., 2004; Abdalla et al., 2004; Rama et al., 2009; Saito et al., 2002).

13.5.1 Resectable Metastases

At this time, curative surgery is reserved for hepatic or pulmonary metastases. While the management of un-resectable metastatic disease is somewhat simplified by the availability of limited options, the approach to the patient with a resectable primary and potentially resectable metastases is more complicated and is ideally considered within a multidisciplinary tumour board to achieve the best possible outcome.

Patients who present with metastases concurrent with their primary cancer may be considered for immediate surgery if the metastases are pulmonary or hepatic, if each tumour is resectable, and if the burden of disease is minimal at each site (NCCN Clinical Practice Guidelines in Oncology, 2009). In the unique situation where the primary cancer is right-sided and the metastases are confined to the liver and require no more than a minor hepatectomy, both the primary and metastases may be removed synchronously in one operation. This approach has been suggested to minimize morbidity by subjecting patients to one major operation rather than two (Martin et al., 2009; Lyass et al., 2001). It also shortens the delay to adjuvant systemic treatment. Combining more extensive colonic or hepatic resections, however, is associated with increased risk of complications (Reddy et al., 2007; Tanaka et al.,

2004); more commonly, staged resection is performed, whereby two operations for the primary cancer and metastasis are separated by an adequate recovery period, usually about 4–6 weeks. Chemotherapy may be given in the interval.

When the primary tumour is resectable, but metastases are un-resectable, treatment decision-making must balance the risk of metastatic progression with potential complications of the primary disease. Most studies have suggested that such patients have resection of their primary cancer as the initial step in their treatment; however, it is controversial whether this is the most beneficial approach (Benoist and Nordlinger, 2009). When the primary tumour is asymptomatic and unlikely to result in obstruction, perforation, or hemorrhage in the short-term, primary treatment with systemic chemotherapy may be preferable for several reasons. First, not only does this approach produce a reduction in metastases in up to 50% of patients, but there is often also a response by the primary tumour. In up to a third of patients, un-resectable metastases become resectable (Adam et al., 2009; Ychou et al., 2008; Barone et al., 2007; Masi et al., 2006). Second, colorectal cancer surgery can be associated with morbidity; administration of chemotherapy before surgical intervention minimizes the chances of treatment delay secondary to complications or prolonged recovery. Third, response to neo-adjuvant chemotherapy has been correlated with lower likelihood of disease progression after metastasectomy and is used by some clinicians as a test of which patients are most likely to benefit from surgery (Adam et al., 2008; Allen et al., 2003). Alternatively, surgery as the initial intervention may be necessary when the colorectal tumour is symptomatic or likely to cause imminent complications. In the specific case of symptomatic rectal cancer with hepatic metastases, neo-adjuvant chemo-radiotherapy may be indicated, but can further postpone systemic therapy and is likely only appropriate in the setting of low volume metastases (NCCN Clinical Practice Guidelines in Oncology, 2009).

The choice, combination, and sequence of drugs most effective in the neo-adjuvant treatment of metastases have yet to be defined. Current recommendations are derived from regimens established to have efficacy in metastatic CRC (NCCN Clinical Practice Guidelines in Oncology, 2009). Available options include the same drugs utilized in the adjuvant setting, with the addition of irinotecan and monoclonal antibodies. Some agents such as oxaliplatin and bevacizumab provide a benefit only when used in conjunction with other drugs; others, like the fluoropyrimidines and cetuximab, are effective as monotherapy but achieve significantly better outcomes when used with other agents. Combinations most often used include FOLFOX (5-FU/LV plus oxaliplatin) and FOLFIRI (5-FU/LV plus irinotecan), both of which have shown a significant and equivalent survival benefit in trials for metastatic CRC (Goldberg et al., 2004; Colucci et al., 2005; Tournigand et al., 2004). Capecitabine has been demonstrated as a safe and effective oral alternative to 5-FU and may be used in its place with oxaliplatin (CAPOX or XELOX) (Cassidy et al., 2008; Diaz-Rubio et al., 2007). The same does not apply to the combination of capecitabine with irinotecan (CAPIRI or XELIRI). Because of the overlapping toxicity profiles of the two drugs, CAPIRI is less tolerable than FOLFIRI, but offers no survival advantage and is not an accepted regimen at this time (Fuchs et al., 2007). A less-commonly administered but newly-accepted neo-adjuvant option is the triple combination of

5-FU/LV with oxaliplatin and irinotecan (FOLFOXIRI), which does not definitely improve survival, but may make a greater proportion of un-resectable metastases eligible for surgery (Falcone et al., 2007).

Survival can be further prolonged in the palliative setting with the addition of either bevacizumab or cetuximab to conventional chemotherapy (Hurwitz et al., 2004; Hochster et al., 2008; Saltz et al., 2008; Kabbinavar et al., 2003; Sobrero et al., 2008; Bokemeyer et al., 2009), though in the latter case the benefit does not apply to all patients. Disappointing response rates to cetuximab on initial evaluation in chemo-refractory metastatic CRC drove efforts to identify markers predictive of response. Activating mutations of the K-RAS oncogene lead to un-regulated cellular proliferation and impaired differentiation (Arteaga, 2002). It is now well-proven that K-RAS mutation status is associated with response to EGFR inhibitors; only patients with wild type K-Ras benefit from cetuximab (Lievre et al., 2006; Karapetis et al., 2008; Van Cutsem et al., 2009a; Bokemeyer et al., 2009). Therefore, current guidelines recommend verification of tumour K-RAS status before initiation of treatment with cetuximab (Allegra et al., 2009). Mutations in BRAF, another proto-oncogene which functions through the same signalling pathway, are found in a subset of patients with wild-type K-RAS and are also associated with resistance to anti-EGFR agents (Di Nicolantonio et al., 2008) (please see Chapter 3 by A.M. Kaz and W.M. Grady and Chapter 8 by C. Saucier and N. Rivard, in this book). Identification of additional molecular markers may allow biologic therapy to be even more precisely tailored. For example, tumour microsatelllite instability status is associated with lack of clinical benefit from 5-FU-based adjuvant chemotherapy (Ribic et al., 2003). Readers are encouraged to consult Chapter 4 by F.J. Carmona and M. Esteller, in this book.

Evidence that adjuvant therapy improves survival after complete resection of metastases is weak (Mitry et al., 2008), leading some experts to advocate starting with neo-adjuvant chemotherapy for all metastatic disease, whether resectable or not (Benoist and Nordlinger, 2009). In addition to the advantages discussed above, they cite the potential for more conservative surgery if tumours respond, and fewer futile operations. However, this strategy is limited by a number of factors, including the potential for lack of response leading some resectable metastases to progress to become un-resectable (Nordlinger et al., 2008), increased cost, adverse drug effects, and the possibility of a complete radiologic (but not pathological) response making metastases difficult to find (Benoist et al., 2006). When given with the aim of subsequent hepatectomy, chemotherapy-associated hepatotoxicity becomes a consideration. Oxaliplatin has been noted to increase the number of vascular liver lesions, resulting in increased peri-operative bleeding (Rubbia-Brandt et al., 2004; Aloia et al., 2006). Steatosis and steatohepatitis are associated with 5-FU and irinotecan, respectively (Zorzi et al., 2007; Pawlik et al., 2007; Vauthey et al., 2006), although the clinical impact of these pathologic findings are controversial (Scoggins et al., 2009; Kooby et al., 2003). These risks appear to be related to the duration of chemotherapy administration, with current evidence indicating that up to six cycles of neo-adjuvant chemotherapy appear to be safe (Welsh et al., 2007; Karoui et al., 2006). An increased risk of operative bleeding and impaired wound healing are also known consequences of bevacizumab, but can be obviated by discontinuation of the drug 6–8 weeks before any surgery (Reddy et al., 2008).

While the majority of chemotherapy trials have focused on systemic treatment, the observation that CRC spread is frequently isolated to the liver has driven interest in regional chemotherapy for hepatic metastases. Chemotherapy infused directly into the hepatic artery (hepatic intra-arterial or HIA chemotherapy) offers the theoretical advantage of maximal local delivery with minimal systemic side effects. It has been studied in both the neo-adjuvant and adjuvant settings, but appears to be inferior to systemic therapy when used alone (Mocellin et al., 2009). There is some evidence that it may prolong survival beyond that achieved by systemic chemotherapy when the two are used together; this role remains to be confirmed in an ongoing NSABP trial.

13.5.2 Un-resectable Metastases

Overall, only a small fraction of patients with metastatic disease will be eligible for surgery. When the disease is inoperable, the chance of long-term cure is low, and the focus of treatment becomes to prolong survival and maintain quality of life.

The only treatment modality with a proven survival benefit in disseminated CRC is systemic chemotherapy. In the research setting, the wide variety of treatment algorithms has limited the capacity of clinical trials to identify individual 'optimal' strategies. What has emerged, however, is that patients who receive all core drug classes – fluoropyrimidines, oxaliplatin, and irinotecan – derive the longest survival benefit, greater than 2 years on average (Goldberg et al., 2007). North American guidelines for the management of metastatic CRC have therefore shifted from the concept of distinct lines of therapy to a 'continuum of care' model, emphasizing individualized schedules that maximize exposure to all active agents while minimizing non-beneficial treatments (NCCN Clinical Practice Guidelines in Oncology). This appears to be best achieved by initiating chemotherapy using one of the accepted effective combinations (e.g. FOLFOX or FOLFIRI) with or without bevacizumab and subsequently switching to previously unused active agents upon disease progression. Unlike bevacizumab, which has a demonstrated survival benefit as first line therapy with any of the standard combinations, cetuximab has a less certain impact on survival and is usually reserved for failure of initial treatment.

When metastatic spread appears to be limited to the liver, local ablative techniques, particularly radiofrequency ablation (RFA), may be considered. RFA involves the image-guided insertion of an electrode into the tumour and the generation of heat through a radiofrequency current to induce tissue destruction. At this time, it is most appropriate for small, potentially resectable lesions (<5 cm) in patients who are otherwise non-surgical candidates (Solbiati et al., 2001; Siperstein et al., 2007).

13.5.3 Resistance to Chemotherapy

It is clear that not all patients with metastatic CRC benefit from existing chemotherapy drugs. Most develop progression of their disease on chemotherapy, in some cases after showing an initial response. Chemo-resistance may be inherent to the tumour or may be acquired following exposure to chemotherapy. Proposed mechanisms for the development of chemo-resistance include decreased drug delivery due to disorganized blood supply in tumours, properties of the tumour microenvironment, hypoxia in tumour cells, increased drug efflux, and proteins involved in the regulation of apoptosis (Prabhudesai et al., 2007). The last of these appears to be particularly important as most chemotherapy drugs function through induction of apoptosis, either directly or indirectly. Mutated or altered expression of apoptotic proteins can lead to dysregulation of apoptosis and reduced efficacy of chemotherapy agents (Shimkets et al., 2005). The most notable examples of these include p53, Bcl-2, TNF-related apoptosis induced ligand (TRAIL), and survivin. Modulators of these proteins are under investigation and may allow a greater proportion of patients to benefit from chemotherapy. For example, oblimeresen sodium, an antisense oligonucleotide targeting the anti-apoptotic protein Bcl-2, has been tested in small studies of patients with metastatic CRC and produced varying degrees of disease stability. Profiling the expressions of these proteins has also been suggested to be of utility in tailoring chemotherapy regimens to each patient, but this approach remains to be investigated (Prabhudesai et al., 2007).

13.6 Palliative Therapy

Patients with advanced CRC who cannot tolerate or do not respond to chemotherapy can still benefit from a number of other treatment modalities. Radiotherapy can alleviate pain from bone metastases and reduce pressure and neurological symptoms secondary to brain metastases. In those who can tolerate surgery, resection of symptomatic metastases to the ovaries or peritoneum can offer relief. Resection with a palliative intent is also a reasonable option both to relieve symptoms and to prevent complications of primary colonic lesions. When removal of the tumour is not possible or risky due to its location, extent, or the patient's overall medical condition, surgical bypass can manage actual or impending obstruction. Finally, endoscopic techniques such as intra-luminal stent placement, electro-fulguration, or laser ablation can provide short-term relief of obstructing and/or bleeding tumours in patients who are not surgical candidates (Karoui et al., 2007; Spinelli et al., 1995).

13.7 Overall Conclusion

The past two decades have yielded major progress in the treatment of CRC with advances in all disciplines including surgical, medical and radiation oncology. Despite this, cure remains unattainable in most cases due to local and systemic spread of the disease. Future investigations will likely target the role of cancer stem cells in both early and metastatic disease, and strategies focusing on molecular profiling of CRC in individual patients may help maximize the benefit of existing and future chemotherapy drugs.

Abbreviations and Acronyms

APR	Abdominoperineal resection
CAPIRI	Capecitabine/irinotecan
CEA	Carcinoembryonic antigen
CRC	Colorectal cancer
EGFR	Epidermal growth factor receptor
FAP	Familial adenomatous polyposis
FOLFIRI	5-FU/LV/irinotecan
FOLFOX	5-FU/LV/oxaliplatin
5-FU	5-Fluorouracil
HNPCC	Hereditary non-polyposis colorectal cancer
IFN-α	Interferon-alpha
IHA	Hepatic intra-arterial
IL-2	Interleukin-2
IMA	Inferior mesenteric arteries
IMPACT	International multi-center pooled analysis of colon cancer trials
IMV	Inferior mesenteric vein
LAR	Low anterior resection
LV	Leucovorin: folinic acid
MOF	Semustine, vincristine, 5-FU
MRI	Magnetic resonance imaging
NACCP	Netherlands adjuvant colon cancer project
NCCN	National comprehensive cancer network
NSABP	National surgical adjuvant breast and bowel project
RFA	Radiofrequency ablation
RCT	Randomized controlled trial
SMA	Superior mesenteric arteries
SMV	Superior mesenteric vein
TME	Total mesorectal excision
TNFα	Tumour necrosis factor α
VEGF	Vascular endothelial growth factor

References

Abdalla EK, Vauthey JN, Ellis LM, Ellis V, Pollock R, Broglio KR, Hess K, Curley SA (2004). Recurrence and outcomes following hepatic resection, radiofrequency ablation, and combined resection/ablation for colorectal liver metastases. *Ann Surg* **239**: 818–25; discussion 825–27.

Abdi EA, Hanson J, Harbora DE, Young DG, McPherson TA (1989). Adjuvant chemoimmuno- and immunotherapy in Dukes' stage B2 and C colorectal carcinoma: a 7-year follow-up analysis. *J Surg Oncol* **40**: 205–13.

Adam R, Wicherts DA, de Haas RJ, Aloia T, Levi F, Paule B et al. (2008). Complete pathologic response after preoperative chemotherapy for colorectal liver metastases: myth or reality? *J Clin Oncol* **26**: 1635–41.

Adam R, Wicherts DA, de Haas RJ, Ciacio O, Levi F, Paule B et al. (2009). Patients with initially unresectable colorectal liver metastases: is there a possibility of cure? *J Clin Oncol* **27**: 1829–35.

Adams GP, Weiner LM (2005). Monoclonal antibody therapy of cancer. *Nat Biotechnol* **23**: 1147–57.

Allegra CJ, Jessup JM, Somerfield MR, Hamilton SR, Hammond EH, Hayes DF et al. (2009). American Society of Clinical Oncology provisional clinical opinion: testing for KRAS gene mutations in patients with metastatic colorectal carcinoma to predict response to anti-epidermal growth factor receptor monoclonal antibody therapy. *J Clin Oncol* **27**: 2091–96.

Allen PJ, Kemeny N, Jarnagin W, DeMatteo R, Blumgart L, Fong Y (2003). Importance of response to neoadjuvant chemotherapy in patients undergoing resection of synchronous colorectal liver metastases. *J Gastrointest Surg* **7**: 109–15.

Aloia T, Sebagh M, Plasse M, Karam V, Levi F, Giacchetti S et al. (2006). Liver histology and surgical outcomes after preoperative chemotherapy with fluorouracil plus oxaliplatin in colorectal cancer liver metastases. *J Clin Oncol* **24**: 4983–90.

Amos EH, Mendenhall WM, McCarty PJ, Gage JO, Emlet JL, Lowrey GC et al. (1996). Postoperative radiotherapy for locally advanced colon cancer. *Ann Surg Oncol* **3**: 431–36.

André T, Boni C, Mounedji-Boudiaf L, Navarro M, Tabernero J, Hickish T et al. (2004). Oxaliplatin, fluorouracil, and leucovorin as adjuvant treatment for colon cancer. *N Engl J Med* **23**: 2343–51.

André T, Boni C, Navarro M, Tabernero J, Hickish T, Topham C et al. (2009). Improved overall survival with oxaliplatin, fluorouracil, and leucovorin as adjuvant treatment in stage II or III colon cancer in the MOSAIC trial. *J Clin Oncol* 27: 3109–16.

Araujo SE, da Silva eSousa AH Jr, de Campos FG, Habr-Gama A, Dumarco RB, Caravatto PP et al. (2003). Conventional approach x laparoscopic abdominoperineal resection for rectal cancer treatment after neoadjuvant chemoradiation: results of a prospective randomized trial. *Rev Hosp Clin Fac Med Sao Paulo* **58**: 133–40.

Arteaga CL (2002). Overview of epidermal growth factor receptor biology and its role as a therapeutic target in human neoplasia. *Semin Oncol* **29**: 3–9.

Averbach AM, Chung D, Koslowe P, Sugarbaker PH (1996). Anastomotic leak after double-stapled low colorectal resection: analysis of risk factors. *Dis Colon Rectum* **39**: 780–87.

Barone C, Nuzzo G, Cassano A, Basso M, Schinzari G, Giuliante F et al. (2007). Final analysis of colorectal cancer patients treated with irinotecan and 5-fluorouracil plus folinic acid neoadjuvant chemotherapy for unresectable liver metastases. *Br J Cancer* **97**: 1035–39.

Baselga J (2001). The EGFR as a target for anticancer therapy – focus on cetuximab. *Eur J Cancer* **37**: S16–22.

Benoist S, Brouquet A, Penna C, Julie C, El Hajjam M, Chagnon S et al. (2006). Complete response of colorectal liver metastases after chemotherapy: does it mean cure? *J Clin Oncol* **24**: 3939–45.

Benoist S, Nordlinger B (2009). The role of pre-operative chemotherapy in patients with resectable colorectal liver metastases. *Ann Surg Oncol* **16**: 2385–2390.

Bentrem DJ, Okabe S, Wong WD, Guillem JG, Weiser MR, Temple LK et al. (2005). T1 adenocarcinoma of the rectum: transanal excision or radical surgery? *Ann Surg* **242**: 472–77.

Bidard FC, Tournigand C, André T, Mabro M, Figer A, Cervantes A et al. (2009). Efficacy of FOLFIRI-3 (irinotecan D1, D3 combined with LV5-FU) or other irinotecan-based regimens in oxaliplatin-pretreated metastatic colorectal cancer in the GERCOR OPTIMOX1 study. *Ann Oncol* **20**: 1042–47.

Black WA, Waugh JM (1948). The intramural extension of carcinoma of the descending colon, sigmoid, and rectosigmoid: a pathologic study. *Surg Gynecol Obstet* **87**. 457–64.

Bleday R, Breen E, Jessup JM, Burgess A, Sentovich SM, Steele G (1997). Prospective evaluation of local excision for small rectal cancers. *Dis Colon Rectum* **40**: 388–92.

Blumberg D, Paty PB, Guillem JG, Picon AI, Minsky BD, Wong WD et al. (1999). All patients with small intramural rectal cancers are at risk for lymph node metastasis. *Dis Colon Rectum* **42**: 881–85.

Bokemeyer C, Bondarenko I, Makhson A, Hartmann JT, Aparicio J, de Braud F et al. (2009). Fluorouracil, leucovorin, and oxaliplatin with and without cetuximab in the first-line treatment of metastatic colorectal cancer. *J Clin Oncol* **27**: 663–71.

Braga M, Frasson M, Vignali A, Zuliani W, Civelli V, Di Carlo V (2005). Laparoscopic versus open colectomy in cancer patients: long-term complications, quality of life, and survival. *Dis Colon Rectum* **48**: 2217–23.

Brodsky JT, Richard GK, Cohen AM, Minsky BD (1992). Variables correlated with the risk of lymph node metastasis in early rectal cancer. *Cancer* **69**: 322–26.

Bulow S, Svendsen LB, Mellemgaard A (1990). Metachronous colorectal carcinoma. *Br J Surg* **77**: 502–5.

Buyse M, Zeleniuch-Jacquotte A, Chalmers TC (1988). Adjuvant therapy of colorectal cancer: why we still don't know. *J Am Med Assoc* **259**: 3571–78.

Cali RL, Pitsch RM, Thorson AG, Watson P, Tapia P, Blatchford GJ et al. (1993). Cumulative incidence of metachronous colorectal cancer. *Dis Colon Rectum* **36**: 388–98.

Cassidy J, Clarke S, Diaz-Rubio E, Scheithauer W, Figer A, Wong R et al. (2008). Randomized phase III study of capecitabine plus oxaliplatin compared with fluorouracil/folinic acid plus oxaliplatin as first-line therapy for metastatic colorectal cancer. *J Clin Oncol* **26**: 2006–12.

Cassidy J, Twelves C, Van Cutsem E, Hoff P, Bajetta E, Boyer M et al. (2002). First-line oral capecitabine therapy in metastatic colorectal cancer: a favorable safety profile compared with intravenous 5-fluorouracil/leucovorin. *Ann Oncol* **13**: 566–75.

Ceelen WP, Van Nieuwenhove Y, Fierens K (2009). Preoperative chemoradiation versus radiation alone for stage II and III resectable rectal cancer. In: *Cochrane Database of Systematic Reviews*, Issue 1. Art. No.: CD006041. DOI: 10.1002/14651858.CD006041.pub2.

Chessin D, Guillem J (2005). Abdominoperineal resection for rectal cancer: historic perspective and current issues. *Surg Oncol Clin North Am* **14**: 569–86.

Choi PW, Yu CS, Jang SJ, Jung SH, Kim HC, Kim JC (2008). Risk factors for lymph node metastasis in submucosal invasive colorectal cancer. *World J Surg* **32**: 2089–94.

Clinical Outcomes of Surgical Therapy Group (2004). A comparison of laparoscopically assisted and open colectomy for cancer. *N Engl J Med* **350**: 2050–59.

Colorectal Cancer Collaborative Group (2001). Adjuvant radiotherapy for rectal cancer: a systematic overview of 8,507 patients from 22 randomised trials. *Lancet* **358**: 1291–304.

Colucci G, Gebbia V, Paoletti G, Giuliani F, Caruso M, Gebbia N et al. (2005). Phase III randomized trial of FOLFIRI versus FOLFOX4 in the treatment of advanced colorectal cancer: a multicenter study of the Gruppo Oncologico Dell'Italia Meridionale. *J Clin Oncol* **23**: 4866–75.

Comella P, Massidda B, Filippelli G, Farris A, Natale D, Barberis G et al. (2009). Randomised trial comparing biweekly oxaliplatin plus oral capecitabine versus oxaliplatin plus i.v. bolus fluorouracil/leucovorin in metastatic colorectal cancer patients: results of the Southern Italy Cooperative Oncology study 0401. *J Cancer Res Clin Oncol* **135**: 217–26.

Cunningham D, Humblet Y, Siena S, Khayat D, Bleiberg H, Santoro A et al. (2004). Cetuximab monotherapy and cetuximab plus irinotecan in irinotecan-refractory metastatic colorectal cancer. *N Engl J Med* **351**: 337–45.

Cunningham D, Pyrhönen S, James RD, Punt CJ, Hickish TF, Heikkila R et al. (1998). Randomised trial of irinotecan plus supportive care versus supportive care alone after fluorouracil failure for patients with metastatic colorectal cancer. *Lancet* **352**: 1413–18.

Curet MJ, Putrakul K, Pitcher DE, Josloff RK, Zucker KA (2000). Laparoscopically assisted colon resection for colon carcinoma: perioperative results and long-term outcome. *Surg Endosc* **14**: 1062–66.

Dahl O, Fluge O, Carlsen E, Wiig JN, Myrvold HE, Vonen B et al. (2009). Final results of a randomised phase III study on adjuvant chemotherapy with 5 FU and levamisol in colon and rectum cancer stage II and III by the Norwegian Gastrointestinal Cancer Group. *Acta Oncol* **48**: 368–76.

de la Torre A, García-Berrocal MI, Arias F, Mariño A, Valcárcel F, Magallón R et al. (2008). Preoperative chemoradiotherapy for rectal cancer: randomized trial comparing oral uracil and tegafur and oral leucovorin vs. intravenous 5-fluorouracil and leucovorin. *Int J Radiat Oncol Biol Phys* **70**: 102–10.

Desch CE, Benson AB 3rd, Somerfield MR, Flynn PJ, Krause C, Loprinzi CL et al. (2005). Colorectal cancer surveillance: 2005 update of an American Society of Clinical Oncology practice guideline. *J Clin Oncol* **23**: 8512–19.

Di Nicolantonio F, Martini M, Molinari F, Sartore-Bianchi A, Arena S, Saletti P et al. (2008). Wild-type BRAF is required for response to panitumumab or cetuximab in metastatic colorectal cancer. *J Clin Oncol* **26**: 5705–12.

Diaz-Rubio E, Tabernero J, Gomez-Espana A, Massuti B, Sastre J, Chaves M et al. (2007). Phase III study of capecitabine plus oxaliplatin compared with continuous-infusion fluorouracil plus oxaliplatin as first-line therapy in metastatic colorectal cancer: final report of the Spanish Cooperative Group for the Treatment of Digestive Tumors Trial. *J Clin Oncol* **25**: 4224–30.

Dixon CF (1939). Surgical removal of lesions occurring in the sigmoid and rectosigmoid. *Am J Surg* **46**: 12–17.

Douillard JY, Cunningham D, Roth AD, Navarro M, James RD, Karasek P et al. (2000). Irinotecan combined with fluorouracil compared with fluorouracil alone as first-line treatment for metastatic colorectal cancer: a multicentre randomised trial. *Lancet* **355**: 1041–47.

Enblad P, Adami H-O, Glimelius B, Kruesmo U, Pahlman L (1990). The risk of subsequent primary malignant diseases after cancers of the colon and rectum. A nationwide cohort study. *Cancer* **65**: 2091–100.

Endreseth BH, Myrvold HE, Romundstad P, Hestvik UE, Bjerkeset T, Wibe A (2005). Transanal excision vs. major surgery for T1 rectal cancer. *Dis Colon Rectum* **48**: 1380–88.

Enker EW, Merchant N, Cohen AM, Lanouette NM, Swallow C, Guillem J et al. (1999). Safety and efficacy of low anterior resection for rectal cancer: 681 consecutive cases from a specialty service. *Ann Surg* **230**: 544–52.

Fain SN, Patin S, Morganstern L (1975). Use of mechanical apparatus in low colorectal anastomosis. *Arch Surg* **110**: 1079–82.

Falcone A, Ricci S, Brunetti I, Pfanner E, Allegrini G, Barbara C et al. (2007). Phase III trial of infusional fluorouracil, leucovorin, oxaliplatin, and irinotecan (FOLFOXIRI) compared with infusional fluorouracil, leucovorin, and irinotecan (FOLFIRI) as first-line treatment for metastatic colorectal cancer: the Gruppo Oncologico Nord Ovest. *J Clin Oncol* **25**: 1670–76.

Fang WL, Chang SC, Lin JK, Wang HS, Yang SH, Jiang JK et al. (2005). Metastatic potential in T1 and T2 colorectal cancer. *Hepatogastroenterology* **52**: 1688–91.

Fernandez FG, Drebin JA, Linehan DC, Dehdashti F, Siegel BA, Strasberg SM (2004). Five-year survival after resection of hepatic metastases from colorectal cancer in patients screened by positron emission tomography with F-18 fluorodeoxyglucose (FDG-PET). *Ann Surg* **240**: 438–47; discussion 447–50.

Figueredo A, Charette ML, Maroun J, Brouwers MC, Zuraw L (2004). Adjuvant therapy for stage II colon cancer: a systematic review from the Cancer Care Ontario Program in evidence-based care's gastrointestinal cancer disease site group. *J Clin Oncol* **22**: 3395–407.

Figueredo A, Rumble RB, Maroun J, Earle CC, Cummings B, McLeod R et al. (2003). Follow-up of patients with curatively resected colorectal cancer: a practice guideline. *BMC Cancer* **3**: 26.

Fisher B, Wolmark N, Rockette H, Redmond C, Deutsch M, Wickerham DL et al. (1988). Postoperative adjuvant chemotherapy or radiation therapy for rectal cancer: results from NSABP protocol R-01. *J Natl Cancer Inst* **80**: 21–29.

Francini G, Petrioli R, Lorenzini L, Mancini S, Armenio S, Tanzini G et al. (1994). Folinic acid and 5-fluorouracil as adjuvant chemotherapy in colon cancer. *Gastroenterology* **106**: 899–906.

Frykholm GJ, Glimelius B, Pahlman L (1993). Preoperative or postoperative irradiation in adenocarcinoma of the rectum: final treatment results of a randomized trial and an evaluation of late secondary effects. *Dis Colon Rectum* **36**: 564–72.

Fuchs CS, Marshall J, Mitchell E, Wierzbicki R, Ganju V, Jeffery M et al. (2007). Randomized, controlled trial of irinotecan plus infusional, bolus, or oral fluoropyrimidines in first-line treatment of metastatic colorectal cancer: results from the BICC-C Study. *J Clin Oncol* **25**: 4779–86.

Galandiuk S, Wieand HS, Moertel CG, Cha SS, Fitzgibbons RJ Jr, Pemberton JH et al. (1992). Patterns of recurrence after curative resection of carcinoma of the colon and rectum. *Surg Gynecol Obstet* **174**: 27–32.

Gastrointestinal Tumor Study Group (1985). Prolongation of the disease-free interval in surgically treated rectal carcinoma. *N Engl J Med* **312**: 1465–72.

Gibson TB, Ranganathan A, Grothey A (2006). Randomized phase III trial results of panitumumab, a fully human anti-epidermal growth factor receptor monoclonal antibody, in metastatic colorectal cancer. *Clin Colorectal Cancer* **6**: 29–31.

Gill S, Loprinzi CL, Sargent DJ, Thome SD, Alberts SR, Haller DG et al. (2004). Pooled analysis of fluorouracil-based adjuvant therapy for stage II and III colon cancer: who benefits and by how much? *J Clin Oncol* **22**: 1797–806.

Goldberg RM, Rothenberg ML, Van Cutsem E, Benson AB 3rd, Blanke CD, Diasio RB et al. (2007). The continuum of care: a paradigm for the management of metastatic colorectal cancer. *Oncologist* **12**: 38–50.

Goldberg RM, Sargent DJ, Morton RF, Fuchs CS, Ramanathan RK, Williamson SK et al. (2004). A randomized controlled trial of fluorouracil plus leucovorin, irinotecan, and oxaliplatin combinations in patients with previously untreated metastatic colorectal cancer. *J Clin Oncol* **22**: 23–30.

Greenberg JA, Shibata D, Herndon JE, Steele GD, Mayer R, Bleday R (2008). Local excision of distal rectal cancer: an update of cancer and leukemia group B 8984. *Dis Colon Rectum* **51**: 1185–91.

Grinnell RS (1954). Distal intramural spread of carcinoma of the rectum and rectosigmoid. *Surg Gynecol Obstet* **99**: 421–30.

Gunderson LL, Sosin H (1974). Areas of failure found at reoperation (second or symptomatic look) following "curative" surgery for adenocarcinoma of the rectum: Clinicopathologic correlation and implications for adjuvant therapy. *Cancer* **34**: 1278–92.

Hahn RG, Moertel CG, Schutt AJ, Bruckner HW (1975). A double-blind comparison of intensive course 5-flourouracil by oral vs. intravenous route in the treatment of colorectal carcinoma. *Cancer* 35: 1031–35.

Heald RJ, Husband EM, Ryall RD (1982). The mesorectum in rectal cancer surgery: the clue to pelvic recurrence? *Br J Surg* **69**: 613–16.

Heald RJ, Ryall RD (1986). Recurrence and survival after total mesorectal excision for rectal cancer. *Lancet* **1**: 1479–82.

Ho DH, Pazdur R, Covington W, Brown N, Huo YY, Lassere Y et al. (1998). Comparison of 5-fluorouracil pharmacokinetics in patients receiving continuous 5-fluorouracil infusion and oral uracil plus N1-(2′-tetrahydrofuryl)-5-fluorouracil. *Clin Cancer Res* **4**: 2085–88.

Hochster HS, Hart LL, Ramanathan RK, Childs BH, Hainsworth JD, Cohn AL et al. (2008). Safety and efficacy of oxaliplatin and fluoropyrimidine regimens with or without bevacizumab as first-line treatment of metastatic colorectal cancer: results of the TREE Study. *J Clin Oncol* **26**: 3523–29.

Hoff PM, Ansari R, Batist G, Cox J, Kocha W, Kuperminc M et al. (2001). Comparison of oral capecitabine versus intravenous fluorouracil plus leucovorin as first-line treatment in 605 patients with metastatic colorectal cancer: results of a randomized phase III study. *J Clin Oncol* **19**: 2282–92.

Hurwitz H, Fehrenbacher L, Novotny W, Cartwright T, Hainsworth J, Heim W et al. (2004). Bevacizumab plus irinotecan, fluorouracil, and leucovorin for metastatic colorectal cancer. *N Engl J Med* **350**: 2335–42.

International Multicentre Pooled Analysis of Colon Cancer Trials (IMPACT) investigators (1995). Efficacy of adjuvant fluorouracil and folinic acid in colon cancer. *Lancet* **345**: 939–44.

Ishikawa T, Fukase Y, Yamamoto T, Sekiguchi F, Ishitsuka H (1998). Antitumor activities of a novel fluoropyrimidine, N4-pentyloxycarbonyl-5′-deoxy-5-fluorocytidine (capecitabine). *Biol Pharm Bull* **21**: 713–17.

Iyer L, Ratain MJ (1998). Clinical pharmacology of camptothecins. *Cancer Chemother Pharmacol* **42(Suppl)**: S31–43.

Jayne DG, Guillou PJ, Thorpe H, Quirke P, Copeland J, Smith A et al. (2007). Randomized trial of laparoscopic-assisted resection of colorectal carcinoma: 3-year results of the UK MRC CLASICC Trial Group. *J Clin Oncol* **25**: 3061–68.

Jeffery M, Hickey BE, Hider PN (2007). Follow-up strategies for patients treated for non-metastatic colorectal cancer. In: *Cochrane Database of Systematic Reviews*, Issue 1. Art. No.: CD002200. DOI: 10.1002/14651858.CD002200.pub2.

Jonker DJ, O'Callaghan CJ, Karapetis CS, Zalcberg JR, Tu D, Au HJ et al. (2007). Cetuximab for the treatment of colorectal cancer. *N Engl J Med* **357**: 2040–48.

Kabbinavar F, Hurwitz HI, Fehrenbacher L, Meropol NJ, Novotny WF, Lieberman G et al. (2003). Phase II, randomized trial comparing bevacizumab plus fluorouracil (FU)/leucovorin (LV) with FU/LV alone in patients with metastatic colorectal cancer. *J Clin Oncol* **21**: 60–65.

Kaiser AM, Kang JC, Chan LS, Vukasin P, Beart RW Jr (2004). Laparoscopic-assisted vs. open colectomy for colon cancer: a prospective randomized trial. *J Laparoendosc Adv Surg Tech A* **14**: 329–34.

Kapiteijn E, Marijnen CA, Nagtegaal ID, Putter H, Steup WH, Wiggers T et al. (2001). Preoperative radiotherapy combined with total mesorectal excision for resectable rectal cancer. *N Engl J Med* **345**: 638–46.

Karapetis CS, Khambata-Ford S, Jonker DJ, O'Callaghan CJ, Tu D, Tebbutt NC et al. (2008). K-ras mutations and benefit from cetuximab in advanced colorectal cancer. *N Engl J Med* **359**: 1757–65.

Karoui M, Charachon A, Delbaldo C, Loriau J, Laurent A, Sobhani I et al. (2007). Stents for palliation of obstructive metastatic colon cancer: impact on management and chemotherapy administration. *Arch Surg* **142**: 619–23.

Karoui M, Penna C, Amin-Hashem M, Mitry E, Benoist S, Franc B et al. (2006). Influence of preoperative chemotherapy on the risk of major hepatectomy for colorectal liver metastases. *Ann Surg* **243**: 1–7.

Kim DG, Madoff RD (1998). Transanal treatment of rectal cancer: ablative methods and open resection. *Semin Surg Oncol* **15**: 101–13.

Kim CJ, Yeatman TJ, Coppola D, Trotti A, Williams B, Barthel JS et al. (2001). Local excision of T2 and T3 rectal cancers after downstaging chemoradiation. *Ann Surg* **234**: 352–58.

Kooby DA, Fong Y, Suriawinata A, Gonen M, Allen PJ, Klimstra DS et al. (2003). Impact of steatosis on perioperative outcome following hepatic resection. *J Gastrointest Surg* **7**: 1034–44.

Krook JE, Moertel CG, Gunderson LL, Wieand HS, Collins RT, Beart RW et al. (1991). Effective surgical adjuvant therapy for high-risk rectal carcinoma. *N Engl J Med* **324**: 709–15.

Kuebler JP, Wieand HS, O'Connell MJ, Smith RE, Colangelo LH, Yothers G et al. (2007). Oxaliplatin combined with weekly bolus fluorouracil and leucovorin as surgical adjuvant chemotherapy for stage II and III colon cancer: results from NSABP C-07. *J Clin Oncol* **25**: 2198–204.

Kuhry E, Schwenk W, Gaupset R, Romild U, Bonjer HJ (2008). Long-term results of laparoscopic colorectal cancer resection. In: *Cochrane Database of Systematic Reviews*, Issue 2. Art. No.: CD003432. DOI: 10.1002/14651858.CD003432.pub2.

Lacy AM, Garcia Valdecasas JC, Delgado S, Castells A, Taura P, Pique JM, et al. (2002). Laparoscopic-assisted colectomy versus open colectomy for treatment of non-metastatic colon-cancer: a randomised clinical trial. *Lancet* **359**: 2224–29.

Laurie JA, Moertel CG, Fleming TR, Wieand HS, Leigh JE, Rubin J et al. (1989). Surgical adjuvant therapy of large-bowel carcinoma: an evaluation of levamisole and the combination of levamisole and fluorouracil. The North Central Cancer Treatment Group and the Mayo Clinic. *J Clin Oncol* **7**: 1447–56.

Lee SJ, Park YS (1998). Serial evaluation of anorectal function following low anterior resection of the rectum. *Int J Colorectal Dis* **13**: 241–46.

Lembersky BC, Wieand HS, Petrelli NJ, O'Connell MJ, Colangelo LH, Smith RE et al. (2006). Oral uracil and tegafur plus leucovorin compared with intravenous fluorouracil and leucovorin in stage II and III carcinoma of the colon: results from National Surgical Adjuvant Breast and Bowel Project Protocol C-06. *J Clin Oncol* **24**: 2059–64.

Leo E, Belli F, Andreola S, Baldini MT, Gallino GF, Giovanazzi R et al. (1996). Total rectal resection, mesorectum excision, and coloendoanal anastomosis: a therapeutic option for the treatment of low rectal cancer. *Ann Surg Oncol* **3**: 336–43.

Leung KL, Kwok SP, Lam SC, Lee JF, Yiu RY, Ng SS et al. (2004). Laparoscopic resection of rectosigmoid carcinoma: prospective randomized trial. *Lancet* **363**: 1187–92.

Liang JT, Huang KC, Lai HS, Lee PH, Jeng YM (2007). Oncologic results of laparoscopic versus conventional open surgery for stage II or III left-sided colon cancers: a randomized controlled trial. *Ann Surg* **14**: 109–17.

Lievre A, Bachet J, Le Corre D, Boige V, Landi B, Emile JF et al. (2006). KRAS mutation status is predictive of response to cetuximab therapy in colorectal cancer. *Cancer Res* **66**: 3992–95.

Lyass S, Zamir G, Matot I, Goitein D, Eid A, Jurim O (2001). Combined colon and hepatic resection for synchronous colorectal liver metastases. *J Surg Oncol* **78**: 17–21.

Martin RC 2nd, Augenstein V, Reuter NP, Scoggins CR, McMasters KM (2009). Simultaneous versus staged resection for synchronous colorectal cancer liver metastases. *J Am Coll Surg* **208**: 842–50; discussion 850–52.

Martoni AA, Pinto C, Di Fabio F, Lelli G, Rojas Llimpe FL, Gentile AL et al. (2006). Capecitabine plus oxaliplatin (xelox) versus protracted 5-fluorouracil venous infusion plus oxaliplatin (pvifox) as first-line treatment in advanced colorectal cancer: a GOAM phase II randomised study (FOCA trial). *Eur J Cancer* **42**: 3161–68.

Masi G, Cupini S, Marcucci L, Cerri E, Loupakis F, Allegrini G, et al. (2006). Treatment with 5-fluorouracil/folinic acid, oxaliplatin, and irinotecan enables surgical resection of metastases in patients with initially unresectable metastatic colorectal cancer. *Ann Surg Oncol* **13**: 58–65.

Mealy K, Burke P, Hyland J (1992). Anterior resection without a defunctioning colostomy: questions of safety. *Br J Surg* **79**: 305–7.

Mellgren A, Sirivongs P, Rothenberger DA, Madoff RD, Garcia-Aguilar J (2000). Is local excision adequate therapy for early rectal cancer? *Dis Colon Rectum* **43**: 1064–71.

Merchant NB, Guillem JG, Paty PB, Enker WE, Minsky BD, Quan SH et al. (1999). T3N0 rectal cancer: results following sharp mesorectal excision and no adjuvant therapy. *J Gastrointest Surg* **3**: 642–47.

Meredith KL, Hoffe SE, Shibata D (2009). The multidisciplinary management of rectal cancer. *Surg Clin N Am* **89**: 177–215.

Middleton PF, Sutherland LM, Maddern GJ (2005). Transanal endoscopic microsurgery: a systematic review. *Dis Colon Rectum* **48**: 270–84.

Miles EW (1908). A method of performing abdominoperineal excision for carcinoma of the rectum and the terminal portion of the pelvic colon. *Lancet* **2**: 1812–13.

Miller K, Moritz E (1996). Circular stapling techniques for low anterior resection of rectal carcinoma. *Hepatogastroenterology* **43**: 823–31.

Milsom JW, Bohm B, Hammerhofer KA, Fazio Z, Steiger E, Elson P (1998). A prospective randomized trial comparing laparoscopic versus conventional techniques in colorectal cancer surgery: a preliminary report. *J Am Coll Surg* **187**: 46–54.

Minsky BD, Mies C, Recht A, Rich TA, Chaffey JT (1988). Resectable adenocarcinoma of the rectosigmoid and rectum. I. Patterns of failure and survival. *Cancer* **61**: 1408–16.

Mitry E, Fields A, Bleiberg H, Labianca R, Portier G, Tu D et al. (2008). Adjuvant chemotherapy after potentially curative resection of metastases from colorectal cancer: a pooled analysis of two randomized trials. *J Clin Oncol* **26**: 4906–11.

Mocellin S, Pasquali S, Nitti D (2009). Fluoropyrimidine-HAI (hepatic arterial infusion) versus systemic chemotherapy (SCT) for unresectable liver metastases from colorectal cancer. In: *Cochrane Database of Systematic Reviews*, Issue 3. Art. No.: CD007823. DOI: 10.1002/14651858.CD007823.pub2.

Moertel CG, Fleming TR, Macdonald JS, Haller DG, Laurie JA, Tangen CM et al. (1995). Intergroup study of fluorouracil plus levamisole as adjuvant therapy for stage II/Dukes' B2 colon cancer. *J Clin Oncol* **13**: 2936–43.

Moore HG, Guillem JG (2002). Local therapy for rectal cancer. *Surg Clin North Am* **82**: 967–81.

Murra JJ, Stahl TJ (1993). Sphincter-saving alternatives for treatment of adenocarcinoma involving distal rectum. *Surg Clin North Am* **73**: 131–43.

Nair RM, Siegel EM, Chen DT, Fulp WJ, Yeatman TJ, Malafa MP (2008). Long-term results of transanal excision after neoadjuvant chemoradiation for T2 and T3 adenocarcinomas of the rectum. *J Gastrointest Surg* **12**: 1797–805.

Nascimbeni R, Burgart LJ, Nivatvongs S, Larson DR (2002). Risk of lymph node metastasis in T1 carcinoma of the colon and rectum. *Dis Colon Rectum* **45**: 200–6.

National Comprehensive Cancer Network (NCCN) (2009). Clinical practice guidelines in oncology. Available at http://www.nccn.org/professionals/physician_gls/f_guidelines.asp (Accessed July 15, 2009).

Neary P, Makin GB, White TJ, White E, Hartley J, MacDonald A et al. (2003). Transanal endoscopic microsurgery: a viable operative alternative in selected patients with rectal lesions. *Ann Surg Oncol* **10**: 1106–11.

Nogué M, Salud A, Batiste-Alentorn E, Saigí E, Losa F, Cirera L et al. (2005). Randomised study of tegafur and oral leucovorin versus intravenous 5-fluorouracil and leucovorin in patients with advanced colorectal cancer. *Eur J Cancer* **41**: 2241–49.

Nordlinger B, Sorbye H, Glimelius B, Poston GJ, Schlag PM, Rougier P et al. (2008). Perioperative chemotherapy with FOLFOX4 and surgery versus surgery alone for resectable liver metastases from colorectal cancer (EORTC Intergroup trial 40983): a randomized controlled trial. *Lancet* **371**: 1007–16.

O'Connell MJ, Laurie JA, Kahn M, Fitzgibbons RJ Jr, Erlichman C, Shepherd L et al. (1998). Prospectively randomized trial of postoperative adjuvant chemotherapy in patients with high-risk colon cancer. *J Clin Oncol* **16**: 295–300.

O'Connell MJ, Mailliard JA, Kahn MJ, Macdonald JS, Haller DG, Mayer RJ et al. (1997). Controlled trial of fluorouracil and low-dose leucovorin given for 6 months as postoperative adjuvant therapy for colon cancer. *J Clin Oncol* **15**: 246–50.

Pakkastie TE, Luukkonen PE, Jarvinen HJ (1994). Anastomotic leakage after anterior resetion of the rectum. *Eur J Surg* **160**: 293–97.

Panettiere FJ, Goodman PJ, Costanzi JJ, Cruz AB Jr, Vaitkevicius VK, McCracken JD et al. (1988). Adjuvant therapy in large bowel adenocarcinoma: long-term results of a Southwest Oncology Group Study. *J Clin Oncol* **6**: 947–54.

Paty PB, Nash GM, Baron P, Zakowski M, Minsky BD, Blumberg D et al. (2002). Long-term results of local excision for rectal cancer. *Ann Surg* **236**: 522–30.

Pawlik TM, Olino K, Gleisner AL, Torbenson M, Schulick R, Choti MA (2007). Preoperative chemotherapy for colorectal liver metastases: impact on hepatic histology and postoperative outcome. *J Gastrointest Surg* **11**: 860–68.

Perretta S, Guerrero V, Garcia-Aguilar J (2006). Surgical treatment of rectal cancer: local resection. *Surg Oncol Clin N Am* **15**: 67–93.

Petrelli NJ, Nagel S, Rodriguez-Bigas M, Piedmonte M, Herrera L (1993). Morbidity and mortality following abdominoperineal resection for rectal adenocarcinoma. *Am Surg* **59**: 400–4.

Pfeiffer P, Mortensen JP, Bjerregaard B, Eckhoff L, Schønnemann K, Sandberg E et al. (2006). Patient preference for oral or intravenous chemotherapy: a randomised cross-over trial comparing capecitabine and Nordic fluorouracil/leucovorin in patients with colorectal cancer. *Eur J Cancer* **42**: 2738–43.

Pietra N, Sarli L, Costi R, Ouchemi C, Grattarola M, Peracchia A (1998). Role of follow-up in management of local recurrences of colorectal cancer: a prospective, randomized study. *Dis Colon Rectum* **41**: 1127–33.

Pilipshen SJ, Heilweil M, Quan SQ, Sternberg SS, Enker WE (1984). Patterns of pelvic recurrence following definitive resections of rectal cancer. *Cancer* **53**: 1354–62.

Pollett WG, Nicholls RJ (1983). The relationship between the extent of distal clearance and survival and local recurrence rates after curative anterior resection for carcinoma of the rectum. *Ann Surg* **198**: 159–63.

Prabhudesai SG, Rekhraj S, Roberts G, Darzi AW, Ziprin P (2007). Apoptosis and chemoresistance in colorectal cancer. *J Surg Oncol* **96**: 77–88.

Quer EA, Dahlin DC, Mayo CW (1953). Retrograde intramural spread of carcinoma of the rectum and rectosigmoid. *Surg Gynecol Obstet* **96**: 24–30.

Rama N, Monteiro A, Bernardo JE, Eugenio L, Antunes MJ (2009). Lung metastases from colorectal cancer: surgical resection and prognostic factors. *Eur J Cardiothorac Surg* **35**: 444–49.

Rasheed S, Bowley DM, Aziz O, Tekkis PP, Sadat AE, Guenther T et al. (2008). Can depth of tumour invasion predict lymph node positivity in patients undergoing resection for early rectal cancer? A comparative study between T1 and T2 cancers. *Colorectal Dis* **10**: 231–38.

Reddy SK, Morse MA, Hurwitz HI, Bendell JC, Gan TJ, Hill SE et al. (2008). Addition of bevacizumab to irinotecan- and oxaliplatin-based preoperative chemotherapy regimens does not increase morbidity after resection of colorectal liver metastases. *J Am Coll Surg* **206**: 96–106.

Reddy SK, Pawlik TM, Zorzi D, Gleisner AL, Ribero D, Assumpcao L et al. (2007). Simultaneous resections of colorectal cancer and synchronous liver metastases: a multi-institutional analysis. *Ann Surg Oncol* **14**: 3481–91.

Renehan AG, Egger M, Saunders MP, O'Dwyer ST (2002). Impact on survival of intense follow-up after curative resection of colorectal cancer: systematic review and met-analysis of randomized trials. *Br Med J* **324**: 1–8.

Ribic CM, Sargent DJ, Moore MJ, Thibodeau SN, French AJ, Goldberg RM et al. (2003). Tumor microsatellite-instability status as a predictor of benefit from fluorouracil-based adjuvant chemotherapy for colon cancer. *N Engl J Med* **349**: 247–57.

Ricciardi R, Madoff R, Rothenberger D, Baxter N (2006). Population-based analyses of lymph node netastases in colorectal cancer. *Clin Gastroenterol Hepatol* **4**: 1522–27.

Rodriguez-Moranta F, Salo J, Arcusa A, Boadas J, Pinol V, Bessa X et al. (2005). Postoperative surveillance in patients with colorectal cancer who have undergone curative resection: a prospective, multicenter, randomized, controlled trial. *J Clin Oncol* 24: 386–93.

Rothenberg ML, Cox JV, Butts C, Navarro M, Bang YJ, Goel R et al. (2008). Capecitabine plus oxaliplatin (XELOX) versus 5-fluorouracil/folinic acid plus oxaliplatin (FOLFOX-4) as second-line therapy in metastatic colorectal cancer: a randomized phase III noninferiority study. *Ann Oncol* **19**: 1720–26.

Rothenberger DA, Wong WD (1992). Abdominoperineal resection for adenocarcinoma of the low rectum. *World J Surg* **16**: 478–85.

Rubbia-Brandt L, Audard V, Sartoretti P, Roth AD, Brezault C, Le Charpentier M et al. (2004). Severe hepatic sinusoidal obstruction associated with oxaliplatin-based chemotherapy in patients with metastatic colorectal cancer. *Ann Oncol* **15**: 460–66.

Saito Y, Omiya H, Kohno K, Kobayashi T, Itoi K, Teramachi M et al. (2002). Pulmonary metastasectomy for 165 patients with colorectal carcinoma: A prognostic assessment. *J Thorac Cardiovasc Surg* **124**: 1007–13.

Saltz LB, Clarke S, Diaz-Rubio E, Scheithauer W, Figer A, Wong R et al. (2008). Bevacizumab in combination with oxaliplatin-based chemotherapy as first-line therapy in metastatic colorectal cancer: a randomized phase III study. *J Clin Oncol* **26**: 2013–19.

Saltz LB, Cox JV, Blanke C, Rosen LS, Fehrenbacher L, Moore MJ et al. (2000). Irinotecan plus fluorouracil and leucovorin for metastatic colorectal cancer. *N Engl J Med* **343**: 905–14.

Saltz LB, Lenz HJ, Kindler HL, Hochster HS, Wadler S, Hoff PM et al. (2007a). Randomized phase II trial of cetuximab, bevacizumab, and irinotecan compared with cetuximab and bevacizumab alone in irinotecan-refractory colorectal cancer: the BOND-2 study. *J Clin Oncol* **25**: 4557–61.

Saltz LB, Niedzwiecki D, Hollis D, Goldberg RM, Hantel A, Thomas JP et al. (2007b). Irinotecan fluorouracil plus leucovorin is not superior to fluorouracil plus leucovorin alone as adjuvant treatment for stage III colon cancer: results of CALGB 89803. *J Clin Oncol* **25**: 3456–61.

Sastre J, Aranda E, Massutí B, Tabernero J, Chaves M, Abad A et al. (2009). Elderly patients with advanced colorectal cancer derive similar benefit without excessive toxicity after first-line chemotherapy with oxaliplatin-based combinations: comparative outcomes from the 03-TTD-01 phase III study. *Crit Rev Oncol Hematol* **70**: 134–44.

Sauer R, Becker H, Hohenberger W, Rodel C, Wittekind C, Fietkau R et al. (2004). Preoperative versus postoperative chemoradiotherapy for rectal cancer. *N Engl J Med* **351**: 1731–40.

Scheithauer W, Kornek G, Rosen H, Sebesta C, Marcell A, Kwasny W et al. (1995). Combined intraperitoneal plus intravenous chemotherapy after curative resection for colonic adenocarcinoma. *Eur J Cancer* **31A**: 1981–86.

Scoggins CR, Campbell ML, Landry CS, Slomiany BA, Woodall CE, McMasters KM et al. (2009). Preoperative chemotherapy does not increase morbidity or mortality of hepatic resection for colorectal cancer metastases. *Ann Surg Oncol* **16**: 35–41.

Sengupta S, Tjandra JJ (2001). Local excision of rectal cancer: what is the evidence? *Dis Colon Rectum* **44**: 1245–61.

Shimkets RA, LaRochelle WJ, Teicher BA (eds) (2005). *Oncogenomics Handbook Understanding and Treating Cancer in the 21st Century*. Humana Press: Totowa, NJ.

Siperstein AE, Berber E, Ballem N, Parikh RT (2007). Survival after radiofrequency ablation of colorectal liver metastases: 10-year experience. *Ann Surg* **246**: 559–65; discussion 565–67.

Sitzler PJ, Seow-Choen F, Ho YH, Leong AP (1997). Lymph node involvement and tumor depth in rectal cancers: an analysis of 805 patients. *Dis Colon Rectum* **40**: 1472–76.

Smith RE, Colangelo L, Wieand HS, Begovic M, Wolmark N (2004). Randomized trial of adjuvant therapy in colon carcinoma: 10-year results of NSABP protocol C-01. *J Natl Cancer Inst* **96**: 1128–32.

Sobrero AF, Maurel J, Fehrenbacher L, Scheithauer W, Abubakr YA, Lutz MP et al. (2008). EPIC: phase III trial of cetuximab plus irinotecan after fluoropyrimidine and oxaliplatin failure in patients with metastatic colorectal cancer. *J Clin Oncol* **26**: 2311–19.

Solbiati L, Livraghi T, Goldberg SN, Ierace T, Meloni F, Dellanoce M et al. (2001). Percutaneous radio-frequency ablation of hepatic metastases from colorectal cancer: long-term results in 117 patients. *Radiology* **221**: 159–66.

Spinelli P, Mancini A, Dal Fante M (1995). Endoscopic treatment of gastrointestinal tumors: indications and results of laser photocoagulation and photodynamic therapy. *Semin Surg Oncol* **11**: 307–18.

Steele GD Jr, Herndon JE, Bleday R, Russell A, Benson A 3rd, Hussain M et al. (1999). Sphincter-sparing treatment for distal rectal adenocarcinoma. *Ann Surg Oncol* **6**: 433–41.

Taal BG, Van Tinteren H, Zoetmulder FA (2001). Adjuvant 5FU plus levamisole in colonic or rectal cancer: improved survival in stage II and III. *Br J Cancer* **85**: 1437–43.

Tan WS, Tang CL, Shi L, Eu KW (2009). Meta-analysis of defunctioning stomas in low anterior resection for rectal cancer. *Br J Surg* **96**: 462–72.

Tanaka K, Shimada H, Matsuo K, Nagano Y, Endo I, Sekido H et al. (2004). Outcome after simultaneous colorectal and hepatic resection for colorectal cancer with synchronous metastases. *Surgery* **136**: 650–59.

Thomas B, Daniel W, Markus M, Heinz S, Theodor J (2008). Neoadjuvant chemoradiation and local excision for T2-3 rectal cancer. *Ann Surg Oncol* **15**: 712–20.

Thomas PR, Lindblad AS (1988). Adjuvant postoperative radiotherapy and chemotherapy in rectal carcinoma: a review of the Gastrointestinal Tumor Study Group experience. *Radiother Oncol* **13**: 245–52.

Tol J, Koopman M, Cats A, Rodenburg CJ, Creemers GJ, Schrama JG et al. (2009). Chemotherapy, bevacizumab, and cetuximab in metastatic colorectal cancer. *N Engl J Med* **360**: 563–72.

Tournigand C, Andre T, Achille E, Lledo G, Flesh M, Mery-Mignard D et al. (2004). FOLFIRI followed by FOLFOX6 or the reverse sequence in advanced colorectal cancer: a randomized GERCOR study. *J Clin Oncol* **22**: 229–37.

Tsikitis VL, Malireddy K, Green EA, Christensen B, Whelan R, Hyder J et al. (2009). Postoperative surveillance recommendations for early stage colon cancer based on results from the clinical outcomes of surgical therapy trial. *J Clin Oncol* **27**: 3671–76.

Twelves C, Wong A, Nowacki MP, Abt M, Burris H 3rd, Carrato A et al. (2005). Capecitabine as adjuvant treatment for stage III colon cancer. *N Engl J Med* 352: 2696–704.

Unemi N, Takeda S (1981). Studies on combination therapy with 1-(tetrahydro-2-furanyl)-5-fluorouracil plus uracil. Effects of uracil on in vitro metabolism of 1-(tetrahydro-2-furanyl)-5-fluorouracil and 5-fluorouracil. *Chemotherapy* 29: 176–84.

Van Cutsem E, Hoff PM, Harper P, Bukowski RM, Cunningham D, Dufour P et al. (2004). Oral capecitabine vs. intravenous 5-fluorouracil and leucovorin: integrated efficacy data and novel analyses from two large, randomised, phase III trials. *Br J Cancer* **90**: 1190–97.

Van Cutsem E, Köhne CH, Hitre E, Zaluski J, Chang Chien CR, Makhson A et al. (2009a). Cetuximab and chemotherapy as initial treatment for metastatic colorectal cancer. *N Engl J Med* **360**: 1408–17.

Van Cutsem E, Labianca R, Bodoky G, Barone C, Aranda E, Nordlinger B et al. (2009b). Randomized phase III trial comparing biweekly infusional fluorouracil/leucovorin alone or with irinotecan in the adjuvant treatment of stage III colon cancer: PETACC-3. *J Clin Oncol* **27**: 3117–25.

Van Cutsem E, Twelves C, Cassidy J, Allman D, Bajetta E, Boyer M et al. (2001). Oral capecitabine compared with intravenous fluorouracil plus leucovorin in patients with metastatic colorectal cancer: results of a large phase III study. *J Clin Oncol* 19: 4097–106.

Vauthey JN, Pawlik TM, Ribero D, Wu TT, Zorzi D, Hoff PM et al. (2006). Chemotherapy regimen predicts steatohepatitis and an increase in 90-day mortality after surgery for hepatic colorectal metastases. *J Clin Oncol* **24**: 2065–72.

Wei AC, Greig PD, Grant D, Taylor B, Langer B, Gallinger S (2006). Survival after hepatic resection for colorectal metastases: a 10-year experience. *Ann Surg Oncol* **13**: 668–76.

Welsh FK, Tilney HS, Tekkis PP, John TG, Rees M (2007). Safe liver resection following chemotherapy for colorectal metastases is a matter of timing. *Br J Cancer* **96**: 1037–42.

Willett CG, Fung CY, Kaufman DS, Efird J, Shellito PC (1993). Postoperative radiation therapy for high-risk colon carcinoma. *J Clin Oncol* **11**: 1112–17.

Williams NS, Dixon MF, Johnson D (1983). Reappraisal of the 5 cm rule of distal excision for carcinoma of the rectum; a study of distal intramural spread and of patients' survival. *Br J Surg* **70**: 150–54.

Williamson ME, Lewis WG, Finan PJ, Miller AS, Holdsworth PJ, Johnston D (1995). Recovery of physiologic and clinical function after low anterior resection of the rectum for carcinoma: myth or reality? *Dis Colon Rectum* **38**: 411–18.

Winslow ER, Fleshman JW, Birnbaum EH, Brunt LM (2002). Wound complications of laparocopic vs open colectomy. *Surg Endosc* **16**: 1420–25.

Wolmark N, Fisher B, Rockette H, Redmond C, Wickerham DL, Fisher ER et al. (1988). Postoperative adjuvant chemotherapy or BCG for colon cancer: results from NSABP protocol C-01. *J Natl Cancer Inst* **80**: 30–36.

Wolmark N, Rockette H, Fisher B, Wickerham DL, Redmond C, Fisher ER et al. (1993). The benefit of leucovorin-modulated fluorouracil as postoperative adjuvant therapy for primary colon cancer: results from National Surgical Adjuvant Breast and Bowel Project protocol C-03. *J Clin Oncol* **11**: 1879–87.

Wolmark N, Rockette H, Mamounas E, Jones J, Wieand S, Wickerham DL et al. (1999). Clinical trial to assess the relative efficacy of fluorouracil and leucovorin, fluorouracil and levamisole, and fluorouracil, leucovorin, and levamisole in patients with Dukes' B and C carcinoma of the colon: results from National Surgical Adjuvant Breast and Bowel Project C-04. *J Clin Oncol* **17**: 3553–59.

Yamamoto T, Matsumoto K, Iriyama K (1998). Potent effects of adjuvant chemotherapy using 5-fluorouracil + leucovorin on DNA aneuploid colorectal cancer. *Int J Clin Oncol* **3**: 165–170.

Yamamoto S, Watanabe M, Hasegawa H, Baba H, Yoshinare K, Shiraishi J et al. (2004). The risk of lymph node metastasis in T1 colorectal carcinoma. *Hepatogastroenterology* **51**: 998–1000.

Ychou M, Raoul JL, Douillard JY, Gourgou-Bourgade S, Bugat R, Mineur L et al. (2009). A phase III randomised trial of LV5FU2 + irinotecan versus LV5FU2 alone in adjuvant high-risk colon cancer. *Ann Oncol* **20**: 674–80.

Ychou M, Viret F, Kramar A, Desseigne F, Mitry E, Guimbaud R et al. (2008). Tritherapy with fluorouracil/leucovorin, irinotecan and oxaliplatin (FOLFIRINOX): a phase II study in colorectal cancer patients with non-resectable liver metastases. *Cancer Chemother Pharmacol* **62**: 195–201.

Zalcberg JR, Siderov J, Simes J (1996). The role of 5-fluorouracil dose in the adjuvant therapy of colorectal cancer. *Ann Oncol* **7**: 41–46.

Zaniboni A, Labianca R, Marsoni S, Torri V, Mosconi P, Grilli R et al. (1998). GIVIO-SITAC 01: A randomized trial of adjuvant 5-fluorouracil and folinic acid administered to patients with colon carcinoma – long term results and evaluation of the indicators of health-related quality of life. *Cancer* **82**: 2135–44.

Zenni GC, Abraham K, Harford FJ, Potocki DM, Herman C, Dobrin PB (1998). Characteristics of rectal carcinomas that predict the presence of lymph node metastases: Implications for patient selection for local therapy. *J Surg Oncol* **67**: 99–103.

Zhou ZG, Hu M, Lei WZ, Yu YY, Cheng Z, Li L et al. (2004). Laparoscopic versus open total mesorectal excision with anal sphincter preservation for low rectal cancer. *Surg Endosc* **18**: 1211–15.

Zorzi D, Laurent A, Pawlik TM, Lauwers GY, Vauthey JN, Abdalla EK (2007). Chemotherapy-associated hepatotoxicity and surgery for colorectal liver metastases. *Br J Surg* **94**: 274–86.

Chapter 14

DIAGNOSIS AND TREATMENT OF RECTAL CANCER

Té Vuong[1], Tamim Niazi[2], Sender Liberman[3], Polymnia Galiatsatos[4] and Slobodan Devic[5]

[1] Department of Radiation Oncology, Jewish General Hospital, McGill University, Montréal, QC, Canada, H3T 1E2, e-mail: tvuong@jgh.mcgill.ca
[2] Department of Radiation Oncology, Jewish General Hospital, McGill University, Montréal, QC, Canada, H3T 1E2
[3] Department of Surgery, McGill University Health Centre, McGill University, Montréal, QC, Canada
[4] Department of Gastroenterology, Jewish General Hospital, McGill University, Montréal, QC, Canada
[5] Department of Medical Physics, Jewish General Hospital, McGill University, Montréal, QC, Canada

Abstract: Carcinoma of the rectum, a common malignancy in developed countries, accounts for approximately one third of colorectal cancers. Although majority of the localized rectal cancers are potentially curable, local recurrence remains a serious problem with severe disability and impaired quality of life. Rectal cancer, which was a surgically-managed tumour, now requires the coordinated efforts of multidisciplinary team, colorectal surgery, radiation oncology, medical oncology, radiology and others. In addition to the staging workup, pre-treatment evaluation of the local disease, by endorectal ultrasound (EUS) and multislice computer tomography (CT) and magnetic resonance imaging (MRI), is utmost important to determine the surgical approach and the need for the various other treatment modalities: radiation and chemotherapy (ChT). The introduction of Total Mesorectal Excision (TME) and neoadjuvant Radiation Therapy (RT) have led to significant improvement in the loco-regional control of the rectal cancer, 90–94%. TME is now widely accepted as the standard surgical technique for rectal cancer. Local recurrence rates have been shown to decrease significantly with TME alone. However, the addition of radiation therapy has furthered this improvement, especially in patients having a circumferential resection margin (CRM) that is involved with tumour on pre-operative imaging. There are two radiation modalities used in the treatment of patients with solid tumours, external beam radiation (EBRT) and brachytherapy (BT). In rectal cancer EBRT is primarily used to optimize the rate of local control achieved by surgery. Numerous clinical trials have confirmed its benefit, with or without chemotherapy, in improving local control. However, the survival advantage and the impact on distant metastasis are controversial. In view of normal organ toxicity associated with EBRT, newer radiation delivery techniques have been explored. High dose rate brachytherapy (HDRB) delivers radiation by an endoluminal approach, avoiding the delivery through other organs, and as such, decreases normal organ toxicity. The emerging prospective data are very promising and an international phase III study is being conducted. Despite significant improvement in local control, over the last decade, one third of the patients continue to fail at distance, with metastases. The role of chemotherapy in conjunction with radiation therapy as a neo-adjuvant modality to TME has been, mostly, accepted as routine in North America. However, to date, evidence from Phase III-randomized studies in rectal cancer fails to demonstrate any benefit from additional post-operative adjuvant 5-fluorouracil (FU)-based chemotherapy in terms of disease-free or overall survival in locally advanced rectal cancer. There have been significant achievements in the treatment of rectal cancer over the past decade with multidisciplinary approach becoming the standard of care. Such approach allows for the selection of those patients who are cured with surgery alone, as well as those at risk for failing locally, thus achieving a balance between treatment toxicity risks and tumour control gains.

Key words: Rectal cancer · External beam radiation therapy · High dose rate brachytherapy · Total mesorectal excision · Chemotherapy

14.1 Introduction

Carcinoma of the rectum is a common malignancy in developed countries and represents, along with colon cancer, the third most common cancer worldwide. In many parts of the western world, it is the first and second cause of cancer death (Canadian Cancer Statistics, 2008). Approximately one third of colorectal cancers arise in the rectum.

Upon initial assessment, 3–5% of patients present with early, localized tumours and preservation of the rectum can be achieved by local excision of the growth. From 15 to 20% of all patients will have metastases, while the remaining 75–80% patients are potentially curable. Local recurrence is a serious problem and is made worse in part because of the limited access to the rectum caused by the presence of pelvic bone, resulting in a smaller likelihood of achieving negative resection margins. Local recurrence causes disabling symptoms that impair quality of life and are difficult to treat. Therefore, unlike colon cancer, treatment of rectal cancer involves radiation therapy in addition to chemotherapy and surgery.

The management of this disease has evolved significantly over the past decade. Initially a surgically managed disease, it now requires the coordinated efforts of a highly skilled multidisciplinary team. Local regional tumour control in rectal surgery has dramatically changed with the recognition of the importance of the circumferential margin by tumour cells (Nagtegaal and Quirke, 2008). It has led to the use of a surgical technique called total mesorectal excision (TME) in which the entire mesorectum is enveloped and resected by precise, sharp dissection (Heald, 1998; Heald et al., 1998; Enker et al., 1995; MacFarlane et al., 1993; Martling et al., 2000). In addition to this key factor in local control, radiation therapy given pre-operatively has been shown, in randomized trials to improve the surgical success by half. Together both modalities have resulted in a reduction in the local recurrence rate from 25–30% to 6–12% (Kapiteijn et al., 2001; Peeters et al., 2007).

Systemic overview and meta-analyses have confirmed the superiority of pre-operative to post-operative radiotherapy (Camma et al., 2000; Colorectal Cancer Collaborative Group: Lancet 2001; Glimelius et al., 2003; Wong et al., 2007), and optimal quality staging is therefore now regarded as a prerequisite for treatment decision making. It allows for the selection of those patients who are cured with surgery alone, as well as those at risk for failing locally, thus achieving a balance between treatment toxicity risks and tumour control gains.

A broad spectrum of radiation treatment strategies are presently used either alone or in combination with drugs in different parts of the world. The aims of this chapter are to review the evidence and discuss the main advantages that a particular approach promotes for different tumour stage presentations.

14.2 Diagnosis and Staging of Rectal Cancer

Pre-treatment evaluation and staging are essential in determining the surgical approach to rectal cancer, as well as the sequencing of the various treatment modalities: radiation, chemotherapy and surgery. The determination of local disease extension (tumour (T), node (N) status) as well as the presence or absence of systemic disease, are the most critical factors. The initial assessment starts with the clinical examination and patient performance evaluation, this is especially critical in the elderly population, while the diagnosis is based on the biopsy examination. A colonoscopy is done to identify metachronous tumour or polyps and includes a precise determination of the distal tumour edge to the anal verge using a rigid proctoscopy.

In the past, local staging was based on digital examination and was the most reliable evaluation tool to determine local disease. Today, imaging modalities include

(Garcia-Aguilar et al., 2002; Gualdi et al., 2000; MacKay et al., 2003; Solomon and McLeoad, 1993; Akasu et al., 2000) endorectal ultrasound (EUS), multi-slice computer tomography (CT) and magnetic resonance imaging (MRI). The extent of local tumour is classified with the pathological T and N staging system, in which T3 and T4 tumour are considered to have a higher risk for local recurrence. The circumferential radial margin (CRM) is now a recognized major factor in predicting for local and distant metastases (Nagtegaal and Quirke, 2008). The CRM represents the retroperitoneal or peritoneal soft tissue margin closest to the deepest penetration of tumour or peri-rectal lymph node metastasis. It is regarded as positive if the distance between the deepest extent of the tumour and the closest CRM measures 0–1 mm on microscopic examination and the local recurrence risk is closely related to this distance.

EUS is a very accurate modality for assessing the depth of tumour penetration through the layers of the bowel wall (T stage), but is less accurate for evaluating the CRM. Its performance is operator-dependent and is technically limited to non-stenotic tumours with an overall accuracy for T stage of 76–93% and for N stage of 61–88% (MacKay et al., 2003; Solomon and McLeoad, 1993). It is likely the best imaging tool for small lesions (Akasu et al., 2000).

In locally advanced cases, MRI is the only modality capable of predicting the CRM (Brown et al., 2003a; Beets-Tan et al., 2001; Mercury, 2007) and providing anatomical information of the entire pelvic region, a major asset for the radiation oncologist and surgeon. The advantage of an intrinsic high soft tissue contrast resolution combined with new technical developments with faster acquisitions, dedicated external coils, and contrast agents, has made MRI the most attractive technique for local staging of rectal cancer.

Presently, CT scan, EUS and MRI are not reliable for the determination of lymph node evaluation (N stage). Ninety percent of positive nodes are within one mm. CT does not accurately distinguish between malignant and benign lymph nodes, which depend on size and shape criteria. EUS performs better using both size and echogenic features, especially when combined with EUS-guided fine needle aspiration. MRI is more reliable, using criteria based on the outline of the node and features of signal intensity (Brown et al., 2003b). It has been suggested that in the future, the predictive accuracy of MRI for involved mesorectal nodes might be increased with the addition of ultra-small super paramagnetic iron oxide (UPSO, Koh et al., 2004). For pre-operative treatment decisions, it is commonly recommended to use the highest tumour or nodal category found by any of the imaging modalities (Cutsem et al., 2008). CT scan is the standard modality for assessing liver or other distant metastases, and is preferred over ultrasound. It is also the preferred technique to screen lung metastasis, especially for the middle and lower third tumours. However, plain chest radiography is still considered acceptable. CT predictive accuracy for T and N staging is low. Finally, the use of PET CT is not standard for patients with newly diagnosed rectal cancer and is presently indicated primarily when there is suspicion of metastasis or recurrent tumours (Herbertson et al., 2007).

14.3 The Role of Radiotherapy in the Treatment of Rectal Cancer

Two radiation modalities are available in the treatment of patients with solid tumour cancers: external beam radiation (EBRT) and brachytherapy (BT).

14.3.1 External Beam Radiation Therapy in Combination with Surgery

14.3.1.1 To Prevent Local Recurrence

External beam radiation therapy (Fig. 14.1) is primarily used in combination with surgery to optimize local control. The treatment is given transcutaneously to the primary tumour and to subclinical pelvic nodal deposits in order to sterilize subclinical disease and surgical margins. More than 15 randomized trials with or without chemotherapy, two meta-analyses (Camma et al., 2000; Lancet, 2001) and a Cochrane review (Wong et al., 2007) support the benefits of radiation for local control. However, the survival advantage is controversial.

The Dutch CKVO 95-04 study (Kapiteijn et al., 2001; Peeters et al., 2007) randomized 1,861 rectal cancer patients, to TME alone versus neo-adjuvant EBRT using 25 Gy in five fractions followed by TME. The results showed that the addition of neo-adjuvant EBRT significantly decreases the local recurrence rate (12% versus 5.6%, Peeters et al., 2007).

These benefits were confirmed by the MRC CR-O7 trial in patients with clear circumferential margins regardless of the quality level of surgery.

14.3.1.2 To Promote Tumour Down-Staging

The second role of radiation therapy is to down-stage the tumour to promote clear circumferential margins and cure.

In the MRC CR-O7 trial (Sebag-Montefiore et al., 2009), high quality surgery was achieved in 53% of the cases. Incomplete cancer cell excision resulted from either technical failure secondary to the patient's anatomy or tumour extension. Increasing the interval time from the end of radiation to surgery was suggested as a prerequisite factor ($p = 0.05$) in the Lyon R90-01 trial with 201 patients randomized to surgery either less than 2 weeks or 5–7 weeks after radiation therapy (François et al., 1999).

14.3.1.3 To Facilitate Sphincter Preservation Surgery

Radiation therapy is not only effective in tumour down-staging and down-sizing but also plays an important third role in promoting sphincter preservation surgery.

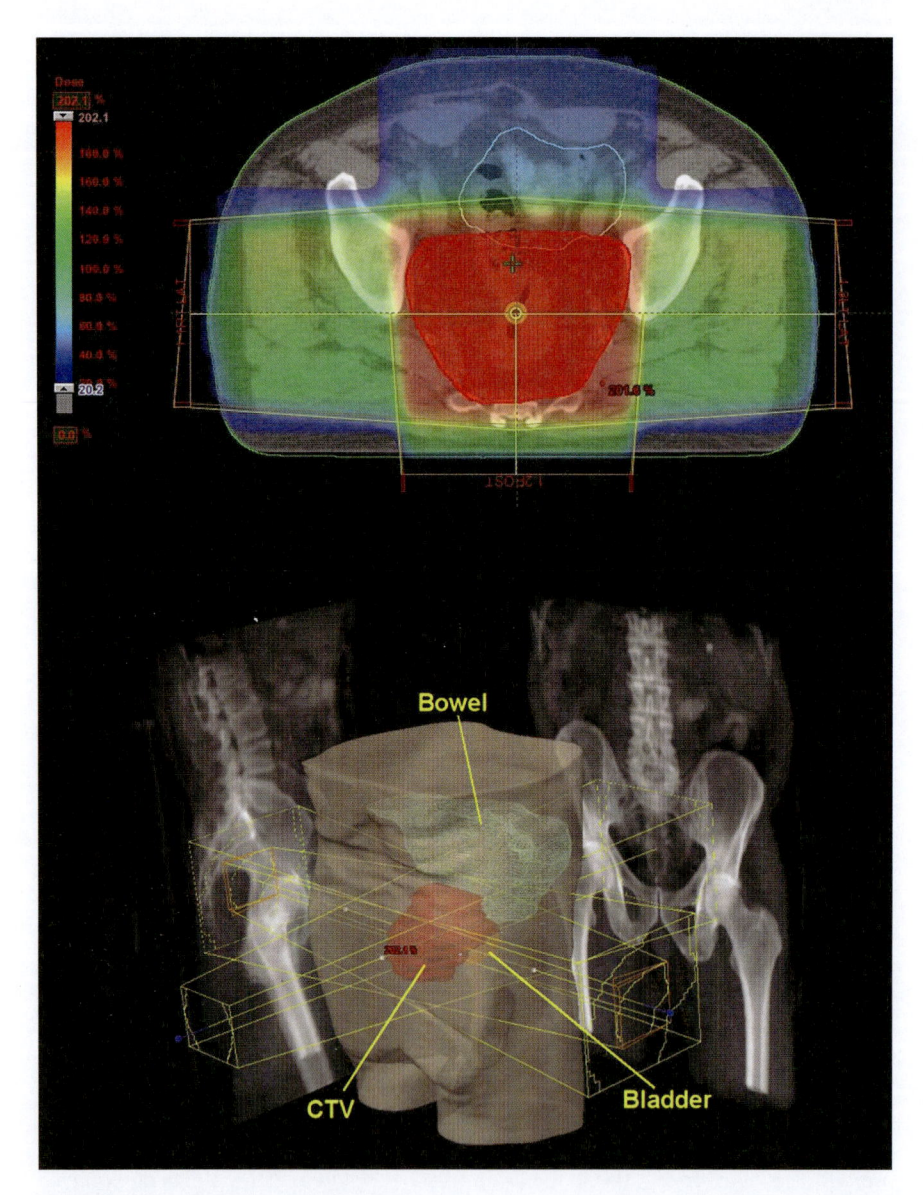

Fig. 14.1 External beam radiation therapy. *Upper picture* shows the axial CT-slice of patient pelvis with superimposed dose distribution achieved within a typical clinical target volume (CTV marked in *red*). Plan was created using a classic 3-field technique employing one lower energy posterior and 2 higher energy lateral wedged beams. Such beam arrangement provides concentrated (higher) dose around target and lower dose to the surrounding healthy tissues. *Lower picture* displays the spatial arrangement of the classic 3-field technique with respect to the patient anatomy and digitally reconstructed radiographs (DRRs) for posterior and one of the lateral beams. DRRs are calculated from CT data, organ contours and radiation fields used on treatment planning station to be subsequently used for patient treatment verification

Table 14.1 Results of endocavitary radiation therapy alone in adenocarcinoma of the rectum treated with curative intent

Author	City (country), years	No. patients	Technique machine	Dose/fraction (Gy)	Local failure (%) (before salvage)	Survival (years)
Papillon (1982)	Lyon (Fr), 1951–1987	312	RT 50 ± Ir	80–130/4–7	9	75%, OS 5
Horiot et al. (1990)	Dijon (Fr), 1970–1996	129	RT 50 ± Ir	90–150/3–5	15	60% OS 5
Tasbas and Sischy (1996)	Rochester (US), 1973–1993	227	RT 50	110/4	5	96%, SpS 5
Gerard et al. (1996)	Lyon-Sud (Fr), 1980–1995	106	RT 50	80–110/4–6	13	83%, OS 5

There are nine randomized trials published using different dose fractionation schedules. Sphincter preservation was specifically addressed in only two of these studies. Pooled data were not statistically significant to support preoperative radiotherapy either alone or with modern chemotherapy regimens (Table 14.1). The Lyon R96-02 randomized trial testing the value of dose escalation is a unique study for patients with low rectal cancer. It shows the value of dose escalation using a boost dose of 85 Gy in three fractions with contact therapy after 39 Gy in 13 fractions of external radiation therapy leading to a sphincter preservation rate of 76% instead of 44% ($p = 0.004$) (Gerard et al., 2004).

14.3.1.4 To Provide Local Control Either with Curative or Palliative Intent

Contact X-therapy or superficial orthovoltage therapy (Fig. 14.2) was introduced more than half a century ago to deliver high dose (80–100 Gy in 3–4 fractions) by small volume radiation (less than 3–4 cm) to early favorable T1 and selected T2 rectal tumours, and is a curative single modality. This technique is limited to tumours

Fig. 14.2 Contact X-ray therapy. The figure depicts the anatomical position of the patient and actual position of the X-ray tube, which has to be held by tradition oncologist during irradiation. Technique developed by Papillon uses short SSD (4 cm) X-ray tube and is used to treat shallow lesions close to the anal sphincter

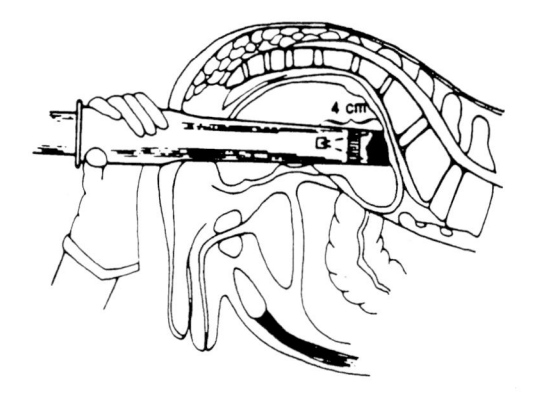

Table 14.2 Sphincter preservation in six trials with pre-operative radiotherapy and delayed surgery compared to immediate surgery, chemotherapy or surgery alone, respectively

Trial	Type of treatment	Preserved sphincters	p-value
Lyon[a]	Preop. Irrad., immediate/delayed surgery	68/76%	ns
Polish[b]	Preop. Chemorad./preop. Short-course	58/61%	ns
EORTC[c]	Preop. Chemorad./preop. irrad.	56/53%	ns
French[d]	Preop. Chemorad./preop. irrad.	52/52%	ns
German[e]	Preop. Chemorad./postop. chemorad.	69/71%	ns
NSABP[f]	Preop. Chemorad./postop. chemorad.	44/34%	ns

[a]François et al. (1999).
[b]Bujko et al. (2006).
[c]Bosset et al. (2006).
[d]Gerard et al. (2006).
[e]Sauer et al. (2004).
[f]Salerno et al. (2009).

10 cm from the anal verge and delivers a total dose varying from 80 to 120 Gy at the mucosa, with a dose fall-off to 25% at 1 cm and 10% at 2 cm. Table 14.2 shows an overview of the results associated with this treatment in series with more than 100 treated patients (Papillon, 1982; Horiot et al., 1990; Tasbas and Sischy, 1996; Gerard et al., 1996).

As rectal cancers penetrate to a greater depth through the rectal wall, the risk of positive regional nodes increases: for T1 tumours the risk is 6–14%, for T2 tumours 17–23% and for T3 tumours 49–66%. Consequently, external beam radiation is necessary in order to encompass the rectum and adjacent nodes and allow for the treatment of both the primary tumour bed together with the mesorectal nodes at risk. For the remaining more advanced T2-3 rectal tumours, external beam radiation alone is considered as an option, usually for either elderly or medically compromised patients. At the Princess Margaret Hospital in Toronto, ON, local control was 30% for partially fixed tumours using a dose of 52 Gy in 20 fractions on a cohort of 229 patients (Brierly et al., 1995). Any consideration of further local gains through radiation dose escalation is limited by the tolerance of normal surrounding structures (genito-urinary tract, soft tissues and bone) in the external beam radiation-treated volume. Nevertheless, limited rectal volumes can tolerate high doses of radiation and can be achieved using a combined approach with external beam and brachytherapy. Usually the treatment starts with external beam radiation, which results in tumour shrinkage, thus permitting a more limited treatment volume at the time of brachytherapy.

Brachytherapy is a unique targeted form of radiation therapy that delivers a localized high dose treatment with a rapid fall-off dose to the tumour and excellent sparing of adjacent normal tissues.

At present, three brachytherapy techniques allow dose supplementing (called boost) to the tumour bed:

a. Contact therapy delivers 50 kv X-rays through an endoluminal approach using a rigid hand-held tube. The treatment volume is determined by direct endoscopic visualization, limited to tumours less than 4 cm in diameter and 10 cm from the anal verge. The depth dose is 100% at 0 mm, 44% at 5 mm and 10% at 2 mm, thus allowing excellent protection of normal tissues, but limiting treatment to superficial lesions. No special shielded room is necessary. Minor anesthesia is required (Fig. 14.2)
b. Interstitial implant uses hollow steel needles through a dedicated crescent-shaped plastic template by direct implant in the perineal area. Iridium 192 wires are inserted in the needles. The treatment volume is determined by clinical examination and limited to tumours below 10 cm from the anal verge. Deeper lesions are well covered by this approach. A shielded room is required. Spinal anesthesia is mandatory (Fig. 14.3)
c. High dose rate brachytherapy is given by an endoluminal approach using a flexible multi-channel rectal applicator 2 cm in diameter. It employs a remote after loading system with Iridium 192 in a shielded room (Vuong et al., 2005). The treatment volume is determined by MRI imaging and a 3D CT based planning system. Both superficial and deep lesions can be treated. A shielded room is required. Minor anesthesia is occasionally needed (Fig. 14.4)

Fig. 14.3 Interstitial brachytherapy. The implant uses hollow steel needles through a dedicated crescent-shaped plastic template by direct implant in the perineal area followed by insertion of Iridium 192 wires. Treatment volume is determined by clinical examination and limited to tumours below 10 cm from the anal verge

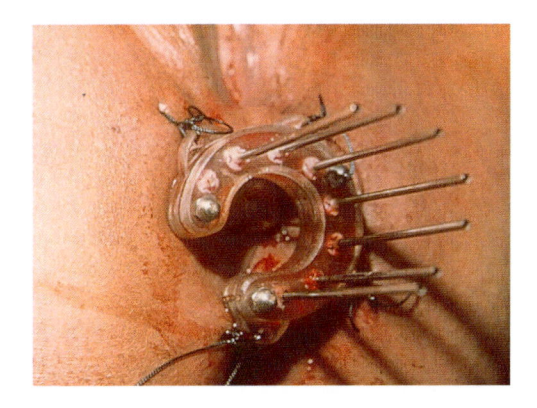

14.3.2 Timing of Radiation Therapy

Sauer et al. (2004) randomized 823 patients with T3-4 rectal cancer to pre- or post-operative chemo radiotherapy (ChTRT, 50.4 Gy and concurrent 5 FU/LV). All

Fig. 14.4 Comparison of Dose distributions achieved with High dose rate endorectal brachytherapy (upper picture) and external beam radiation therapy (lower picture). High dose rate brachytherapy is given by an endoluminal approach using a flexible multi-channel rectal applicator having 2 cm in diameter and a remote after loading system with Iridium 192. The treatment volume is determined by MRI imaging and a 3D CT-based treatment planning system

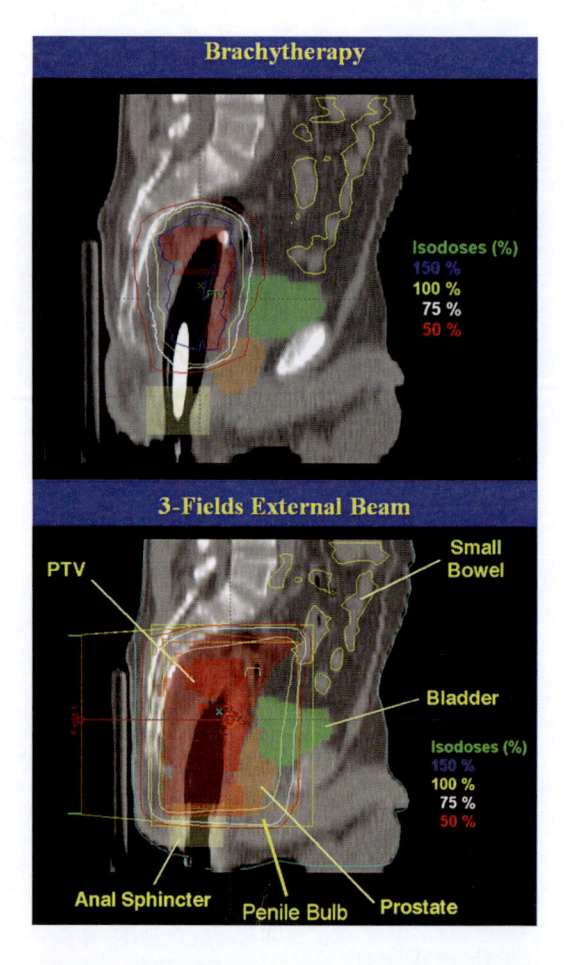

patients received adjuvant chemotherapy (ChT). In the pre-operative arm, significant benefits ($p = 0.004$) in local tumour recurrence (6%) with less acute (27%) and long-term (14%) grade 3 and 4 toxicity were observed. This outweighed the LR rate (13%), and higher acute (40%) and long-term (24%) grade 3 and 4 toxicity of the post-operative arm. With a median follow-up of 40 months, there was no difference in 5-year survival rates (74% versus 76%). MRC C07 (Sebag-Montefiore et al., 2009) compared short course pre-operative radiotherapy (25 Gy in 5 fractions) with selective post-operative radiotherapy (45 Gy in 25 fractions with 5 FU) for patients with positive radial margins defined as ≤ 1 mm. The primary outcome measure was local recurrence. A reduction of 61% in the relative risk of local recurrence for patients receiving the pre-operative radiotherapy (hazard ratio [HR] 0.39, 95% CI 0.27–0.58, $p < 0.0001$) was demonstrated. As well, an absolute difference at 3 years of 6.2% (95% CI 5.3–7.1) (4.4% preoperative radiotherapy versus 10.6% selective postoperative chemo-radiotherapy) was observed. A relative improvement in disease-free survival of 24% was noticed for patients receiving pre-operative radiotherapy (HR 0.76, 95% CI 0.62–0.94, $p = 0.013$), and an absolute difference at 3 years of 6.0% (95% CI 5.3–6.8) (77.5% versus 71.5%) was achieved. Overall survival was not different between the groups (HR 0.91, 95% CI 0.73–1.13, $p = 0.40$). Therefore, pre-operative radiotherapy short course or long course, with chemotherapy is clearly more advantageous for local control than post-operative chemo-radiotherapy.

14.3.3 Radiation Therapy Alone or with Chemotherapy?

Bosset et al. (2006) used a 2 × 2 factorial design, comparing 45 Gy in 25 fractions with 45 Gy in 25 fractions and 5 FU on weeks 1 and 5, plus or minus post-operative ChT. There was no difference in overall survival (OAS), (HR 1.02, 95% CI 0.83–1.26; favoring preoperative RT) or disease-free survival (DFS) 0.84 (95% CI 0.78–1.13; favoring preoperative ChTRT). Local Relapse as the first site of recurrence was higher with the pre-operative RT alone arm, 17%, versus 8.7% for pre-operative ChTRT, 9.6% for pre-operative RT with post-operative ChT and 7.6% for pre-operative ChTRT with post-operative ChT. This suggests that the addition of ChT, regardless of whether it is given before or after surgery, confers a significant local control (LC) benefit.

Gerard et al. (2006) compared pre-operative RT (45 Gy in 25 fractions) with and without 5-FU and Leucovorin (LV). All patients received post-operative adjuvant FU LV × 4, for T3-4 M0 rectal cancers. Acute toxicity was significantly higher in the ChTRT arm (14.6 versus 2.7% grade 3–4 toxicity; $p < 0.0001$). Tumour sterilization rate was 3.7% after RT versus 11.7% for ChTRT. There was a significant decrease in LR (16.5% for RT versus 8% in the ChTRT). However, at 5 years, there were no significant differences in OAS or rate of sphincter-preserving surgery (SPS). The addition of 5-FU-based chemotherapy to pre-operative RT improves local control but is not translated into improvement in disease-free and overall survival. Pre-operative chemo-radiation also resulted in a higher acute grade 3 and 4 toxicity compared to radiotherapy alone.

Thus, pre-operative combined chemotherapy and radiation therapy is currently the treatment of choice, and is widely accepted when long course treatment is used as standard therapy for rectal cancer.

14.3.4 Dose Fractionation

There are two most commonly used dose fractionation regimens: the short course (25 Gy in five fractions) and the long course (45 Gy in 25 fractions). The short course is mainly a standard of care for northern European countries, while the long course is the preferred regimen in North America and southern European countries.

A Polish trial (Bujko et al., 2006) is the only randomized-controlled trial that compared 25 Gy in five fractions (BED 37.5 Gy–10, 5 Gy/fractions) with 50.4 Gy in 28 fractions with 5 FU. In this trial, there was no difference in OAS (67.2% versus 66.2%, $p = 0.960$) or DFS at 4 years (58.4% for RT versus 55.6% for ChTRT, $p = 0.820$).

Moreover, there was no difference in LR rate (9.0% versus 14.2%, $p = 0.170$). Complete pathological response rates were 0.7% after RT alone and 14% after pre-operative ChTRT. There was an increase in early radiation toxicity (18.2% versus 3.2%, $p < 0.001$) with ChTRT and no difference in severe late toxicity with 10.1% versus 7.1% ($p = 0.360$).

With large tumours, the goal of downstaging is crucial to ensure a CRM-negative resection and the long course of pre-operative chemo-radiation therapy is preferable followed by surgery at 6–8 weeks. The short course is used for small tumours with clear CRM.

14.3.5 Immediate or Delayed Surgery

The time interval between pre-operative chemo-radiotherapy and surgery is 6–8 weeks. After short course radiotherapy, immediate surgery is performed. For the long course treatment, the basis for this interval is to avoid the acute inflammatory phase related to normal tissue reaction and to allow for tumour downstaging. The impact of this interval is presently validated by an ongoing Swedish trial where patients are randomized either to a short (less than a week) or long interval (4–6 weeks) between short course radiotherapy and surgery.

14.4 Surgery for Rectal Cancer

Surgical management of rectal cancers is often challenging. Surgical procedures aim to provide the best oncologic outcomes and sphincter preservation rates, while trying to minimize sexual dysfunction and post-operative complications.

Appropriate pre-operative evaluation and staging are crucial to planning and executing surgery for rectal cancers. Since many patients will undergo neo-adjuvant treatment, the treating surgeon should examine the tumour before and after the treatment. The final decisions about surgical procedures are done in the operating room, especially for low rectal tumours. Rigid proctosigmoidoscopy is the most accurate method of assessing the distance of the tumour from the anal verge. Digital examination is also useful in evaluating the fixity of the tumour, and its relationship to the anorectal ring. Pelvic MRI has become increasingly useful both for staging rectal tumours and evaluating the relationship between the tumour and the pelvic structures such as the prostate, vagina and pelvic floor muscles (Salerno et al., 2009). Invasion of these structures may require their removal at the time of surgery.

It is now widely accepted that rectal resection for cancer should be done using the technique of total mesorectal excision (TME). Local recurrence rates have been shown to decrease to as low as 6.4% with TME alone. TME is defined as complete excision of all the mesorectal tissue enveloped in an intact layer of the endopelvic fascia. Anteriorly, Denovilliers' fascia is resected with the specimen, although this may be left when the tumour is on the posterior wall of the rectum, thereby decreasing the risk to the neurovascular bundles. Posteriorly, a smooth, bilobed mesorectum is sharply dissected off the sacral fascia, preserving the inferior hypogastric nerve plexuses (Nagtegaal and Quirke, 2008). For upper rectal tumours, selective mesorectal excision may be performed. It is important, however, to avoid 'coning in' on the mesorectum, and division of the mesorectum must be at a level distal to the tumour.

There has been debate over the necessary distal margin length. Traditionally, 5 cm distal margins were thought to be necessary. Examination of surgical specimens, however, shows that downward sub-mucosal spread of tumour is rare beyond 1 cm in well- to moderately-well differentiated tumours, and that recurrence rates do not change with a larger distal margin. The widespread use of neo-adjuvant chemo-radiation is felt to play a role in the lack of distal spread (Mezhir et al., 2005). It has also been shown more recently that the circumferential resection margin (CRM) plays a more important role in predicting local recurrence rates (Quirke et al., 1986). Patients having a CRM that is involved with tumour on pre-operative imaging often benefit from neo-adjuvant down-staging modalities, in order to increase R0 resection rates. The two most common surgical procedures performed for rectal cancer are the low anterior resection (LAR) and abdominoperineal resection (APR). LAR involves the division of the rectum and the creation of an anastomosis between the colon and the rectal stump. Division of the rectum is usually performed using a linear of curvilinear stapler. An anastomosis can then be created using a circular stapler. When division of the rectum is performed higher up, as in upper rectal tumours, hand-sewn anastomoses can also be created. For tumours that are very low in the rectum, stapling the rectum may not be an option because the distal margin will be compromised. In these cases, trans-anal division of the rectum may be done, followed by a hand-sewn coloanal anastomosis (CAA). Proper patient selection is important, since patients with impaired sphincter function before radiation and inter-sphincteric dissection will most likely aggravate their incontinence issue after undergoing CAA.

In order to improve functional results with ultra-low LAR or CAA, a coloplasty or a colonic J-pouch can be fashioned, thereby creating a reservoir for stool. The benefits of these procedures include decreases in stool frequency, urgency and nighttime bowel movements (Remzi et al., 2005). APR involves TME with the addition of excision of the anal sphincter complex and levator muscles. A perineal dissection is performed, gaining access to the ischiorectal spaces laterally, and the retrorectal space is entered anterior to the coccyx. Anteriorly, the rectum is mobilized at the level of the recto-vaginal septum or the prostatic capsule. APR leaves a defect in the perineum, which is then closed in layers. Drains are usually left through the perineum, or in the pelvis from above. In patients where a large defect is expected, flaps can be used (rectus, gracilis etc.) to close the defect and bring in fresh tissue, especially in the case of a radiated pelvis.

In the case of locally advanced tumours involving other pelvic organs (vagina, uterus, ovary, prostate, bladder, sacrum, ureter), these structures often have to be resected en bloc. It is important to be aware of these issues prior to surgery so that the patient can give the appropriate consent, and the surgery can be well planned, especially when other surgeons may be needed to assist. In borderline cases, where it is unclear whether an organ is involved, repeat imaging is useful after neo-adjuvant therapy is given.

14.4.1 Laparoscopy

Laparoscopic colectomy (LC) for colon cancer has been shown in several trials to provide comparable oncologic outcomes to open colectomy, with modest benefits in terms of post-op narcotic use, recovery of bowel function and hospital length of stay. The role of laparoscopy in rectal cancer surgery is still being evaluated in randomized controlled trials. As was the case in laparoscopic colectomy, the steep learning curve may be an impediment to widespread adoption of laparoscopic rectal cancer surgery should the trials underway show benefits with the procedure.

14.4.2 Local Treatment for Early Rectal Cancer

Patients with early rectal cancers may be treated with local excision techniques. Trans-anal excision (TAE) can be performed using retractors to expose the lower rectum, or by trans-anal endoscopic microsurgery (TEM), which uses laparoscopic-like instruments and can reach higher rectal tumours.

Appropriate staging is important, since local excision techniques do not excise the nodes in the mesorectum. The risk of nodal metastases ranges from 10 to 34% for all T1 tumours. This can be subdivided into high risk and low risk tumours, which have different chances of node metastases. Tumours without lymphovascular invasion (LVI) have positive nodes in 11% versus 32% with LVI. Tumours confined to sm1 and sm2 levels of the submucosa carry risks of 3 and 8% respectively, while sm3 tumours will have nodal metastases in 23% of the cases (Nascimbeni et al., 2002).

A recent series looking at long-term survival after TAE for T1 rectal cancer shows a local recurrence rate of 13.2% versus 2.7% for rectal resection, with disease-specific survival of 87% versus 96% for rectal resection. The authors concluded that TAE should be restricted to patients who have medical prohibitive contraindications to major surgery or have made an informed decision to accept oncologic risks of local excision and avoid the functional consequences of rectal resection (Nash et al., 2009).

It has been suggested that adjuvant chemo-radiotherapy should be given when T2 rectal cancers have been excised locally, assuming that further surgery is not an option, as the risk of recurrence is unacceptably high (Chakravarti et al., 1999).

TME is now widely accepted as the standard surgical technique for rectal cancer patients. However, patients with early rectal cancer have minimal risk of lymph node involvement, as such, these patients can be treated with transanal local excision.

Regardless of the technique all patients with rectal cancer should be managed with multidisciplinary approach.

14.5 Adjuvant Chemotherapy

Over the last decade, the introduction of TME surgery together with pre-operative radiotherapy with (long course radiation) or without chemotherapy (short course) have dramatically improved local control in patients with rectal cancer with a local relapse rate of 6–8%. Nevertheless, meta-analysis and Cochrane review failed to show an impact on the incidence of metastases, and disease-free and overall survival. Thirty to thirty-five percent of patients continue to fail at distance, with metastases.

14.5.1 Before the Era of TME Surgery

In North America, three randomized trials examined chemotherapy alone or in combination with post-operative chemo-radiation to a control arm with surgery alone (Gastrointestinal Tumor Study Group, 1985; Krook et al., 1991; Wolmark et al., 2000). All showed a benefit with the combination of chemotherapy and radiation. Consequently, these results led to the 1990 consensus of the National Institutes of Health that recommended post-operative adjuvant chemo-radiotherapy as standard treatment for patients with rectal cancer classified as AJCC stage II (T3N0) or stage III (any tumour with regional nodes) (Hyams et al., 1997). The schedule started 4–8 weeks after resection with two cycles of bolus 5-FU (without leucovorin). Radiotherapy was started at cycle 3 and 4 with bolus 5-FU, followed by two more cycles of bolus 5-FU post-chemo-radiation therapy. Later, a randomized Korean study indicated the benefits of a shorter interval after resection on disease-free survival when compared to a later start (Lee et al., 2002).

14.5.2 Neo-Adjuvant Chemo-Radiation Therapy and TME Era

The German study AIO/CAO/ARO 94 introduced a new standard in the combined treatment modality approach to patients with rectal cancer (NIH, 1990). The pre-operative strategy with combined chemo-radiation therapy is less toxic and favours sphincter preservation (p value was not significant however). Most importantly, local failure is significantly lower (6%, $p < 0.006$) when compared to the 13% in the post-operative chemo-radiation group). All patients received adjuvant chemotherapy that was given with four cycles of 5-FU. There was no difference in disease-free and overall survival with 35% of metastases observed in both arms.

To date, evidence from Phase III randomized studies in rectal cancer fails to demonstrate any benefit from additional post-operative adjuvant 5-FU-based chemotherapy following either pre-operative radiotherapy or chemo-radiotherapy in terms of disease-free or overall survival in locally advanced rectal cancer. Whether this is related to the low compliance rate following 5-FU-based chemo-radiation reported in phase III randomized studies remains to be clarified.

On the other hand, the role of adjuvant chemotherapy in patients with colon cancer is clearly established as beneficial for disease-free and overall survival especially with the introduction of the modern chemotherapy oxaliplatin-based regimen.

There is no randomized phase III trial to support the routine use of oxaliplatin-based therapies (CAPOX, FOLFOX) in the adjuvant setting for patients with rectal cancer. However, in North America, for the high-risk patients (presence of positive nodes (stage III) or CRM-positive defined by pathological examination), FOLFOX is the commonly used adjuvant regimen based upon the results of adjuvant colon studies and the efficacy of these new drug regimens in the metastatic setting (readers will find more information in Chapter 13, in this book). For patients with complete response after neo-adjuvant ChTRT and stage II disease, without any neo-adjuvant therapy, the practice is even less established.

Unfortunately, it is unlikely that such a question will be answered in America. On-going randomized trials on adjuvant chemotherapy for patients with rectal cancer used FOLFOX in the standard arm and chemotherapy is given to all patients after pre-operative chemo-radiation on the basis of pre-operative staging (despite the known unreliable predictive value of nodal staging) whereas in Europe, adjuvant treatment recommendations are based upon pathological staging. Thus, there is a need to develop better risk stratification criteria and tailored treatment recommendations for adjuvant chemotherapy.

In conclusion, adjuvant chemotherapy for rectal cancer following neoadjuvant chemo-radiotherapy is presently recommended for patients at high risk. It continues to vary significantly in the western world, unlike treatment for colon cancer.

14.6 Conclusion

The management of rectal cancer has evolved significantly over the past decade. Patients with locally advanced rectal cancer are treated with neo-adjuvant radiation therapy, with or without chemotherapy, followed by total mesorectal excision. The new technique of delivering local radiation therapy intra-lumenally, high dose rate brachytherapy, appears very promising. However, further phase III clinical trials will help establish its role as one of the standard approaches. There is significant controversy as to the recommended chemotherapy for locally advanced rectal cancer patients with pathological complete response. As such, all patients with rectal cancer, especially patient with locally advanced tumours should be managed with a multidisciplinary approach.

Abbreviations and Acronyms

APR	Abdominoperineal resection
BT	Brachytherapy
CAA	Coloanal anastomosis

CAPOX	Capecitabine and oxaliplatin
CKVO	Commissie Klinisch Vergelijkend Onderzoek
CRM	Circumferential resection margin
CTRT	Chemotherapy radiotherapy
CT	Computer tomography
ChT	Chemotherapy
DFS	Disease-free survival
EBRT	External beam radiation
EUS	Endorectal ultrasound
FOLFOX	Folinic acid, oxaliplatin and fluorouracil
FU	5-Fluorouracil
HDRB	High dose rate brachytherapy
HR	Hazard ratio
LAR	Low anterior resection
LC	Laparoscopic colectomy
LV	Leucovorin
LVI	Lymphovascular invasion
MRI	Magnetic resonance imaging
N	Node
OAS	Overall survival
RT	Radiation therapy
SPS	Sphincter-preserving surgery
T	Tumour
TAE	Trans-anal excision
TME	Total mesorectal excision
UPSO	Ultra-small super paramagnetic iron oxide

References

Akasu T, Kondo H, Moriya Y et al. (2000). Endorectal ultrasonography and treatment of early stage rectal cancer. *World J Surg* **34**: 1061–68.

Beets-Tan RG, Beets GI, Vliegen RF et al. (2001). Accuracy of magnetic resonance imaging in prediction of tumour-free resection margin in rectal cancer surgery. *Lancet* **357**: 497–504.

Bosset JF, Collette L, Calais G et al. (2006). Chemotherapy with pre-operative radiotherapy in rectal cancer. *N Engl J Med* **355**: 1114–23.

Brierly J, Cummings BJ, Wong WS et al. (1995). Adecarcinoma of the rectum treated with by radical external beam therapy. *Int J Radiat Oncol Biol Phys* **31**(2) 255–59.

Brown G, Radcliffe AG, Newcombe RG et al. (2003a). Pre-operative assessment of prognostic factors in rectal cancer using high-resolution magnetic imaging. *Br J Surg* **90**: 355–64.

Brown G, Richard CJ, Bourne MW et al. (2003b). Morphologic predictors of lymph node status in rectal cancer with the use of high-spatial resolution MR imaging with histopathological comparison. *Radiology* **227**(2): 371–77.

Bujko K, Nowacki MP, Nasierowska-Guttmejer A et al. (2006). Long-term results of a randomized trial comparing pre-operative short-course radiotherapy with pre-operative conventionally fractionated chemoradiation for rectal cancer. *Br J Surg* **93**: 1215–23.

Camma C, Giunta M, Fiorica F et al. (2000). Pre-operative radiotherapy for resectable rectal cancer: A meta-analysis. *J Am Med Assoc* **284**: 1008–15.

Canadian Cancer Statistics (2008). Toronto ISSN 0835-2976: Canadian Cancer Society/National Cancer Institute of Canada.

Chakravarti A, Compton CC, Shellito PC et al. (1999). Long-term follow-up of patients with rectal cancer managed by local excision with and without adjuvant irradiation. *Ann Surg* **230**: 49–54.

Colorectal Cancer Collaborative Group (2001). Adjuvant radiotherapy for rectal cancer: A systematic overview of 8,507 patients from 22 randomised trials. *Lancet* **358**: 1291-304.

Cutsem EV, Dicato M, Haustermans K et al. (2008). The diagnosis and management of rectal cancers: expert discussion and recommendations derived from the 9th World Congress on Gastrointestinal cancer, Barcelona, 2007. *Ann Oncol* **19(Suppl. 6)**: v1–6.

Enker WE, Thaler HT, Cranor ML, Polyak T (1995). Total mesorectal excision in the operative treatment of carcinoma of the rectum. *J Am Coll Surg* **181**: 335–46.

François Y, Nemoz CJ, Beaulieux J et al. (1999). Influence of the interval between pre-operative radiation therapy and surgery on downstaging and the rate of sphincter preservation surgery for rectal cancer: the Lyon R90-01 randomized trial. *J Clin Oncol* **17**: 2396–402.

Garcia-Aguilar J, Pollark J, Lee SH et al. (2002). Accuracy of endorectal ultrasonography in pre-operative staging of rectal tumours. *Dis Colon Rectum* **45**: 10–15.

Gastrointestinal Tumor Study Group (1985). Prolongation of the disease free interval in surgically treated rectal carcinoma. *N Engl J Med* **312**: 1465–72

Gerard JP, Ayzac L, Coquard R et al. (1996). Endocavitary irradiation for early rectal carcinomas T1 (T2): a series of 101 patients treated with the Papillon technique. *Int J Radiat Oncol Biol Phys* **36**: 775–83.

Gerard JP, Chapet O, Nemoz C et al. (2004). Improved sphincter preservation in low rectal cancer with high dose pre-operative radiotherapy: the Lyon R96-02 randomized trial. *J Clin Oncol* **22**: 2404–9.

Gerard JP, Conroy T, Bonnetain F et al. (2006). Pre-operative radiotherapy with or without concurrent fluorouracil and leucovorin in T3-4 rectal cancers: results of FFCD 9203. *J Clin Oncol* **24**: 4620–25.

Glimelius B, Gronberg H, Jarhult J et al. (2003). A systematic overview of radiation therapy effects in rectal cancer. *Acta Oncol* **42**: 476–92.

Gualdi GF, Casciani E, Guadalaxara A et al. (2000). Local staging of rectal cancer with transrectal ultrasound and endorectal magnetic resonance imaging: comparaison with histologic findings. *Dis Colon Rectum* **43**: 338–45.

Heald RJ (1998). The 'Holy Plane' of rectal surgery. *J R Soc Med* **81**: 503–8

Heald RJ, Moran BJ, Ryall RD et al. (1998). Rectal cancer: the Basingstoke experience of total mesorectal excision, 1978–1997. *Arch Surg* **133**: 894–99.

Herbertson RA, Lee ST, Tebbutt N, Scott AM (2007). The expanding role of PET technology in the management of patients with colorectal cancer. *Ann Oncol* **18**: 1774–81.

Horiot JC, Roth SL, Calais G et al. (1990). The Dijon clinical staging system for early rectal carcinomas amenable to intracavitary treatment techniques. *Radiother Oncol* **18(4)**: 329–337.

Hyams DM, Mamounas EP, Petrelli N et al. (1997). A clinical trial to evaluate the worth of pre-operative multimodality therapy in patients with operable carcinoma of the rectum: a progress report of the National Surgical Breast and Bowel Project Protocol R-03. *Dis Colon Rectum* **40**: 131–39.

Kapiteijn E, Marijnen CA, Nagtegaal ID et al. (2001). Pre-operative radiotherapy combined with total mesorectal excision for resectable rectal cancer. *N Engl J Med* **345**: 638–46.

Koh DM, Brown G, Temple L et al. (2004). Rectal cancer: mesorectal lymph nodes at MR imaging with USPIO versus histopathologic findings–initial observations. *Radiology* **231**: 91–99.

Krook J, Moertel C, Gunderson L et al. (1991). Effective surgical adjuvant therapy for high risk rectal carcinoma. *N Engl J Med* **324**: 709–15.

Lee JH, Lee JH, Ahn JH et al. (2002). Randomized trial of postoperative adjuvant therapy in stage II and III rectal cancer to define the optimal sequence of chemotherapy and radiotherapy: A preliminary report. *J Clin Oncol* **20**: 1751–58.

MacFarlane JK, Ryall RD, Heald RJ (1993). Mesorectal excision for rectal cancer. *Lancet* **341**: 457–60.

MacKay SG, Pager CK, Joseph D et al. (2003). Assessment of the accuracy of transrectal ultrasonography in anorectal neoplasia. *Br J Surg* **90**: 346–50.

Martling AL, Holm T, Rutqvist LE et al. (2000). Effect of a surgical training programme on outcome of rectal cancer in the County of Stockholm. Stockholm Colorectal Cancer Study Group, Basingstoke Bowel Cancer Research Project. *Lancet* **356**: 93–96.

Mercury study group (2007). Extramural depth of tumour invasion at thin-section MR in patients with rectal cancer. Results of the Mercury study. *Radiology* **1**: 132–39.

Mezhir JJ, Smith KD, Fichera A et al. (2005). Presence of distal intramural spread after pre-operative combined-modality therapy for adenocarcinoma of the rectum: what is now the appropriate distal resection margin? *Surgery* **138**(4): 658–63; discussion 663–64.

Nagtegaal ID, Quirke P (2008). What is the role for the circumferential margin in the modern treatment of rectal cancer? *J Clin Oncol* **26**: 303–12.

Nascimbeni R, Burgart LJ, Nivatvongs S et al. (2002). Risk of lymph node metastasis in T1 carcinoma of the colon and rectum. *Dis Colon Rectum* **45**(2): 200–6.

Nash G, Weiser MR, Guillem JG et al. (2009). Long-term survival after transanal excision of T1 rectal cancer. *Dis Colon Rectum* **52**(4): 577–82.

NIH (1990). NIH consensus conference: Adjuvant therapy for patients with colon and rectal cancer. *J Am Med Assoc* **264**: 1444–50.

Papillon J (1982). *Rectal and Anal Cancer: Conservative Treatment by Irradiation: An Alternative to Radical Surgery*. Springer: New York, NY.

Peeters KC, Marijnen CA, Nagtegaal ID et al. (2007). The TME trial after a median follow-up of 6 years: increased local control but no survival benefit in irradiated patients with resectable rectal carcinoma. *Ann Surg* **246**: 693–701.

Quirke P, Durdey P, Dixon MF et al. (1986). Local recurrence of rectal adenocarcinoma due to inadequate surgical resection: Histologic study of lateral tumour spread and surgical excision. *Lancet* **2**: 996–99.

Remzi FH, Fazio VW, Gorgun E et al. (2005). Quality of life, functional outcome, and complications of coloplasty pouch after low anterior resection. *Dis Colon Rectum* **48**: 735–43.

Salerno GV, Daniels IR, Moran BJ et al. (2009). Magnetic resonance imaging prediction of an involved surgical resection margin in low rectal cancer. *Dis Colon Rectum* **52**(4): 632–39.

Sauer R, Becker H, Hohenberger W et al. (2004). Pre-operative versus post-operative chemoradiotherapy for rectal cancer. *N Engl J Med* **351**: 1731–40.

Sebag-Montefiore D, Stephens RJ, Steele R et al. (2009). Pre-operative radiotherapy versus selective post-operative chemo-radiotherapy in patients with rectal cancer (MRC CR07 and NCIC-CTG C016): a multicentre, randomized trial. *Lancet* **373**: 811–20.

Solomon MJ, McLeod RS (1993). Endoluminal transrectal ultrasonography: accuracy, reliability and validity. *Dis Colon Rectum* **36**: 200–5.

Tasbas M, Sischy B (1996). Endocavitary radiation for treatment of distal rectal carcinoma and 20 years experience. *Int J Radiat Oncol Biol Phys* **36**: 211 (abstract).

Vuong T, Devic S, Moftah B et al. (2005). High-dose-rate endorectal brachytherapy in the treatment of locally advanced rectal carcinoma: technical aspects. *Brachytherapy* **4**: 230–35.

Wolmark N, Wieand S, Hyams D et al. (2000). Randomized trial of postoperative adjuvant chemotherapy with or without radiotherapy for carcinoma of the rectum: National surgical adjuvant breast and Bowel project Protocol R-02. *J Natl Canc Inst* **92**: 388–96.

Wong RKS, Tandan V, De Silva S, Figueredo A (2007). Pre-operative radiotherapy and curative surgery for the management of localized rectal carcinoma. In: *Cochrane Database of Systematic Reviews*, Issue 2. Wiley: New York, NY.

Chapter 15

FUTURE DIRECTIONS

Jacques Huot[1] and Nicole Beauchemin[2]
[1]*Le Centre de recherche en cancérologie de l'Université Laval et Centre de recherche du CHUQ, l'Hôtel-Dieu de Québec, Québec, QC, Canada, G1R 2J6,*
e-mail: Jacques.Huot@fmed.ulaval.ca
[2]*Rosalind and Morris Goodman Cancer Research Centre, McGill University, 3655 Promenade Sir-William-Osler, Lab 708, Montreal, QC, Canada, H3G 1Y6,*
e-mail: nicole.beauchemin@mcgill.ca

Abstract: Colorectal cancer is a prevalent cancer worldwide. Patients suffering from this disease usually develop liver metastases. Significant therapeutic advances have increased 5-year survival rates to over 50%. We present a summary of the highlights of the various chapters relative to new therapies and research developments in treating this debilitating disease.

Key words: Survival · Liver metastases · Chemotherapy · Anti-angiogenenic agents · Diet · Diagnostic tests · miRNA

Colorectal cancer is the third most common cancer worldwide. It represents 10% of all cancer-related deaths in North America, and in many parts of the western world, it is the second leading cause of cancer deaths. In most cases, death results as the consequence of the formation of liver metastases. In fact, hepatic metastases develop in 50% of the patients and are responsible for two thirds of colorectal cancer patient deaths (Shimada et al., 2009). Nevertheless, recent clinical observations developed on the basic findings reported in this book indicate that the situation is changing. Indeed, multidisciplinary management of patients on clinical trials now results in 5-year survival rates of over 50%. A cure of certain patients is even a realistic goal (Gallagher and Kemeny, 2009).

The standard curative treatment of patients with colorectal cancer is liver resection or local ablative treatment using radio frequency or cytoablation. These approaches result in a 5-year survival rate of 25–58%. In addition, the use of new drug combinations such as 5-FU/folinic acid with oxaliplatin or irinotecan has increased the overall survival up to 20 months. More importantly, these drug combinations have down-sized tumours to levels that enable resection, thereby increasing the 5-year survival rate. The success of this multi-drug chemotherapeutic approach is still further enhanced when anti-angiogenic agents such as bevacizumab are added to the regimen. Similarly, the use of anti-EGFR antibodies such as cetuximab or panitumumab allows individualizing of treatments in patients harbouring K-Ras mutations (Langerak et al., 2009; Shimada et al., 2009; van Krieken et al., 2008).

The therapeutic gains obtained during the recent years are encouraging and highlight that further therapeutic progresses can be expected in the near future by following similar experimental and translational strategies. In particular, therapeutic gains will be obtained by further refining surgical liver resection. Therapeutic gains will also be obtained by discovering new effective drugs and drug combinations. In particular, great hopes are placed on tailored therapies such as those using cetuximab. In that context, it is obvious that the identification of novel putative targets for chemotherapy will be a great asset. Important therapeutic breakthroughs can also be expected from studies aimed at developing colon-specific delivery systems (McConnell et al., 2009). On the other hand, resistance to chemotherapy still represents a major obstacle to treatment efficacy. It limits the efficacy not only of drugs such as 5-FU and oxaliplatin but also of bevacizumab (Ellis and Hicklin, 2008). Along these lines, the identification of clinically valid biomarkers of resistance to anti-cancer treatments is a critical medical need with vast therapeutic potential. It will allow individualizing the treatment and avoid administering inappropriate drugs to resistant patients.

Intriguingly, colon cancer is well recognized as associated with obesity. In particular, insulin resistance associated with obesity promotes colonocyte proliferation and suppresses apoptosis (Murthy et al., 2009; Vanamala et al., 2008). This raises the possibility that the incidence of colon cancer can be prevented by diet manipulation. Notably, diet rich in fruits and vegetables seems to prevent colon cancer (Michels et al., 2006). However, this field of research is still in its infancy and much remains to be discovered since most studies have not yet identified the targets of nutritional intervention (Marshall, 2009). Nevertheless, prevention remains an important goal for reducing colon cancer burden. Refining colon cancer screening procedures is another means to reduce its incidence. Recently, new promising diagnostic tests have been developed that permit early detection and therapeutic intervention. They include, sigmoidoscopy, colonoscopy, computed tomographic colonography and guaiac-based faecal occult blood tests (Lieberman, 2009). miRNA expression profiles in tissue and blood also has potential in detection, screening and surveillance of colorectal cancer. For example, a high tumour/normal expression ratio of miR-20a, miR-21, miR-106a, miR-181b and miR-203 is associated with poor survival. When used in combination with serum CEA, the miRNA expression profile may accurately predict disease-free survival and response to chemotherapy (Aslam et al., 2009). In addition, it can be expected that within the next few years, populations and individuals harbouring susceptibility genes to the development of colon cancer will readily be clinically identified and provided with the necessary follow-up to prevent the development of this debilitating disease (Tomlinson et al., 2007, 2008; Tenesa et al., 2008).

In conclusion, important progress has been achieved during the last decade in the understanding and the treatment of colorectal cancer and liver metastases. This progress has been attained through multidisciplinary efforts designed to tackle the disease and through the quick translation of basic knowledge towards treatment. We hope that our book will encourage students, basic researchers and clinicians to work together to still further improve the quality of life and life expectancy of colon cancer patients. This will be our greatest reward.

Abbreviations and Acronyms

CEA	Carcinoembryonic antigen
EGFR	Epidermal growth factor receptor
5-FU	5-fluoro uracil
miRNA	micro RNA

References

Aslam MI, Taylor K, Pringle JH, Jameson JS (2009). MicroRNAs are novel biomarkers of colorectal cancer. *Br J Surg* **96**: 702–10.

Ellis LM, Hicklin DJ (2008). Pathways mediating resistance to vascular endothelial growth factor-targeted therapy. *Clin Cancer Res* **14**: 6371–75.

Gallagher D, Kemeny N (2009). Treatment of patients with colorectal cancer: emphasis on liver metastases. *Expert Opin Pharmacother* **10**: 109–24.

Langerak A, River G, Mitchell E, Cheema P, Shing M (2009). Panitumumab monotherapy in patients with metastatic colorectal cancer and cetuximab infusion reactions: a series of four case reports. *Clin Colorectal Cancer* **8**: 49–54.

Lieberman D (2009). Colon cancer screening and surveillance controversies. *Curr Opin Gastroenterol* **25**: 422–27.

Marshall JR (2009). Nutrition and colon cancer prevention. *Curr Opin Clin Nutr Metab Care* **12**: 539–43.

McConnell EL, Liu F, Basit AW (2009). Colonic treatments and targets: issues and opportunities. *J Drug Target* **17**: 335–63.

Michels KB, Giovannucci E, Chan AT, Singhania R, Fuchs CS, Willett WC (2006). Fruit and vegetable consumption and colorectal adenomas in the Nurses' Health Study. *Cancer Res* **66**: 3942–53.

Murthy NS, Mukherjee S, Ray G, Ray A (2009). Dietary factors and cancer chemoprevention: an overview of obesity-related malignancies. *J Postgrad Med* **55**: 45–54.

Shimada H, Tanaka K, Endou I, Ichikawa Y (2009). Treatment for colorectal liver metastases: a review. *Langenbecks Arch Surg* **394**: 973–83.

Tenesa A, Farrington SM, Prendergast JG, Porteous ME, Walker M, Haq N et al. (2008). Genome-wide association scan identifies a colorectal cancer susceptibility locus on 11q23 and replicates risk loci at 8q24 and 18q21. *Nat Genet* **40**: 631–37.

Tomlinson IP, Webb E, Carvajal-Carmona L, Broderick P, Howarth K, Pittman AM et al. (2008). A genome-wide association study identifies colorectal cancer susceptibility loci on chromosomes 10p14 and 8q23.3. *Nat Genet* **40**: 623–30.

Tomlinson I, Webb E, Carvajal-Carmona L, Broderick P, Kemp Z, Spain S et al. (2007). A genome-wide association scan of tag SNPs identifies a susceptibility variant for colorectal cancer at 8q24.21. *Nat Genet* **39(8)**: 984–88.

van Krieken JH, Jung A, Kirchner T, Carneiro F, Seruca R, Bosman FT et al. (2008). KRAS mutation testing for predicting response to anti-EGFR therapy for colorectal carcinoma: proposal for an European quality assurance program. *Virchows Arch* **453**: 417–31.

Vanamala J, Tarver CC, Murano PS (2008). Obesity-enhanced colon cancer: functional food compounds and their mechanisms of action. *Curr Cancer Drug Targets* **8**: 611–33.

INDEX

A

Acetylation, 102, 113–114
Activin, 71, 83–84, 88–89
Adenoma, 9, 66–69, 71–73, 75–78, 80, 82, 86, 88, 90, 110–111, 117, 141–143, 150–151, 158, 162, 175–178, 182, 191, 215, 217, 220, 222, 226, 257–258, 264, 266–267, 272, 291, 294, 300, 322, 324, 330, 331, 336–337, 363, 377
Adherens junction, 148, 151–152, 158, 218–219
Adhesion, 11–14, 16–20, 22–25, 37, 41, 43–44, 47, 51, 54, 57, 74–75, 84, 110, 113, 132, 143, 150–151, 156, 158, 173–194, 218–220, 222–225, 248, 257, 290, 298, 302, 304–305, 307–311, 324
Adjuvant chemotherapy, 52, 83, 149, 324–325, 327, 334, 344, 354, 365, 367, 370–371, 373–374, 398, 403–404
Aneuploidy, 68
Angiostatin, 259, 265
Apoptosis, 2, 11, 17–18, 22, 37–39, 44, 51, 55, 66, 77–80, 83–84, 106, 110–111, 115, 117, 153, 156, 207, 214, 217, 223–224, 296–297, 302, 310, 328, 330, 332, 336, 376, 410
Arresten, 256, 259

B

Base excision repair, 69, 72–73, 88–89
E-cadherin, 13–14, 22–23, 74–75, 109, 147–148, 150–152, 156, 158–161, 176, 179–182
Bevacizumab, 15, 42, 211, 243, 254, 269, 271, 332–335, 368, 373–375, 409–410
Bone morphogenetic protein, 83, 89

C

Capecitabine, 333, 367, 373, 377, 405
Carcinoembryonic antigen, 190–194, 228, 302, 310, 371, 377, 411
β-Catenin, 11, 13, 22, 71, 73–75, 89, 110, 138–139, 141, 148, 150–162, 179, 181, 210, 220–221, 307
Cell adhesion molecules, 13, 23–25, 41, 57, 143, 156, 173–194, 220, 298, 304, 308–309, 311, 324
Cdk4, 80, 89
Cetuximab, 52, 76, 211, 271, 330–332, 334–336, 368, 373–375, 410
Chemokines, 10, 15–17, 20, 23–24, 36–37, 40, 46–47, 56–57, 115, 137, 143, 224, 257, 259–260, 273, 291–294, 298–301, 309, 333
  receptors, 15–17, 23, 36–37, 46, 56, 299–301
Chemotherapy, 15, 52, 83, 127, 130, 136, 139, 140, 142, 149, 193, 269, 324–325, 327–329, 331, 334, 344, 354–355, 365–367, 371, 373–377, 390–391, 393, 395–396, 398–399, 403–405, 410
Chromatin, 2, 9, 101–103, 114, 117, 334
  immunoprecipitation, 103, 117
Chromosome
  instability, 67–69
  translocation, 67, 79, 156, 158, 211–212, 256
Cimetidine, 188–189, 194, 310
Circulating tumour cells, 19–20, 33, 38, 45, 56, 223, 301
Clonal evolution model, 3
Coagulation, 37, 40, 47, 50–51, 186, 243–244, 261–263
Coagulopathy, 47, 256, 261

Collagen, 10–11, 22, 46, 174, 177–178, 182, 207, 211, 218, 220–221, 228, 233
Collagenases, 22
Colon cancer initiating cells, 130–135
Colon cancer metastasis, 9, 15, 20, 23, 173–194, 243–274, 309
Colonization, 9, 21–23, 34–36, 39, 45–46, 180, 185, 301, 304, 308–309
Colorectal carcinoma, 21, 104, 115, 174–176, 178–181, 183–184, 186–189, 191–193, 209–210, 214, 217, 220, 222, 224, 290, 302, 304, 310, 323–325
Cox-2, 110, 188, 226, 264, 267, 270, 273, 298, 308, 310, 331–332
Cytokeratins, 49
Cytokines, 10–11, 20, 40, 46–47, 53–55, 79, 152, 157, 187, 189–190, 192, 210, 220, 257, 259–260, 290–297, 299, 302, 304, 307–309

D
Demethylation, 5, 105
Dll-4, 248, 250, 252, 273
DNA
  methylation, 9, 67, 74, 102–107, 109, 112–116
  methyltransferases, 102, 114, 117
  microarrays, 103, 335
  mismatch repair, 68–72, 90, 322
Dukes staging, 34, 215

E
Early oncogenesis model, 4–5, 7
E-cadherin, 13–14, 22–23, 74–75, 109, 148, 150–152, 156, 158–161, 176, 179–182, 210, 218, 252, 260, 307
Endostatin, 256, 259, 265
Endothelium, 16, 18–20, 22, 45, 51, 188, 192, 223–224, 244, 262
Epigenetic, 2–3, 5, 9–10, 66–67, 81, 89, 101–118, 159, 257, 322, 333, 336
Epigenome, 109
Epithelial-mesenchymal transition, 12–14, 147–163, 179, 181, 207, 218, 228
EpCAM, 13, 24, 133, 143
E-selectin, 20–22, 44, 47, 184, 186–189, 194, 224–225, 302–308, 310–311
Etanercept, 310
External Beam Radiation therapy, 393–398
Extracellular matrix, 10–12, 24, 39, 45–46, 51, 56, 80, 113, 155, 158, 173, 182, 184, 220–222, 226, 244, 247, 259, 273, 290, 297, 299, 309, 311

Extravasation, 8–9, 18–22, 37, 40, 43–45, 51, 54, 184, 186–188, 190–192, 224–225, 275, 290, 301–309

F
Factor VIIa, 261
Familial adenomatous polyposis, 73, 86, 90, 150, 322, 337, 363, 377
FAS, 37, 44, 78, 296, 311
Fibrin, 10, 50, 221, 261–261
Fibronectin, 11, 22, 40, 46, 80, 174, 176–177, 179, 182, 218
Fluoropyrimidine, 327, 366–368, 370–371, 373, 375
5-Fluorouracil, 134, 327, 334, 337, 366, 377, 390, 405
Fusion model, 3, 5–6

G
Gene
  transfer model, 4, 6
  tumour suppressor, 2, 9, 66, 71, 77, 79, 81–84, 89, 102–104, 106–112, 116–117, 161, 181, 216, 257–258, 324–325, 333–334
Genetic predisposition model, 4, 6–7
Genetics, 65–90, 104
Genomic instability, 66–73, 105, 324–327, 336

H
Hereditary non-polyposis colorectal cancer, 326, 377
High dose rate brachytherapy, 397–398, 404–405
Histones, 2, 101–103, 113–114, 116–117, 334
  modifiers, 2
Homing, 2, 19–21, 43, 182, 187
Hyaluronan, 11, 244, 248, 253
Hypermethylation, 2, 13, 104–111, 114–116, 159, 180–181, 326, 334
Hypomethylation, 13, 104–107, 115

I
Iatrogenic factors, 54–56
Immunoglobulin, 18, 174, 176, 189, 273
Inflammation, 2, 11, 18, 54, 106, 189, 226, 249, 253, 257, 290–292, 298–300, 309, 331
Infliximab, 310
Insulin-like growth factors, 2, 24, 107, 208, 228, 254, 265, 273
Integrin, 11–13, 16, 18, 20, 22, 24, 37, 40, 47, 54, 85, 158, 174–181, 189, 193, 218–219, 221, 223, 225, 247–248, 252–253, 262

Index

Intravasation, 8–9, 11, 15–17, 34, 38, 155, 184, 186, 220–223, 244
Irinotecan, 135, 327, 334–335, 337, 368–369, 373–375, 377, 409

K

Kupffer cells, 20–21, 39, 47, 57, 190–192, 291, 298, 302–304

L

Laminin, 2, 11–12, 22, 156, 162, 174–175, 218, 220–221, 223
Leucovorin, 327, 334–335, 337, 354, 356, 367, 369–370, 377, 399, 403, 405
Leukocyte, 5, 8, 18, 40, 174, 182, 184–190, 194, 260, 292–293, 300, 305, 311
Levamisole, 366–367
Linear progression model, 3
Liver, 12, 15–16, 18–24, 34–37, 39–41, 43–57, 85, 89, 90, 115, 149, 161, 175–181, 186, 188, 190–193, 209–210, 212, 217, 223–225, 228, 244, 246, 250, 263, 265–269, 273, 289–311, 329, 361, 369, 371–372, 374–376, 390, 392, 395–397, 404, 409–410
Liver metastasis, 15, 33, 40, 47–48, 51, 54, 56, 115, 161, 177, 188, 209, 217, 265–267, 281, 289–311
Lung, 7, 11, 19–20, 22, 37, 41, 44, 46, 48–49, 51–52, 107, 129, 132, 149, 182, 185–188, 210, 213, 268, 289, 300, 302–306, 361, 371–372, 392
Lymphangiogenesis, 14–17, 36, 243–274
Lymphatics, 254, 264, 266–268, 270, 273, 300, 344, 353–354, 361

M

Macrometastases, 9, 23, 309
Mesenchyme, 175, 246
Metaanalysis, 264, 325, 329, 347, 352, 366–367, 403
Metalloproteinases, 12, 15, 24, 155, 162, 177, 194, 220, 228, 259, 273, 292, 295–296, 299, 311
Metastasis
 adhesion to endothelial cells/homing concept, 19–21
 colon cancer
  epigenetic contribution, 115–116
  cell adhesion molecules, 173–194
  epithelial cell signaling, 205–228
  angiogenesis and lymphangiogenesis, 243–274

 host inflammatory response, role of, 289–311
 colorectal, physiopathology of, 33–57
 genes, 85–89
 microRNAS as switches, 112–113
 model, 3–7, 191, 217
Methylation
 inhibitors, 116
 signatures, 102, 104, 115
Microenvironment, 2, 5, 9–11, 18–19, 21, 23–24, 40, 42–43, 45, 49, 52, 54, 56, 156–157, 174, 184, 187, 209, 220, 225, 254–263, 272, 290, 292–293, 299, 309, 376
Micrometastases, 9, 22–23, 34–35, 40, 42, 44, 49, 51, 54–55, 217, 353–355
MicroRNAs, 102, 112–113
Microsatellite instability, 67–72, 89–91, 112, 215
Microvesicles, 6, 243, 256–257, 260, 272
Mitomycin C, 368–369
Mutations
 APC, 73–76, 158
 CTNNB1, 75
 DNA, 66
 gene, 9, 71, 81, 85, 181
 germline, 52, 70, 72–73, 75, 82–83, 86–88, 322, 331
 K-Ras, 158, 219–221, 258, 330–331, 374, 410
 somatic, 3–7, 69, 74, 85, 87–88
 TGFBR2, 66, 71–73, 79–83, 87–88, 90

N

Necrosis, 47, 54, 57, 159, 224, 255, 291, 296, 298, 311, 377
Neo-angiogenesis, 38, 156–157

O

Obesity, 53, 410
Oncogenes, 2, 4–7, 9, 24, 66, 71, 75–76, 78, 84, 89–90
Oncosome, 3, 6, 257
Osteopontin, 85
Oxaliplatin, 134, 333–335, 337, 354, 356, 368, 370, 373–375, 377, 404–405, 409–410

P

p15, 80
p21, 78, 80, 90, 295
p27, 80

p53, 2, 7, 9, 66, 69, 72–73, 77–78, 84, 87, 90, 181, 256–258, 264, 322, 324–325, 334, 376
Panitumumab, 76, 211, 330–331, 336, 368, 410
Parallel progression model, 3
Pericyte, 34, 246–251, 253, 259
Peritoneum, 41, 48–49, 371–372, 376
Phosphatidyl-inositol-3 (PI-3) kinase, 51, 57
Phospho-EGFR, 51
Phosphorylation, 13, 15, 74, 79–80, 102, 206–207, 209, 211–213, 215–217, 250, 295
PIK3CA mutations, 78, 216–217
Plasminogen activator, 15, 25, 80, 115, 155, 162, 220–221, 228
Platelets, 8, 18, 24, 37–38, 40–41, 57, 174, 184–188, 208, 228, 248, 260–262, 265, 272–273
Predictive markers, 327, 330
PRL3, 85
Prognostic markers, 139, 222, 321–337
Prostaglandins, 157, 226, 267, 298, 331
Proteoglycan, 11, 22, 46
Proto-oncogene, 2, 9, 76, 374

R

Radiation therapy, 129, 380, 391, 393–395, 397–400, 403–405
Rb, 37, 53, 80
Rectal cancer, 35, 38, 77, 209, 330, 346, 354, 363–367, 369–371, 373, 389–405
Rectum, 19, 34, 38, 48, 289, 326, 347–353, 359–361, 363–365, 390, 395–396, 401–402
Replication, 68–71, 78, 90, 102, 325–326, 369
Resection, 42–43, 49–50, 55–56, 149, 183, 193, 290, 310, 324, 330, 361–367, 369–374, 376–377, 389, 391, 400–405, 409–410

S

Seed and soil hypothesis, 19–20
Selectin, 18, 20–22, 34, 37, 40, 44, 47, 174, 182–189, 194, 224–225, 302–308, 310–311
Sentinel lymph node, 343–356
Sialyl-Lewis, 20, 184–185, 187–188
Signalling pathways, 11, 66, 73–84, 150, 156, 182, 206–207, 212–217, 219, 223, 226, 255, 262, 267, 298, 322, 325, 331, 374

SMAD4, 13, 66, 73, 79, 81–84, 87, 294, 324–325
Staging of neoplasms, 353
Steatosis, 53–54, 374
Stroma, 9–10, 12, 14, 23, 40, 49, 52, 57, 137, 143, 147–148, 156, 158–159, 209, 221, 223, 246, 255, 259–260, 262, 264, 273, 290–291, 293, 296, 299, 308–309
Surgery, 34, 42–43, 48–50, 53–55, 193, 260, 290, 324, 326, 334, 344–345, 361, 363–367, 369, 371–376, 390–391, 393–397, 399–403, 405
Surveillance, 17, 37–39, 44–45, 53, 80, 311, 371–372, 410

T

T-cell factor/lymphoid enhancer factor, 74–75, 90, 151, 162
Telomerase, 2
Tenascin, 80, 156, 162
Thrombin, 50, 261–262
Thrombospondin-1, 226, 265
Tissue factor, 37–38, 50–51, 57, 256, 261, 273
Toll-like receptor-4 (TLR4), 37, 53
Topoisomerase I, 369
Total mesorectal excision, 364, 377, 391, 400, 404–405
Transcriptome, 101
Transforming growth factor-α, 2, 25, 208, 218
Transient compartment model, 3, 5
Trichostatin A, 117
Trousseau's syndrome, 261
Tumour dormancy, 42, 55, 260
Tumour-host interactions, 193
Tumour necrosis factor-α, 54, 57, 224, 296, 298, 311, 377
Tumstatin, 256, 259
Tyrosine kinases, 84, 90, 206–214, 216, 228, 250, 254, 270–271, 273
Tyrosine phosphatases, 46, 84–85, 207, 212

U

Ubiquitination, 102, 208, 256

V

VE-cadherin, 22, 252, 260, 307
VEGF, 14–17, 25, 36–37, 40, 42, 46, 54, 57, 115, 136, 143, 156–157, 162–163, 209–210, 213, 225–226, 248–257, 259–260, 262–268, 270–272, 292–294, 299, 300, 308–309, 311, 332–333, 336–337, 368, 377